Front Office Management
for the Veterinary Team

Second Edition

Heather Prendergast, BS, AS, RVT, CVPM

Certified Veterinary Practice Manager
Synergie Consulting
Las Cruces, New Mexico

SAUNDERS
ELSEVIER

3251 Riverport Lane
St. Louis, MO 63043

FRONT OFFICE MANAGEMENT FOR THE VETERINARY TEAM, EDITION 2   ISBN: 978-0-323-26185-2
Copyright © 2015, 2011 by Saunders, an imprint of Elsevier Inc.

All rights reserved. No part of this publication may be reproduced or transmitted in any form or by any means, electronic or mechanical, including photocopying, recording, or any information storage and retrieval system, without permission in writing from the publisher. Details on how to seek permission, further information about the Publisher's permissions policies and our arrangements with organizations such as the Copyright Clearance Center and the Copyright Licensing Agency, can be found at our website: www.elsevier.com/permissions.

This book and the individual contributions contained in it are protected under copyright by the Publisher (other than as may be noted herein).

Notices

Knowledge and best practice in this field are constantly changing. As new research and experience broaden our understanding, changes in research methods, professional practices, or medical treatment may become necessary.

Practitioners and researchers must always rely on their own experience and knowledge in evaluating and using any information, methods, compounds, or experiments described herein. In using such information or methods they should be mindful of their own safety and the safety of others, including parties for whom they have a professional responsibility.

With respect to any drug or pharmaceutical products identified, readers are advised to check the most current information provided (i) on procedures featured or (ii) by the manufacturer of each product to be administered, to verify the recommended dose or formula, the method and duration of administration, and contraindications. It is the responsibility of practitioners, relying on their own experience and knowledge of their patients, to make diagnoses, to determine dosages and the best treatment for each individual patient, and to take all appropriate safety precautions.

To the fullest extent of the law, neither the Publisher nor the authors, contributors, or editors, assume any liability for any injury and/or damage to persons or property as a matter of products liability, negligence or otherwise, or from any use or operation of any methods, products, instructions, or ideas contained in the material herein.

Library of Congress Cataloging-in-Publication Data

Prendergast, Heather, author.
  Front office management for the veterinary team / Heather Prendergast. -- 2nd edition.
      p. cm.
  Includes bibliographical references and index.
  ISBN 978-0-323-26185-2 (pbk. : alk. paper) 1. Veterinary services--Administration. 2. Animal health technicians. 3. Office management. I. Title.
  [DNLM: 1. Veterinary Medicine--organization & administration--United States. 2. Animal Technicians--United States. 3. Office Management--organization & administration--United States. 4. Practice Management, Medical--organization & administration--United States. 5. Veterinarians--United States. SF 756.4]
  SF756.4.P74 2015
  636.089068--dc23   2013042884

Vice President and Publisher: Linda Duncan
Content Strategist: Shelly Stringer
Associate Content Development Specialist: Katie Starke
Publishing Services Manager: Jeffrey Patterson
Senior Project Manager: Tracey Schriefer
Designer: Ashley Miner

Printed in China

Last digit is the print number: 9   8   7   6   5   4   3   2   1

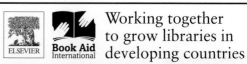

Working together
to grow libraries in
developing countries

www.elsevier.com • www.bookaid.org

To my mother ~the wind beneath my wings ~ who has guided and given me inspiration,
motivation and empowerment. You have been a truly amazing woman.
I miss you dearly.

Preface

Veterinary assistants and technicians are an essential component to every practice. Practice managers and hospital administrators help guide the team and continue the progression of excellent medicine and customer service. All team members fulfill an ever-expanding role in the veterinary practice, both clinically and administratively. These increased responsibilities require a greater need for professional knowledge and skill. This text has been designed to provide the basics of administrative skills as well as a guide for more advanced practice management philosophies. Many technicians step into the role of practice management and learn as they go; this book will aid the understanding and application that you will face as your professional career grows.

New to This Edition

The Veterinary Hospital Managers Association (VHMA) created *Critical Competencies: A Guide for Veterinary Practice Management Professionals* as an overview of the skills needed to be an effective practice manager. The VHMA has identified five performance domains that relate to the job of a veterinary practice manager: human resources, law and ethics, marketing and client relations, organization of the practice, and financial management. To be successful in each of the performance domains, certain knowledge requirements must be met and a set of critical competencies must be achieved. The critical competencies that must be achieved to master each performance domain are listed at the beginning of the chapter along with the knowledge requirements for developing your career in each aspect of veterinary practice management. These critical competencies include: *decision-making, integrity, critical and strategic thinking, planning and prioritizing, oral communication and comprehension, and writing and verbal skills.* As you read the chapter, you will be reminded of these critical competencies when you see this icon. Read the description of a

 typical task that is required of a practice manager, and think about which critical competency is needed to complete this task. When is it important to practice good decision making? What knowledge requirements would you need to conduct staff meetings or handle a client complaint? The goal of outlining these critical competencies and knowledge requirements within each job domain is to help you connect the dots between the skills required to be the best practice manager you can, and show you how to practice these skills in the real world.

Features in This Textbook

Important Features Include the Following:

- **Learning Objectives** and **Key Terms** at the beginning of each chapter guide you in your study and enable you to check your mastery of the content in each chapter.

KEY TERMS

16 Personality Factors
Campbell Interest and Skill Survey
Career Planning
Cover Letter
Myers-Briggs Type Indicator
Personal Skills
Resume
Transferable Skills

LEARNING OBJECTIVES

When you have completed this chapter, you should be able to:

1. Identify the importance of professional development.
2. Identify skills that one possesses.
3. Discuss career fields that are available.
4. Explain how to develop an effective cover letter.
5. Explain how to develop an effective resume.
6. Discuss how to email cover letters and resumes.
7. List methods used to prepare for an interview.
8. List questions to ask a potential employer.
9. Discuss how to follow up after an interview.
10. Differentiate offers of employment.
11. Discuss retirement savings.

- **Critical Competencies** as described by the VHMA are listed at the beginning of each chapter to indicate important skills as they relate to each job domain, and critical competency tasks are highlighted throughout the text to reinforce the knowledge requirements of a practice manager.

CRITICAL COMPETENCIES

1. **Analytical Skills** - the ability to analyze information and use logic to address problems; the ability to quickly and accurately grasp complex information and concepts and to make correct inferences.
2. **Critical and Strategic Thinking** - the ability to think critically about situations and to understand the relevance of information for different problems; use critical reasoning to generate and evaluate alternative courses of action or points of view relevant to an issue.
3. **Decision Making** - the ability to make good decisions, solve problems, and decide on important matters; the ability to gather and analyze relevant data and choose decisively between alternatives.
4. **Integrity** - honesty, trustworthiness, and adherence to high standards of ethical conduct.
5. **Resourcefulness** - the ability to understand what it takes to complete the job; apply knowledge, skills, and expertise to perform tasks quickly and efficiently.
6. **Writing and Verbal Skills** - the ability to comprehend written material easily and accurately; ability to express thoughts clearly and succinctly in writing.

In the law and ethics domain, practice managers monitor procedures and policies of the practice to determine whether events or processes comply with laws, regulations, and standards.

Knowledge Requirements

The tasks related to legal and ethical standards require knowledge of state/provincial and federal laws, legal codes, government regulations, professional standards, and agency rules.

reports should list the amounts due in current, 30-, 60-, and 90-day increments. Clients who owe practices money after 90 days not only are unlikely to pay, but also prevent practices from being able to pay their own accounts and employees. The practice must implement a no-charge policy to prevent AR from growing rapidly and hurting the practice's revenue. *Current AR should never be more than 1.5% of the gross revenue.*

Veterinary practice managers manage accounts receivable and accounts payable.

Figure 20-3 is an AR report that shows that the largest balance of the accounts receivable is the current amount due, followed by the total of 90 days past due. The current balance must be monitored; if this balance does not decrease within 30 days, strategies must be implemented to prevent past due amounts from rolling over to 60 and 90 days past due. The sum of $3661.32 (90 days past due) is unlikely to be collected, and the AR manager must determine appropriate strategies to collect these funds as soon as possible. Chapter 18 discusses AR in more detail.

the ARPP. Benchmarks are not yet available for ARPP; however, internal benchmarks can be created from internal historical data.

Average Client Transactions

Average client transactions (ACTs) include all transactions a client makes in the hospital: exams, diagnostics, diets, and medication refills. When a client returns for a recheck, diet, or medication refill, it causes the ACT to drop; unless each transaction is monitored, managers may become alerted to a declining ACT. When transactions are investigated, managers can see client follow-up is the cause, and the alert is justified.

Historically, the average client transaction has been a key KPI. It was monitored to ensure that team members were making recommendations, and clients were accepting them. If the average client transaction was consistently low, leaders should have determined why and developed a solution to increase the low figure.

Recently, ACTs have fallen out of favor, because practices have consistently increased ACTs without increasing the value to client. As a result, the veterinary industry has created "sticker shock" and decreased the consumer confidence in veterinary medicine. In addition, ACTs can vary

- **Veterinary Practice and the Law** boxes provide specific details regarding laws and regulations that pertain to each chapter. These boxes link directly to the critical competencies described at the beginning of the chapter.

⚖ VETERINARY PRACTICE and the LAW

It is the responsibility of the team to recognize animal abuse when it is presented to the veterinary hospital. AVMA considers it the responsibility of veterinarian to report such cases to the appropriate authorities, whether or not state law mandates reporting. Veterinary team members are responsible to protect the health and welfare of animals and people; in fact, animal abuse is linked to domestic violence. Reporting animal abuse may not only save a patient's life, but a family member's as well.

- **What Would You Do/Not Do?** boxes present real-life situations that occur in the veterinary practice and guide you through the appropriate responses.

WHAT WOULD YOU DO/NOT DO?

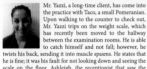 Mr. Yazzi, a long-time client, has come into the practice with Taco, a small Pomeranian. Upon walking to the counter to check out, Mr. Yazzi trips on the weight scale, which has recently been moved to the hallway between the examination rooms. He is able to catch himself and not fall; however, he twists his back, sending it into muscle spasms. He states that he is fine; it was his fault for not looking down and seeing the scale on the floor. Ashleigh, the receptionist that saw the incident offers him a chair to sit on, and rest until his back relaxes. He declines to sit down, stating he just needs to get home and lay down on the bed.

Ashleigh is afraid that the client may sue the practice.

What Should Ashleigh Do?
Ashleigh should first notify the owner and practice manager of the incident and write down the entire incident, before fine details are forgotten. Pictures should be taken of the scale, and how the client tripped. If the client calls and threatens the practice, the professional liability company should be called and informed of the incident.

Second, the practice should invest in some large protective barriers that clients can see, preventing them from tripping on the low lying scale. Pictures of the barriers should also be taken, indicating the corrective action the practice has taken, to prevent incidents such as this from occurring again. If it is feasible, the practice can sink the scale into the floor creating a flat surface (simply cut a space out of the concrete that will tightly fit the scale). Place a mat or rug over the scale for a nice appearance.

- **Practice Point** boxes spotlight important tips to running a successful practice.

Discounts per Veterinarian
This is a very important number to track. Discounting, which is described later in detail, has significant impact on the profits of the hospital. Tracking discounts by DVM can put this number into perspective. It helps manage who is responsible for discounting and what is being given away.

> **PRACTICE POINT** Every team member, not just DVMs, should be held accountable for unplanned discounts given to clients.

DVM Expenses, as a Percent of Gross Income
It is important to know how much a veterinarian is costing the hospital, especially in relation to how much they are producing. On average, a veterinarian should be producing five times (5×) the amount of his or her salary. If the expense is higher than what is being produced, alternative pay strategies may be considered.

Income Centers, as a Percentage of Gross Income
Income center management is imperative. Goals must be created and obtained. Showing these percentages will put these numbers into perspective, and gives the manager the tools to identify which income centers need further develop-

Accounts payable should be monitored on a monthly basis to ensure that there is not more spending than receiving. If the practice spends more money than it takes in, the practice will be in serious financial deficit in the upcoming months. Small practices that are relatively new may experience months that produce less than others, and a plan should be implemented in case this occurs. Spending must decrease, practice income must increase, and the practice employees should be held accountable for wastage. The fee structure may be re-evaluated, and practice managers should ensure charges are not being missed. If a line of credit is needed to keep the practice floating during the slow months, then a plan must be implemented to pay back the loan as soon as possible.

Client Surveys
Client surveys are an easy monitoring solution to understand the satisfaction and level of client comfort with the services the practice provides (Figure 20-4). Clients maintain the business; therefore it is imperative to make sure they are satisfied and perceive the value of the service provided. If clients are unsatisfied, practices want to be notified and given the opportunity to address the problem. Hospitals do not want to lose clients or have negative comments made about them throughout the community. It is very important to strive for a high level of satisfaction from every client.

- **Review Questions** ensure that you have mastered complete comprehension of each chapter.
- **Recommended Readings** provide additional sources of detailed information on important topics.

Evolve Resources

The instructor Evolve site (for instructors only) includes:
- A test bank including 500 multiple-choice questions with rationales for the correct and incorrect answer options.
- An image collection containing all the images from the book (approximately 400 images).
- PowerPoint presentations for each chapter to assist with lecturing.

The student and instructor Evolve site includes:
- Interactive working forms to allow students to practice. These forms include sample checks and deposit slips, incident reports, history-taking forms, laboratory submission forms, patient medical records, a master problem list, a boarding admission form, a histopathology form, a stock supply list, a radiology checkout log, and several different types of logs necessary for inventory and practice management.
- Interactive activities, including word searches and video case studies, to help you master important terms.
- End-of-chapter quizzes taken from the book.

Acknowledgments

The completion of this text permits the opportunity to relay appreciation to the many individuals who contributed their time and efforts. The completion would not have been possible without any of them.

The photographs in the textbook were taken by Clint Derk. I am indebted to him for his careful precision and patience in taking the photos, thus enhancing the value of this book. Clint has always said, "Life is too short to *not* enjoy what you do; *make the best of everything you do!*"

The team at Jornada Veterinary Clinic donated their time, skills, and smiles. Dr. Nancy Soules and Dr. Katie Larsen, my mentors and friends, have encouraged me and inspired me to take it to the next level. Without them, this hobby and career would not be as enjoyable as it has been. Brooke Lockridge: this edition would never have been possible without your help, expertise, and opinions; thank you does not begin to cover how much I appreciate everything you do.

To each of my past, present, and future students: we know this career can be rewarding. ***Find a practice that allows you to shine and that will shine the light on you! Enjoy life while you can.***

Contents

PART I VETERINARY PRACTICE AS A BUSINESS, 1

1 Veterinary Health Care Team Members, 2
2 The Receptionist Team, 13
3 Team Leadership, 47
4 Veterinary Ethics and Legal Issues, 72
5 Human Resources, 86
6 Stress, Burnout, and Compassion Fatigue, 137
7 Practice Design, 146
8 Technology in the Office, 155
9 Outside Diagnostic Laboratory Services, 166
10 Marketing, 181

PART II COMMUNICATION MANAGEMENT, 209

11 Client Communication and Customer Service, 210
12 Interacting with a Grieving Client, 228

PART III VETERINARY PRACTICE SYSTEMS, 237

13 Appointment Management, 239
14 Medical Records Management, 255
15 Inventory Management, 274
16 Controlled Substances, 291
17 Logs, 301
18 Accounts Receivable, 307
19 Pet Health Insurance and Wellness Plans, 317
20 Finance Management, 329
21 Safety in the Veterinary Practice, 358
22 Security, 392

PART IV CLINICAL ASSISTING IN THE VETERINARY PRACTICE, 399

23 Clinical Assisting, 400
24 Calculations and Conversions, 434
25 Professional Development, 446

Appendix: Abbreviations, 457
Glossary, 459

Contents

PART I VETERINARY PRACTICE AS A BUSINESS

1. Veterinary Health Care Team Members, 2
2. Management, 18
3. Leadership
4. Value ... and Local Laws, 22
5. Human Resources, 51
6. ...
7. Practice Design, 111
8. Technology in the Office, 136
9. ...
10. Marketing, 162

PART II COMMUNICATION MANAGEMENT

11. Client Communication and Customer Service, 200
12. Working with a Grieving Client, 222

PART III VETERINARY PRACTICE SYSTEMS

13. Appointment Management, 219
14. Medical Records Management, 234
15. Inventory Management
16. Controlled Substances, 291
17. Logs, 300
18. Accounts Receivable, 305
19. Preventive Insurance and Wellness Plans, 316
20. Finance Management, 320
21. Safety in the Veterinary Practice, 353
22. Security, 392

PART IV CLINICAL ASSISTING IN THE VETERINARY PRACTICE

23. Client Assisting, 400
24. Calculations and Conversions, 414
25. Professional Development, 426

Appendix Abbreviations, 455
Glossary, 456

## PART I

Veterinary Practice as a Business

The veterinary health care team is what makes the practice a success. The team is made up of individuals with different qualities and intellectual levels. One team member may be great as an assistant, but may lack the patience to work with clients in the reception area. A veterinarian may be a great surgeon, but may have a less than desirable bedside manner. A great team is made of different individuals with different strengths and weaknesses that develop respect and rapport for one another. Each helps another team member at any time and is willing to help increase the knowledge of others.

Leadership is critical in the practice. A leader leads the team to success, developing policies to guide the team, not micromanage. Successful leaders lead by behavior and actions, not words or demands.

Every team member lives by a code of ethics. Ethics are developed by society and are generally considered the cultural norm. Veterinary ethics are developed by the profession, which each team member must adhere to. The American Veterinary Medical Association, Veterinary Hospital Managers Association, and the National Association of Veterinary Technicians in America have developed a Code of Ethics for each member to follow. The AVMA's code of ethics has been adopted by many state veterinary boards and is the basis for many Practice Acts.

Laws have been established for the protection of employer and employees. Practice managers and owners must be familiar with federal and state laws, as penalties can be high for those in violation. Employee manuals and job descriptions should be developed for the protection of both the practice and the employees. A manual allows team members to understand what is expected of them once they are hired, policies of the practice, and termination procedures, should they ever be needed. Procedural manuals outline all of the procedures the practice follows; a simple guideline allows new team members to excel at their position, while providing a refresher for those long-term employees that do not practice the procedure often.

Team training is essential to the success of a team; it must occur often, even for long-term team members. Continuing education (CE) revitalizes everyone, igniting passion and enthusiasm, preventing burnout. A CE budget must be created, allowing teams to continue developing on a yearly basis (at minimum).

For new team members, the creation of a structured training plan is a must. Training in phases prevents the new team member(s) from becoming overwhelmed, as many procedures and tasks are learned in one day. It also prevents the skipping of procedures and tasks and allows the task to be mastered before moving onto the next skill level. Training in phases and regulation of employee hours can prevent stress and burnout that is so strongly associated with veterinary technology.

Practice design is essential to the efficiency of the practice. Items needed for a task should be placed as close together as possible to decrease the time to complete tasks. Team members must use correct posture and lifting movements to prevent injury while on the job. Overuse and inappropriate lifting can injure the back over time; measures must be taken to prevent injuries before they happen.

Marketing occurs every day, intentionally or not. The internal team must be fully trained and ready to produce before any marketing plan can be created or implemented. This includes brushing up on client service, client education and facility maintenance. While these areas are being mastered, Web page design and social media should be developed and implemented. The Web page has taken the place of the yellow pages; it makes the first impression for potential clients and enhances the relationship with existing clients.

Seize the opportunity to incorporate all of these components to be a creative, successful practice model.

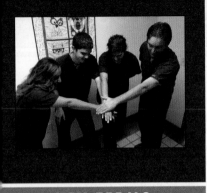

Veterinary Health Care Team Members

KEY TERMS

American Veterinary
  Medical Association
  (AVMA)
Groomer
Kennel Assistant
National Association of
  Veterinary Technicians
  in America (NAVTA)
Office Manager
Practice Manager
Receptionist
Veterinarian
Veterinary Assistant
Veterinary Practice Act
Veterinary Support
  Personnel Network
  (VSPN)
Veterinary Technician
Veterinary Technician
  National Examination
  Committee (VTNE)

OUTLINE

Students, 3
Groomers, 4
Kennel Assistants, 5
Veterinary Assistants, 5
Veterinary Technicians, 6
Veterinary Technologists, 7
Veterinary Technician Specialties, 7

Receptionists, 8
Office Managers, 8
Veterinarians, 9
Practice Managers, 9
Hospital Administrators, 10
Team, 10
Programs to Enhance Staff Education, 11

LEARNING OBJECTIVES

When you have completed this chapter, you should be able to:

1. Define various positions within a veterinary practice.
2. Describe job duties associated with each
   position in the hospital.
3. Discuss the advantages of a "team"
   environment.
4. Identify courses of study to enhance the
   education of each position.

The veterinary practice can be a highly structured environment that provides an excellent career for all team members. The goal of every practice should be to provide excellent medical care to patients and outstanding customer service to clients while providing a workplace that is friendly, efficient, and safe. Each team member contributes to the success of the practice. Veterinarians are responsible for providing the guidelines of medical care, and veterinary assistants and technicians are responsible for following these guidelines to provide excellent client and patient care.

In-hospital patients receive care from all team members—from kennel assistants to veterinarians—and all team members are responsible for ensuring patient safety and comfort. Patients can never be left in feces and urine; they must always have access to water and food when allowed and be hospitalized in a warm, comfortable environment. Team members share responsibilities for these hospitalized patients, and all must take initiative to provide the best care, whatever their positions are in the practice. Any team member who sees a patient in a dirty cage must clean it immediately.

Outpatients include those that visit the practice for examinations, vaccinations, lab work, or services that do not require hospitalization. The entire team provides service to these clients, and it is each team member's responsibility to ensure the client receives the necessary services in a timely and professional manner. Medications, client instructions, and handouts should be supplied to the client when needed. Clients are often overwhelmed with information they obtain while at a veterinary hospital; therefore client handouts are pertinent for excellent customer service.

Clients are turning to the Internet more than ever to educate themselves about diseases, products, and veterinary procedures. The Internet has a vast amount of information, but not all of it is correct. Veterinary practices must provide accurate and supplemental information to clients who have questions. The Internet should not be looked at negatively, but incorporated appropriately as a means to educate clients. Once clients find new information on products and procedures, they should be encouraged to contact the practice with questions. Team members can use this opportunity to strengthen the client-patient-practice relationship.

Clients expect excellent customer service from veterinary practices. It can take weeks to receive laboratory results in human medicine, and many times the physician never calls the patient with results, but rather the patient has to visit the office to receive results. In veterinary medicine, clients expect veterinarians to call the following day with results and often are upset if the results are not available sooner. Many opinion polls conducted in the past have placed veterinarians higher than physicians when respondents were asked to rank professions and the value they place on each. Some individuals value their veterinarians more than their physicians because the level of care they receive from their veterinary practice far exceeds the care they receive from their own physicians. This is a goal every team member should strive for.

Team members have rights and responsibilities in practices, including a safe work environment. Practices are not completely hazard free. Dogs and cats will bite, but practices can ensure that the proper equipment is available to prevent or reduce those hazards from occurring. Team members must use proper equipment when needed, and all should receive proper training on when and how to use personal protective equipment. A safe work environment can lead to a fun, interactive workplace that results in a satisfying career.

A key ingredient to teamwork is open and honest communication among employees, managers, and owners. The second ingredient to a successful team is developing and embracing respect for one another. When teamwork is evident, clients notice and recommend the friendly, honest, genuine service that a veterinary practice can provide.

> **PRACTICE POINT** Every team member has a responsibility and is a contributing factor to the veterinary practice.

The veterinary health care team involves all members of the staff. Each team member plays a significant role in a successful practice. Roles and duties vary by practice and typically are defined in the job description section of an employment manual. Team members working together as a group to provide better patient and client care than those who work as individuals. Team members may include, but are not limited to students, groomers, kennel assistants, veterinary assistants, credentialed veterinary technicians, veterinary technologists, receptionists, veterinarians, office managers, and practice managers. Many practices also have specializations within each team member position. Having a team leader can significantly improve communication and accountability.

Larger practices may have a structured hierarchy, with each team member having a specific role in the practice. Technicians may be limited to hospitalized patients, surgical recovery, or laboratory, whereas others may be assigned to outpatient visits. Smaller practices have assistants and technicians assigned to all areas of the practice. Each area of the hospital requires special knowledge and training, all of which contribute to the success of the practice.

Each new team member must become familiar with a number of topics in each practice. Because many practices use different products and equipment or perform procedures with different methods, a list of questions has been developed that each team member should be familiar with when starting a new position (Box 1-1).

Students

Students may function as observers or hold paid positions within a hospital. Many students must complete externships as part of a program. High school students can earn grades while completing a required number of hours at the job site, and veterinary assistant and technician students

BOX 1-1	Common Questions for the New Team Member

- What are the common emergencies seen at the practice?
- Are emergencies accepted after hours? If not, where are clients advised to go?
- What species are seen by the practice?
- What are the common diseases seen in the practice's geographic area?
- What are local vaccination protocols?
- Which heartworm/flea/tick preventive is recommended?
- Which nutritional products and food are sold at the practice?
- What routine surgeries are performed in the practice?
- What postoperative pain protocols are available for each species?
- What specialty procedures are performed in the practice?
- Is the hospital accredited by the American Animal Hospital Association?
- Does the practice board animals? If not, who is recommended?
- Does the practice have a groomer? If not, who is recommended?
- At what age are pets recommended to be altered?

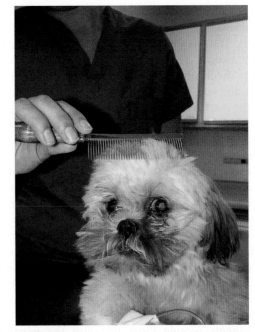

FIGURE 1-1 Groomers play an important role in the veterinary practice.

may fulfill hours required for their coursework. Students may be assigned tasks by the school that must be performed before course completion, which aids in the training process. Task lists can be used as a guide for both the practice and the student. Many practices consider externships as a form of a working interview. Students are encouraged to perform beyond expectations and employers are encouraged to train as if this student is a potential candidate.

Many veterinary schools have in-clinic prerequisites that must be completed before application and/or admission. Veterinary students can also complete an externship in a private practice to obtain more experience before graduating from a professional program.

Groomers

Groomers perform technical skills that they have acquired in order to care for patients and satisfy clients. This takes patience. They must take precautions to prevent injury to animals as well as themselves. Animals can become scared and aggressive while being groomed. Clippers are loud and tables can scare pets, causing them to become more aggressive than usual (Figure 1-1).

Several courses are available to learn how to groom; on-the-job training is also available. The National Dog Groomers Association works with groomers throughout the country to promote and encourage professionalism and education to maintain the image of the pet grooming profession. Their goal is to unite groomers through membership, promote communication with colleagues, set recognized grooming standards, and offer those seeking a higher level of professional recognition the opportunity to have their grooming

BOX 1-2	Responsibilities of Groomers

Successful groomers must:
- Have patience with clients and pets, and have excellent customer service skills
- Communicate clearly with clients; use professional words and enunciate clearly
- Show compassion for the pet and empathize with the client
- Be flexible and able to work around client schedules
- Stay abreast of new product releases, their mechanism, and benefits of use
- Receive continuing education regarding skin diseases, infections and common internal and external parasites
- Be aware of communicable and zoonotic diseases

skills certified. In some states licensure or certification is required.

At times, groomers are the first to recognize abnormalities that should be further investigated by a veterinarian. Groomers often detect abnormal anal glands, skin tags, masses, and ear infections while they care for pets. Owners appreciate and respect groomers' opinions when these abnormalities are found and often follow up with a visit to a veterinary practice (Box 1-2).

Groomers need to communicate clearly and professionally as a part of retaining clients. Many clients require extra time because they expect the best for their pets. Many times pets become uncooperative, producing a less than perfect cut; this can upset clients. Any grooming mistakes reflect on the groomers, who must be able to communicate well to handle dissatisfied clients.

Grooming can be an extremely satisfying career for many team members because results of an excellent job can be viewed immediately.

BOX 1-3	Responsibilities of Kennel Assistants

Successful kennel assistants must:
- Have patience with clients and pets, and have excellent customer service skills
- Be able to release patients to clients with the veterinarians directions
- Provide compassionate care to patients
- Provide clean bedding, water, and food as directed by veterinary team members
- Communicate well with team members
- Understand the importance of prioritizing tasks that have been assigned
- Accept tasks willingly
- Bathe patients as directed
- Lift patients up to 50 lb
- Have knowledge of communicable diseases
- Understand the transmission potential of zoonotic diseases
- Assist the veterinarian and veterinary technician with medicating patients
- Understand nutrition and the importance of a proper diet
- Maintains cleanliness of the hospital
- Know when to report an emergency situation
- Safely use cleaning chemicals

BOX 1-4	Responsibilities of Veterinary Assistants

Successful veterinary assistants must:
- Have patience with clients and pets, and have excellent customer service skills
- Maintain legible and accurate medical records
- Provide compassionate care to patients
- Provide clean bedding, water, and food as directed by veterinary team members
- Prepare and maintain exam rooms and treatment areas
- Communicate clearly with team members and clients
- Accept tasks willingly
- Bathe patients as directed
- Have knowledge of communicable diseases and methods of prevention
- Understand the transmission potential of zoonotic diseases
- Assist the veterinarian and veterinary technician with medicating patients
- Prepare and explain treatment plans for medical procedures to clients
- Understand nutrition and the importance of a proper diet
- Release patients and clearly communicate directions provided by veterinarian
- Maintain cleanliness of the hospital
- Perform laboratory analysis on samples as instructed by a veterinary team
- Know when to report an emergency situation
- Excel at animal restraint, and be able to lift patients up to 50 lb
- Effectively position patients for diagnostic radiographs
- Understand common procedures performed in the practice
- Have knowledge of common drugs used in the practice
- Understand the importance of prioritizing tasks
- Have initiative to learn and raise the practice to the next level of care

Kennel Assistants

Kennel assistants (also referred to as animal care attendant) are critical to the health care team. Kennel assistants keep the patients clean and alert the team of any changes in patient status. Most kennel assistants receive on-the-job training, learning procedures and protocols while they gain proficiency.

Kennel assistants should become familiar with cleaning protocols as well as any harmful and potentially fatal cleaning products. Mixing cleaning chemicals should be against hospital policy because of the possibility of creating toxic fumes. Many team members are unfamiliar with chemical reactions that can cause harm to both employees and patients.

Kennel assistants should be trained to detect emergency situations that may occur while a patient is hospitalized, including anaphylactic shock and seizures. They must also be trained on the prevention of disease transmission. Many diseases can be transmitted by fomites (e.g., bowls, litter pans) that are not cleaned completely. Cages can also retain aerosolized droplets of disease organisms when not cleaned properly. Cages are considered to have seven sides: the front cage door (two sides) and the five sides of the interior of the cage. All sides should be cleaned with a safe disinfectant approved for killing viruses and fungi.

Kennel assistants must be able to interpret correct nutritional instructions, feed the correct diet and amount, and remove food from preoperative patients. Soiled blankets must be removed immediately, and the soiling (urine, bowel movement or vomitus) should be recorded in the medical treatment sheet.

Appropriate safety precautions should be taken when moving patients to another cage or when walking patients outdoors. This important team member reports any and all behavior and condition changes to the immediate patient supervisor (Box 1-3).

Veterinary Assistants

Veterinary assistants are a strong asset to the team. Veterinary assistants may help a veterinary technician and/or veterinarian. They should excel at physical restraint, laboratory skills, patient care, and client relations (Box 1-4). Veterinary assistants often are key to clinics that excel in client satisfaction and patient care. Kennel assistants may report to a veterinary assistant, who in turn reports critical patient information to either a veterinary technician or veterinarian (Figure 1-2). Assistants can be trained on the job by veterinary technicians or practice managers or attend veterinary assistant programs. Veterinary assistants are encouraged to become approved veterinary assistants, receiving the designation of AVA. AVAs are overseen by the National Association of

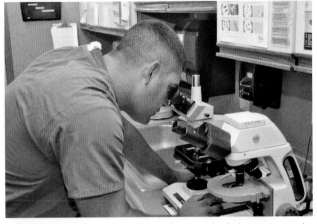

FIGURE 1-2 Veterinary assistants play a vital role by increasing the efficiency of veterinary technicians. This assistant is preparing a urinalysis for the veterinarian to read.

BOX 1-5	Continuing Education Requirements for Veterinary Technicians
Alabama	8 hours per 1 year
Alaska	10 hours per 2 years
Arizona	10 hours per 2 years
Arkansas	6 hours per 1 year
California	20 hours per 2 years
Colorado	16 hours per 2 years
Connecticut	Not required
Delaware	12 hours per 2 years
Florida	15 hours per 2 years
Georgia	15 hours per 2 years
Hawaii	Does not license
Idaho	14 hours per 2 years
Illinois	15 hours per 2 years
Indiana	16 hours per 2 years
Iowa	30 hours per 3 years
Kansas	Not required
Kentucky	6 hours per year
Louisiana	Not required
Maine	Not required
Maryland	24 hours per 3 years
Massachusetts	12 hours per year
Michigan	Not required
Minnesota	10 hours per 2 years
Mississippi	10 hours per year
Missouri	5 hours per year
Montana	Does not license
Nebraska	16 hours per 2 years
Nevada	10 hours per 2 years
New Hampshire	12 hours per year
New Jersey	Does not license
New Mexico	8 hours per year
New York	Not required
North Carolina	12 hours per 2 years
North Dakota	8 hours per 2 years
Ohio	10 hours per 2 years
Oklahoma	10 hours per year
Oregon	15 hours per 2 years
Pennsylvania	16 hours per 2 years
Rhode Island	12 hours per year
South Carolina	10 hours per 2 years
South Dakota	12 hours per 2 years
Tennessee	12 hours per year
Texas	10 hours per year
Utah	Does not license
Vermont	18 hours per 2 years
Virginia	6 hours per year
Washington	30 hours per 3 years
Washington, DC	Does not license
West Virginia	8 hours per year
Wisconsin	15 hours per 2 years
Wyoming	10 hours per 2 years

Veterinary Technicians in America (NAVTA), and must qualify through the completion of an approved program, and sit for an examination. Visit www.NAVTA.org for more information on becoming an AVA.

It has been recognized that credentialed veterinary technicians work more effectively when they have a trained assistant who can aid them in the completion of their responsibilities. Practices can then enhance the client relationships, further driving the client bonding and compliance rates.

Veterinary Technicians

Veterinary technicians are critical to the health care team. A credentialed technician is a graduate of a 2-year veterinary technology program approved by the American Veterinary Medical Association (AVMA). A technician must pass an examination given by the state and the Veterinary Technician National Examination Committee (VTNE) before receiving a license. Depending on the state, the graduate may be considered registered (RVT), certified (CVT), or licensed (LVT), or may be called an animal health technologist (AHT).

Credentialed technicians are allowed to perform certain duties under the direct supervision of a veterinarian. *Direct supervision* is defined as having a licensed veterinarian on premises and readily available while a veterinary technician completes certain duties. These duties vary from state to state; therefore each state veterinary practice act must be evaluated individually. Credentialed technicians may be required to attend continuing education to maintain licensure; states vary regarding the minimal number of credits required (Box 1-5).

The veterinarian generally assigns a patient to veterinary technicians. The technician follows all instructions for a treatment protocol, including medication, nutrition, laboratory tests, and exercise (Box 1-6). Technicians must document all treatments given to the patient and include any observations, such as bowel movements or urination, in the record or on a hospital sheet. This allows the veterinarian to follow the treatment progress of patients. Veterinary technicians are critical for client interaction as well. An informed staff member should update clients daily regarding the progress of their pets. Clients appreciate updates throughout the day as well as any educational materials regarding their pets' disease or conditions.

> **PRACTICE POINT** National Veterinary Technician Week is held the 3rd week of October, as designated by NAVTA.

BOX 1-6	Responsibilities of Veterinary Technicians and Technologists

In addition to all of the skills outlined for kennel and veterinary assistants, successful veterinary technicians and technologists must:

- Perform physical assessments
- Comprehend vaccines and vaccinations protocols, and be able to explain vaccine recommendations to clients
- Understand and teach clients the significance of disease prevention, nutrition and preventative care
- Provide treatments to patients, including SQ, IM, and IV injections
- Comprehend the mechanism of action for drugs and their potential complications and side effects
- Calculate dosage of drugs
- Develop safety protocols for assistants
- Perform common procedures and laboratory analyses
- Become proficient at obtaining samples for laboratory analysis
- Perform dental prophylaxis
- Monitor patients perioperatively and postoperatively
- Properly care for all surgical materials, sterilize packs, and maintain surgical facilities
- Effectively place and secure IV catheters
- Perform electrocardiograms

WHAT WOULD YOU DO/NOT DO?

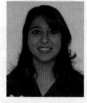 Sabrina, a veterinary assistant of 5 years has interest in furthering her career by attending a credentialed veterinary technician program to receive her license. She has seen the tasks and procedures credentialed technicians at other practices can complete, and wonders if she would be able to complete them in her practice as well. Currently, her practice does not have a credentialed technician, so her scope of the level of activities is limited. She also wonders if she would receive any raises in her practice for her schooling, as well as added responsibilities. She cannot decide if she should attend a campus or distance program.

What Should Sabrina Do?

Sabrina should first address her enthusiasm for the profession with the owner of the practice. The veterinarian may be completely oblivious as to how much a credentialed technician could help out the practice. Sabrina should mention the tasks and procedures other credentialed technicians complete and how it benefits their practices; an analogy can be made as to how Sabrina will benefit the current practice: "The typical veterinarian's gross income will be increased by $93,311 for each additional credentialed technician per veterinarian in the practice" (*Fanning J, Shepherd AJ, 2010*).

Second, Sabrina may ask about the possibility of promotion and added responsibilities, along with a potential raise for the future, should she complete her degree. Should Sabrina receive satisfied answers, she can decide if a distance or campus program would be best for her; finances, location and the scope of the program should all be considered.

Veterinary Technologists

A veterinary technologist can be a graduate of a 4-year Bachelor of Science program in veterinary technology accredited by the AVMA. A veterinary technologist may also hold an associate's degree in veterinary technology along with a bachelor's degree in another program, such as business, management, or health science. Technologists tend to work in positions that require a higher level of education and may hold teaching positions within technology programs or veterinary schools.

The head veterinary technician or technologist is responsible for overseeing veterinary technicians, assistants, and kennel personnel. They are responsible for training employees, implementing new and/or updated protocols and procedures, as well as maintaining inventory and ordering products.

Veterinary Technician Specialties

Veterinary technicians may decide to focus on a specific area of care, currently consisting of 14 specialty academies and 1 society. A society is defined as a group of individuals, veterinary technicians, hospital staff, and veterinarians interested in a specific discipline or area of veterinary medicine. An academy is the term selected by the NAVTA to designate a group receiving recognition as a specialty (Box 1-7).

BOX 1-7	Veterinary Technician Specialties and Societies

- Academy of Veterinary Emergency and Critical Care Technicians (AVECCT): www.avecct.org
- Academy of Veterinary Technician Anesthetists (AVTA): www.avta-vts.org
- Academy of Veterinary Dental Technicians (AVDT): www.avdt.us
- Academy of Internal Medicine for Veterinary Technicians (AIMVT): www.aimvt.com
- American Association of Equine Veterinary Technicians and Assistants (AAEVT): www.aaevt.org
- Academy of Equine Veterinary Nursing Technicians (AEVNT): www.aaevt.org
- Society of Veterinary Behavior Technicians (SVBT): www.svbt.org
- Academy of Veterinary Behavior Technicians (AVBT): www.avbt.net
- Academy of Veterinary Zoological Medicine Technicians (AVZMT): www.avzmt.org
- Academy of Veterinary Surgical Technicians (AVST): www.avst-vts.org
- Academy of Veterinary Technicians in Clinical Practice (AVTCP): http://avtcp.org
- Academy of Veterinary Nutrition Technicians (AVNT): http://nutritiontechs.org
- Academy of Veterinary Clinical Pathology Technicians (AVCPT): www.avcpt.net
- Association of Zoo Veterinary Technicians (AZVT): www.azvt.org

Technicians who choose to specialize must accumulate a specific number of hours within a particular specialty during a set number of years. For example, The Academy of Internal Medicine for Veterinary Technicians requires a minimum of 3 years' experience, with 6000 hours of experience as a credentialed veterinary technician in the field of internal medicine. All experience must be completed within 5 years before application. Candidates are also expected to have a minimum of 40 hours of continuing education on internal medicine before application submission.

Whether a veterinary assistant, veterinary technician, or technologist, every team member should be educated in basic laboratory work performed in a hospital. Veterinary technicians and technologists must be able to prepare and read blood smears, cytology preparations, urine samples, and fecal smears. Veterinary assistants may become proficient at running chemistry panels and complete blood cell counts on in-house laboratory equipment. All assistants and technicians should become proficient at radiology and learn the safety issues associated with all laboratory equipment, including the radiology machines. A veterinarian's productivity increases by delegating tasks associated with patient care to veterinary technicians and assistants. This allows the veterinarian to concentrate on diagnosing, prescribing medication, and performing surgeries.

Receptionists

Receptionists are often the "face" of the veterinary practice (Box 1-8). They play a significant role in the success of a practice and must appear professional, polite, and caring. They must listen to client stories, show empathy when needed, and be able to collect money from clients under difficult circumstances.

Receptionists (Figure 1-3) greet clients, detail and clarify invoices, and receive money. They answer the phone and can turn an inquiring phone call into an appointment.

BOX 1-8 | Responsibilities of Receptionists

Successful receptionists must:
- Have patience, empathy, and compassion for clients and patients
- Communicate well with team members and clients in a professional, respectful manner
- Provide exceptional client service to every client by identifying their needs and wants
- Answers phones efficiently, with a positive tone of voice
- Turn phone shoppers into appointments
- Educate clients on basic animal care, parasites, and routine procedures
- Listen to clients
- Interpret patient medical records
- Prepare client transactions, accept payment and/or explain payment policy to clients
- Minimize chaos at the front desk
- Maintain an effective appointment system

Receptionists acknowledge clients when they walk in and out of the practice. They make the first impression on a client, whether on the phone or at the front desk.

Receptionists are critical to the success of the hospital. They may or may not make a good first impression, succeed or fail at scheduling appointments, and enhance or devalue the client experience. Receptionists have a difficult job; however with proper training and communication skills, this position can be very rewarding at the end of the day.

Office Managers

The office manager is generally responsible for overseeing the front office staff as well as training receptionists to excel at customer service and public relations (Box 1-9). An office manager may allow a client to charge services and generally oversees accounts receivable. An office manager's realm of authority and decision making may be quite broad or limited depending on the administrative needs and criteria established by the practice. Many office managers are responsible for bank deposit preparation and performance. An office manager is courteous, friendly, and professional. His or her demeanor, whether positive or negative, trickles down through the rest of the team.

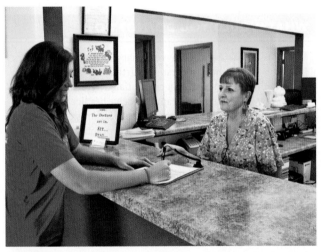

FIGURE 1-3 Receptionists should greet clients as they enter the practice.

BOX 1-9 | Responsibilities of Office Managers

In addition to all of the skills outlined for receptionists, successful office managers must:
- Train and oversee duties of receptionists
- Develop coping strategies to handle angry clients
- Determine if and when clients may charge for services rendered; manage accounts receivable, statements, and collections
- Review client satisfaction surveys
- Review medical records, invoices, and daily bank deposits for accuracy

Veterinarians

Veterinarians are the only members of the team allowed to diagnose, prescribe medications, and perform surgery on patients (Box 1-10). They have completed 4 years of a professional, AVMA-accredited school of veterinary medicine (Box 1-11). Veterinarians must be licensed in the state where they work and must pass both national and state examinations before receiving licensure. Veterinarians are required to complete a minimum number of hours in continuing education each year and must report their hours to the state veterinary board. These requirements ensure veterinarians offer the best medical care available to patients and clients (Figure 1-4).

Practice Managers

A practice manager helps keep the entire team working together and often reports to a hospital administrator. Practice managers generally handle client and personnel issues, supervise training sessions for team members, and hold team members accountable for their actions. Duties may also include reviewing records for completeness, observing for missed charges, and ensuring that policies are followed correctly (Figure 1-5). New strategies may be implemented by the practice manager, with the goal of increasing business as well as introducing new products to the clinic. Most practice managers hold a bachelor's degree in science or business administration; others hold an associate's degree in veterinary technology. Practice manager's benefit from either type of degree, which allows them to excel at managing a veterinary hospital.

BOX 1-10	Responsibilities of Veterinarians

Successful veterinarians must:
- Practice quality and current medicine with empathy and compassion
- Communicate well with clients and team members
- Educate clients and team members
- Motivate team members, build and maintain team moral, and uphold core values of the practice
- Attend continuing education seminars on a regular basis
- Have patience and a positive attitude
- Successfully delegate tasks
- Diagnose, prescribe medication, and perform surgery
- Accurately and legibly enter data into medical records in a timely manner

BOX 1-11	Veterinary Schools

- Auburn University College of Veterinary Medicine: www.vetmed.auburn.edu
- Colorado State University College of Veterinary Medicine and Biomedical Sciences: www.cvmbs.colostate.edu
- Cornell University College of Veterinary Medicine: www.vet.cornell.edu
- Cummings School of Veterinary Medicine at Tufts University: www.tufts.edu/vet
- Iowa State University College of Veterinary Medicine: www.vetmed.iastate.edu
- Kansas State University College of Veterinary Medicine: www.vet.ksu.edu
- Louisiana State University School of Veterinary Medicine: www.vetmed.lsu.edu
- Michigan State University College of Veterinary Medicine: www.cvm.msu.edu
- Mississippi State University College of Veterinary Medicine: www.cvm.msstate.edu
- North Carolina State University College of Veterinary Medicine: www.cvm.ncsu.edu
- Ohio State University College of Veterinary Medicine: www.vet.ohio-state.edu
- Oklahoma State University Center for Veterinary Health Sciences: www.cvm.okstate.edu
- Oregon State University College of Veterinary Medicine: www.vet.orst.edu
- Purdue University School of Veterinary Medicine: www.vet.purdue.edu
- Texas A&M University College of Veterinary Medicine & Biomedical Sciences: www.cvm.tamu.edu
- Tufts University School of Veterinary Medicine: www.tufts.edu/vet
- Tuskegee University College of Veterinary Medicine, Nursing & Allied Health: www.tuskegee.edu/academics/colleges/cvmnah.aspx
- University of California School of Veterinary Medicine: www.vetmed.ucdavis.edu
- University of Florida College of Veterinary Medicine: www.vetmed.ufl.edu
- University of Georgia College of Veterinary Medicine: www.vet.uga.edu
- University of Illinois College of Veterinary Medicine: www.cvm.uiuc.edu
- University of Minnesota College of Veterinary Medicine: www.cvm.umn.edu
- University of Missouri College of Veterinary Medicine: www.cvm.missouri.edu
- University of Pennsylvania School of Veterinary Medicine: www.vet.upenn.edu
- University of Tennessee College of Veterinary Medicine: www.vet.utk.edu
- University of Wisconsin-Madison School of Veterinary Medicine: www.vetmed.wisc.edu
- Virginia Tech Virginia-Maryland Regional College of Veterinary Medicine: www.vetmed.vt.edu
- Washington State University College of Veterinary Medicine: www.vetmed.wsu.edu
- Western University of Health Sciences College of Veterinary Medicine: www.westernu.edu/veterinary

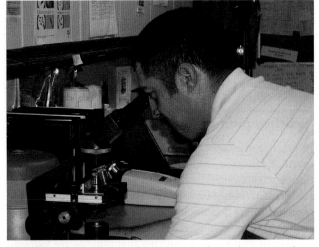

FIGURE 1-4 Veterinarians diagnose, prescribe medications, and perform surgery.

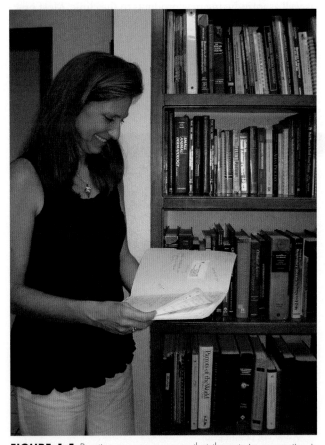

FIGURE 1-5 Practice managers ensure that the veterinary practice is operating effectively. They must display a friendly attitude and maintain a professional appearance.

> *PRACTICE POINT* Visit www.vhma.org for more educational opportunities for office and practice managers

A practice manager may have to wear many hats while on the job: copier repair technician, computer technician, plumber, veterinary technician, kennel assistant, and/or counselor. Just as with the office manager, the practice manager must have a positive, friendly attitude with an open-door

---

BOX 1-12 | **Responsibilities of Practice Managers**

Successful practice managers must:
- Have patience
- Lead the team in a positive manner
- Address conflict immediately, and provide consistent discipline to avoid discrimination claims
- Oversee team schedules, maximizing use during busy times, and making alternative plans during slower times
- Develop training protocols and performance evaluations, and provide coaching for the entire team
- Oversee building maintenance, including parking lot, lighting, and interior and exterior structures
- Oversee inventory, controlled substance, and safety programs
- Develop communication pieces for clients
- Develop sales strategies to increase revenue
- Hire, fire, and train in a legal manner
- Develop and maintain employee benefits program
- Determine efficient methods for completion of tasks and procedures for all positions in the practice
- Develop and maintain budget for hospital, reconcile accounts, track and measure income
- Strategically plan and create goals for future purchases

policy for all team members. Great attitudes encourage a professional and successful atmosphere (Box 1-12).

Hospital Administrators

A hospital administrator may be a veterinarian, technician, or a business manager. He or she generally has complete authority over the operation of the business and practice. This position is responsible for setting budgets, paying bills, creating organizational structure, and planning events. A typical administrator is responsible for all the duties of the office manager and practice manager. Although a hospital administrator may not be a veterinarian, this person should have general knowledge of quality assurance and performance in veterinary medicine and may act in an advisory role in helping establish and supervise protocols of the practice. A hospital administrator may report to the owner or shareholders if multiple members own the practice. Hospital administrators often make the final purchasing decisions.

Team

All roles on a veterinary team are important. All members contribute significantly. As is commonly said, there is no "I" in "team." Each team member must help others complete tasks in the most efficient manner (Box 1-13). Kennel assistants may need to help a technician restrain a patient for laboratory work, and a technician may need to clean kennels; a veterinarian may need to answer the phone when all receptionists are working actively with clients. This is why cross-training team members in all areas of the practice is crucial. Information and communication can be accessed and shared easier when team members are knowledgeable in several areas of the practice. When a team environment is

BOX 1-13	Characteristics of Successful Team Environments

- Team members understand one another's priorities and difficulties and offer help when the opportunity arises.
- Open communication exists among all employees, managers, and owners.
- Problem solving occurs as a team.
- The team is recognized for outstanding results, as are individuals for personal contributions.
- Team members are encouraged to make suggestions and test their abilities to improve the quality and quantity of work

BOX 1-14	National Veterinary Technician Organizations

- National Association of Veterinary Technicians in America (NAVTA): www.navta.net
- Canadian Association of Animal Health Technologists and Technicians: (CAAHTT) www.caahtt-acttsa.ca

created, any role in the veterinary health care team is rewarding. Patients receive better care, clients receive better customer service, and employees enjoy coming to work. When team members enjoy their jobs, they are accountable, more efficient and strive to achieve higher goals. Every practice can benefit from a team attitude.

Programs to Enhance Staff Education

Several programs are available online and at community colleges across the United States to enhance staff education. Veterinary assistant courses are available to help teach the basics of animal restraint, disease development, and client communication. Veterinary technician courses are available on campus and through distance learning. Distance programs give students the advantage of working in a practice while attending classes in the evening or on weekends via the Internet. Students can practice techniques learned in class under the direct supervision of their employing veterinarians and credentialed veterinary technicians. Distance education technology schools must be accredited by the AVMA in order for the students to take the licensing examination (VTNE) upon graduation from the program.

Students physically attending veterinary technology programs participate in clinics that are either on campus or organized through local veterinary hospitals, allowing students to obtain the direct experience needed to graduate from the program. Once students graduate, state and national technician organizations offer continuing education opportunities (Box 1-14), in addition to regional and national meetings hosted by large organizations.

VetMedTeam is an online continuing education resource that offers both free and fee-based courses. Courses offered cover a variety of subjects (veterinary assistant, veterinary technology, veterinary and practice management) and vary in depths of knowledge (basic principles, advanced principles and advanced concepts). The advantage of VetMedTeam courses is that they are all asynchronous; therefore students do not have to meet at an exact time for class. Participants work at their own pace and when they have time (after work and on the weekends). To access all of the benefits that VetMedTeam offers, visit their homepage at www.VetMedTeam.com.

The Veterinary Support Personnel Network (VSPN) is a group dedicated to veterinary technicians and assistants, receptionists, office managers, and other support staff who work with, for, or in the field of veterinary medicine. To access all VSPN's features (message boards, chat forums, continuing education, etc.), team members can register at www.vspn.org. Membership to VSPN is free. The VSPN community brings together members from all over the world to interact, teach, and learn. Members of VSPN have access to thousands of colleagues worldwide who want to help each other become a success.

Local specialty and emergency centers may offer continuing education for staff members of surrounding veterinary clinics. These seminars are generally free and cover a broad range of topics, including law and liability, emergency care, and practice management issues. In addition, local and regional veterinary technician organizations often offer continuing education at reasonable prices.

Manufacturer and distributor representatives are other excellent resources for continuing education for staff members. They have educational information available and are always willing to give presentations to staff.

VETERINARY PRACTICE and the LAW

It is the responsibility of the team to recognize animal abuse when it is presented to the veterinary hospital. AVMA considers it the responsibility of the veterinarian to report such cases to the appropriate authorities, whether or not state law mandates reporting. Veterinary team members are responsible to protect the health and welfare of animals and people; in fact, animal abuse is linked to domestic violence. Reporting animal abuse may not only save a patient's life, but a family member's as well.

REVIEW QUESTIONS

1. List the main duties associated with a groomer.
2. List the main duties associated with a kennel assistant.
3. List the main duties associated with a veterinary assistant.
4. List the main duties associated with a veterinary technician.
5. Define a technician specialty.
6. What is the purpose of continuing education?
7. Where do you see yourself in 5 years? 10 years?
8. What qualities will you bring to the veterinary practice?

9. Which of the following is a requirement for becoming a credentialed Veterinary Technician?
   a. Passing only the state licensing exam
   b. Graduating from a 2-year veterinary technology program approved by the AVMA
   c. Obtaining at least 5 years of experience in the related field then passing licensure exam
   d. None of the above

10. Which of the following is a responsibility of a veterinary assistant?
    a. Restraint of animals
    b. Client satisfaction
    c. Laboratory skills
    d. All of the above
    e. Both A and C

11. What does NAVTA stand for?
    a. Nationally Accredited Veterinary Technologist of America
    b. National Association of Veterinary Teams of America
    c. National Association of Veterinary Technicians in America
    d. None of the above

12. Which of the following are responsibilities of a Practice Manager?
    a. Overseeing the front office staff only
    b. Only managing the finances of the practice
    c. Ensuring the correct staff members are hired for team management
    d. Having multiple responsibilities covering all employees, client relations, finances, and overall maintenance of practice.

13. Which of the following are requirements of a veterinarian?
    a. Obtaining continuing education requirements each year.
    b. Passing both national and state licensing exams
    c. Graduating from an AVMA-accredited school of veterinary medicine
    d. All of the above

References

Fanning J, Shepherd AJ: Contribution of veterinary technicians to veterinary business revenue, *JAVMA* 236:846, 2010.

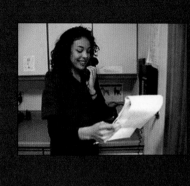

The Receptionist Team

OUTLINE

Managing the Reception Area, *14*
Team Etiquette, *15*
Developing Effective Phone Techniques, *16*
Managing Multiple Phone Lines, *18*
Turning Phone Calls into
  Appointments, *19*
Taking Messages for Veterinarians
  and Technicians, *20*
Liability of Telephone Calls, *20*
Personal Phone Calls, *21*
Managing and Processing Mail, *21*
Client Relations, *21*
Forms Commonly Used in Veterinary
  Practice, *22*
  The Medical Record, *22*
  Consent Forms, *23*

Patient History, *24*
Health Certificates, *25*
Medical Records Release Form, *28*
Boarding, *29*
Handling Special Situations
  with Clients, *29*
Reviewing Invoices with Owners, *33*
Payment for Services, *33*
  Declined Transactions, *38*
  Daily Reconciliation, *39*
  Deposits, *41*
  Petty Cash, *41*
Creating a "WOW" Service, *42*
  Front Desk Chaos, *42*
  The Waiting Clients, *42*
  Creating an Exceptional Finale!, *43*

LEARNING OBJECTIVES

When you have completed this chapter, you should be able to:

1. Define staff etiquette.
2. Develop effective phone techniques.
3. Develop frequently asked questions for the reception team.
4. Describe how to control telephone conversations with clients.
5. Identify techniques for handling multiple phone lines.
6. Identify techniques used to turn a phone "shopper" into an appointment.
7. Define the liability associated with giving medical advice over the phone.
8. Describe methods to greet clients effectively.
9. Differentiate forms used in the veterinary practice.
10. Identify a veterinary health certificate.
11. Effectively discuss invoices with clients.
12. List methods to accept payments on client accounts.
13. Handle declined credit card transactions comfortably.
14. Explain how to reconcile the end-of-day transactions and totals.
15. Explain how to make daily deposits.

CRITICAL COMPETENCIES

1. **Adaptability** - being open to change and flexible work methods; the ability to adapt behavior to changing conditions or new information.
2. **Compliance** - being reliable, thorough, and conscientious in carrying out work assignments; has an appreciation for the importance of organizational rules and policies.
3. **Critical and Strategic Thinking** - the ability to think critically about situations and to understand the relevance

of information for different problems; use critical reasoning to generate and evaluate alternative courses of action or points of view relevant to an issue.
4. **Decision Making** - the ability to make good decisions, solve problems, and decide on important matters; the ability to gather and analyze relevant data and choose decisively between alternatives.
5. **Integrity** - honesty, trustworthiness, and adherence to high standards of ethical conduct.

KEY TERMS

Anesthetic Release Form
Client Patient
  Information Sheet
Debit Transactions
Deposit
End-of-Day
  Reconciliation
Etiquette
Euthanasia Release Form
International Health
  Certificates
Intrastate Health
  Certificates
Liability
Master Problem List
Medical Records
Petty Cash
Privacy Act
Rabies Certificates
Rabies Neutralizing
  Antibody Titer
Reception Area
Role-Playing
Species

6. **Oral Communication and Comprehension** - the ability to express one's thoughts verbally in a clear and understandable manner, and the ability to actively listen and attend to what others are saying; must have good group presentation skills.
7. **Persuasion** - the ability to change the attitudes and opinions of others and to persuade them to accept recommendations and change behavior.

8. **Resourcefulness** - the ability to understand what it takes to complete the job; apply knowledge, skills, and expertise to perform tasks quickly and efficiently.
9. **Writing and Verbal Skills** - the ability to comprehend written material easily and accurately; ability to express thoughts clearly and succinctly in writing.

The ultimate goal of the receptionist team is to provide immediate, consistent, dependable, and courteous service to the client. The receptionists are the front line of any veterinary health care team. These team members are responsible for clients' first impressions (which start on the phone); creating a positive first impression helps improve client retention, increases client referrals, and ultimately drives client compliance. Therefore receptionists should greet clients in a friendly manner as soon as they walk in the door. They are also the last members of the team to take care of clients; therefore the need to make a lasting positive impression is a must.

Receptionists should have a professional demeanor and appearance; this includes professional hair, ironed clothing, and limited facial piercings and tattoos. Clients are not likely to take recommendations from someone they perceive as less than professional.

A second crucial goal is to support quality client and patient care through effective communication with team members. Clients often call throughout the day requesting updates on their pets. The receptionist team is responsible for either relaying the information to the owner or transferring the call to a knowledgeable team member. Clients may also call for suggestions or advice relating to their pets. It should be the goal of the receptionist to provide the most current, correct information available on the subject. If a receptionist does not know the answer, he or she is responsible for finding it.

Often, receptionists are responsible for creating and/or presenting treatment plans (estimates) for clients. Be sure to review Chapter 11 regarding client communications and the delivery of estimates. Understanding effective delivery techniques will help drive client acceptance of the recommendations being made.

Last, but not least, receptionists have the task of creating a "WOW" experience for the client. This WOW experience is what keeps clients returning and referring their friends and family. Review the end of this chapter for ideas to help create the "WOW" experience (Figure 2-1).

Managing the Reception Area

Many activities occur in the reception area; clients engage in conversation, pets may interact, and children may be in danger. The reception team monitors this area and must be able to control situations that may arise.

> **PRACTICE POINT** The reception area is often the first visual impression a client has of a practice; it must be spotless and chaos free.

Clients often attempt to share knowledge with each other; however, on occasion the information is not accurate or appropriate. Receptionists should try to monitor conversations and may need to move a client into a room sooner than anticipated because of the topic being addressed. "Toxic" topics include a poor experience the client is having at the practice or has had in the past, incorrect information regarding diseases or treatments, and offensive topics and language. It can be easier to isolate the offender and apologize to the victim than to remove the victim and let the offender repeat the conversation with another client arriving at the practice.

Pets may interact in smaller reception areas, which may result in tragedy. Dogs may try to attack each other, and cats may escape if they are not in a carrier. Receptionists should ensure every dog is on a leash and provide one when necessary. If cats are not in a carrier, the receptionist may offer to

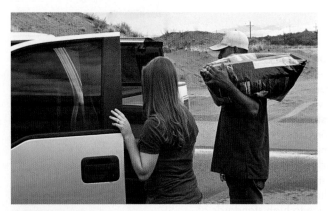

FIGURE 2-1 Creating a "WOW" experience. A team member assists a client to their car with food.

place the cat in a cage until a room is ready. Team members may also lend carriers to clients to prevent injury and escape.

Children occasionally attempt to pet the other animals in the waiting room. This can be dangerous to the child and encourages the spread of contagious disease. Receptionists may need to remind parents to control their children while in the waiting room because not all pets are fond of children. Creating a child play area can reduce these attempted interactions.

A receptionist may also need to triage patients as they arrive. Triage is prioritizing patients according to the severity of their conditions. If a patient arrives with symptoms of any contagious disease, such as the parvovirus, the patient should be immediately placed in isolation or kept in the car away from other animals in the reception area. If a patient arrives with an emergency, the pet may need to be rushed to the treatment area (without the client) to be further evaluated by the team. If a client feels it is an emergency, always have a veterinary technician evaluate the patient for stability. What clients consider an emergency is not always an emergency to team members, but must be treated as one (to enhance a positive client perception).

Basic animal instinct is just as important with the receptionist team as it is with technicians. Team members must not place their faces in the immediate face of an animal or behave aggressively with trained police or narcotics dogs. Receptionists must realize that not every animal is friendly and fearless. New smells, other animals, and unfamiliar people may place animals on alert and make them fearful.

Most clients do not inform veterinary team members when their pet has urinated in the waiting room, or do not notice when they have urinated. Receptionists are the closest team member to this area, and should scan the waiting room several times an hour to prevent urine from sitting on the floor. Several scenarios can occur when urine remains: clients slip and fall, odor permeates the practice, or clients form a negative perception of the hospital. These can all be prevented with a diligent receptionist.

Team Etiquette

Etiquette is defined as the rules that society has set for the proper way to behave around other people. The most obvious facet of etiquette is being kind and polite to others; therefore every team member must appear professional and treat both clients and other team members with respect.

Clients, visitors, and fellow employees observe actions of team members. The potential for veterinary practice growth, client acceptance, and compliance is based on team member etiquette. The failure to use etiquette among team members can be detrimental. Clients perceive the stress associated with poor etiquette, ultimately leading to decreased communication, client noncompliance, and poor profits (Box 2-1).

Team etiquette contributes to a positive team culture within the hospital. As mentioned above, clients (as well as others) perceive negative environments and cultures. Characteristics of a negative work culture include teams that do not work well together and employees that are not team players, gossip about one another, and form cliques. Characteristics of a positive culture include pride, ownership and accountability of the hospital, and client care that exceeds expectations. When team members have respect for one another, and practice etiquette as they should, a positive culture is formed. Negative cultures must be corrected and prevented in order for clients to continue returning to the hospital, and recommending friends and family. See Chapter 3 for more ideas on creating positive team environments.

> **PRACTICE POINT** Build etiquette into every conversation with team members and clients. Consider respect, empathy, and communication skills while building rapport with others.

Etiquette must also be recognized when a client's pet is being euthanized. This is an extremely difficult time for clients, and the receptionist can make the experience less painful. The receptionist should notify all team members that a euthanasia is planned so everyone can be sensitive to the atmosphere of the clinic (e.g., no laughing or giggling in the halls). A sign can also be posted on the door to the room where the euthanasia is occurring or lights can be turned off in the hallway in front of the exam room door; this helps ensure all team members are aware of the event.

Take care of all business transactions for euthanasia's before the procedure is performed. This includes choosing disposal options, presenting an invoice, and collecting fees. This allows a client to leave the building when they are ready, and not have to stop at the reception desk on the way out.

Team members should always wear name tags to identify themselves to the clients. Clients appreciate knowing who is caring for their pets. If a technician is credentialed, the appropriate abbreviation should be on the badge as well. Veterinarians should also have name badges. Clients may assume a technician is still treating their pet when, in fact,

---

BOX 2-1 | Ideas to Encourage Staff Etiquette

- Greet team members with a smile every morning. Happiness is contagious.
- Introduce team members when they are not acquainted with visitors and clients.
- Greet clients with a smile when they arrive.
- Always say goodbye to both clients and team members as they leave the practice—and mean it.
- Be a team player.
- Dress and act professionally.
- Do not criticize. Take the opportunity to educate team members instead of reprimanding.
- Have respect for each team member and client.
- Do not gossip.

the veterinarian has entered the room. Identification can be in the form of a pin, a magnet, or an embroidered name on the team member's scrubs.

Developing Effective Phone Techniques

The human voice has four components: volume, tone, rate, and quality. The volume of the receptionist's voice should make listeners comfortable, increasing the quality of the conversation. If a person's voice is too loud, listeners (in this case, clients) may pull the phone away from their ear, preventing them from hearing all of a conversation. If a receptionist's volume is too low, clients may be too embarrassed to ask for clarification on something they did not hear well. Correct volume is essential to a successful phone experience.

The tone of a voice is also referred to as *pitch*. Some speakers have a low, comforting tone, which increases the quality of the conversation. Others may have a high, squeaky pitch. Some clients may be unable to understand a squeaky voice and become irritated. The tone of voice a receptionist uses to answer the phone can give a client a lasting impression. Team members should have a pleasant, confident, and understandable voice. Tones can indicate "I am too busy to take your call right now" or "I am at your service today; how may I help you?" Team members should smile as they answer the phone; the tone of that smile will come across the phone line (Figure 2-2).

The rate of speaking can greatly affect a conversation. Speaking too quickly can leave the listener confused and unable to follow instructions. People who naturally speak fast should often remind themselves to slow their speaking rate. The receptionist must be efficient and knowledgeable and speak slowly and clearly. Many older clients cannot hear well and may not be able to understand a team member who is speaking rapidly. This can also imply that the practice is busy and that the receptionist does not have time for the client.

The quality of voice is a combination of clarity, volume, rate, and tone. Word choice and enunciation contribute to the clarity of a phone conversation. Poor word choice and enunciation devalues the professionalism and decreases the confidence the client has in the practice. Review Chapter 11 for methods to enhance word choices and enunciation.

All four factors are interrelated and have compounding effects on each other. Recording telephone conversations can help team members realize what they sound like on a phone and help improve skills and telephone etiquette. Hearing one's own voice can be an eye opener. *If you do not know what your voice sounds like, you cannot correct it.* Since tone of voice can make or break a conversation (and make or break a new client for the hospital), training of this sort should be implemented. It is also advised that recordings of team members occur randomly; knowing that a recording is taking places can alter ones behavior (it is advised to let team members and clients know they will be recorded for training purposes only).

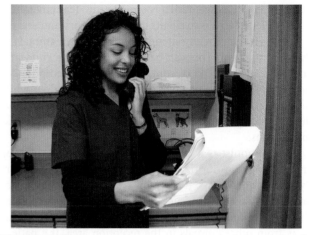

FIGURE 2-2 Answering the phone with a smile projects a friendly attitude that can be detected by the listener.

Team members should answer the phone by introducing themselves; this notifies the client with whom they are speaking and quickly develops a relationship. *"Good morning, ABC Animal Clinic, this is Teresa. How may I help you?"* is a good example. Often, long time clients feel guilty or embarrassed when they call and cannot identify whom they are speaking with; an introduction will help eliminate this.

It is important to write down the client and patient name when the caller has given this information. This prevents team members from having to ask for names to be repeated and possibly appearing disorganized. A call that has been placed on hold allows the team member to address the client personally when resuming the conversation. *"Thank you for holding, Mrs. Jones. Sparky's record indicates that he is due for vaccines …"*

Guidelines should be developed covering what to say and what not to say on the telephone. Many times, the same topic said with different words can have a very different meaning to the caller. For example, a client may call the hospital to request an appointment, believing that Fluffy's ear infection is a sudden emergency. The receptionist may respond, *"There are no appointments available until next week; however, you can come in as a walk-in and wait to be seen."* A client only hears *"we have no appointments,"* and they disengage in the conversation.

A better response would be, *"It sounds like we need to see Fluffy today, Mrs. Smith. We can accept you as a walk in, because our appointments are booked today. We can work Fluffy in between our appointments if you don't mind waiting."* By rewording the conversation, the client feels that it is important to come today, and the practice is willing to schedule her in. This helps build rapport and respect between the practice and the client.

Office managers may also develop a list of frequently asked questions and appropriate responses for topics such as:
- Setting up appointments
- Clients wanting to talk with the veterinarian immediately
- Clients asking for an update on a hospitalized pet
- A client asking questions regarding a statement or invoice

- Price shopping
- Angry and abusive callers
- Placing callers on hold
- Creating estimates
- Refill requests for food and medications
- Emergency calls
- Confirming upcoming surgeries and general appointments

Role-playing can facilitate correct responses to these potentially difficult situations. Role-playing places team members out of their comfort zone, as they feel that other team members may cast judgment on them. However, in a positive culture, team members help one another form excellent responses. Practicing (role-playing) together makes these situations more comfortable, and easy to handle when presented by clients.

> *PRACTICE POINT* Role-play (with team members) difficult scenarios that may occur with clients, to build confidence in personal responses.

Team members must learn not to say certain phrases. Expressions such as *"I don't know"* can imply the team member is not knowledgeable or does not care to get the correct information for the client. Instead of saying *"I don't know,"* team members should reply, *"that is a great question, let me find out."* Rather than saying a hurried *"just a second,"* a team member might say *"give me just a moment to get that [information or product]."* The combination of words and tone can have a powerful effect on clients. Words and phrases such as *"absolutely!", "I know how much you care,"* and *"I understand"* are powerful words that help create empathy with clients (Box 2-2).

Some clients enjoy casual phone conversations with the staff. Clients enjoy talking about their pets, and veterinary professionals are ideal listeners. However, the receptionist may need to control the conversation. Team members want to let clients know they are listening, caring, and compassionate, but another phone line may be ringing or another client may be waiting to pick up a pet (Figure 2-3). A few options exist to help control this conversation. It is acceptable to let the client know that there is another client waiting and that someone will call the client back with more information in approximately 10 minutes (then follow the general rule and call back in 5 minutes). Otherwise, ask closed-ended (yes or no) questions only, such as *"Is Fluffy vomiting?"* or *"Does Fluffy have diarrhea?"* (closed-ended questions are not ideal when taking an accurate history from clients; it is only made as a suggestion here, to help control prolonged conversations). Some clients may still attempt to prolong the conversation, but team members usually can get an appointment scheduled and end the conversation. It can be difficult to end a conversation without making the client perceive that the team member does not care. However, with practice and role-playing, team members can learn to convey sincerity. Receptionists often hear the same questions repeatedly when answering phones at a veterinary practice. Frequently asked

BOX 2-2	Powerful Words and Phrases

- "I understand"
- "I know you love your pet"
- "Unconditionally"
- "Extremely"
- "Absolutely"
- "Enormously"
- "Unquestionably"

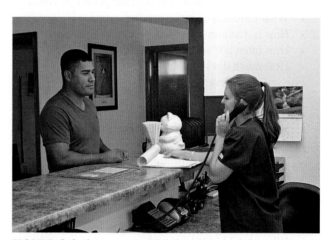

FIGURE 2-3 The receptionist must be able to multitask in a friendly and polite manner.

questions (FAQs) can be compiled to enhance the knowledge of the receptionist team, allowing questions to be answered immediately.

> Veterinary practice managers respond to client questions.

Technicians and veterinarians may be unable to take a phone call to answer simple questions if they are with a client or patient. The receptionist team can enhance the client's experience by being able to answer simple questions such as:
- Vaccine protocols
  - How old do puppies and kittens have to be to start vaccinations?
  - What vaccinations are recommended?
  - What vaccinations are included?
  - How often are vaccinations given?
  - What is included in the initial puppy or kitten examination?
  - How much do vaccinations cost?
- Spaying and neutering pets
  - How old do pets have to be to be altered?
  - Do vaccinations have to be current?
  - What does the surgical procedure entail?
  - Is pain medication included?
  - When do pets need to arrive at the practice?
  - When are they usually ready to go home?

- Do they need to be held off food and water?
- How much does the procedure cost?
- What lab work is required? Are IV fluids required?
- Sick pets
  - Is the pet vomiting? If yes, for how long?
  - Does the pet have diarrhea? If yes, for how long?
  - Does the pet have an appetite?
  - Is the pet current on vaccinations?
- Heartworm preventative
  - What is it?
  - What tests are required to start the pet on preventive?
  - What products does the practice carry?
  - How is it administered?
  - How often is it administered?
  - How much does it cost?
- Flea and tick preventive
  - What diseases do fleas and ticks carry?
  - Can people catch these diseases?
  - What products does the practice carry?
  - How are these products administered?
  - How often are these products administered?
  - How much do they cost?
- Diets
  - What special diets does the practice carry?
  - What maintenance diets does the practice carry?
  - What should I feed my pet?

New team members may be overwhelmed with new information. FAQ sheets can help new team members answer questions almost as well as those with experience.

Managing Multiple Phone Lines

Receptionists have clients to greet as they walk in and out of the practice, invoices or charges to enter, and multiple phone lines to answer at the same time (Figure 2-4). As a general rule, phones should not ring more than two times before being answered. In today's world, most clients call on a cell phone verses a landline. Often, the phone rings on the client's cell phone at least one time before the practice phone rings; therefore, if it has rung twice in the practice, it has rang three times for the client. Too many rings on the clients phone can create a negative perception to the client.

> **PRACTICE POINT** Respect clients' time when placing them on hold.

If a receptionist is with another client or on another line, it is acceptable to ask the client to hold momentarily because another phone line is ringing. For example, *"Good morning, ABC Animal Clinic, this is Teresa. I am on the other line [or with another client], are you able to hold one moment?"* Once the client answers yes (and they must be given time to answer), the team member should say, *"thank you."* This allows the receptionist to finish with the first client.

Asking a client *"Are you able to hold one moment?"* does exactly that; it *asks* the client politely. A short *"can you*

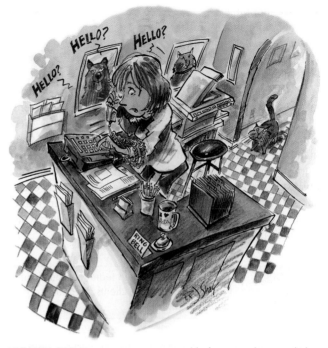

FIGURE 2-4 Receptionists are responsible for many duties, including managing multiple telephone lines and greeting incoming clients.

hold?" becomes a demand rather than a question. *"Thank you for holding, how may I help you?"* can then resume the conversation. If multiple lines continue ringing, a receptionist may also ask clients if a return call is possible instead of waiting on hold. *"Thank you for holding, this is Teresa. I have a client waiting for me, do you mind if I call you back in 10 minutes so you do not have to continue to hold?"* Once again, the client should be called back ASAP, or no more than 5 minutes later.

It is important not to leave callers on hold for more than 1 minute. Most current phone systems sound an alert after 1 minute; at this time clients should be told that the team member helping them would return momentarily. Do not continue to place clients on hold each time the alarm sounds. If the client will be on hold more than 1 or 2 minutes, the client should be asked if a team member could return the call as soon as the requested information is available. One minute on hold seems like 5 minutes to a client.

The time a client is on hold can be a valuable marketing resource time. Special on-hold systems can generate specific messages about the veterinary practice or specific diseases that may be a concern to the geographic area. Clients can be educated on a variety of topics while they are on hold. This information can include practice hours, history of the veterinarians, or specialties or products that the practice offers. (See Chapter 10 for more information regarding marketing for the veterinary practice.) If the caller has something to listen to, the wait time does not seem as long. Recordings can also assure the client that the phone line has not been disconnected. It can be difficult to determine if a call has been disconnected if the line is silent (especially while on cell phones).

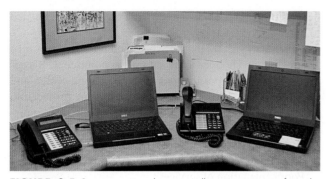

FIGURE 2-5 Some practices have a call center separate from the reception area.

BOX 2-3 | Labor Versus Service

- If 20 clients are seen in one day and a receptionist increases the average transaction of each client by $10, the receptionist has added $200 to the income for the day ($20 × $10 = $200).
- If the employee is paid $9 per hour and works an 8-hour day, she would be paid $72 per day. The labor formula of 20% is added for tax purposes ($72 × 20%) = $14.40. $72 + $14.40 = $86.40. The employee costs the employer $86.40.
- $200 − $86.40 = $113.60 of additional income per day. $113.60 × 5 days = $568 of additional income per week!

Receptionists should also be able to call on cross-trained team members to help assist when the phone lines continue to ring. Team members should also realize that if a phone line has rung more than two times, the receptionist team needs help. This is an ideal time for cross-trained employees to make a difference. Telephone calls are one of the first impressions made to a client, whether new or existing. If a client believes he or she was rushed through a conversation or that a call was never answered, the client may go to another practice.

Veterinary practices should never have an answering machine on during the day to catch an overflow of phone calls. The majority of new clients will not leave a message and will call another practice. If a receptionist is too busy to check the messages, return phone calls may not be made until much later in the shift. Every phone call must be answered during business hours. Current trends indicate clients dislike answering machines and automated phone services and want to talk to a live person. Prevent this potential irritant by having several team members available to answer the phone.

Practices may also find that all phone lines are always busy. If this is the case, it is imperative to add additional phone lines and team members to help answer the additional calls. If clients call a practice and always get a busy signal, they may chose to find another veterinary practice.

An ideal scenario is to have a call center located separately from the reception area (Figure 2-5). This allows the receptionist to give clients full attention as they enter and leave the practice. Mistakes are decreased when team members can concentrate on one client at a time. The team member(s) in the call center can concentrate on answering calls promptly and can review patient histories without other clients overhearing conversations. Some practice owners may argue that this will increase labor costs; however, if a receptionist can increase an average transaction by $10 either by catching a missed charge or by selling a client an extra $10 of service, then one receptionist has covered the cost of the labor and increased the profits at the end of the day (Box 2-3). Ultimately, clients are satisfied and will return because they experienced superior customer service within the veterinary practice. A continued interruption in client service builds a negative perception of the practice.

Turning Phone Calls into Appointments

A receptionist has the potential to turn every inquiring phone call into a client. A friendly and genuine voice makes a potential client feel comfortable and encourages the caller to ask questions. When the receptionist can answer questions in a polite, educated, and unhurried manner, the caller is inclined to make an appointment with the veterinary practice. The receptionist should ask open-ended questions to generate conversation. Open-ended questions do not require a yes or no answer; they open the door for discussion. The more education and value a team member can provide a potential client, the more likely the practice will gain a new client. Receptionists should always ask if they could make an appointment at the end of a phone conversation and end the discussion with *"Mr. Jones, have I answered all of your questions today? My name is Emma, and please call back anytime with any other questions you may have."*

Anytime a client (or potential client) asks questions regarding the price of the service, team members should be able to educate the client on service itself, and "WOW" the client with the value they will receive when coming to the practice. For example, a client calling to obtain the price of a neuter should not just receive the dollar amount. Compare the following examples, and determine which conversation will secure an appointment:

Example 1:

    Receptionist: *"Good morning, XYZ Animal Hospital. How can I help you?"*
    Client: *"Can you tell me the price of a spay for my dog?"*
    Receptionist: *"How big is your dog?"*
    Client: *"22 pounds."*
    Receptionist: *"That will be $100.99."*
    Client: *"OK, thank you."*

Example 2:

    Receptionist: *"Good morning, ABC Animal Hospital. This is Carol, how may I help you?"*
    Client: *"Can you tell me the price of a spay for my dog?"*
    Receptionist: *"Of course I can. I need to ask a few questions, which will help me give you the best estimate. First, what is your dog's name?"*
    Client: *"Rosy."*

Receptionist: *"How old is Rosy, and what breed is she?"*

Client: *"She is 6 months old and is a basset hound."*

Receptionist: *"Oh, bassets are so cute at this age! Tell me, how much does Rosy weigh, approximately?"*

Client: *"22 pounds."*

Receptionist: *"Now that I have this information, let me give you some information about the spay procedure for Rosy, and what you can expect postoperatively. First, it is best to spay her at a young age; this will help her recover quicker and helps prevent cancer associated with heat cycles later in her life. Here at ABC Veterinary Hospital, we perform a preoperative examination and listen to her heart and lungs, and look for any abnormalities that may alter our anesthesia plan. We also perform blood work, ensuring Rosy's liver and kidneys are functioning normally, as this can also alter our anesthetic plan. Each patient is different, and must be evaluated as such. Before Rosy's anesthesia, she is given pain medication and a tranquilizer to help her feel more comfortable. When Rosy is under anesthesia, we monitor her blood pressure, ECG, heart rate, respiratory rate, and temperature, among other vitals. When she awakes from anesthesia, she is kept in our recovery room with our veterinary technicians, where we continue to monitor her vitals. Rosy will go home with pain medication for you to start that evening, along with a complete set of discharge instructions. Do you have any questions about the procedure itself?"*

Client: *"Not about the procedure. How much does it cost?"*

Receptionist: *"The exam, blood work, preoperative pain medication, anesthesia, surgery, and pain medication for you to take home is all included in our price of $159.89. I have an appointment available for Rosy on Tuesday, would you be able to bring her in between 8 and 9 in the morning?"*

A conversation of this nature has established several points.

- A relationship has being established by the receptionist. She obtains Rosy's name, allowing her to use it in the conversation.
- She makes a personal comment about the breed. (The comment does not have to be breed specific; it may be a comment about the pets name or age.) The point is to make a specific, positive comment about the pet itself, continuing to build the relationship.
- By explaining the procedure itself, the receptionist is showing value in the service being provided. Perhaps ABC Veterinary Clinic is more expensive than XYZ Animal Hospital, however she explains why. She is also educating the client on why specific procedures are important
- At the end of the conversation, she offers the client an appointment date right away; many times receptionists will end a conversation with "Would you like to make an appointment?" This allows the client to say, *"No, I will call back later."* When a specific time slot is offered, client acceptance is much higher.

Always show value in the service being offered. Clients do not know good medicine from bad medicine, and they depend on team members to provide the education needed to make a good decision.

Benchmarks show that practices should be able to turn 70% of phone-shopped calls into an appointment. Receptionists should keep a logbook near the phone center, and track incoming calls. If 70% of calls are not turned into appointments, managers should determine why and implement training to increase this number. Potential reasons for a low percentage of acceptances include the following:

- Team member tone of voice or word choice
- Poor explanation of services
- Lack of training: unable to answer client questions
- Lack of recommending a specific time to set an appointment

> **PRACTICE POINT** 70% of phone shoppers should become a client. Maintain a log to track and improve numbers.

Taking Messages for Veterinarians and Technicians

Clients often call and want to speak to a doctor as soon as possible. The receptionist should be able to determine if a technician would be able to answer a client's questions. Technicians have many answers and can verify any additional information with the veterinarian. This allows the veterinarian(s) to continue providing service for clients and patients that are currently on the premises. Receptionists should always pull the applicable medical records for either the technician or veterinarian taking the call; this allows the team member to review the case before answering questions. Once the team member has answered the client's question, comments regarding the telephone conversation must be documented in the medical record. This allows the next team member to be able to follow the case if the client comes to the veterinary practice for an appointment or follow up with another phone call. It is important that every conversation with clients be documented in the medical record. Every case should be treated as if it will go to court. Simply speaking, if something is not documented in the record, legally it never happened. (See Chapter 4 for more information on documentation and the law.)

Messages need to be legible and contain accurate information. Team members should ask for a current phone number and repeat the number back to the client. Mild dyslexia is common, and team members will transpose numbers when writing down the client's phone number. Repeating the number prevents this error, which causes a loss of valuable time for the team. Messages can be written on a duplicate message pad; if a message is lost or misplaced, a copy is available for referral (Figure 2-6).

Liability of Telephone Calls

Team members can be held accountable for incorrect verbal communication. Misunderstood conversations can be held against the veterinary practice. Every telephone call must be

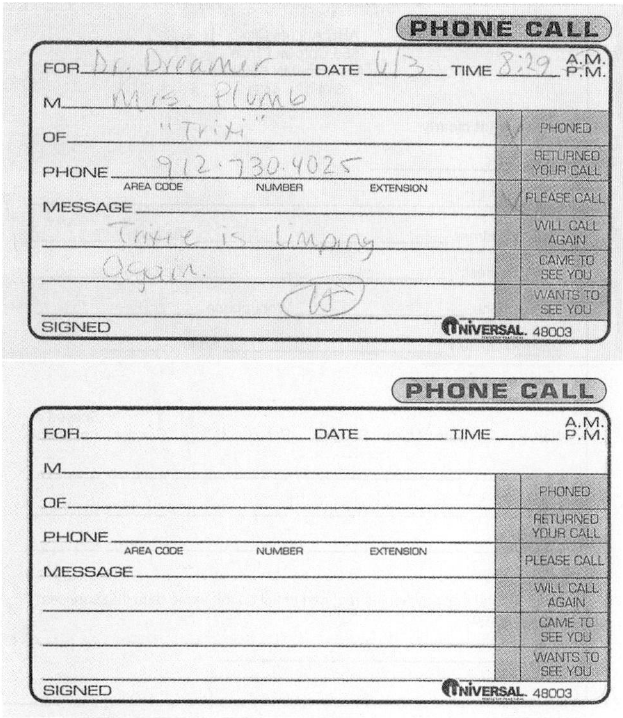

FIGURE 2-6 Duplicate message pads prevent lost messages.

documented in the patient's record, with details regarding the conversation. Only the veterinarian should give health care advice over the phone. Advice from another staff member is inappropriate and can be considered malpractice. Phrases such as *"you may want to wait and watch," "this does not sound like an emergency,"* or *"you can just give some Pepto-Bismol if your pet is vomiting"* **must never be said.** If the pet happens to die overnight, have complications, or be seen at an emergency clinic, the veterinary practice can be held liable. Always advise clients that if they are concerned about their pet's health, they should bring the animal in for an examination. Then document this call in the medical record. They have called for a service; offer to solve it with an appointment.

> **PRACTICE POINT** Clients call the hospital because they are concerned about their pet. Schedule them an appointment, versus advising them to *"wait and watch"*.

Veterinarians can also be held liable for giving medical advice over the phone if something happens to the patient. Malpractice lawsuits may have fewer consequences if the veterinarian gives advice compared with staff giving advice; however, the potential still exists. Veterinarians must also remember to document the conversation immediately; many veterinarians rush into the next appointment and forget to write the conversation in the medical record.

Personal Phone Calls

Business lines must be available for business use at all times. The employee manual should clearly state that personal phone calls are limited to emergencies only. If a personal call occurs, it must be kept short and to the point to keep lines available for clients. Potential clients who cannot reach the office may dial the next veterinary practice listed in their search, or clients with emergencies may panic if they cannot reach the practice immediately.

Cell phone policies should exist in veterinary practices (and be documented in the employee manual). Cell phones disengage team members from clients and decrease productivity.

Managing and Processing Mail

Veterinary practices receive many pieces of literature on a daily basis. Some is junk, but the majority consists of statements, laboratory reports, information on upcoming continuing education opportunities, or ads for the release of new products and books. All mail must be given to the person to whom it is addressed. Some veterinarians and technicians may like their mail to be opened, allowing greater efficiency in sorting, but others may prefer to keep their privacy. Statements and invoices should be given to the manager in charge of paying bills; all statements must be reviewed for correct charges. All laboratory reports should be placed within the clients' records and placed on the veterinarian's desk for review. Magazines and journals must be given to the subscriber. Continuing education brochures should be posted, allowing the entire team to note the opportunities available to further their knowledge.

Client Relations

Clients draw preliminary opinions about a practice within the first 2 to 5 minutes of entering the building. This perception (especially if it is negative) can continue through the rest of the visit. Team members should always greet clients as they enter the facility, regardless of what other tasks they may be doing. If a receptionist is on the phone, acknowledging clients with a smile and a wave is acceptable. If a receptionist is helping another client, greet the entering client with a smile and say, *"Hello, I will be with you in a moment."* If the receptionist is working with another team member, that task should be put aside and the client should receive the full attention of both team members.

Greeting clients by their names and addressing their pets create a positive first impression (Figure 2-7). This can be difficult with first-time clients; however, if team members can find something to compliment the owner or patient about, this can be overcome. Conversation starters such as *"Fluffy is such a beautiful girl,"* or *"Your necklace is beautiful, Mrs. Jones,"* make clients feel acknowledged. Small comments help provide exceptional service. Many clients prefer to be addressed as Mr., Mrs., or Dr. Once the initial appointment has began, team members may ask the new client how they wish to be addressed. A notation can be made in the record, allowing team members to address clients appropriately each time they arrive at the practice.

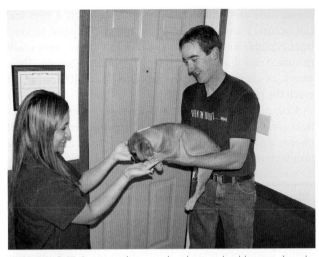

FIGURE 2-7 Greeting clients at the door and addressing them by name makes them feel they are getting personalized attention.

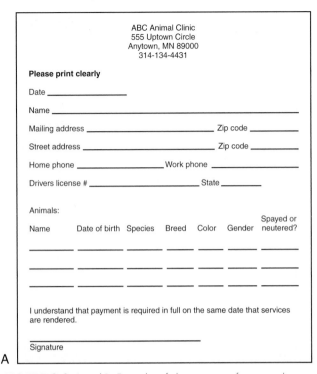

FIGURE 2-8 A and B, Examples of client patient information sheets.

When a client has been provided a service at the veterinary hospital, a follow-up appointment may be needed. It is very important to schedule that appointment while the client is still in the practice, and prior to accepting payment for services. Once payment has been rendered, the client closes down and is ready to leave the hospital. Creating the appointment before payment will have higher compliance. Most clients return for follow-up appointments when they are previously scheduled. If the patient is recovering well and the client has to initiate the phone call to make an appointment, it may not get done. Vaccines that need boosters and to be given within a certain time must be scheduled because clients "forget" and do not call to make an appointment. Receptionists should give the client an appointment card with the scheduled time on it as a friendly reminder. (See Chapter 13 for examples of appointment cards.)

Forms Commonly Used in Veterinary Practice

Clients may be asked to fill out various forms regarding their personal contact information (Figure 2-8), their pet's information and history, or a variety of release forms. Receptionists need to be sure all forms are filled out completely when a new client enters information. Obviously, contact information is vital in order to call the owner with updates regarding his or her pet's health. Address information must be current so that reminders may be mailed for vaccines, tests, and medication refills. Anytime a client returns to the clinic, the receptionist must verify that the contact information in the record is still current. It is also important that the client sign the bottom of the form, which should state that he or she (the client) is responsible for any charges regarding the listed patients.

> **PRACTICE POINT**   Become familiar with every consent form the practice uses, and be able to explain them in detail to clients.

The pet's information is an essential portion of the record. Details should include species, gender, date of birth, breed, color, and alteration status. *Species* refers to the classification: dog, cat, bird, rabbit, reptile, and so forth (Box 2-4). Team members must learn about breeds within a species; owners can be easily offended when team members are unfamiliar with their pet's breed. Purebred animals are generally easy to classify; mixed breeds can be referred to by the breed they most resemble. Mixed-breed cats can be difficult to classify and are generally described by their hair coat. Domestic shorthair (DSH) refers to a short-haired cat, domestic medium hair (DMH) refers to a cat with medium-length hair, and domestic longhair (DLH) refers to a long-haired cat.

The Medical Record

Each animal should have its own medical record as part of the overall record (Figure 2-9). The medical record should be dated each time an entry is made, listing the presenting problems and the author's initials. Practices may use paper medical records, be paperless, or paper light. Paper medical records must be kept on 8½ × 11 inch sheets of paper (index cards are no longer acceptable). Regardless of the type of medical records, every client conversation, consent form, lab report, consultation, physical exam, medication administered and dispensed, must be documented in the medical record. Paperless practices have the benefit of being able to access client records, laboratory results, and radiographs at any computer station. Paperless records allow space to be used for profit producing centers (versus space once used to hold medical records); they also result in decreased numbers of lost files and results. Review Chapter 14 for a complete medical records discussion.

Arroyo Vista Animal Clinic
2303 Inspiration Lane

Owner's name _____ Spouse _____

Address _____

Home telephone _____ Work telephone _____

Employer's name and address _____

Spouse's employer and address _____

Best time to call regarding your pet _____ Phone number _____

In case of emergency, please call _____

WRITTEN ESTIMATES ARE AVAILABLE UPON REQUEST. Please ask the receptionist if an estimate is needed. **ALL FEES ARE DUE AT THE TIME SERVICES ARE RENDERED.** If you plan to pay with a check or credit card, please complete the following:

MC ___ Visa ___ Exp Date _____ Driver's License Number _____ State ____ Expires _____

How did you hear of Arroyo Vista Animal Clinic? Yellow Pages ___ Referral (Name) _____ Other _____

Number and type of pets in your household? _____

Pet's origin: Humane Society ____ Pet Shop ____ Kennel ____ Breeder ____ Friend ____ Stray ____ Other ____

	Pet #1	Pet #2	Pet #3
Name			
Species (dog, cat)			
Breed			
Color			
Age			
Date of birth			
Sex			
Length of time owned			
Spayed or neutered			
Vitamins? (type)			
Diet (kind of food)			
Type of grooming products			
Inside or outside?			
Last rabies vaccine?			
Last DHLP vaccine? (Dog)			
Last parvo vaccine? (Dog)			
Last FVRCP vaccine? (Cat)			
Last FeLV vaccine? (Cat)			
Last leukemia test? (Cat)			
Last heartworm test? (Dog)			
Heartworm prevention?			
Last fecal exam?			
Last dental?			
Prior illness?			
Prior surgery?			

B

FIGURE 2-8, cont'd

BOX 2-4 | Species Identification

SPECIES	COMMONLY REFERRED TO AS	ABBREVIATION
Canine	Dog	K-9
Feline	Cat	Fe
Avian	Bird	Av
Iguanas, snakes, etc.	Reptiles	Re
Lagomorph	Rabbit	Ra
Equine	Horse	Eq
Bovine	Cow	Bo

Consent Forms

Clients may be asked to sign a variety of consent forms before various treatments and procedures can be performed on their pets (Figure 2-10, *A-K*). Every member of the team must be able to explain the meaning of any form a client is asked to sign. The forms are self-explanatory, however, team members must read the consent forms aloud to the client, helping to ensure the client understands what he or she is signing. Law does not require consent forms; their purpose is to protect the veterinary health care team. If the form is documented in the record, it can be submitted if a court case arises. If it is not documented, the assumption is that it was never discussed. All consents should contain the owner's and patient's names along with the date and the initials of the team member helping the client sign the forms.

Information included on consent forms should include known risks, alternatives, prognosis, and possible complications. Anesthetic release forms clearly indicate that anesthesia could result in death. Vaccination release forms (see Figure 2-10, *G*) state the risks and benefits of vaccinating pets along with the possibility of anaphylactic reaction, which may result in death. Euthanasia release forms (see Figure 2-10, *H* and *I*) state that the owner is presenting the pet for a painless, humane death (and should state that *euthanasia results in death*). Owners declining treatment or recommended diagnostic tests may also need to sign a release based on practice policies. Owners can refuse to vaccinate their pets, prevent heartworm disease,

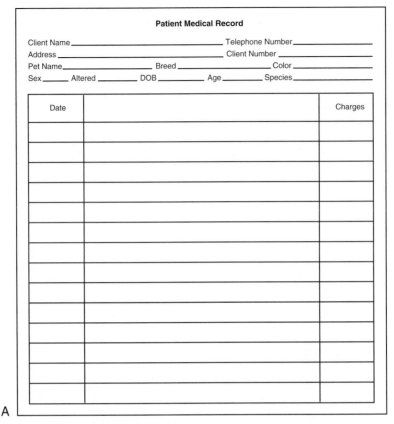

Patient Medical Record

Client Name _____   Telephone Number _____
Address _____   Client Number _____
Pet Name _____ Breed _____ Color _____
Sex _____ Altered _____ DOB _____ Age _____ Species _____

Date		Charges

A

FIGURE 2-9 A and B, Sample medical record sheet.

or test for heartworm disease. For the best interests of the practice, the owner should sign a release indicating that he or she, the client, does not hold the hospital, veterinarian, or any team member liable for any disease the client's pet may encounter when not accepting preventive measures recommended by the veterinarian and/or practice. When clients decline services of this nature, brochures and educational material should be sent home with clients. Sometimes, clients just need more information to make a decision (always document any literature that was sent home with the client in the medical record). This provides proof of additional information that was sent with client, and if the client calls and asks questions about the handout, team members know which handout is being referred to.

Patient History

Comprehensive patient medical history forms are essential when collecting information about new patients. Clients should fill out a form answering questions regarding the pet's health history. This helps the veterinary team diagnostically if any problems arise. History forms can also include an area for the owner to sign that allows the practice to treat the patient and acknowledges that the owner agrees to pay for services rendered (on the day the service is provided).

Rabies certificates are often printed by veterinary software systems. The team member enters the rabies tag bumber, lot number, and manufacturer of the vaccine. Lot numbers or

serial numbers of vaccines are critical information that must be entered in the event of a recall. If this information is not identified on the certificate or in the medical record, practices would not be able to identify who received the recalled vaccine. Client and patient information are automatically populated by the practice management software; veterinary signature and license numbers must be added to all printed certificates.

If a rabies vaccine book (handwritten verses computer generated) is used, the correct owner and patient information must be legible. The date and the owner's name, address, and phone numbers are required. The patient's name, age, breed, and gender are also required. The rabies tag number and lot number are then entered, along with the veterinarian's signature and license number. The rabies tag number often identifies lost animals; therefore it is important to ensure the information has been added correctly and legibly.

Spay and neuter certificates are generated once a pet has been altered. This provides the owner with proof that the pet was altered if such proof is ever needed. This certificate may also be required when ordinances require pets to be registered with a city or county. Many city and county agencies require pets to be licensed, capping the number of pets allowed per household. All pets may be required to be licensed, including dogs, cats, rabbits, and ferrets, as well as some exotic species. Practices should be familiar with local laws regarding pet licensing. Local chapters of the Humane

SANDIA RESORT AND CASINO CLINIC
30 Rainbow Road NE, Albuquerque, NM
(505) 555-1212

DVM		Date:
DVM		Owner:
		Patient:

Presenting Complaint:_____

Temp.:_____ Pulse:_____ Resp. Rate:_____

Wt.:_____ Ideal Wt.:_____ Current Rx _____

Findings:

	Normal	Abnormal	Not exam.		Normal	Abnormal	Not exam.
General Appearance				Lymph Nodes			
Skeletal System				Mucous Membranes			
Heart				Eyes			
Lungs				Ears			
Abdomen				Mammary Glands			
Testicles				Skin			

Skin Chart   (L) Dorsal   (R)   (R) Ventral (L)

1. ABSCESS
2. SKIN TUMORS
3. SKIN CYSTS
4. DRY/FLAKING
5. OILY
6. HAIR LOSS
7. FLEAS
8. TICKS
9. WOUND

Vaccinations:	
DHLPP	
DHLPP/Corona	
Bordetella	
Rabies (1 yr.)	
Rabies (3 yr.)	
FVRCP	
FVRCP/Leukemia	

<u>Heartworm</u>: Neg.   Pos.   Result Pending   Not Done   <u>Fecal</u>: Neg.   Pos.   Result Pending   Not Done

Objective/Additional Findings:_____

_____
_____
_____
_____
_____
_____
_____

Diagnosis/Prognosis:_____

Plan/Treatment:_____

_____
_____
_____
_____

Laboratory/Medical/Surgical Recommendations: _____

Follow-up Comments: Date:_____ _____

_____
_____
_____

B

FIGURE 2-9, cont'd

Society of the United States and animal shelters are excellent sources of information regarding laws and ordinances pertaining to pets.

A master problem list is a summary of the patient's health status (Figure 2-11). Vaccinations, laboratory tests, acute and chronic diseases, and current medications can be listed on one sheet. Master lists can increase efficiency when team members do not have to search through the entire record to find medication refill information. The list can clearly indicate when a patient is overdue for an examination, vaccinations, or laboratory work. Master problem lists should also include any vaccine, medication,

or anesthetic reaction the pet may have had in the past. The use of electronic medical records is reducing the need for master sheets, because these are automatically produced by the software.

Health Certificates

Health certificates are required by airlines, as well as some state and federal agencies, when traveling with pets. Airlines want to ensure the pet is in healthy condition before accepting it for transport, and states want to ensure the pet is not importing any diseases. Both federal and state agencies are responsible for the prevention of disease and have various regulations

ABC Veterinary Clinic

Surgery/Anesthesia Consent Form

Client Name_____ Date _____

Pet's Name_____

Your pet has been scheduled for a procedure requiring sedation or anesthesia. By signing this form, you authorize ABC Veterinary Clinic and its agents to administer tranquilizers, anesthetics, and/or analgesics that are deemed appropriate for your pet. Please be aware that all drugs have the potential for adverse side effects in any particular animal. The chances of such occurrence are extremely low.

I am aware that staff is not on premises after hours, and I agree to indemnify ABC Veterinary Clinic and its agents harmless from and against any and all liability arising from the care that is provided.

In an effort to ensure your pet's safety and to anticipate any problems before they may occur, we have available preanesthetic electrocardiogram and blood testing capabilities to detect hidden heart, liver, kidney, or other problems that may increase the risk to your pet. This testing is available for an additional charge. If abnormalities are detected, we will attempt to notify you, and the anesthetic procedure may be delayed or modified. Please verify the procedures being performed and indicate your wishes concerning the option of preanesthetic testing. If you have any questions, please ask BEFORE signing this form.

Procedures scheduled:_____

Routine surgical procedures are painful. We recommend postoperative pain medication for each procedure. Pain medication is automatically dispensed for each patient. If you **decline postoperative pain medication, please sign here:**_____

How may we contact you **today?**_____

Home phone _____ Work phone_____

Cell phone/pager _____ Client signature_____

A

Arroyo Vista Animal Clinic

2303 Inspiration Lane, Anywhere, USA
Dr. Larsen, Dr. Cooke, and Dr. Thompson
Hospitalization/Surgical Consent Form

Owner's Name_____

Pet's Name_____ Breed_____ Sex_____ Age_____ Color_____

I certify that I own the above described animal and do hereby consent and authorize Dr. Larsen or her associates to hospitalize and/or administer vaccinations, medication, tests, surgical procedures, or treatments the doctor and her associates deem necessary for the health, safety, or well-being of the above animal while it is under their care and supervision.

If the pet should injure itself in an escape attempt, refuse food, urinate or defecate on itself, become ill or die while in the hospital, I will hold Dr. Larsen and her associates, along with the staff of Arroyo Vista Animal Clinic, free of any responsibility and/or liability in the absence of gross negligence.

I realize that my pet will only be discharged during regular office hours and when the doctor or her associates are present, and the fee due for its care will be paid in full at that time. If I neglect to pick up my pet within five (5) days of written notice, you may assume the animal is abandoned and you are thereby authorized to dispose of it as you see fit. I further realize that should I not pay the amount due at the time of pickup, I will be responsible for reasonable costs of collection, including court costs and reasonable attorney's fees.

In the event that I become ill, move, or change my address, it shall be my duty to inform the hospital of such changes.

I hereby acknowledge that I have read the foregoing and fully understand the terms and conditions set forth.

Signed_____ Dated_____

Staff Member Signature_____ Dated_____

B

FIGURE 2-10 A to K, Examples of various release forms. A, Surgery/anesthesia consent form. B, Hospitalization/surgical consent form.

{CLINICNAME}
{CLINICADDRESS1}
{CLINICADDRESS2}
{CLINICCITY} , {CLINICSTATE} {CLINICPOSTALCODE}
{CLINICPHONE}

Standard Consent Form
{CURRENTDATE[SHORT]}

Client ID: {ID}   Patient ID: {PATIENTID}
Client Name: {FULLNAME}   Name: {NAME}
Address: {ADDRESS1}   Species: {SPECIES}
                    {ADDRESS2}   Breed: {BREED}
                    {CITY} , {STATE} {POSTALCODE}   Sex: {SEX}
Telephone: {PHONENUMBER}   Color: {COLOR}
                                                        Markings: {MARKINGS}
                                                        Birth Date: {BIRTHDATE[SHORT]}

I hereby certify that I am the owner of the above-named animal or am responsible for it and have the authority to execute this consent.

I hereby authorize the performance of the following procedure(s):

_____

_____

I hereby also authorize the use of such anesthetics as you deem advisable and performance of such surgical or therapeutic procedures as you determine to be indicated. I understand that conditions not known may make it advisable that other surgical/treatments be done. {CLINICNAME} will try to contact me before doing added treatments, should they not be able to contact me, I authorize such treatments/anesthetics/surgeries, etc. when and if they are deemed necessary.

I agree to indemnify and hold {CLINICNAME} harmless from and against any and all liability arising out of the performance of any of the procedures referred to above.

All charges including boarding costs will be paid when the pet is released from the hospital. If the pet is not called for within 10 (ten) days after the specified time for return and if the doctor/clinic is not notified of an alternate date within this ten day period, the pet will be considered ABANDONED. {CLINICNAME} is given the right to dispose of the animal as the doctor/clinic sees fit -- including giving the animal away or euthanasia. It is understood that abandonment does not relieve me of my responsibility for all costs of services, medication, and boarding.

_____
(Signature of legal owner or responsible person)

AT WHAT NUMBER CAN YOU BE CONTACTED TODAY?

C

Pre-Surgery Questionnaire

	Yes	No
1. Has your pet eaten within the last twelve hours?	____	____
2. Has your pet had anything to drink within the last four hours?	____	____
3. Has your pet vomited or had any diarrhea within the last week?	____	____
4. Have you noticed any rashes or itching?	____	____
5. Any history of trauma in the last week?	____	____
6. Any previous problems with anesthesia?	____	____
7. Is your pet current on all vaccinations?	____	____
8. Has your dog been tested for heartworms in the last twelve months?	____	____
9. Is your dog currently on heartworm prevention?	____	____
10. Is your cat feline leukemia negative?	____	____
11. Is your pet currently on medication?	____	____

If so, please list:_____

12. Does your pet have any other medical problems or conditions?	____	____

If so, please explain:_____

13. Would you like your pet's nails trimmed at no additional cost?	____	____

14. Purebred cats may require an alternate anesthesia protocol to lessen the anesthetic risk. Please initial the line to the right that you understand there will be additional charges.   ____

15. Would you like an Elizabethan collar to take home? (If the patient starts licking while in our care, we will automatically send home a collar.)   ____   ____

16. Is your pet microchipped?	____	____

Signature: _____ Date: _____

If you are not certain about the questions above, please consult a veterinary technician prior to admission for advice.

D

FIGURE 2-10, cont'd C, Standard consent form. D, Pre-surgery questionnaire.

Continued

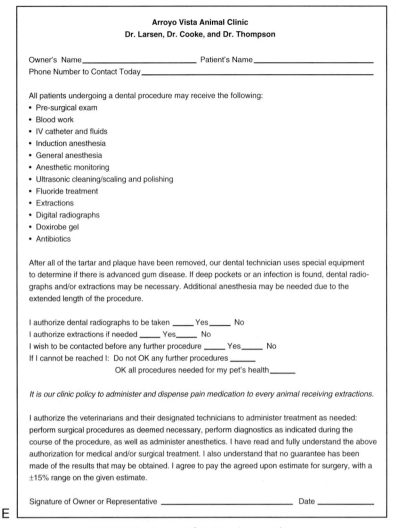

Arroyo Vista Animal Clinic
Dr. Larsen, Dr. Cooke, and Dr. Thompson

Owner's Name_____ Patient's Name_____
Phone Number to Contact Today_____

All patients undergoing a dental procedure may receive the following:
• Pre-surgical exam
• Blood work
• IV catheter and fluids
• Induction anesthesia
• General anesthesia
• Anesthetic monitoring
• Ultrasonic cleaning/scaling and polishing
• Fluoride treatment
• Extractions
• Digital radiographs
• Doxirobe gel
• Antibiotics

After all of the tartar and plaque have been removed, our dental technician uses special equipment to determine if there is advanced gum disease. If deep pockets or an infection is found, dental radiographs and/or extractions may be necessary. Additional anesthesia may be needed due to the extended length of the procedure.

I authorize dental radiographs to be taken _____ Yes_____ No
I authorize extractions if needed _____ Yes_____ No
I wish to be contacted before any further procedure _____ Yes_____ No
If I cannot be reached I: Do not OK any further procedures _____
                    OK all procedures needed for my pet's health_____

It is our clinic policy to administer and dispense pain medication to every animal receiving extractions.

I authorize the veterinarians and their designated technicians to administer treatment as needed: perform surgical procedures as deemed necessary, perform diagnostics as indicated during the course of the procedure, as well as administer anesthetics. I have read and fully understand the above authorization for medical and/or surgical treatment. I also understand that no guarantee has been made of the results that may be obtained. I agree to pay the agreed upon estimate for surgery, with a ±15% range on the given estimate.

Signature of Owner or Representative _____ Date _____

E

FIGURE 2-10, cont'd E, Dental consent form.

regarding the entry of animals. Interstate health certificates are generally good for 10 days before shipment (Figures 2-12).

The pet must be fully examined by a veterinarian before the certificate is issued. Most states require submission of a copy of the health certificate. International health certificates are generally good for 30 days and require the signature of the state veterinarian. These certificates are for shipment of pets out of the United States. Both forms of health certificates require the owner's name, address, and phone number along with the name, address, and phone number of the person who will be accepting and taking responsibility of the pet. All of the animal's identifying information must be included, including age, breed, gender, and microchip or tattoo number. The animal's vaccines must be current and the vaccination information clearly stated. Small animal and large animal health certificates differ; large animal certificates should indicate tests that are required (by state law) and completed, with the results stated. Before shipment to any state or country, regulations must be verified. Some countries have strict regulations regarding the importation of animals, mostly to limit disease transmission.

Some countries require a series of rabies vaccines and a rabies titer to import animals. The rabies neutralizing antibody titer test (RNATT) is a general term for the methods that measure rabies virus neutralizing antibody (RVNA) titers. Other countries may require a microchip before importation, along with deworming and the application of flea and tick preventive immediately before shipment. Visit the U.S. Department of Agriculture at www.aphis.usda.gov/regulations/vs/iregs/animals/ for the most current information regarding animal importation procedures.

Medical Records Release Form

A signed consent form to release medical records may be required by some states. It is important to understand the Privacy Act and not release any records without the client's authorization. The Privacy Act of 1974 states, in part:

No agency shall disclose any record which is contained in a system of records by any means of communication to any person, or to another agency, except pursuant to a written request by, or with the prior written consent of, the individual to whom the record pertains.

Many practices have owners fill out medical release forms and return them to the clinic either by mail, email, or fax.

Arroyo Vista Animal Clinic
Dr. Larsen, Dr. Cooke, and Dr. Thompson

Owner's Name _____ Patient's Name _____
Phone Number to Contact Today _____

Pre-Anesthesia Blood Work

Under 2 Years of Age	2-7 Years of Age	Above 7 Years of Age
ALT, BUN, CREA, ALK Phos, Glucose, TP **Total: $39.91**	ALT, BUN, CREA, ALK Phos, Glucose, TP, Electrolytes **Total: $55.67**	Comprehensive blood work: ALT, ALB, AMY, BUN, Ca, CREA, ALK Phos, Glob, Bili, Glucose, TP, Electrolytes, CBC **Total: $117.35**

I choose the appropriate blood work for my pet's age. _____ (initial)
I decline the recommended blood work and assume anesthetic risk. _____ (initial)

Your pet's health is our primary concern. Our most effective and safest anesthetic drugs require the use of an intravenous catheter (IV) placed on the forearm of your pet's leg. This requires a small area to be shaved and disinfectant applied. Your pet will receive IV fluids during and after the anesthetic period, which provides for safer anesthesia, a quicker recovery, and better pain management. An IV also gives the ability to provide emergency drugs if needed. An additional $39.11 will be applied to your account.

I give permission for my pet to receive IV fluids. _____ (initial)
I do not give permission for my pet to receive IV fluids. _____ (initial)

It is our belief that pain control is necessary for patients that have surgery. Not only is it humane to prevent pain, it has been scientifically proven that pets recover faster with pain medication. Additional pain medication ranges from $15.00 to $30.00 based on the size of your pet.
I request that my pet receive pain medication. _____ (initial)
I decline pain medication for my pet. _____ (initial)

I am the owner or caretaker of the pet, and I assume all responsibility of care after surgery. I understand that all anesthesia and surgical procedures involve a degree of risk and realize results cannot be guaranteed. While performing the surgery, should the veterinarian find the procedure to involve more than originally estimated, I will be contacted prior to continuation. If I cannot be contacted, I authorize the veterinarian to continue with the procedure deemed appropriate for my pet. I understand that I will be responsible for full payment upon patient discharge.

Signature of owner/caretaker _____
Contact phone number _____
Signature of staff member _____

F

FIGURE 2-10, cont'd F, Anesthesia consent form.

Continued

Medical records release forms should also give an estimated time of when records will be available for pickup or fax so the client will know when to expect them. Some practices charge a fee for copying records; this price must be included on the release.

> **PRACTICE POINT** Always ask clients to sign a medical records release form in order to comply with the Privacy Act of 1974.

Boarding

Boarding consent forms may list services offered by veterinarians that clients might need to be reminded of (Figure 2-13). When admitting a pet for boarding, it is important to document the names and dosages of medication(s) the pet will be receiving as well as what kind of food the animal eats (including at what frequency and times). It must also contain emergency contact information in case of an emergency as well as an authorization to treat the pet according to veterinary recommendations.

Many practice management software systems include consent forms that can be modified. When these consent forms are chosen by a team member, the client and patient information is automatically populated; the form can then be printed and reviewed with the owner.

Handling Special Situations with Clients

Clients can be pleasant or difficult, depending on the kind of person they are, the type of day they have had, or the type of situation presented to them once they arrive at the practice. If a client has had a bad day, the team may take the brunt of the person's frustration. Team members should remember not to take the comments of these clients personally and instead try to make it a better day for the client.

Pet Immunization Information/Consent
ABC Veterinary Clinic

Immunizing your pet is an important procedure that in most cases will provide protection against an illness that may be life threatening. In past years, veterinarians have followed the vaccine manufacturer's guidelines and recommended annual revaccination for diseases that were believed to be a threat to our patients. Recent studies have shown that annual revaccination may not be necessary for some diseases because many pets are protected for three years or longer when vaccinated. Although most pets do not react adversely to vaccination, some have had allergic or other systemic reactions after receiving a vaccine. Rarely, the allergic reaction can be so profound that it may be life threatening. Certain immune-mediated diseases such as hemolytic anemia (anemia caused by red blood cell destruction), thrombocytopenia (low blood platelet numbers), and polyarthritis (joint inflammation and pain) in dogs may be triggered by the body's immune response to a vaccine. A serious additional concern has been a lump forming at the site of the vaccination. Why this occurs in cats is controversial at best, but it is considered extremely rare. In some cats, if these lumps persist, a tumor known as a fibrosarcoma may form that may have grave consequences if ignored. If your cat develops a lump under the skin after a vaccination that persists for longer than four weeks, you should have it examined as soon as possible.

Vaccinating your pet should not be taken lightly. Failure to vaccinate could result in your pet contracting a serious preventable disease. However, unnecessary vaccinations should be avoided. A decision to vaccinate should only come after you and your veterinarian consider your pet's age and the risk of exposure to disease. Vaccinations given at the appropriate age and at the appropriate intervals will greatly benefit your pet and protect it against some life-threatening diseases.

I understand the risks and benefits associated with vaccinating my pet. I hereby release ABC Veterinary Clinic of all liabilities associated with vaccinating my pet.

Owner _____ Date _____

G

Euthanasia Release

I, the undersigned, do hereby certify that I am the owner of the animal, and hereby give ABC Veterinary Clinic full and complete authority to euthanize the animal in whatever manner the doctor shall deem fit. I hereby release the doctors and staff from any and all liabilities for euthanizing said animal. I understand that euthanasia results in death.

I do also certify that the said animal has not bitten any person or animal during the last 15 days and to the best of my knowledge has not been exposed to rabies.

Owner _____ Date _____

H

{CLINICNAME}
{CLINICADDRESS1}
{CLINICADDRESS2}
{CLINICCITY}, {CLINICSTATE} {CLINICPOSTALCODE}
{CLINICPHONE}

Euthanasia Authorization
{CURRENTDATE[SHORT]}

Client ID:	{ID}	Patient ID:	{PATIENTID}
Client Name:	{FULLNAME}	Name:	{NAME}
Address:	{ADDRESS1}	Species:	{SPECIES}
	{ADDRESS2}	Breed:	{BREED}
	{CITY}, {STATE}	Sex:	{SEX}
	{POSTALCODE}		
Telephone:	{PHONENUMBER}	Color:	{COLOR}
		Markings:	{MARKINGS}
		Birth Date:	{BIRTHDATE[SHORT]}

I, the undersigned, do hereby certify that I am the owner (duly authorized agent for the owner) of the animal described above, that I do hereby give the doctors of {CLINICNAME} permission to euthanize and dispose of said animal in whatever manner the said doctors of {CLINICNAME}, their agents, servants or representatives deem fit. I also release the doctors, {CLINICNAME} , their agents, servants and representatives for any and all liability for so euthanizing and disposing of said animal. I do also certify that to the best of my knowlege the said animal has not bitten any person or animal during the last ten (10) days and has not been exposed to rabies.

SIGNED _____

I

FIGURE 2-10, cont'd G, Immunization information and consent form. H, Euthanasia release form. I, Euthanasia authorization form.

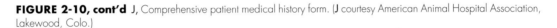

AAHA
AMERICAN
ANIMAL
HOSPITAL
ASSOCIATION

Comprehensive Patient Medical History Form

	Yes	No
Are your address and phone still correct?		
Do you have pet health insurance?		
Are your pet's vaccinations up to date?		
Is your pet spayed or neutered?		
Was there a heartworm test in the last year?		
Is your pet taking heartworm prevention Rx?		
Has your pet been tested for worms in the last year?		
Have you seen your pet passing any worms?		
Has your pet had any illness/injury in the last year?		
Has your pet ever had a seizure?		
Does your pet get table scraps?		
Did your pet eat in the last four hours?		
Does your pet ever strain to urinate?		
Has there been any recent vomiting?		
Has your pet been coughing?		
Has your pet been sneezing?		
Has your pet been gagging?		
Any listlessness?		
Any weakness?		
Any lameness? Circle leg: RF LF RR LR		
Shaking of the head?		
Scratching? Where?		
Significant hair loss?		
Scooting of rear?		
Unusual lumps or bumps?		
Bad breath?		
Unusual discharge?		
Diarrhea?		
Constipation?		
Stiffness?		
Behavior changes?		

	Increased	Decreased
Drinking?		
Appetite?		
Urination?		
Defecation?		
Weight?		

Reason for visit today?
_____
_____
_____

Has your pet been examined elsewhere for the same condition?   Yes   No

If so, where?_____

What medication is your pet now taking?
_____
_____

Is your pet allergic to any food or Rx?   Y   N

If yes, please describe _____

What flea control is used?

Anything else we need to know?
_____
_____
_____
_____
_____
_____

I hereby authorize the hospital to prescribe for and treat the conditions presented on this form for the pet presented by me. The hospital and staff will not be held liable for any problems that develop provided that reasonable care is provided. Furthermore, I agree to pay fees in full for services rendered when pet is discharged from the hospital's care unless other prior arrangements have been agreed upon by both parties.

_____   _____
Signature   Date

J

FIGURE 2-10, cont'd J, Comprehensive patient medical history form. (J courtesy American Animal Hospital Association, Lakewood, Colo.)

Continued

Receptionists must effectively handle hostile clients on the phone. Although clients may call and be angry at the practice for some reason, the receptionist handling the conversation can turn the call into a positive experience. First, the receptionist should listen to the client. Once the client has finished his or her portion of the conversation, the receptionist should review the facts, ensuring that a miscommunication does not occur. If possible, the receptionist should identify the client's needs, and provide a solution, in turn, making the client happy.

If the situation is above what a receptionist can handle, and a manager is available to take the telephone call, the manager and client can discuss the case. If a supervisor is not available, the receptionist can politely state that the manager who can handle the situation is not available at the moment but he or she will return the call as soon as possible. A delay in the conversation may either infuriate the client that the situation cannot be immediately resolved, or allow the client to calm down before a manager returns the call. All team members should have some authority to make a client happy, immediately, especially when a supervisor is unable to aid in the satisfaction process.

Angry clients that are at the practice should be taken into an exam room and allowed to vent in private. A team member who simply listens to the client often diffuses the situation. The team member can try to offer a solution that is satisfactory to the client to resolve the problem. If the fault lies with the practice, the mistake must be admitted and apologized for. Many times this repairs the situation immediately. (See Chapter 11 for more resolution techniques for angry clients.)

Grieving clients can be difficult because they have just suffered an emotional loss, sometimes similar to that experienced when losing a family member. Depending on the situation, clients may be in shock and disbelief; others have accepted the situation and are sad. Clients in shock and disbelief may be angry (the pet may have just been hit by a car, and they are angry at the driver as well as at the practice for not doing more to save their pet). On occasion, a poor prognosis has been given for a patient, but the client believes that more could be done to save the pet. The client may leave quickly, ask for a copy of the animal's records, and go to another veterinarian for a second opinion.

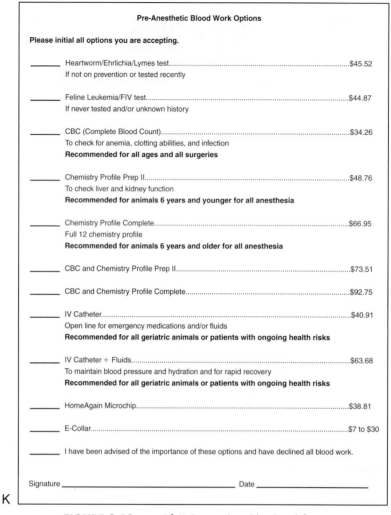

FIGURE 2-10, cont'd K, Pre-anesthetic blood work form.

In all of these situations, clients must be taken to an isolated area to discuss their pet's condition; the reception area is not appropriate for providing sensitive information. The clients must be allowed to vent their anger (only verbally, *not* physically) before they leave the practice. Once they have been able to discuss the situation with a team member, the situation will likely calm down. Chapter 12 discusses the stages of grief in detail and provides more information on how team members can help clients cope with a traumatic situation.

> **PRACTICE POINT** Always place angry clients in a private room (away from other clients), then begin diffusing the situation.

Clients who arrive at the practice under the influence of drugs or alcohol can be dangerous to team members and other clients. Impaired individuals cannot reason because their ability to comprehend information is decreased. Drugs and alcohol distort thought processes; trying to hold a rational conversation can be dangerous. The client should be asked

to leave, and the practice manager or veterinarian can call the client at a later time. If the client refuses to leave, the police should be called. The situation should not be allowed to progress, and the team should not make an effort to satisfy the client. Satisfaction will not occur when drugs have influenced the person's mental state.

Clients may slip and fall in the practice, presenting a significant liability. Signs must be posted when the floor is wet, and a team member should be available to direct clients around the wet area until it is dry. Clients may trip on rugs, shelving units, or any other object that sits on the floor. Wall-to-wall carpets should not curl up at the seams, and area rugs should have anti-skid material on the back to prevent tripping and slipping. Objects such as scales should have large warning barriers at the corners to prevent tripping (Figure 2-14). Team members should rush to the side of any client who has fallen in the practice. Many times team members are in shock when a client falls, and they stop and stare. The client should be asked if he or she feels any pain and where it is coming from. If needed, stabilize the patient in the same location until an ambulance arrives. Once the client feels stable

Master Problem List

Client name_____ Telephone number_____

Address _____ Client number _____

Pet name_____ Breed _____ Color_____

Sex _____ Altered _____ DOB _____ Age _____

	Date received	Date received	Date received	Date recieved
DHLPP				
FVRCP				
FeLV				
Rabies				
HWT				
FeLV/FIV				

Chronic diseases/date of onset:_____

_____

_____

_____

Current medications and directions:_____

_____

_____

_____

_____

FIGURE 2-11 Example of master problem list.

enough to leave independently or the ambulance leaves for the hospital, pictures of the area should be taken. All team members who witnessed the accident should immediately write down the facts of the accident. If time passes before members write out the events, details will be forgotten. It may be advised to call the liability insurance company to inform it of the accident in case a lawsuit is brought against the practice. Chapter 21 discusses a variety of safety issues within the practice that should be addressed.

Reviewing Invoices with Owners

A team member should always review invoices with owners before collecting money. Services that have been provided should be detailed, and the receptionist should be knowledgeable enough to answer questions easily (cross-training helps in this area) (Figure 2-15). An invoice of the services should be detailed to include every facet of the service. The client should be able to review the invoice while the team member explains the charges (Figure 2-16). Following is a detailed example.

Scruffy had surgery at ABC Animal Clinic, and the client has arrived to pick her up. The receptionist greets the client, *"Hello, Mrs. Rogers, are you here to pick up Scruffy? I have her invoice ready for you. Today she had a preoperative exam at no charge; preoperative blood work for $45.99; a preoperative ECG for $49.99; and IV fluids for $54.85, which includes the IV catheter, IV administrative set, and the fluids. Her anesthesia, which included pre-operative pain medication and vital monitoring was $101.20; the ovariohysterectomy, which*

included the surgery pack and materials was $97.89; and her post operative pain medication which was given after surgery and for you to take home is $24.99. Scruffy's total is $398.34. Do you have any questions for me?"

This detailed presentation allows the client to read and understand the services provided. The value of the service has increased to the client once all procedures that have been provided are explained. An alternative conversation would be, *"Hello, Mrs. Rogers. I have Scruffy's invoice ready. The total is $398.34. How would you like to pay for that today?"* In this situation, the client does not know what she is paying for and may have a sense of sticker shock at the cost of a "simple spay." She will not perceive the value of the services her pet was provided and may respond, *"My, that is expensive!"* She may look for a cheaper clinic for her next veterinary visit.

Payment for Services

The most common forms of payment are by cash (including debit card), check, or credit card. The practice manager may choose which credit cards to accept. Practices pay a percentage of the total credit card transaction to the bank issuing the card. Most machines are very simple to operate; a team member slides the card and enters the expiration date and charge amount, and the machine connects to a designated terminal and either approves or declines the transaction (Figure 2-17). Debit transactions are quite similar, except the client enters a personal identification number (PIN) code before the transaction is approved.

carrier for transportation in commerce, unless accompanied by a health certificate executed and issued by a licensed veterinarian (7 USC 2143: 9 CFR, Subchapter A, Part 2).

(See reverse for additional OMB statement)

FORM APPROVED
OMB NO. 0579-0036)

U.S. DEPARTMENT OF AGRICULTURE
ANIMAL AND PLANT HEALTH INSPECTION SERVICE

UNITED STATES INTERSTATE AND INTERNATIONAL CERTIFICATE OF HEALTH EXAMINATION FOR SMALL ANIMALS

WARNING: Anyone who makes a false, fictitious, or fraudulent statement on this document, or uses such document knowing it to be false, fictitious or fraudulent may be subject to a fine of not more than $10,000 or imprisonment of not more than 5 years or both (18 U.S.C 1001).

1. TYPE OF ANIMAL SHIPPED ☐ Dog ☐ Cat ☐ Other ☐ Nonhuman Primate

CERTIFICATE NUMBER P132195

2. TOTAL NUMBER OF ANIMALS

PAGE

3. NAME, ADDRESS AND TELEPHONE NUMBER OF OWNER/CONSIGNOR

USDA License/or Registration No. if applicable Telephone:

4. NAME, ADDRESS AND TELEPHONE NUMBER OF CONSIGNEE

USDA License/or Registration No. if applicable Telephone:

5. ANIMAL IDENTIFICATION *(To be completed by owner/consignor)*

6. VACCINATION HISTORY *(To be completed by veterinarian)* *attach original signature rabies certificate here*

COMPLETE USDA TAG COLLAR AND/OR TATTOO NUMBER	BREED - COMMON OR SCIENTIFIC NAME	AGE	SEX	COLOR OR DISTINCTIVE MARKS	RABIES ☐ Killed Virus ☐ Live Virus		D-H-L		OTHER VACCINATIONS, TESTS OR TREATMENT	
					Date	Product	Date	Product	Date	Type/Result
(1)										
(2)										
(3)										
(4)										
(5)										
(6)										
(7)										
(8)										
(9)										
(10)										

"X" applicable statements

☐ OWNER/CONSIGNOR CERTIFICATION: I certify that the information concerning the animals described above in Item 5 is true and correct, and that I am the owner/consignor of such described animals and that I have physical and legal custody of such animal (s).

☐ I hereby certify that the animal(s) in this shipment is (are), to the best of my knowledge acclimated to air temperatures lower than 7.2º c, (45º f).

SIGNATURE DATE

VETERINARY CERTIFICATION: I certify that the animal (s) described in item 5 have been examined by me this date, that the information provided in item 6 is true and accurate to the best of my knowledge, and that the following findings have been made "X" applicable statements.

☐ I certify that the animal (s) described and on continuation sheet(s) if applicable, have been inspected by me this date and appear to be free of any infectious or contagious diseases and to the best of my knowledge, exposure there to, which would endanger the animal or other animals or would endanger public health.

☐ I certify that the animal (s) described above, and on continuation sheet(s) if applicable, have been inspected by me this date and appear to be free of physical abnormalities which would endanger the animal.

☐ To my knowledge the animal (s) described above, and on continuation sheet(s) if applicable, originated from an area not quarantined for rabies and have not been exposed to rabies.

ENDORSEMENT FOR INTERNATIONAL EXPORT (WARNING: International Shipments require certification by an accredited veterinarian. States may also require such certification).

Apply USDA Seal or Stamp here

SIGNATURE OF USDA VETERINARIAN DATE

NAME, ADDRESS AND TELEPHONE NUMBER

Telephone:

LICENSE NO.

Accredited ☐ Yes ☐ No

LICENSING STATE

SIGNATURE DATE

APHIS FORM 7001 (AUG 2001) Replaces edition of (Aug 94) which may be used This certificate is valid for 30 days after issuance

PART 1 - TO ACCOMPANY SHIPMENT

A

No. 82137

OFFICIAL HEALTH CERTIFICATE
(COVERING CANINE, FELINE AND OTHER SMALL ANIMALS ONLY)

INTERSTATE ☐
EXHIBITION ☐
SALE ☐

OWNER OR CONSIGNOR ______ CONSIGNEE ______

ADDRESS ______ (STREET) DESTINATION ______ (STREET)

______ (CITY) (STATE) ______ (CITY) (STATE)

DESCRIPTION OF ANIMALS

SPECIES	BREED	SEX	AGE	COLOR AND MARKINGS	VACCINATION TAG NO.

IMMUNIZATION DATA

RABIES VACCINATION ______ TYPE USED ______ DATE ______

DISTEMPER IMMUNIZATION (PERMANENT OR ANTI-SERUM) ______ TYPE USED ______ DATE ______

HEPATITIS IMMUNIZATION (PERMANENT OR ANTI-SERUM) ______ TYPE USED ______ DATE ______

I hereby certify that I have examined the above described animals and find same to be free from symptoms of contagious or infectious diseases, and to the best of my knowledge and belief the above animals have not been exposed to infectious or contagious diseases. I also certify that I am licensed by the State of New Mexico and accredited by the New Mexico Livestock Board and U.S. Department of Agriculture for the issuance of Health Certificates for interstate and international shipments. NOTE: Subject to requirements of state of destination.

______ CLINIC NAME ______ DATE ISSUED ______ SIGNATURE ACCREDITED VETERINARIAN

B FORM NO. 15 4/04

FIGURE 2-12 A, International health certificate. B, Interstate health certificate. (A Courtesy U.S. Department of Agriculture.)

Arroyo Vista Animal Clinic
2303 Inspiration Lane, Anywhere, USA
Dr. Larsen, Dr. Cooke, and Dr. Thompson
Boarding Admission Form

Owner's Name _____ Date _____

Address _____ Phone _____

City _____ In case of emergency, please call _____

Pet's Name _____ Breed _____ Sex ____ Age ____ Color _____

Date of last vaccine _____ Please circle which vaccine: DHPP   FVRCP   FeLV

Date of last rabies vaccine _____ Date of last Bordetella vaccine _____

Medications while boarding _____

Belongings _____

Pet's Name _____ Breed _____ Sex ____ Age ____ Color _____

Date of last vaccine _____ Please circle which vaccine: DHPP   FVRCP   FeLV

Date of last rabies vaccine _____ Date of last Bordetella vaccine _____

Medications while boarding _____

Belongings _____

Pet's Name _____ Breed _____ Sex ____ Age ____ Color _____

Date of last vaccine _____ Please circle which vaccine: DHPP   FVRCP   FeLV

Date of last rabies vaccine _____ Date of last Bordetella vaccine _____

Medications while boarding _____

Belongings _____

While boarding, please perform the following procedures:

Physical exam _____ Vaccinations _____

Heartworm test _____ Bath _____ Dip _____ Nail trim _____

Other: _____

_____

_____

_____

All animals entering the hospital must be up to date on vaccinations and free of external
parasites (fleas, ticks) or they will be treated upon admission at the owner's expense.
I authorize Arroyo Vista Animal Clinic to treat my pet(s) in case an emergency situation should
arise.
Pets are released only during the regular office hours. It is my responsibility to inform the
hospital if I will be delayed in picking up my pets; I will assume all costs associated with an
extended stay.

Owner's signature _____ Date _____

A

FIGURE 2-13 A, Sample boarding admission form.

Continued

> **PRACTICE POINT**   Always show the clients the value of the services provided when presenting an invoice (or estimate/treatment plan).

If a client will use their card as a debit transaction (verses credit), the practice will pay less in credit cards fees. Team members are encouraged to ask clients if they would like to enter their debit number for the transaction (if the practice accepts debit). If a practice does not currently accept debit, managers are encouraged to investigate options, and implement this feature. While investigating, managers may also find that the credit cards rates they are paying are exceptionally high. This is a service that must be managed, because these fees can eat into the profits of the hospital. Benchmarks show that credit card fees average 1.5% of gross revenue.

The signature on the credit card must match the signature on the slip. According to the Red Flags Rule established by the Federal Trade Commission, any credit card transaction should be verified with a picture ID. The Red Flags Rule has been developed to help decrease fraud and the use of stolen credit cards. At the time of publishing this edition, the Red Flags Rule does not apply to veterinary clinics; however, this could change in the near future. It would be wise for practices to implement this safety feature, regardless. Visit the Federal Trade Commission at www.ftc.gov/bcp/edu/microsites/redflagsrule/index.shtml to stay abreast of any changes.

CareCredit is a credit card used exclusively for veterinary medicine. Other divisions of CareCredit are available for human medical care. Clients can apply either online or while at the practice. A receptionist can enter the information online or through a telephone operator, and approval can be received in as little as 10 minutes. CareCredit generally runs specials with the first-time use of the card. Visit www.carecredit.com for current information. Many

Boarding Admission Form

Please read the following statements and sign below.

All animals entering the hospital for boarding must be current on vaccinations and free of parasites. If not, they will be treated upon entering at the owner's expense.

All dogs that have boarded five days or more will be bathed prior to discharge unless the animal's health or temperament makes it hazardous to the animal or handlers. If tranquilizers are necessary for treatment/handling, permission is granted.

Pets are released only during regular clinic hours.

I expect to pick up my pet(s) on _____ (date).

If I neglect to contact/pick up my pet(s) within 7 days of said date, Arroyo Veterinary Clinic may assume my pet has been abandoned and is hereby authorized to dispose of the pet(s) as it deems best (including euthanasia).

I authorize Arroyo Veterinary Clinic to treat as needed _____

OR

I request Arroyo Veterinary Clinic to treat, but not to exceed $ _____

Signed _____

Dated _____ Emergency # _____

I request Arroyo Veterinary Clinic to walk my pet daily for exercise. I understand that Arroyo Veterinary Clinic and its staff will do all that is possible to prevent the escape of my pet. But if my pet slips out of its collar/leash and is NOT retrievable (runs off), I will not hold Arroyo Veterinary Clinic responsible for negligence or punitive damages.

Signed _____

Belongings: _____

Medications: _____

Feeding schedule: _____

B

FIGURE 2-13, cont'd B, Sample boarding admission form.

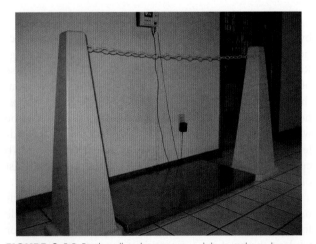

FIGURE 2-14 Bright yellow barriers around the weight scale prevent clients and team members from tripping.

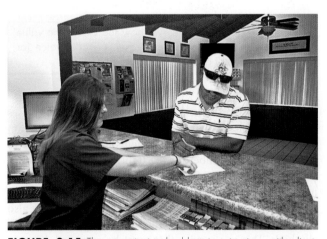

FIGURE 2-15 The receptionist should review invoices with clients before accepting payment.

ABC Animal Clinic
134 Uptown Circle
Anytown, MN 89000
800-555-5555

Maria Rogers
6454 Downtown Circle
Anytown, MN 89001   Account # 21312

"Scruffy" Rogers
Age: 9 years
Weight: 45#
Reminders: DHPP due 5/10/15
              Rabies due 5/10/16
              Heartworm Test due 5/10/14

Invoice Number: 10090
Date: 04/28/13
Dr. Nancy Dreamer

Date	Service	Unit	Extended Cost
04/28/13	Pre-Anesthetic Exam	1	0.00
04/28/13	Pre-Anesthetic Blood Work	1	$45.99
04/28/13	CBC/Chemistry	1	
04/28/13	Electrolytes	1	
04/28/13	Pre-Anesthetic ECG	1	$49.99
04/28/13	IV Fluids – Surgery	1	$54.85
04/28/13	IV Catheter	1	
04/28/13	IV Administration Set	1	
04/28/13	Normosol 1 Liter	1	
04/28/13	General Anesthesia	1	$101.20
04/28/13	Pre-Anesthetic	1	
04/28/13	Sevoflurane	1	
04/28/13	K-9 OVH under 50#	1	$97.89
04/28/13	OVH Pack	1	
04/28/13	Suture Material	2	
04/28/13	Biohazard Fee	1	
04/28/13	Surgical Monitoring	1	
04/28/13	Post-Operative Pain Medication	1	$24.99

	Subtotal	$374.91
	Tax 6.25%	23.43
	Invoice Total	$398.34

FIGURE 2-16 Sample invoice.

veterinary clinics in the United States accept CareCredit, allowing clients to charge veterinary care costs if their pet has an emergency while traveling.

Accepting cash has associated risks. Cash can be counterfeit. A local bank should be consulted regarding tips to recognize counterfeit money. Counterfeit money has no value, and detecting the passer can be difficult. Ask the local police department if it alerts local businesses to the passing of counterfeit money.

Large amounts of cash should be kept in a separate, locked safe, out of the sight of clients. It only takes a second for a client or person off the street to reach over the counter and grab money from the drawer. Cash drawers should have a lock and be locked immediately after it has been closed. Drawers should never be left unattended, especially if left unlocked. One moment of inattention can result in the loss of hundreds of dollars.

Many clinics also use check machines. Once checks are swiped through the terminal and the transaction has been approved, the money is automatically withdrawn from the customer's account and deposited into the clinic's bank

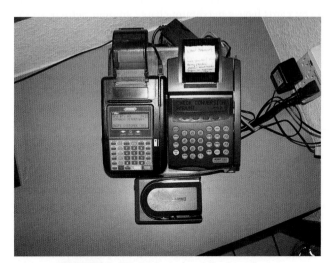

FIGURE 2-17 Credit card and check machine.

account. If the client has insufficient funds in the account, the transaction will be declined and the client will need to use another source of payment.

When accepting checks, the receptionist must always make sure the check is signed, dated, and written for the correct amount. Second, always make sure the check is in the team member's hand or the cash drawer, not still in the client's checkbook.

A cashier's check is a check from the bank itself and represents guaranteed funds. Traveler's checks are similar to cashier's checks but must be signed and completed in front of a team member. The signature must match the person's identification and the previous signature on the face of the traveler's check. Cashier's and traveler's checks are much less risky than personal checks (for practices that do not use a check authorization service).

Receptionists should always verify identification when processing payments. Team members must protect the clinic against consumer fraud and stolen checks or credit cards. Most check reader terminals require a driver's license number to be entered into the machine before accepting the transaction.

> **PRACTICE POINT** Always verify identification when accepting checks or credit cards.

Pet health insurance is also an option for owners. For a majority of policies, owners pay the practice for services their pet receives and are then reimbursed by the insurance company. See Chapter 19 for more information.

Declined Transactions

If a client's credit card, check, or debit card has been declined, politely and discreetly inform the client of the decline. Ask for an alternative method of payment. Some credit card and debit cards have a maximum charge amount per day, so the overdraft may be unintentional. Do not assume that a client has bad credit because of a refusal; there may be an innocent reason behind the decline.

Hospital policy regarding declined charges should be developed and instituted so that consistency runs throughout the practice. Some clinics allow a client to return to pay on the account; others may keep medication that was to be dispensed until a client can return with payment. Never keep a client's pet because of a declined payment. Practices are then responsible for the upkeep and care of the pet until the owner returns. If it is a sick and debilitated pet, the owner may not return! It is against the law in many states to hold a pet for ransom. Each state has different lien laws regarding holding pets; practice owners and managers should check with their state board of veterinary medicine for clarification.

The practice leadership is responsible for determining if the clinic will allow clients to charge for services rendered. Every member of the team must be familiar with the policy, including the veterinarians. Practice owners,

WHAT WOULD YOU DO/NOT DO

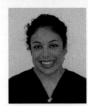

Lori, a receptionist of 5 years, is reviewing an invoice with Mr. DeWitt. Mr. DeWitt had his pet, Furminator, neutered at the practice and has arrived to pick him up. After Lori has reviewed all of the charges and gives Mr. DeWitt his total, he presents a credit card to pay for the transaction. Lori runs the credit card through on the machine, which returns a denied response. Lori quietly informs Mr. DeWitt that his credit card has been denied, and asks for an alternative form of payment. Mr. DeWitt becomes very upset and demands that she run the credit card again, saying, "there must be a mistake!" Lori grants the request and runs the credit card again. Again, the card is denied, which she informs him once more. He becomes even angrier and demands that she call the credit card company and determine why the card has been denied. She informs him that they will not provide the information to her, and she offers to call the company and hand the phone over for him to discuss the situation. After a lengthy, loud conversation with the credit card company, Mr. DeWitt slams down the phone exclaiming how "stupid" the company is and that he is canceling his credit card. Lori again politely asks for payment of services, which increases Mr. DeWitt's frustrations. He says, "I have been a client here for 5 years and you can't even give me the grace of charging one time? I should cancel you just as I am canceling my credit card!"

What Should Lori Have Done?

Lori should have put Mr. DeWitt into a room to discuss the declined credit card. Many clients become embarrassed and act irrational when confronted of such news. Many times, credit or debit cards are simply declined due to the maximum amount of charges allowed per day. Others are declined due to lack of payment received or the credit card has reached the maximum allowed charges.

Perhaps Mr. DeWitt's comment of canceling the credit card came out of frustration, but that is not a comment that needs to be heard by other clients. Clients may only hear part of the conversation and misconstrue the comment.

Mr. DeWitt's account could have been analyzed and determined by the practice manager if he would be allowed to return to the practice to make a payment at a later time; many times, the length of the client-patient relationship and history of payment will aid in the decision.

practice managers, and/or office managers should be the only team members allowed to approve this type of transaction. Often, veterinarians and technicians empathize with the client and wish to extend credit; unfortunately, many clients will not return to make a payment. CareCredit should always be offered to clients wishing to charge services. This allows the practice to give clients an option when they may not be able to pay for services rendered (the practice will receive immediate payment, and the client can make payments to CareCredit). Not all

clients can afford the most expensive services, so several payment options should be available. Clients may elect conservative treatment because of the cost of services and should not be judged for their decisions (on the other hand, do not assume clients cannot afford necessary services).

Daily Reconciliation

Balancing the accounts at the end of the day is a crucial task. Incomplete transactions, errors, and missing money, credit card receipts, or checks can all be found when balancing. It is much easier to find errors at the end of the day than searching for them the next day or following week (Figures 2-18 and 2-19).

Reconciliation is the process of matching and comparing figures from a transaction totals sheet with the actual receipts and funds accepted as payments. The balance of the transaction totals sheet must match the funds. Reconciliation compares account records to uncover any possible discrepancies. Practices may have different methods of ensuring reconciliation, but the goal is the same; the computer daily total transactions must equal the daily flow sheet.

> **PRACTICE POINT**   Receptionists must be held accountable for balancing the drawer at the end of the day or shift. If a discrepancy exists, it must be located before the employee leaves.

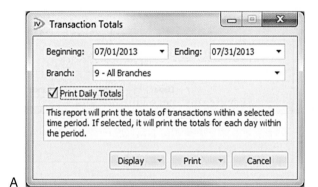

CALCULATION METHOD:

Total Invoices	= (Total Item Amounts) before tax and discount applied
Tax	= (Tax) - (Returned Tax)
Net Services	= (Total Invoice) - (Discount) + (Tax) - (Returns) + (Debit Adj) - (Credit Adj)
Total Payment	= (Cash) - (Change) + (Check) + (Card) - (Refund)

Date	Invoices	Disc.	Tax	Returns	Deb Adj	Cre Adj	Services	Cash	Check	Card	Refund	Payment

FIGURE 2-18 A and B, Transaction totals screen and transaction totals report. (Courtesy IntraVet, Effingham, Ill.)

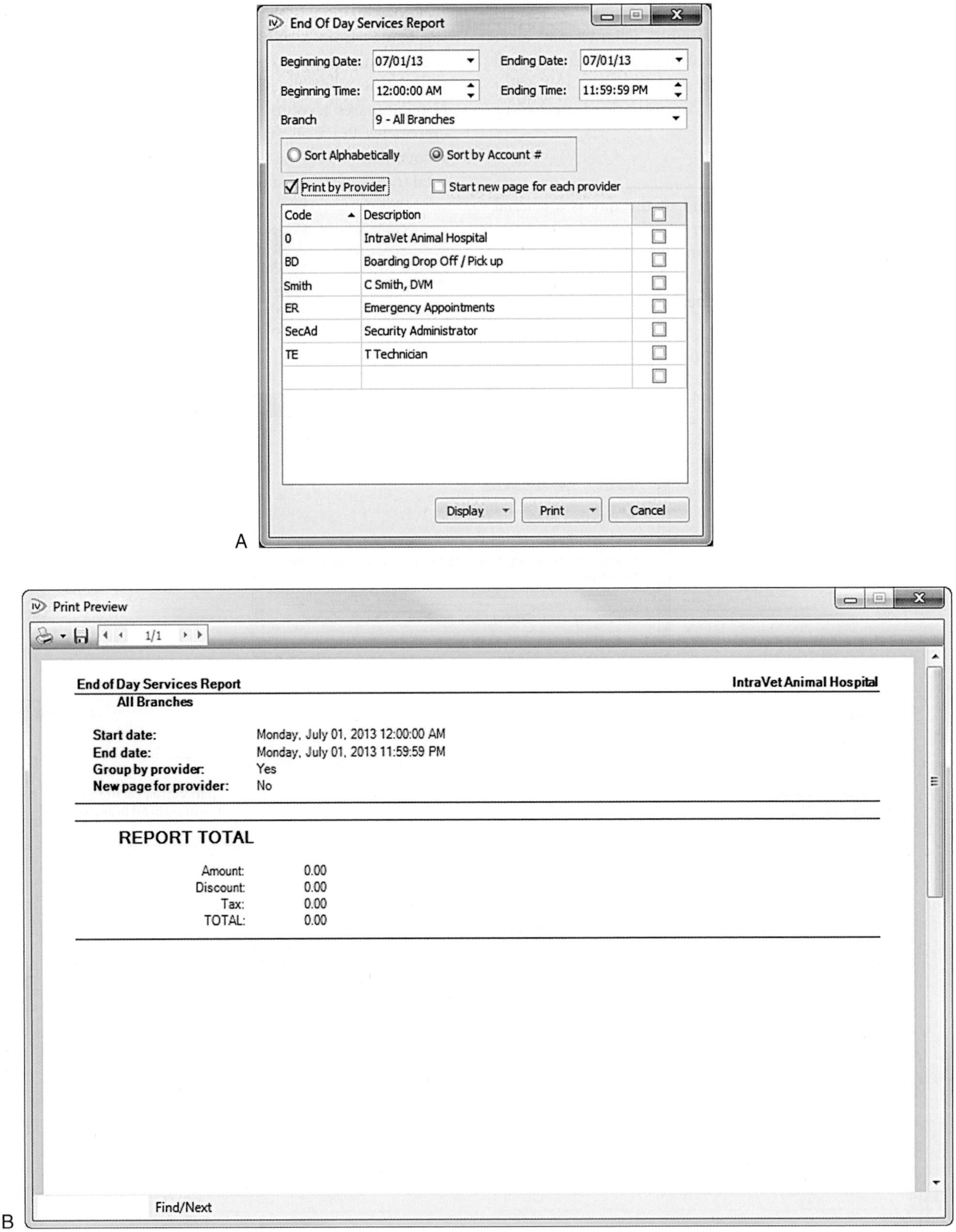

FIGURE 2-19 A, End of day services screen. B, End of day services report. (Courtesy IntraVet, Effingham, Ill.)

Transaction Totals	6/1/2013			ABC Animal Clinic	
Total Invoices	$ 5,497.69				
Total Cash	$ 1,409.65	(A)	Cash Counted	$ 1,209.65	(E)
Total Checks	$ 382.96	(B)	Checks Counted	$ 382.96	(F)
Total Credit Card	$ 4,105.08	(C)	Credit Card Slips Counted	$ 4,105.08	(G)
Total Payment	$ 5,497.69	(D)	Total Counted	$ 5,697.69	(H)

A = E + $200.00
B = F
C = G
D = H − $200.00 (starting cash balance)

FIGURE 2-20 Transaction totals sheet.

The cash drawer or register will contain an opening amount of cash predetermined by the practice management. It should be the same amount every day, comprised of a variety of bills to give change when needed. A recommendation may be $200, broken into one $20 bill, four $10 bills, eight $5 bills, 50 $1 bills, and $50 in quarters, dimes, nickels, and pennies. At the end of the day, the total amount in the cash drawer should be $200 plus any cash payments made by clients (Figure 2-20, A). This cash amount must equal the cash payments on the computer daily total transaction sheet. If the remaining cash does not equal $200, the error must be found. Once the cash balances, the cash from clients should be removed from the cash drawer and placed in a bank bag and set aside in preparation for a deposit.

The checks must also be reconciled and compared against the check totals on the computer daily total transaction sheet (see Figure 2-20, B). If a check machine is used, the machine will require team members to "batch out" at the end of the day. The total on the check batch sheet must match the total of the checks themselves as well as the transaction daily total sheet. If they do not match, the error must be investigated. If a check machine is not used, checks must be totaled and compared; again, if a discrepancy exists, the error must be found.

The credit card slips must also be totaled and matched against the transaction daily total sheet (see Figure 2-20, C). If there are any missing credit card slips or transactions, the error must be identified. Credit card machines will also need to be "batched out" at the end of the day; the total on the batch sheet must match the totals of the credit card slips and the transaction sheet. Finally, the cash, checks, and credit cards must equal the total on the daily transaction total sheet (see Figure 2-20, D). If they do not match, the error must be found.

Credit card slips and checks deposited through an automatic check machine need to be stored in a safe and locked place. It is important that these documents be kept for 7 years (depending on state law) in case a client chooses to dispute a transaction.

As a last check (see Figure 2-20):
- A + B + C = D, and E + F + G = H.
- B = F and C = G.
- Finally, D = H − $200 (the starting cash balance).

If any discrepancies exist, team members must be accountable; the error must be found and corrected before anyone leaves for the day.

Deposits

Deposits to the bank must be recorded on a deposit slip. Cash is entered on the cash line and checks typically are entered individually. If a check machine is used, the checks do not need to be deposited at the end of the day (because they have been electronically deposited). For practices without check machines, checks should be stamped "for deposit only, ABC Veterinary Clinic" on the back, including an account number. The cash and checks are totaled and entered at the bottom of the deposit slip (Figure 2-21). This total must match the cash and check total on the transaction sheet. Deposits should be made on a daily basis because it is unsafe to leave large amounts of cash in the office.

It is important to have a checks and balances system in place. All totals should match and must be double-checked. It is very important to eliminate errors as much as possible; double-checking a team member's work helps. The person checking the transactions as well as the team member double-checking the work should initial each transaction total.

Adding machine tape should be banded around receipts from checks and credit cards in case any questions arise regarding reconciliation. Deposit totals can be recorded in the practice checkbook or in a daily log book maintained by the practice manager. The practice manager should always compare deposits from the bank statement to the log entry.

Petty Cash

Petty cash is a term used to describe cash set aside in the practice to purchase items needed for the business when a check is not available. For example, the veterinarian may need some turkey meat for a special patient that will not eat regular dog food. In this situation, a team member can

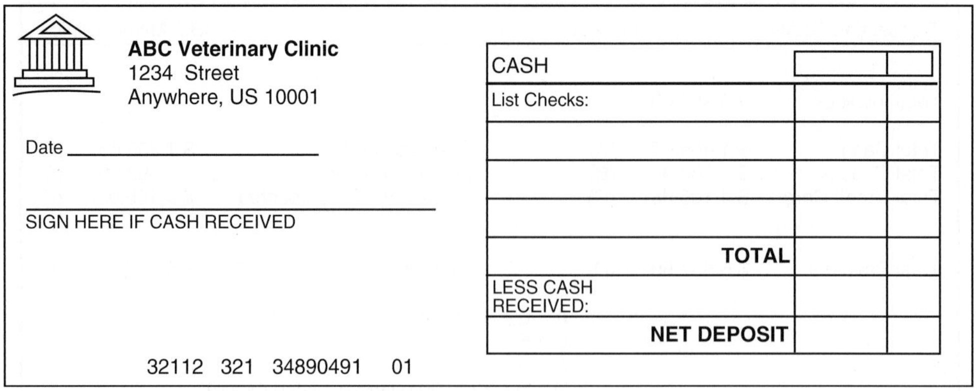

ABC Veterinary Clinic
1234 Street
Anywhere, US 10001

Date ____________________

____
SIGN HERE IF CASH RECEIVED

32112 321 34890491 01

CASH		
List Checks:		
TOTAL		
LESS CASH RECEIVED:		
NET DEPOSIT		

FIGURE 2-21 Deposit slip.

take some money from the petty cash bag and purchase the meat. A receipt must be returned and placed in the bag for balancing and reconciliation purposes. The money should be counted at the end of every shift to ensure that money is not missing and that receipts account for any money spent.

Creating a "WOW" Service

Practices never get a second chance to make a first impression. In fact, if you get a second chance, it can take over 3 years to overcome the negative perception that was built around that visit. In addition, one person (on average) tells 13 people about the bad experience they had. If a practice has one client per day that suffers a bad experience, 260 people could know by the end of the week how bad the service is at ABC Veterinary Clinic. This equates to 3120 people per year! Now throw social media into this equation. How fast does word travel in social media outlets? Creating a "WOW" experience has never been more important.

> PRACTICE POINT Creating a WOW service drives client compliance and referrals.

First impressions come in the tone of voice of team members, appearances, actions, smiles, and word choice, all of which have been described throughout this chapter.

Consider being prepared for each client visit. Prep every medical record before the client arrives. Perform a compliance check. What services is this pet due for? Does he or she need heartworm preventive or flea and tick medication (see Figure 13-15)? Has a wellness plan been discussed with this client (see Chapter 19 on Wellness Plans)? It is time that practices stop thinking about *transactions,* and learn to create *interactions.* Interactions build client relationships, which include trust and rapport. If a client does not have trust in the hospital, they will not accept recommendations. Being prepared for each visit allows team members to have a tailored, individual approach for every client, every time they visit the hospital.

Front Desk Chaos

Stop the chaos at the front desk. Consider walking into a human practitioner's office. If the phone is constantly ringing, team members appear frantic, clients are coming and going without a smile on their face, what impressions are given to those clients sitting in the lobby? One could comment, *"This is a crazy place! It must be that way through the whole practice! Is the doctor going to have time for me?"* Clients cannot see behind the scenes; however, they are very creative at developing scenarios.

In veterinary practices, the above scenario occurs everyday, and this is the client's true perception of the hospital. What can be done to minimize the chaos? Consider a few of these tips:

- Place the call center elsewhere in the hospital. Allow team members to concentrate on the clients in front of them.
- Hire accordingly for the front office. This office makes the first impression; therefore ensure that it runs as smooth as possible
- Have a different desk space for clients that are checking in, and those that are checking out.
- Review appointment times and stagger the schedule to prevent overlapping.

Clients know when customer service is good or bad. Clients rarely know when veterinary medicine is good or bad. However, clients perceive that when customer service is bad, the veterinary medicine is worse, and if customer service is excellent, the doctor(s) can do no wrong.

The Waiting Clients

Inevitably, some days the appointment schedule is going to get backed up. Emergencies and walk-ins flood the practice, even with the best-laid plans. Therefore team members must have a backup plan (both entertainment and communication) for clients that have to wait to be seen.

Receptionists should constantly be monitoring the schedule for delays. How long is a client waiting to be seen? Keep a log, so that anomalies can be addressed and corrected. Client compliance drops the longer clients have to wait (irritated

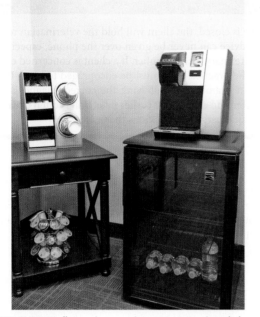

FIGURE 2-22 Coffee and tea machines are a nice benefit for waiting clients.

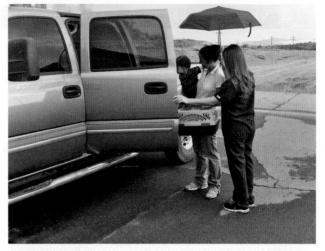

FIGURE 2-23 A team member provides extra service by holding umbrella for a client as they get into car.

clients will not accept all recommendations). If a team member notes the schedule is getting backed up, call clients ahead of time and let them know of the delay. They may choose to reschedule rather than wait for a prolonged period of time (clients appreciate these calls). For those clients that are already in the office, set a timer to continue checking on them every 5 minutes. Remember, 5 minutes in a small room seems like 10! Communication is the absolute key to client happiness in this situation.

Practices may consider having a machine to make coffee and hot tea while clients wait (Figure 2-22). Allowing clients to select their flavor and make the brew can take several minutes. Have some toys for the kids. Children get bored very easily, making the wait seem even longer for the parent. Some practices may have a play room, others may have a simple toy box for kids to pick a toy for entertainment.

Team members can also take the opportunity to educate clients on diseases or preventative care topics. For those that have pet portals, take the client on a tour of the Web site and pet portal, helping them become more aware of the services they can access. Pictures can also be taken of the pet(s) and uploaded to the practice management software. Taking this time to develop a relationship with the client is vital, and not many practices invest in this time wisely. Set your practice apart by going the extra mile.

> **PRACTICE POINT** Use time wisely with waiting clients. Develop and build interactions and relationships (don't allow clients to sit in the exam room alone!)

Creating an Exceptional Finale!

Once patients have been examined and the client visit is complete, he or she will return to the receptionist desk to be checked out. Again, making a lasting impression is vital—service must be prompt, perfect, and chaos free. Review the visit with the client, repeating any recommendations made by the veterinary team. Clients must hear recommendations three times before it sticks, and the receptionist can solidify these plans.

Schedule follow-up appointments before charging out the client (most clients are ready to rush out the door once payment has been made). Ensure the invoice is correct and explain the charges to the client (as previously addressed). Once the transaction is complete (the interaction *is not* done yet), evaluate the client and see if he or she needs help getting to the car (don't ask if help is needed, just do it!). Carry food, pet carriers, or medication for the owner. If it is raining outside, provide an umbrella service; walk the client out holding the umbrella over their head, keeping them dry getting into their car (Figure 2-23).

Follow up with every client. When to follow up depends on what service was provided. If a puppy or kitten received vaccinations, call the client that night, making sure the pet handled the visit without any side effects. This can be a great time to re-address the characteristics associated with mild vaccine reactions, or perhaps any unanswered questions the client may have had while in the practice earlier. If a pet had surgery, or was released from the hospital that day, call the client that night (clients are *most* concerned about their pet the first night of being at home, so make the time to call and check on the patient). Last, but not least, ask clients how the service was. Develop a survey that clients can submit to the practice anonymously (see Chapter 10 for more information on surveys).

Mediocre service sustains a practice; however, outstanding service will build a practice (in more ways than just profits)!

VETERINARY PRACTICE and the LAW

The receptionist position is one of the most vulnerable positions to liability lawsuits. Many clients call because their dog is just not feeling right, or the cat vomits several times a week, but they do not want to bring him or her in. Clients are seeking free advice, and for the receptionist to tell them *"everything will be all right, just wait and watch!"* In reality, if something happens to this pet overnight, or over the weekend while the practice is closed, the client will hold the veterinarian responsible. Advice can never be given over the phone, especially by a nonveterinary team member. If a client is concerned enough to call the practice, they must be encouraged to bring the pet in for an examination, allowing the correct diagnosis to be made. Remind clients that earlier detection is often cheaper to treat than emergency situations that arise.

REVIEW QUESTIONS

1. Record a phone conversation between two team members. One should act as a receptionist; the other should be a client. Have the team member use the following techniques while talking with the "client."
   - Speak loudly
   - Speak softly
   - Speak rapidly
   - Do not smile when answering the phone
   - Smile while answering the phone

   Analyze the recording. What were the differences? Is the call confusing? What changes could improve each call?

2. Identify mistakes and incompleteness on the following client form.

ABC Animal Clinic
555 Uptown Circle
Anytown, MN 89000
314-134-4431

Please print clearly

Date: _____4/30/13_____

Name _____Santiago Garcia_____

Mailing address __1645 Horse Lane, Mesa, AZ____ Zip code ___06070____

Street address _____ Zip code _____

Home phone ___576-895-8576____ Work phone __867-869-8695____

Drivers license # _____ State _____

Animals:

Name	Date of birth	Species	Breed	Color	Gender	Spayed or neutered?
Chuck	12/15/10	Canine	Chih	Black		N

I understand that payment is required in full on the same date that services are rendered.

_____
Signature

---

3. Reconcile the end-of-day report for the veterinary practice below and develop a deposit for your cash and checks.

Total invoices:	$6579.08
Total cash:	$568.90
Total checks:	$2567.78
Total credit cards:	$3442.40

Your opening cash drawer was $200.00

<table>
<tr><td rowspan="9">ABC Veterinary Clinic
1234 Street
Anywhere, US 10001

Date _____

_____
SIGN HERE IF CASH RECEIVED

32112　321　34890491　　01</td><td>CASH</td><td></td><td></td></tr>
<tr><td>List Checks:</td><td></td><td></td></tr>
<tr><td></td><td></td><td></td></tr>
<tr><td></td><td></td><td></td></tr>
<tr><td></td><td></td><td></td></tr>
<tr><td align="right">TOTAL</td><td></td><td></td></tr>
<tr><td>LESS CASH RECEIVED:</td><td></td><td></td></tr>
<tr><td align="right">NET DEPOSIT</td><td></td><td></td></tr>
</table>

4. Determine mistakes on the following end-of-day reconciliation:

Total invoices:	$6798.34
Total cash:	$235.68
Total cash counted:	*$435.68*
Total checks:	$564.67
Total checks counted:	*$480.98*
Total credit card transactions:	$5977.99
Total credit card slips counted:	*$4478.67*
Total payments:	$6798.34
Total counts:	_____

5. Why are health certificates required?
6. What makes the first impression on clients?
7. What information should not be given to clients over the phone?
8. How can a phone shopper be turned into a client?
9. How should a declined credit card be handled?
10. Why should invoices be reviewed with clients, not just given to them?
11. How many components does the human voice contain?
    a. 2
    b. 6
    c. 4
    d. 3
12. Which of the following is a proper phone introduction?
    a. "Hello, this is Brooke, how can I help you"?
    b. "Good Morning, ABC Animal Clinic, this is Teresa. How may I help you"?
    c. "ABC Veterinary Clinic, can I help you"?
    d. "Good afternoon, ABC Animal Clinic. How may I help you"?
13. If the appointment schedule is full the receptionist should say which of the following during a phone conversation?
    a. "Sorry Mrs. Jones, we are unable to see you today; can I schedule you an appointment for next week?"
    b. "You are welcome to drop off Fluffy with us today, or come in as a walk-in, because we do not have any appointments available, but we would be glad to work you in."
    c. "We have had several emergencies and walk-ins already today. Can Bella wait to be seen until tomorrow?"
    d. "Mrs. Smith, you can come in as a walk-in but you will have a very long wait; we are extremely busy today."

14. When should receptionists reconcile the transactions to ensure they are all correct?
    a. Daily at the end of the day
    b. Weekly
    c. Daily at the beginning to the following day
    d. On an as-needed basis
15. What is the purpose of requiring owners to sign consent forms?
    a. To ensure the owner is understanding of why they are leaving their pet
    b. To protect veterinary practices and team members from any issues that may arise and may need to be submitted in the case of a lawsuit.
    c. To satisfy state law
    d. All of the above

Recommended Reading

Finch L: *Telephone courtesy and client service*, ed 4, Fairport, NY, 2009, Axzo Press.
Gearson RF: *Beyond customer service. Keeping clients for life*, ed 3, Fairport, NY, 1998, Axzo Press.
Heinke MM: *Practice made perfect: a guide to veterinary practice management*, ed 2, Lakewood, CO, 2012, AAHA Press.
Wilson JF: *Legal consent forms for the veterinary practice*, ed 4, Yardley, PA, 2006, Priority Press.

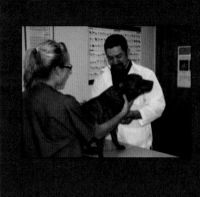

Team Leadership

OUTLINE

Mission, Vision, and Values, *49*
  Mission, *49*
  Vision, *49*
  Values, *49*
Leadership, *49*
  Emotional Intelligence, *51*
  Leadership Styles, *52*
  Leadership Commitment, *52*
  Become an Effective Leader, *52*
  Utilizing Leadership to Set
    Expectations, *53*
Creating Positive Cultures, *53*
  Understanding Diversity, *53*
  Work and Life Balance, *54*
  Preventing Burnout, *54*
The Positive Effects of a Team, *54*
  Troubleshooting and Problem Solving, *55*
The Four *R*'s of Team Management, *55*
Empowering Employees, *55*

Delegation, *56*
  Learning How to Delegate, *56*
Methods of Communication, *57*
  Meetings, *58*
  Team Newsletter, *60*
  Evaluations, *60*
Conflict Management, *63*
Increasing Staff Efficiency, *64*
Time Management of Leaders, *65*
Decreasing Loss, *65*
  Travel Sheet, *66*
  Accountability, *66*
  Inventory Management, *66*
  Appropriate Fee Setting, *66*
**Motivating and Retaining Team
  Members,** *68*
  NAVTA: 2011 Demographics
    Survey, *70*

KEY TERMS

Accountability
Conflict Management
Delegation
Directive Management
Effective Communication
Emotional Inelegance
Empowerment
Evaluation
Mission
Supportive Management
Travel Sheet
Values
Vision

LEARNING OBJECTIVES

When you have completed this chapter, you should be able to:

1. List methods to become an effective leader.
2. Describe and understand various management styles.
3. Discuss the empowerment of team members.
4. Discuss effective delegation.

5. Clarify methods to increase team communication.
6. List methods to resolve conflict.
7. Discuss methods to increase team efficiency.
8. Identify methods to decrease loss in the practice.

CRITICAL COMPETENCIES

1. **Adaptability** - being open to change and flexible work methods; the ability to adapt behavior to changing conditions or new information.
2. **Analytical Skills** - the ability to analyze information and use logic to address problems; the ability to quickly and accurately grasp complex information and concepts and to make correct inferences.
3. **Compliance** - being reliable, thorough, and conscientious in carrying out work assignments; has an appreciation for the importance of organizational rules and policies.

4. **Continuous Learning** - a curiosity for learning; actively seek out new information, technologies, and methods; keep skills updated and apply new knowledge to the job.
5. **Creativity** - the ability to think creatively about situations, to see things in new and different ways; use imagination and creativity to develop innovative solutions to problems.
6. **Critical and Strategic Thinking** - the ability to think critically about situations and to understand the relevance of information for different problems; use critical reasoning to generate and

evaluate alternative courses of action or points of view relevant to an issue.

7. **Decision Making** - the ability to make good decisions, solve problems, and decide on important matters; the ability to gather and analyze relevant data and choose decisively between alternatives.

8. **Integrity** - honesty, trustworthiness, and adherence to high standards of ethical conduct.

9. **Leadership** - a willingness to lead and take charge; the ability to motivate others and mobilize group effort toward common goals.

10. **Oral Communication and Comprehension** - the ability to express one's thoughts verbally in a clear and understandable manner, and the ability to actively listen and attend to what others are saying; must have good group presentation skills.

11. **Persuasion** - the ability to change the attitudes and opinions of others and to persuade them to accept recommendations and change behavior.

12. **Planning and Prioritizing** - the ability to effectively manage time and workload to meet deadlines; the ability to organize work, set priorities, and establish plans for achieving goals.

13. **Relationship Building** - the ability to develop constructive and cooperative working relationships with others and maintain them over time; must also be able to settle disputes, resolve grievances and conflicts, and negotiate with others.

14. **Resilience** - the ability to cope effectively with pressure and setbacks; the ability to handle crisis situations effectively and remain undeterred by obstacles or failure.

15. **Resourcefulness** - the ability to understand what it takes to complete the job; apply knowledge, skills, and expertise to perform tasks quickly and efficiently.

16. **Writing and Verbal Skills** - ability to comprehend written material easily and accurately; ability to express thoughts clearly and succinctly in writing.

Successful management of the veterinary health care team is essential to practice survival. The team attracts new clients, retains clients, educates clients, and satisfies clients. The team includes every member of the veterinary hospital, from the kennel assistants to the veterinarians. Each person contributes significant time and energy to each client and patient. Practice managers and hospital administrators may not have direct contact with clients, but they support the team by developing and providing staff training, client education materials, and excellent managerial structure to help the organizational run smoothly.

In a veterinary practice there are many benefits to employees acting as a team rather than a set of individuals. Team members recognize and understand their interdependence, allowing personal and team goals to be accomplished with mutual support. They feel a sense of pride and ownership in the practice and are committed to reaching goals that they have helped establish. All team members contribute to the success of the practice by applying their unique skills and talents to obtain those goals and by always being willing to accept new challenges. New ideas and challenges can stimulate team members to become strong performers and encourage others to follow. Team members continually work together to improve their service to clients, patients,

and each other, and all of these team qualities make participation in a veterinary practice an excellent and rewarding career. A dedicated and proficient team that understands basic practice management is likely to achieve extraordinary goals and boost the practice's compliance rate. Team building is a continuous process that never ends; the trials and errors that are a part of this process allow each team member to learn and grow from the mistakes made along the way (Box 3-1).

Successful leadership comes with practice, education, and time. Many managers have learned success through trial and error and by finding what works best in their particular practices. What works in one practice may not work in another; continuing education and self-development of each team member can help with the generation of ideas, taking the veterinary hospital to the next level.

Basic management of a veterinary practice includes organizational development and employee development. Organizational development is defined as the development, improvement, and effectiveness of an organization that includes the culture, values, system, and behaviors. Employee development helps improve the vision, empowerment, learning, and problem-solving abilities of team members.

BOX 3-1	Suggestions for Creating Positive Team Interactions

- Help others be right, not wrong.
- Have fun.
- Smile!
- Be enthusiastic.
- Seek ways for new ideas to work, not reasons why they won't.
- Be courageous.
- Maintain a positive attitude.
- Maintain confidentiality.
- Verify information given to you; do not gossip.
- Speak positively of others at all times.
- Say "thank you" for kind gestures.
- If you don't have something positive to say, don't say anything.

Mission, Vision, and Values

A mission, the vision, and the values (MVVs) of a hospital are core competencies that must be integrated in every practice. MVVs set the structure, creating a positive culture, and goals that help define team member expectations. Without these, team members do not have a direction; they simply show up to work and complete the tasks assigned to them. Owners make it day to day, with no clear light at the end of the tunnel, and managers struggle to implement successful goals and policies to increase value in the hospital. The mission and vision should be evaluated every couple of years, ensuring that they are still in alignment with the beliefs of the owner(s).

> **PRACTICE POINT** The mission, vision, and values of the hospital are core competencies every hospital should implement.

Mission

The mission is defined as the purpose of the hospital; it is the fundamental reason that the practice exists. Mission statements are short and simple, and easy to remember. Every team member must live by the mission of the hospital. For example, if the goals for ABC Veterinary Hospital are to provide superior medical services for patients, treat owners with respect, and provide an excellent team environment, one might develop the following mission statement: *"To provide comprehensive high-quality veterinary care with emphasis on exceptional client service and patient care, while providing employees with desirable, fulfilling, and financially rewarding employment."*

Once the mission has been developed, it should be implemented into job descriptions, performance expectations and client materials. This holds the team accountable to both clients and fellow employees.

Vision

A vision is the desired future of the practice. Where does the practice want to be (financially, medically, staffing, etc.)

in 1 year, 5 years, or 10 years? The vision supports the mission and must be attainable. Do the current procedures and/or policies support the vision? If not, what needs to be changed, in order to reach this goal?

Values

Values are guiding principles that are not to be compromised during change; they provide ethical guidance and will not be violated. Violation of values could be considered for grounds of immediate termination, if stated in the employee manual. Compassion, advocacy, respect, and empathy (CARE) for patients and their owners would be a set of values that cannot be compromised.

Once MVVs have clearly been established, goals of the hospital can be set. The following is a short list (although not conclusive) of areas that MVVs have an effect on.

Human resources: Managers cannot hire new employees without knowing what direction the practice is headed. What type of team member is needed, and what skills are essential to help the practice attain the MVVs? If team members are not meeting the expectations created by the MVVs, can they be coached to improvement, or should they be terminated? For high producing team members, what continuing education is needed to help them continue contributing to the success of the practice (and achieving the MVVs)?

Without MVVs, employee turnover is generally high, resulting in decreased client loyalty, compliance and retention. All of the issues just mentioned decrease the goodwill value of the hospital.

Marketing: Where is the practice going? What are the important messages that should be relayed to clients? How will that message be relayed? Is the internal team prepared to handle the key messages?

Finance: What profit centers should be established and/or maintained to meet the MVVs? If the goal is to provide above standard care, what is being done to acquire new and modern medical equipment?

The MVVs play a very important role in the development of the entire practice. If the team knows what direction the practice is going, it is no longer just a job. If the owner wishes to sell the practice in 20 years, MVVs give direction and a goal to meet.

Leadership

Leadership is vital to the success and growth of a practice. Leadership is influence; a leader is one who influences others, motivating them into action and inspiring them to become the best they can be. Leaders in veterinary practice must guide effective communication and create an environment that facilitates teamwork. Through good leadership, team members can appreciate how they contribute to the big picture of exceptional patient and client care.

> **PRACTICE POINT** A leader is one who influences others, motivating them to be the best they can be.

Leadership is about character, behavior, and actions (actions speak louder than words!). Every leader must look in the mirror; are the characteristics and behaviors that one is striving for (within the team) exhibited day in and day out (by oneself)? Through these characteristics, leaders compel individuals to pursue the mission, value, and goals (of the leader[s]).

Leaders must hold themselves to a higher standard of patient care, customer service, performance, and personal behavior. Leading by example has a much more profound effect on team members than leading by directive. Examples show team members what is expected of them when it comes to patient and client care. All team members should be held accountable for providing the best care possible, and leaders can set the stage for this to occur. Leadership that promotes a poor standard of care and professionalism will also affect the team, because team members are only as good as their leaders. Managers of this type should be terminated because they will cause the team to disintegrate and the practice to fail. Owners of this type must re-evaluate themselves and consider self-development if they wish to have successful practices.

In modern society, leaders must strive to achieve short- and long-term goals; create effective, efficient methods to complete tasks; and be proactive instead of reactive to situations. A leader's personal effectiveness can directly influence a hospital's success. Leaders must determine the most effective method to manage team members and be able to recognize their own strengths and weaknesses as well as those of others. A motivating leader generates enthusiasm and excitement, and an organized leader provides the path to achieve goals; the best type of leader does both. A leader sets the practice's vision and goals, communicating the vision to the team so they may help accomplish those goals.

Leadership skills are not developed overnight; they come with patience, education, and trial and error. Managing a practice has both wonderful and terrible days. A leader is sometimes viewed as a "good guy," sometimes as a "bad guy," and sometimes as uncaring and lacking compassion. However, the success of a business can depend on the quality of the leader. Someone who is capable of being either a good guy or bad guy when necessary will keep the team focused so they provide excellent quality of care.

Excellent leaders use human, technical, and conceptual skills to succeed in that role. *Human skill* is the ability to understand people and what motivates them and to be able to direct their behavior through effective leadership. Not all team members respond to leadership, training, or education in the same manner. Characteristics such as shyness, decreased confidence, and poor communication skills make it more difficult to train some team members (but can easily be overcome). Domineering, independent, and strong-willed individuals may also have a hard time accepting training. Effective leaders can determine what motivates these various personality types and have a positive influence on each (Box 3-2).

Technical skill is the ability to apply leadership, skill, and knowledge of equipment, procedures, and hospital policies to team members in an effective, ambitious manner. Leaders must be able to train or provide training to team members

---

BOX 3-2 | **Fundamentals That Build Effective Leadership**

- Trust: Development of a trusting relationship with each team member facilitates open communication.
- Accept change: Effective leaders understand that disruptions occur and are willing to make and accept change to succeed.
- Focus: Leaders have the ability to achieve and direct their time and energy to achieve goals.
- Commitment: Effective leaders work continually to find new ideas to help make policies and procedures succeed. Accepting change helps promote commitment.
- Compassion: Leaders care about and desire to understand team members and their families.
- Integrity: Integrity demands that leaders seek to create quality assurance for their clients, patients, and team members and facilitate a positive relationship with all.
- Endurance: Leaders demonstrate courage, perseverance, and strength when situations, people, or the environment becomes chaotic or difficult.

BOX 3-3 | **Characteristics of Effective Leaders**

- Self-confident
- Sincere
- Enthusiastic
- Effective listener
- Effective communicator
- Accepting of diverse cultures
- Team player
- Problem solver
- Innovator and renovator
- Will admit mistakes

---

on all equipment, maintenance of equipment, functions, and supplies needed to maintain that piece of equipment. Team members need training on policies and procedures that have been developed to have a successful implementation. Policy training can be difficult for some employees, especially long-term employees, as they may be resistant to policy change or implementation.

Conceptual skill is the ability to sense how the leadership style affects the practice and to make change in a positive way. Not all leadership styles have a positive effect on team members. An effective leader can determine when changes are needed and try various leadership styles until success has been attained.

Leaders must possess several qualities to be successful. Self-confidence, sincerity, and enthusiasm for the job are essential. Leaders are effective listeners and accept diverse cultures. To have an effective team, a leader must be a team player and work to solve problems, innovate, and renovate existing policies, procedures, and environments. Leaders explain how to accomplish a task and give a challenge to the team. This allows the team members to think for themselves creatively, which can develop leaders for the future (Box 3-3).

Effective leaders possess self-confidence. They believe they have the ability to complete tasks efficiently and effectively. Leaders accentuate positive personal attributes and do not dwell on negative weaknesses. Self-confident leaders take risks and are able to make recommendations and changes without delay.

Genuineness and sincerity come from within and promote trust and communication. Team members know the suggestions and changes made by sincere leaders enhance the skills of all involved. It is important to show appreciation for employee contributions and create a culture that celebrates values and victories. It is genuine acts of caring that lift people up and create a desire to exceed expectations.

Enthusiasm shows that leaders are interested in their practices and the steps needed to make it successful. Enthusiasm is contagious to fellow team members and should be a part of practice culture. Enthusiastic team members are excited to come to work, enjoy sharing experiences with others, appreciate humor, and enjoy the teamwork environment.

Listening effectively has become a lost skill in today's world; talking has overtaken listening. Listening is the ability to receive, attend to, interpret, and respond to words and body language. Poor listening skills can result in misinterpretation of information, leading to malpractice in the medical field. Poor listening and interpretation can cause a communication breakdown when a leader is trying to manage a practice effectively and lead team members in a positive style.

One of the most important skills for effective leadership is to be an effective communicator. Communications must be done in a clear and pleasant manner. Effective communicators think clearly, talk sparingly, and listen intently. It is imperative to think topics through before jumping to a conclusion. All issues must be understood and interpreted before an action can be taken. Rash decisions should not be made, or devastating results may occur. Time should be taken to interpret the facts and prevent immediate judgments. Talking too much can be a problem itself and greatly inhibits listening. Tone is as important as talking; positive, enthusiastic tones are much more effective than negative, authoritarian tones.

Exceptional leaders create environments where team members are empowered to communicate openly, voice their concerns, and make changes where necessary to produce an improved service. Inhibiting this environment can be detrimental.

Ethnic cultures have different means of communication, and an effective leader must be able to determine the best method of communication for each. Morals and ethics vary among ethnicities, ultimately affecting the learning and training abilities of different team members. Leaders must be accepting of diverse cultures, welcoming the different qualities each possesses, and work with them to provide the best leadership possible.

Veterinary practice is a team business. A team is a simple concept: a group of individuals with different skills and attributes, which contribute the positive culture of the hospital.

Effective leaders build teams that allow the business to succeed at all levels, including providing excellent patient and client care and maintaining a friendly and cohesive work environment, all while being able to create and maintain a profit for the practice. Leaders invite creative thinking from team members, and integrate this creative thinking into daily conversations. Creative thinking facilitates productive, problem solving team members that are not afraid to move outside the box.

> **PRACTICE POINT** Effective leaders build teams that allow the practice to succeed at all levels; every team member contributes to this success.

When building teams, exceptional leaders attract the right people and place them into the right positions. They also integrate personal growth with practice growth, which encourages career development of each team member. Without personal growth and development, the practice growth is stalled.

Leaders must possess skills to solve problems before they arise—to be proactive instead of reactive. Leaders determine the problem; collect, listen, and interpret the facts; and present a variety of solutions to the team. Team members should be asked how they would resolve a situation; their point of view is *critically* important in problem resolution. In addition, problem solvers are accountable and productive.

Managing a practice requires attention to both internal and external forces. Change is required to keep up with modern technology and medicine. Leaders must be aware of innovations available and how they can improve the practice. Pharmacology, equipment, computer technology, and medicine reveal new science every year; flexibility is a must. If one innovation does not work within the practice, another should be tried. Trial and error produces the best results. Practice policies and procedures must undergo refinement on a yearly basis. Review policies that need updating, make a plan, set goals, and implement the change needed.

All people make mistakes. An effective leader must be able to admit mistakes that have been made and correct them. Team philosophy allows mistakes to be made while creating an environment for employees to learn from those mistakes. When environments are created in which team members are not afraid to take on new responsibilities and skills, mistakes are bound to be made. However, effective leaders can help all team members learn from those errors and prevent the mistake from occurring again (allowing mistakes does not allow the team member to complete tasks carelessly; mistakes should be accounted for and learned from).

Amazing leaders consistently seek ways to help team members gain satisfaction from their responsibilities, enhancing the inspiration, excitement, and accountability of each and every employee.

Emotional Intelligence

Emotional intelligence (EI) is defined as the ability to identify, assess, and control one's emotions. Characteristics of EI include self-awareness, self-control, self-motivation and empathy. Self-awareness involves the recognition of one's

emotions, and gives insight into the response that follows a trigger. The more emotions are understood, the easier it is to control ingrained responses. Self-control aids one in managing stressful triggers and can moderate angry responses, helping one maintain perspective and focus. Self-motivation is contagious to others; as a leader, use self-motivation to influence others. Empathy allows one to respond to others with a clear mind, judgment free. If responses include empathy, the speaker is more likely to open up, presenting information that would most likely be held within.

> **PRACTICE POINT** Strong emotional intelligence is a key characteristic of effective leaders.

Leaders must be able to control their emotions, as these are behaviors that influence team members. A strong emotional intelligence is required for exceptional leaders.

Leadership Styles

Leadership and communication styles are essential in the management of people and business. Leadership depends on and results from the behavior of the manager; therefore the most effective form is to lead by example. A solid leader understands what motivates each individual and how he or she will respond, and can direct the employee's behavior to have a desired outcome. Ultimately, leaders must accept the task and responsibility of influencing the behavior of others.

Two theories of effective management are *directive* and *supportive*. Directive management is task oriented, whereas supportive behavior is people oriented. Some managers are task oriented and others are supportive; some leaders may use a combination of the two styles. Effective managers can determine which style will work best with each situation that arises. Directive managers are task oriented and are more interested in achieving results than in discussing how a task will be completed. Supportive managers listen to employees and encourage them to express their thoughts and opinions. Tasks may be discussed in detail to be completed, and leaders provide feedback and recognition as well as an open level of communication.

The best managers are flexible and adapt to the differing needs of different team members. Some employees may need a directive style of management; others may require a supportive environment. A combination may yield the best results. Assigning tasks in a directive fashion allows team members to complete them in their own manner, developing self-confidence and leadership abilities that will benefit the practice in the future. By offering some supportive management, leaders can provide positive feedback on a project and invite the team members to discuss problems that may arise during the project. The style of leadership in a practice can make or break the practice by severely affecting team member performance.

Leadership Commitment

Effective leaders are committed to their jobs, their team members, and themselves. It is imperative that leaders keep commitments that they have made to their team; again, the best leadership style is to lead by example. Commitments are made to others, and others depend on that person to complete them.

> **PRACTICE POINT** Leaders who do not uphold commitments themselves cannot expect their team to uphold commitments.

Leaders who do not uphold commitments cannot expect team members to follow through either. If commitments cannot be followed through, they should not be made in the first place. If commitments are not being held by team members, leaders must re-evaluate themselves first.

Become an Effective Leader

The preceding suggestions will help every leader become more efficient at managing team members. The ideas discussed next will help enhance the skills already developed.

Learn something new every day. Often, managers feel they have mastered the skills to be effective leaders. However, something can be learned from every situation, which helps create an amazing leader. Make it a point at the beginning of each day to look for at least one new thing that can enhance the team. Leaders must continue to challenge themselves to grow; mediocrity does not lead to an innovative, motivated team.

Strive for excellence every day. It is unrealistic to expect perfection on every task and skill, but all team members should perform their best at all times; this includes all owners, leaders, and managers.

Take charge of team morale. Negative environments are difficult to work in, and clients pick up on negative interactions. Improving team morale improves employee performance, enhances client relationships, and creates a wonderful working environment, all of which results in decreased team member turnover and burnout.

Smile every day. Smiling is contagious.

Inspire vision and trust. Influence others through behavior to inspire vision; keep commitments, tell the truth, and say, "I am sorry" to inspire trust.

Accept and embrace suggestions. Some suggestions may not be the best, but do not reject ideas given by team workers. Embrace the suggestion and build on it.

Do not spread gossip or foster rumors. Curtail gossip to improve the quality of the workplace environment. Effective teams are built on trust and respect. Determine the facts and kill the gossip.

Provide motivation. Not all team members are motivated by the same technique. Learn what motivates each individual and foster an environment that will create and maintain motivation for everyone.

Enable others to act. Leaders foster collaboration with trust and delegation. Trust and delegation lead to accountable, productive team members that have a sense of ownership for the hospital.

Remember that actions speak louder than words. Lead by example and the team will follow. Behavior wins respect of

the team. Leaders must live the mission and vision of the hospital; if leaders want to gain respect and commitment from the team, they must model the behavior they expect from others.

Utilizing Leadership to Set Expectations

All of the qualities and characteristics just mentioned are required of effective leaders. It was stated previously that leaders are held to a higher expectation than any other team members, and if team members are expected to perform exceptionally, then leaders must model the way.

Most of the characteristics listed earlier are soft skills that can be woven into job descriptions and performance expectations for all team members. However, the skills must be placed within the documents in order for team members to be held accountable. See Chapter 5 for more details on job descriptions and performance reviews that will raise the bar in veterinary practice management.

Creating Positive Cultures

Positive cultures are created when all of the previously mentioned attitudes and behaviors have been developed in a practice. Negative cultures are those in which practices experience high turnover, individuals (versus team members) show up to complete the tasks assigned to them, and team members have no passion, enthusiasm, integrity, or accountability. Negative cultures affect clients; they have decreased trust in the practice and undeveloped relationships, both of which result in decreased client compliance and retention.

> *PRACTICE POINT* Creating a positive culture in the practice decreases employee turnover rate and drives client compliance.

Positive cultures are ones that produce an excellent work environment that promotes open communication, ingenuity, independence, accountability, and productivity. Positive cultures have decreased team member turnover rates and yields high-producing team members that live the mission, values, and visions of the practice. Team members are accountable for these MVVs and are accountable for achieving the goals associated with them.

Every leader must evaluate the true culture that exists in the practice. *"What is really going on in this hospital?"* Identify changes that are needed to create a positive culture and implement them immediately. Negative cultures are detrimental and steps must be taken to start improving them, immediately

Creating positive cultures starts with the evaluation of the leaders and managers. Are the soft skills previously listed being practiced on a daily basis? Are the MVVs developed and implemented into the "practice way of life"? Is continuing education (CE) provided for all team members, regardless of their position? CE stimulates team members and ignites passion and enthusiasm from within. Creating a positive culture is one of the most important tasks a leader must accomplish when leading a practice.

Understanding Diversity

It was stated previously in a discussion of soft skills that leaders must be able to accept diverse ethnicities and change management styles in order to effectively teach and communicate with each. The same model applies for the different generations that exist in today's workforce. Strong leaders understand and mold as needed for success with each.

Veterans, baby boomers, Generation X, and Generation Y make up the team members in practices today. People are living longer (and may have reduced retirement forcing them into work), creating a unique situation, in that four generations are within the workplace. This unique situation creates a new challenge for managers, as they must understand the different needs, and wants, for each generation (Tables 3-1 and 3-2). To really understand the generations, it's helpful to consider their underlying values, or personal lifestyle characteristics, as shown in Table 3-1. Given these underlying values, it makes it easier to understand the resulting workplace characteristics (see Table 3-2) that are attributed to each generation.

TABLE 3-1	Personal and Lifestyle Characteristics of Various Generations			
PERSONAL/LIFESTYLE CHARACTERISTICS	**VETERANS (1922-1945)**	**BABY BOOMERS (1946-1964)**	**GENERATION X (1965-1980)**	**GENERATION Y (1981-2000)**
Core values	Respect for authority Conformers Discipline	Optimism Involvement	Skepticism Fun Informality	Realism Confidence Extreme fun Social
Family	Traditional Nuclear	Disintegrating	Latch-key kids	Merged families
Education	A dream	A birthright	A way to get there	An incredible expense
Communication/media	Rotary phones One-on-one Write a memo	Touch-tone phones Call me anytime	Cell phones Call me only at work	Internet Smart phones Email
Dealing with money	Put it away Pay cash	Buy now, pay later	Cautious Conservative Save, save, save	Earn to spend

TABLE 3-2 | Workplace Values as Seen by Various Generations

WORKPLACE CHARACTERISTIC	VETERANS (1922-1945)	BABY BOOMERS (1946-1964)	GENERATION X (1965-1980)	GENERATION Y (1981-2000)
Work ethic	Respect authority Hard work Age = seniority Company first	Workaholics Desire quality Question authority	Eliminate the task Self-reliant Want structure and direction Skeptical	What's next? Multitasking Tenacious Entrepreneurial
Work is ...	An obligation	An exciting adventure	A difficult challenge A contract	A means to an end
Leadership style	Directive, command and control	Quality	Everyone is the same Challenge others Ask why	Remains to be seen
Communication	Formal memo	In person	Direct, Immediate	Email Text message
Rewards and feedback	No news is good news Satisfaction in a job well done	Money Title Recognition, Give me something to put on the wall	*"Sorry to interrupt, but how am I doing?"* Freedom is the best reward	Whenever I want it, at the push of a button Meaningful work
Motivated by	Being respected	Being valued and needed	Freedom and removal of rules	Work with other bright people
Work/life balance	Keep them separate	No balance: "Live to work"	Balance: "Work to live"	Balance: "It's 5 PM— I've got another gig"
Technology is ...	Hoover Dam	The microwave	What you can hold in your hand PDA Cell phone	Ethereal, intangible

It is imperative to treat and respond to each generation differently, enhancing the positive culture that each leader strives for.

Work and Life Balance

To be an effective leader, one has to balance work and life. This can be hard, as many leaders are go-getters and work hard to achieve the goals set both personally and professionally. However, to be exceptional, one must create this balance, or burnout will occur. One must also pass this skill onto the team, as the team is what makes the practice a success.

> **PRACTICE POINT** Work and life balance is a requirement when implanting procedures to prevent team member burnout.

Exceptional leaders have learned to delegate responsibility to the team and created a positive culture, which allows team members to make decisions. This allows the manager to walk away from the practice at the end of the day, knowing that everything in the practice "is going to be okay". Because the team can make decisions, there is no need to check in with the hospital or for team members to text asking for approval on various items. Leaving work at the end of the day is exactly that: the work brain is turned off. This then allows the balance to kick in: exercise, family time, reading a book, or going to the movies. If this life balance is not made available, burnout will occur, likely within 5 years. Burnout reduces enthusiasm,

initiative, and productivity. When leaders experience burnout, the team follows (leaders lead by example!).

It is also the responsibility of the manager to ensure every team member has a balance between work and life; without it, team member turnover is high. Many times, payroll is cut and team members work exceptionally long hours. Veterinary medicine is emotionally and physically exhausting. If team members have no energy left at the end of the day to enjoy life, burnout will occur. Review team member schedules, ensuring overtime is not accumulated on a regular basis. Help team members determine what life attributes are important to them, and make sure those attributes are experienced on a daily basis.

Preventing Burnout

Every topic that has been presented before this section prevents team member burnout, when implemented properly.

- Develop a mission, vision, and values
- Look in the mirror and evaluate yourself
- Lead by example
- Investigate practice culture
- Listen to the team
- Implement continuing education
- Encourage balance between work and life

The Positive Effects of a Team

A team can develop realistic and achievable goals. Because each team member contributes to the development of goals,

members will work hard to ensure they are obtained. This contributes to a sense of pride, accountability, and ownership of the practice. Because of this pride, team members recognize the importance of disciplined work habits and ensure their behavior meets team standards. This prevents behaviors such as calling in and leaving the rest of the team short staffed. If team members need time off, they do everything in their power to have their shift covered or provide coverage for the team member who needs time off.

Team members often understand one another's priorities and offer help or support when difficulties arise. This may occur in both the practice and in personal life. Offering a supportive work environment can ease the burden of personal issues; views and opinions from co-workers can help solve personal problems.

A leader of a team is one who guides the group. Leaders do not micromanage or dictate a group; a leader simply guides. They empower their team with resources and techniques to solve issues instead of placing a band aid on the problem. Teams may discuss topics, problems, and solutions and develop and plan to implement a new policies or procedures. An effective leader will help guide the team through the appropriate steps to achieve the goal(s).

Troubleshooting and Problem Solving

A team uses a leader in many ways, one of those being as a troubleshooter. Troubleshooting problems before they occur can prevent a minor problem from becoming a major problem. Excellent managers and practice owners can envision the problem before it becomes one and institute measures of prevention. At the same time, once a problem has developed, a leader needs a team to help solve the problem. All the team members should be included in evaluation of the problem. Once a solution has been developed, the entire team can apply the change, which is likely to be successful with the entire team promoting it.

> **PRACTICE POINT** Teams need leaders to help troubleshoot; leaders need to allow teams to help problem solve.

The Four *R*'s of Team Management

Responsibility, *respect*, *rapport*, and *recognition* contribute to managing a successful team. **Responsibility** denotes a duty or obligation that a team member is expected to uphold. Team members should be delegated responsibilities that they are expected to complete and follow through. Completion should be expected within a set time and may need some guidance; however, team members should be given space to complete the project and not be micromanaged. If a team member cannot be given responsibility, cannot complete a project, or must be micromanaged, it may be questioned why the team member is an employee.

A successful manager establishes a team that can accept delegated tasks and complete those tasks responsibly without the need for micromanaging. Micromanaging decreases the leader's time and efficiency; a leader who chooses to micromanage should be the one who completes the project.

Respect is consideration or esteem given to another person. Each member of the team must respect other team members' education, skills, and values. Without respect for each other, team members' morale and self-esteem drop, producing a negative attitude for the entire team. Team members must learn that not all employees have the same thoughts and philosophies, and many people complete tasks differently based on education or previous skill sets. This can be accepted as long as the same ultimate goal is reached in a timely manner and all team members understand this accepted philosophy. Each member possesses expert skills and credentials that warrant respect.

Rapport is a mutual trust or emotional relationship that exists among team members. Great rapport starts at the top with owners and managers. Magnificent rapport is effused to clients who recognize how well the team works together during busy and stressful times and how they enjoy each other's company. Team members with great rapport have respect for each other and are delegated responsibilities on a daily basis. They complete tasks as a team and seek others' opinions while completing those tasks.

Recognition is achievement. Team members should be recognized for a job well done as soon as it is warranted. Many team members only hear of mistakes they have made and the necessary corrections and never hear about the excellent quality of work they produce. Positive situations need to be recognized and brought to the attention of all team members so they can all benefit. Amazing leaders know that high performing teams are high producing teams, and they succeed together.

Empowering Employees

Employee empowerment is essential to the success of a veterinary practice. *Empower* means to give power or authority to; to authorize; to enable or permit. This entails giving team members the ability and permission to complete tasks and objectives. Empowering is the concept of encouraging and authorizing workers to take initiative to improve operations, reduce costs, and improve the quality and quantity of service. Client education is an essential task that all team members should be allowed to complete. By empowering team members to educate clients with the information the practice has implemented, the staff will work above and beyond its usual level. Team members should be allowed to complete laboratory analysis, answer client questions, and treat patients (as directed by the veterinarian). All tasks require extensive training, which should be provided to obtain the best team possible. Once team members have achieved these skills, they must be allowed to use them in the best way possible. Empowering team members to use their skills brings satisfaction to the employee, veterinarian, and client. The goal is to have team members who can manage themselves individually as well as their own projects. Teams that are engaged in daily operations are proactive and strive for the

highest quality of care for patients and clients while working to increase profits for the business.

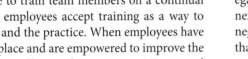

> PRACTICE POINT   Empowering employees is the concept of encouraging and authorizing team members to take initiative to improve operations, reduce costs, and improve the quality and quantity of service.

Empowered employees are only as good as their expertise, and expertise comes from training and exceptional leadership. It is imperative to train team members on a continual basis. The strongest employees accept training as a way to improve themselves and the practice. When employees have pride for their workplace and are empowered to improve the daily operations, they will exceed expectations. Emotional ownership of a practice (versus financial ownership) yields high returns. Team members can never receive enough training. Training motivates team members on a continual basis and also helps retain the strongest employees (while preventing burnout).

Delegation

Independent and strong-willed employees find it hard to delegate tasks to others, often feeling that other team members will not complete the tasks as well as they can. Delegation and empowerment are critical tasks that must be learned and used by all members of management (Figure 3-1). One person cannot possibly manage all aspects of a veterinary practice. A veterinarian or manager cannot see and discharge patients, receive payments, and manage accounts receivable, inventory, and accounts payable while continuing to provide the best treatment possible for hospitalized patients. Delegation and empowerment are the keys to a successful veterinary practice. Delegation frees time, reduces stress, allows a work-life balance, and shows team members they are capable of completing their assigned tasks (builds confidence and future leaders).

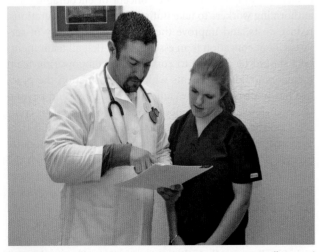

FIGURE 3-1 It is important to delegate tasks, increasing staff use and improving team morale.

Learning How to Delegate

Motivated and enthusiastic team members are eager to accept tasks delegated by a manager. Often, it takes more time to learn to delegate than it takes the team member to complete the task(s) that has been delegated to them. Some managers fear that by delegating tasks, they are admitting failure and the inability to complete all tasks. This is not the case. Delegation increases the efficiency of a manager, while building a stronger, accountable, and productive team.

It is important to take small steps when learning to delegate. One task should be delegated and completed, then the next. Often leaders delegate many projects and then receive negative results from a portion of them. The leader then feels that he or she cannot delegate successfully and stops the delegation process. It is also essential, when delegating large tasks, that the team member is involved in the developing of an action plan. This will help motivate the delegating team member and ensure a complete understanding of the project, enhancing the success of the project.

When choosing to delegate duties, choose an employee who has interest in the task, and the ability to accomplish it. Not all team members have the same strengths; therefore choosing the correct person for the task is essential to the success of the delegation.

The details of the task should be discussed with the team member. Two-way conversations are encouraged (using open-ended questions); this will facilitate a complete understanding on both parts. Use the SMART system (specific, measurable, agreed, realistic, and time bound); this will ensure that all aspects and expectations of the task have been addressed, and both parties are in agreement of the expected results.

> PRACTICE POINT   Use the SMART system to effectively delegate tasks to team members.

Specific: Define the task. Why is it being delegated, why is it important, and what are the expected outcomes?

Measurable: How is this task going to be measured in terms of progress and completion?

Agreed: Based on the previous descriptions, both parties agree on the importance of the task and how the results will be achieved. What resources will be needed to achieve these results? Books, equipment, additional team members?

Realistic: The task that is being delegated and the goals that are sought are realistic, with time constraints in place.

Time bound: How and when will results be expected? Create check-in points (set dates on the calendar, so both parties know when to expect these check-in dates). Creating check-in points prevents micromanagement and keeps the lines of communication open.

To become efficient and understand delegation and empowerment, one must accept error. When empowering and delegating tasks to team members, they will make mistakes. Team members will learn from their mistakes through trial and error. Mistakes offer a learning opportunity for all when

they are shared with the entire team. Effective leadership, delegation, and empowerment help create and motivate other team members to become individual team leaders through personal development, improved self-confidence, and lessons on how to solve problems.

Along with delegation skills, it is imperative that leaders learn to accept help graciously. Again, many leaders will not accept help from others because they believe it makes them appear ineffective or weak. In reality, accepting help when needed is a part of positive, team-oriented culture. Not accepting help and having to make excuses for not finishing tasks or completing them in an unsatisfactory manner carries a greater stigma than accepting help. Asking for help or delegating work to team members shows commitment to the team and leads members to ask for help when needed.

WHAT WOULD YOU DO/NOT DO?

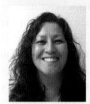 Frances, the practice manager of ABC Veterinary Clinic has been asked to oversee the construction of the new boarding facilities. On top of the new duty, she is also responsible for the accounts receivable, reminders, and recall systems. She also must place orders for products and supplies, monitoring and improving sales during a specified period. Frances becomes overwhelmed at trying to complete all of her assigned tasks; she therefore sends out reminders late and does not complete recalls or callbacks. Statements were also completed incorrectly and did not get recorded in the client accounts. When Frances was confronted by the owner of the practice of the ineffective management strategies, Frances became extremely defensive in stating it was the owners fault for expecting too much of her.

What Should Frances Have Done?

Frances should have delegated tasks to other employees. An office manager can be trained and be able to maintain the accounts receivable, where as a receptionist can be taught to print reminders on a regular basis. A head veterinary technician that works on the floor would be able to oversee inventory and inventory management, potentially improving the management of the products. Inventory can be scrutinized easier by someone who uses the supplies and dispenses products on a daily basis.

By delegating, Frances would still be able to oversee all of the tasks; the person that the tasks were assigned to could provide feedback and ask any questions that may arise. Changes could be made with both Frances and the team member, ensuring maximum efficiency and task completeness. By delegating, Frances could have paid maximum attention to the new project, and used the team to improve the client services.

When Frances was confronted by the owners, instead of becoming defensive, she should have admitted that she had become overwhelmed, and was sorry that she did not admit her mistake earlier. The qualities of a great leader are to admit mistakes, delegate effectively, and train others to follow in a leadership position. A great team aids in making delegation easier and efficient.

Methods of Communication

Communication between and among team members is just as critical as communication with clients. Team members must fully understand policies and procedures as well as any changes that may occur, and it is the leader's responsibility to ensure that.

Communication is the key to the success of any change. Many times changes in policies and procedures fail because of the lack of communication among leadership and team members. Leaders wish to implement a change, and team members may not understand the change, the reason for the change, or what benefit would likely result. When including team members in the discussion, this path of resistance can be avoided.

> **PRACTICE POINT** Leaders must communicate clearly with team members before any change can be expected or implemented.

Leaders and managers should hold staff meetings when they wish to implement change. If team members discuss a change and give their opinions on how a policy or procedure can be updated, they are more likely to accept and implement the change. Team members may have ideas or methods to better implement the change and may have positive or negative thoughts on the process that management had not considered. Employee concerns must be addressed when making changes or the transition will meet resistance.

Several barriers, including poor listening, preoccupation, impatience, and/or resistance to change or new ideas contributes to poor communication among team members and can be exhibited on the part of either the leader or team members. It is imperative that managers not show these qualities and always be mindful of them to prevent them from occurring. Office and practice managers have many duties, tasks, and responsibilities to complete, but employee communication should be the top priority. If team members feel they have not been heard or that the manager was preoccupied, they will follow the example that was set for them.

Good listeners are good problem solvers. It should be a priority for everyone on the team to be a good listener. Listening to clients and team members improves the level of communication at all levels (Box 3-4).

Because of the aforementioned barriers, the information being communicated to a listener may not be received the way it was intended. Practice managers should be aware of misinterpretations, work to overcome barriers, and improve

BOX 3-4	Ideas to Increase Communication in a Practice

- Meetings
- Internal newsletters
- Team member performance/expectations evaluations

channels of communication with team members. Additional channels may be used to ensure complete understanding. Changes to policies and procedures may be discussed at a meeting (with solutions developed by the team) (channel 1); a summary of the notes should then be given to all team members (channel 2); a discussion regarding the success of the change should be on the agenda for the following meeting (channel 3); and an internal newsletter addressing the new change may be circulated 1 month after the change (channel 4). Other channels may be developed by practices to make sure all team members are on board. Managers should periodically evaluate channels and make sure they are understood and used by all team members.

Teams that practice open and honest communication encourage ideas and opinions and are open to disagreements and discussions. Strong teams are likely to have disagreements (which is a healthy part of communication); when disagreements are aired, all opinions can be discussed. Each team member is more likely to accept and understand others thoughts and opinions, and accept them with an open mind. With open communication, members are more likely to resolve conflicts quickly and constructively and will not need the help of management. Open communication is a major component of a successful practice.

Meetings

Regular team meetings should become routine in the veterinary practice. Meetings allow the communication channels to remain open and persuade team members to discuss problems and create solutions as a team (Figure 3-2). They also allow goals for the practice to be developed and reviewed on a regular basis.

 Veterinary practice managers conduct staff meetings.

Meetings raise practice benchmarks, thereby providing for total quality management, increased profits, and improved compliance with staff recommendations and client

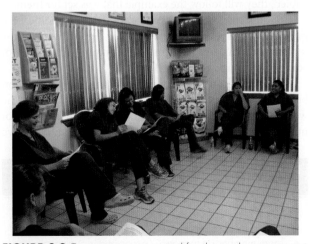

FIGURE 3-2 Team meetings are critical for clear and open communication among all employees.

acceptance. Many practice owners argue the fact that meetings cost money and lose revenue when the business is closed. The fact is that practices cannot afford to *NOT HAVE* meetings, based on the facts just presented. In fact, meetings that are held weekly increase team member communication, problem solving, and contributes to a positive culture.

> **PRACTICE POINT** Practices cannot afford to **not** have meetings.

Employees must be paid for their time, and food may be provided for meetings. An hour-long meeting with 13 staff members and 2 veterinarians costs an average of $462 in wages; this does not account for the cost of food or lost profits from closed doors. However, the accountability of team members and increased production from these meetings far outweighs the costs associated with hosting them. Veterinarians are expected to attend every meeting; they are a leader in the practice, and they lead by example.

A meeting facilitator has a difficult but important job. The facilitator is responsible for starting and ending the meetings on time, controlling the topics, and preventing negativity from overcoming the team (Box 3-5). Facilitating meetings does not come naturally; acquired skills may be needed to run meetings efficiently and with a minimum of stress. Community colleges offer facilitator classes that may benefit those leading meetings, making the job easier and more pleasant.

Some practices choose to have a lunch meeting one day per week; others close for half a day and incorporate training sessions into the meeting. Others may have short daily breakfast meetings at which they discuss the plan for the day and the clients and/or cases that are expected. If meetings are held at lunchtime, team members should be allowed to eat first and decompress from the morning activities. Once a majority of the team has finished eating, the meeting can begin.

Whichever method works best for a given hospital, it is very important to begin and end meetings on time. Employees resent attending meetings that start late and run late. Meetings should begin when they are scheduled, regardless of who is present. Team members who arrive late must take responsibility to find out at a later time what they missed. The meeting should not be stopped and topics repeated for latecomers; this devalues the meeting for those who were on time. Reviews of topics should be avoided at the end of the meeting; these can be typed into a summary and given to team members after the meeting. If tasks were assigned to fellow team members, those assignments should be quickly reviewed before the meeting ends.

BOX 3-5	**Meeting Rules**

- Start and end on time
- Set a maximum length of 45 minutes
- Create an agenda
- Facilitate topic movement

The value of the meeting is lost when team members lose interest and watch the clock instead of the speaker. Meetings should not last for more than 45 minutes. Those that last longer are less productive because of a loss of interest, and active participation in the meeting begins to drop. Larger groups may require longer meeting times so that each member can participate. If longer meetings are needed, breaks should be factored in to allow the team to reenergize so they can fully focus and participate in the discussions. Meetings could possibly be held more frequently, allowing more productive meetings in a shorter time.

Agendas should be created for meetings, which can expedite the meeting process. Team members know what topics are on the list and when to address concerns they have. This helps keep the meeting running on time and prevents getting off topic and further delaying the meeting. Suggestions for meeting topics can be asked of team members. A note board can be placed in a central location of the practice, and team members can add topics that they feel need to be discussed. Topics may include further education on a specific procedure, policy clarification, or education regarding a disease.

The meeting facilitator can take the topics and prioritize them. This ensures that the most important topics are addressed first, allowing ample time for discussion. Other topics must also be addressed, if only briefly. If a topic is left off the agenda, team members may feel that their input was not important, and they may be reluctant to volunteer topics in the future.

Once the agenda has been created, the meeting should adhere to those items. It is vital that the meeting stay on track and on time. If one person dominates the discussions and rambles, employees will soon lose interest in the meeting and it will be a waste of everyone's time. The meeting leader is responsible for not letting this happen and must use tact when guiding the discussion back to the agenda. If a heated discussion begins and emotions run high, it may be suggested that the topic be researched and readdressed at the next meeting. This allows emotions to settle before the next meeting and gives time to find resolution to the problem. The next topic can then be addressed. The same applies to topics that are taking an extensive amount of time to decide or solve. The team members can then be assigned homework; their job would be to provide a solution at the next meeting as well as develop a list of pros and cons regarding the subject. The topic can then be added to the top of the agenda for the next meeting and the remainder of the current agenda can be addressed.

Meetings should not be allowed to become gripe sessions, and it is important that the meeting facilitator prevent this from happening. If team members begin to gripe, the leader can ask how that team member would recommend fixing the problem. The problem can then be opened for discussion to all team members so that a solution can be found as a team. The leader can guide the discussion into a positive frame by using encouraging and exciting words. Positive energy trickles from the top down, with the remaining team members taking nonverbal cues from the management team. This can turn a gripe session into a positive problem-solving meeting. The end result is a team that works better together in a happy and friendly environment.

Always review accomplishments and successes before ending a meeting. Client compliments, employees' personal accomplishments, and successful changes should all be addressed. Meetings ending on a positive note leave team members feeling important, empowered, and willing to continue to work above and beyond the call of duty to make the practice a success.

A summary of the meeting should be provided to team members after the meeting. Many topics are often forgotten about because many ideas and/or changes may be discussed in meetings. Other team members may have been absent or were tardy for the meeting. Notes should be detailed and summarized in a positive fashion, and should not incorporate an authoritarian tone; absent team members may unconsciously reject the information. The notes should be a friendly reminder for those who were in attendance. Meeting notes also serve as a proof of discussion for all team members when they forget a topic has been addressed. Notes from previous meetings can be pulled from the file and handed to employees who need a friendly reminder.

Successful teams discuss problems and use a method of decision making called *consensus*. This means that all team members discuss possible solutions, all voices and opinions are heard, and the entire team works toward a group decision (Figure 3-3). This does not mean that every decision is going to satisfy each team member; however, employees will realize that compromises are necessary. Consensus ensures that every member of the team has agreed to support the decision, and no resentment should be left on the table. Each team member understands that the best decision was made based on the presenting circumstances. If everyone takes responsibility for reaching a consensus, the problem will be solved, the task will be completed, and each team member is more accountable for enforcing the change.

> **PRACTICE POINT** Leaders that implement a consensus style among team members will have greater success at implementing policies.

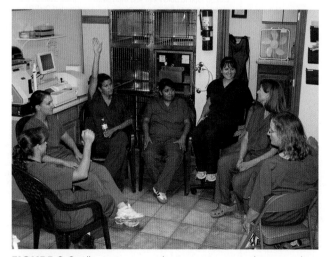

FIGURE 3-3 Allowing team members to participate in decision making improves their acceptance of changes in the practice.

Team members should be asked to participate in meetings and should be held responsible for paying attention and actively listening. To help engage participation, team members can be asked to present topics. This will help create accountability and develop a sense of pride among the staff, along with developing self-confidence and independence. To enhance the education being provided, team members may use learning games, videos, brochures, and team handouts.

Team Newsletter

Team newsletters are an effective form of communication for large veterinary hospitals. Monthly newsletters can inform the teams of birthdays, special anniversaries (employment anniversaries, marriage, stop smoking, etc.), and special events that will occur in the coming months. Changes to procedures and policies can be discussed, as well as in-house continuing education topics. Smaller hospitals can use the same newsletter format; it may only be a two-page newsletter, however it opens the communication channels with employees. It shows respect for one another, adds rapport, and highlights the accomplishments of the team. Fun photos can be included, as well as fun facts and catchy phrases. The goal is team member communication; making it fun for employees adds to the success of the project (Figure 3-4).

Evaluations

Evaluations are a necessity when managing a successful business. However, the quality and quantity of evaluations must be evaluated, critiqued, and updated, allowing the best implementation of practices. Team member coaching must occur throughout the year. This means feedback must be provided every day in order for employees to continue to

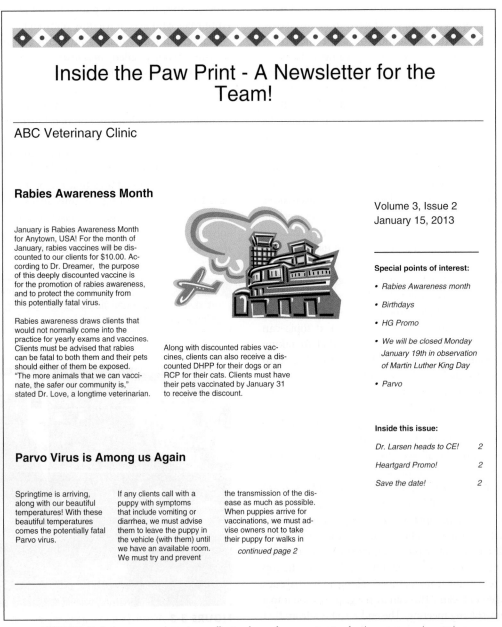

Inside the Paw Print - A Newsletter for the Team!

ABC Veterinary Clinic

Rabies Awareness Month

January is Rabies Awareness Month for Anytown, USA! For the month of January, rabies vaccines will be discounted to our clients for $10.00. According to Dr. Dreamer, the purpose of this deeply discounted vaccine is for the promotion of rabies awareness, and to protect the community from this potentially fatal virus.

Rabies awareness draws clients that would not normally come into the practice for yearly exams and vaccines. Clients must be advised that rabies can be fatal to both them and their pets should either of them be exposed. "The more animals that we can vaccinate, the safer our community is," stated Dr. Love, a longtime veterinarian.

Along with discounted rabies vaccines, clients can also receive a discounted DHPP for their dogs or an RCP for their cats. Clients must have their pets vaccinated by January 31 to receive the discount.

Volume 3, Issue 2
January 15, 2013

Special points of interest:

- Rabies Awareness month
- Birthdays
- HG Promo
- We will be closed Monday January 19th in observation of Martin Luther King Day
- Parvo

Inside this issue:

Dr. Larsen heads to CE!	2
Heartgard Promo!	2
Save the date!	2

Parvo Virus is Among us Again

Springtime is arriving, along with our beautiful temperatures! With these beautiful temperatures comes the potentially fatal Parvo virus.

If any clients call with a puppy with symptoms that include vomiting or diarrhea, we must advise them to leave the puppy in the vehicle (with them) until we have an available room. We must try and prevent

the transmission of the disease as much as possible. When puppies arrive for vaccinations, we must advise owners not to take their puppy for walks in

continued page 2

FIGURE 3-4 A team newsletter is an effective form of communication for the veterinary hospital.

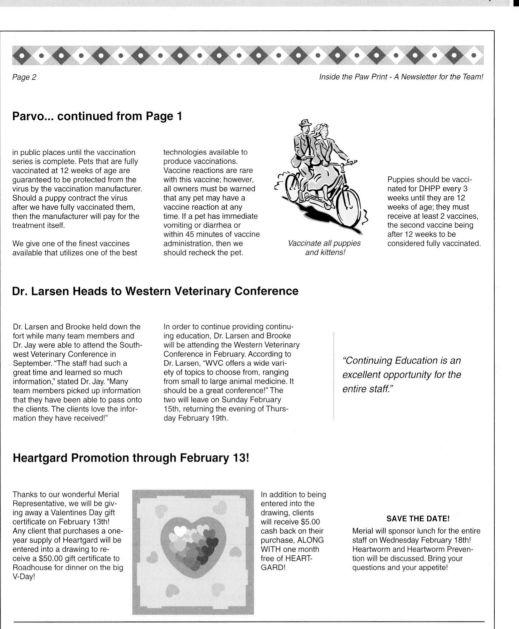

Parvo... continued from Page 1

in public places until the vaccination series is complete. Pets that are fully vaccinated at 12 weeks of age are guaranteed to be protected from the virus by the vaccination manufacturer. Should a puppy contract the virus after we have fully vaccinated them, then the manufacturer will pay for the treatment itself.

We give one of the finest vaccines available that utilizes one of the best technologies available to produce vaccinations. Vaccine reactions are rare with this vaccine; however, all owners must be warned that any pet may have a vaccine reaction at any time. If a pet has immediate vomiting or diarrhea or within 45 minutes of vaccine administration, then we should recheck the pet.

Vaccinate all puppies and kittens!

Puppies should be vaccinated for DHPP every 3 weeks until they are 12 weeks of age; they must receive at least 2 vaccines, the second vaccine being after 12 weeks to be considered fully vaccinated.

Dr. Larsen Heads to Western Veterinary Conference

Dr. Larsen and Brooke held down the fort while many team members and Dr. Jay were able to attend the Southwest Veterinary Conference in September. "The staff had such a great time and learned so much information," stated Dr. Jay. "Many team members picked up information that they have been able to pass onto the clients. The clients love the information they have received!"

In order to continue providing continuing education, Dr. Larsen and Brooke will be attending the Western Veterinary Conference in February. According to Dr. Larsen, "WVC offers a wide variety of topics to choose from, ranging from small to large animal medicine. It should be a great conference!" The two will leave on Sunday February 15th, returning the evening of Thursday February 19th.

"Continuing Education is an excellent opportunity for the entire staff."

Heartgard Promotion through February 13!

Thanks to our wonderful Merial Representative, we will be giving away a Valentines Day gift certificate on February 13th! Any client that purchases a one-year supply of Heartgard will be entered into a drawing to receive a $50.00 gift certificate to Roadhouse for dinner on the big V-Day!

In addition to being entered into the drawing, clients will receive $5.00 cash back on their purchase, ALONG WITH one month free of HEART-GARD!

SAVE THE DATE!

Merial will sponsor lunch for the entire staff on Wednesday February 18th! Heartworm and Heartworm Prevention will be discussed. Bring your questions and your appetite!

FIGURE 3-4, cont'd

improve and exceed expectations. Saving reviews for once a year is detrimental.

 Veterinary practice managers conduct employee performance reviews.

Coaching may come in the form of positive acknowledgment or asking for change (versus reprimand). When asking for change, a negative perception can be avoided, and allows the employee to self-critique and make changes as needed.

> **PRACTICE POINT** Team member coaching should occur year round and not be saved for performance evaluation day.

Evaluations are also known as performance reviews; performance reviews are critical and should be developed from the job description. If the performance expectations are not clear in the job description, team members cannot be held accountable, and evaluations are essentially useless. Review Chapter 5 and develop detailed job descriptions that can be linked to performance expectations. The practices mission, vision, and values must also be a part of a performance review; does the employee live and breathe these three core factors of the practice? Can these three statements be repeated within 5 seconds, if asked what they are? Review the importance and development of the previously discussed mission, vision, and values.

Employee evaluations are an excellent time to address concerns and issues and to open the door for communication between team members and management. Concerns

Employee Survey

Please give your honest, most objective assessment of your performance over the past 12 months of your employment. Please return survey no later than _____ .

Please rate the following from 1 (poor) to 5 (outstanding). Assign NA if not applicable.

1. Accomplishes tasks   _____

2. Enthusiastic and positive attitude   _____

3. Leadership abilities   _____

4. Honest and trustworthy   _____

5. Team player   _____

6. Work ethic   _____

7. Client education and communication skills   _____

8. Provides timely service to clients   _____

9. Attentiveness and response to client needs   _____

10. Observance of practice policies   _____

11. Participation in staff meetings   _____

12. On time for shift   _____

13. Provides innovative ideas for practice improvement   _____

What are your goals for the next 12 months? _____

_____

_____

What can you do to help increase client satisfaction and compliance? _____

_____

_____

_____

What can you do to help your team members improve themselves over the next 12 months?

_____

_____

_____

List any suggestions, comments, or improvements that you feel would help benefit the practice.

_____

_____

_____

FIGURE 3-5 Employee surveys alert management to possible problems in the practice.

can be addressed and documented. Managers can be of assistance to help solve personal and personnel issues and/or address concerns regarding policies or procedures. Some team members may not feel comfortable addressing their concerns in front of other team members and may use evaluation time to do so. Managers should readdress and follow up with concerns throughout the year to ensure problems have been resolved.

Team member accomplishments should also be addressed during evaluations. Many team members complete projects,

receive certifications, and obtain licensure and must be commended for their achievements.

Team members may be encouraged to fill out an employee survey (Figure 3-5). This can help management address issues or topics that may not have surfaced. Management can then be proactive at preventing and solving problems before they arise. Practices can develop their own employee surveys, highlighting policies and procedures within the hospital (Box 3-6); each position should have position-specific evaluations, because goals, tasks, and responsibilities differ.

BOX 3-6	Guidelines for Creating Employee Surveys

- Make them task oriented
- Make them position oriented
- Ask specific questions that relate to the practice's visions and goals
- Provide an area for questions, comments, and suggestions
- Ask team members to state goals (personal and professional) for the following 12 months

---

BOX 3-7	Determining the Extent of Conflicts

- Is this an individual problem?
- Who is involved?
- Does this problem relate to job satisfaction? Why?
- Is patient or client care compromised? How?
- Is poor service the issue? How?
- Does the team need more training? What kind of additional training is needed?
- Is the practice short staffed, resulting in stress and conflicts? Why?

Restraint, client education, and work ethic are a few examples that can be used in a veterinary technician's evaluation. Customer service, phone skills, and client-oriented personality may be examples for a receptionist's evaluation.

Many times, when completing evaluations, leaders focus on the past and not the future. Employees and managers learn to dread evaluations; managers find something else that they feel takes priority, limiting the time spent in this area (because of the low comfort level). When proper coaching is implemented and used daily, evaluations can focus on the future. Team members deserve this feedback (and should receive it, as indicated in the employee manual); turn this dreaded task into a fun, exciting, and motivating experience that everyone can look forward to. Focus on how the performances of each person can contribute to raising the standards of practice.

> **PRACTICE POINT** When completing evaluations, remember to focus on the future, not the past.

Performance feedback with employee surveys is meaningful to team members because they understand what is expected of them and can monitor their performance against expectations. Many times, team members will judge their own actions harder than management and critique themselves severely. Any correction needed is merely a suggestion that the employee takes to the next level. When a team environment such as this has been created and is successful, managing employees becomes a rewarding opportunity.

Conflict Management

Conflicts are normal between team members and occur whenever two or more people work together. Some team members can manage the conflict by themselves, others need a leader to intervene and confront the conflict. Conflicts should be viewed as an opportunity to solve problems. Confidential, open discussions can resolve issues before they become destructive. When conflict is properly handled, it can stimulate new thinking, progress, and growth. Unmanaged conflicts divide team members and should be dealt with as soon as possible.

Practices without conflict can be just as harmful as those with conflict. Employees may be afraid to speak their opinions, or they have learned to work in a culture where they survive best by simply completing orders given to them. A culture of this sort can be detrimental; it prevents creative thinking, innovation, and change. It can also encourage passive resistance because opinions are not permitted. Employees are simply employees in environments such as this, not team members. They may become disgruntled and leave the practice for a more positive, creative environment.

The top three issues that cause conflict in the workplace environment are gossip, lack of training, and lack of communication. Conflicts should be identified and confirmed with all parties involved. A leader does not need to stir the nest when there is no conflict or spread gossip about a possible conflict. Once the problem has been confirmed, leaders should ensure they fully understand the issue(s) by repeating the problem to the presenting team member(s) and express empathy on both parts. Understanding and explaining the other team member's opinion and view of the issue may solve the problem immediately if a simple misunderstanding has occurred. Both team members involved should be aware that the problem is understood and that each of there concerns are valid. Once problems and opinions have been stated and are open for discussion, the emotions are released from the problem and the tension decreases. Team members should not be told how to act or what to think (this does not solve the problem). A caring and empathetic environment makes it easier for honesty and open communication (a normal part of practice culture), allowing conflicts to be resolved relatively easily.

Veterinary practice managers mediate internal disputes between staff personnel.

> **PRACTICE POINT** Conflicts must be addressed ASAP, or the ammunition will be banked (as arsenal) for future use.

When determining the extent of conflict, questions such as those listed in Box 3-7 can be asked. Open-ended questions stimulate discussion. Who, what, when, where, why, and how introduce open-ended questions. Many times, both parties in a conflict have underlying, unmet needs (from the other party). If these needs can be determined, discussed,

BOX 3-8 | Guidelines for Conflict Resolution

- Discuss the problem as soon as possible. A delay in discussion may result in additional conflict or may be interpreted that management is not interested in the problem.
- Listen to all the issues and keep an open mind. Encourage team members to talk with open-ended questions.
- Determine the real issue. Frequently, a complaint is made about a superficial problem when, in reality, a deeper problem exists. For example, a team member may have a workload complaint when a personality conflict is the real problem.

- Exercise control and avoid arguments. Everyone has opinions; let them be stated. Emotional outbursts lead nowhere.
- Avoid a delay in decision making. Unresolved problems spread like wildfire and can add undue stress to the entire team.
- Maintain records of the problem. Document the conflict in case the same problem arises in the future. Recalling details at a later date usually is impossible.

and understood by each other, a positive conflict resolution is in the process.

To help correct conflict, specific facts should be used when discussing the problem (removing all emotion associated with the conflict is a must). As an example, *"Patients did not receive 12 PM treatments today,"* is a statement that only presents the facts. *"Patients did not receive 12 PM treatments today because a personality conflict exists between the two treatment technicians"* is a statement that includes an emotion. This emotion can heighten the conflict and must be removed before resolution can move forward. If a personality conflict exists, facts must be used to determine why and which needs have been unmet by each party. Clear expectations based on the unmet needs can be set and a solution created based on the compromises (Box 3-8).

Occasionally, team members may need to be addressed regarding poor work ethic and performance. Leaders may first ask why the poor performance has begun. Perhaps the employee is having medical issues that had not been revealed, or resentment of "lazy" team members may be to blame. The source of the problem should be identified. Once the problem is identified, the employee should be shown what impact his or her poor performance has on other team members, clients, and patients. When poor performers see the impact they have on others, they may make suggestions for change and be willing to implement their own changes. If suggested changes do not occur, a written warning may be needed.

Some conflicts may involve managers, who can become defensive when confronted with a complaint. Just as with other team members, some will take complaints personally. Facts need to be stated and listened to, internalized, and processed. Some points may be valid; team members often try to help the leader just as the leader has helped team members in the past.

If numerous complaints arise against one team member, a serious problem may exist. Regardless of the nature of the complaint, the details should be reviewed and a resolution should be developed. Unmanaged conflicts can lead to unprofessional behavior and potential workplace violence. Should violence of any sort result, the practice owners and managers may be responsible, because they did not initiate any form of conflict resolution.

Increasing Staff Efficiency

A fine balance often exists between increasing efficiency and not compromising quality of care; however, quality of patient and client care can actually improve with increased team efficiency. Veterinarians only have so many hours in a day; by delegating tasks, veterinarians can see more patients. However, team members must be fully trained to accept the delegated tasks and accomplish them in an efficient manner while maintaining a high quality of care.

 Veterinary practice managers manage daily work assignments.

Therefore protocols and standards of care should be written out and made easily accessible to all team members. New team members may need a reminder of the correct procedure to follow; older team members may need a reminder if they have not performed a procedure in several months. See Chapter 5 for more information on employee procedural manuals.

PRACTICE POINT Increasing staff efficiency can increase the quality of client and patient care.

Leveraging teams increases the profitability and productivity of all team members. Once team members have been trained, they should be used appropriately. Underused team members often leave a practice in search of one that will fully utilize their skills.

To help improve team efficiency and decrease client wait time, several recommendations can be made. The veterinarian is responsible for providing care, diagnostics, prescriptions, and surgery to patients. The receptionist and office manager are responsible for entering charges and collecting money for services rendered (the veterinarian should not have any part of collecting funds or enforcing no-charge policies; this decreases the efficiency of the team and affects clients waiting to be seen). Veterinary technicians and assistants are responsible for client education, treatment plan preparation and presentation, lab procedures, pharmacology, and patient care.

Consider asking all team members (DVMs included) to track the tasks they complete on a daily basis, for 1 week.

Managers can then compile lists associated with each position. Strengths and weaknesses can be identified, helping to determine where inefficiencies lie. Programs can be implemented to ensure staff leveraging occurs to the maximum potential.

Second, travel sheets can eliminate any discrepancy in charge amounts and decrease lost charges (see section titled Decreasing Loss at the end of this chapter). The team schedule should be evaluated next, eliminating any overstaffing or understaffing with the client schedule. Additional team members may be needed during a busy time of the day. For example, at 5 PM, when clients arrive to pick up animals that were dropped off earlier in the day, pick up medications, or arrive for appointments, extra team members may be added to assist in these areas. Fewer team members may be needed when surgery is the only activity occurring in the practice. The team member schedule should be analyzed to match the client schedule. More times than not, inefficient team member schedules affect client service.

Overstaffing causes an increase in payroll and decreases in team efficiency, accountability, and productivity. Understaffing increases loss through missed charges, client relationships, and client compliance. In addition, team members experience burnout, resulting in decreased production and passion, and they may eventually leave the practice.

Common areas of waste include time, money, energy, products, and supplies. Team members must use time efficiently to continue to provide excellent customer service and prevent clients from having to wait. Laboratory analysis should be performed efficiently and without mistakes. Team members may need to learn to multitask and perform several analyses at the same time to increase efficiency. By multitasking, team members can save energy as well. Products and supplies used to provide services to clients are often overlooked. Waste in these areas is generally high in most practices; teams should brainstorm ways to become more efficient, with an ultimate goal of decreasing waste.

Task lists can also be developed for each area of the practice to ensure that all tasks are completed before the end of the shift. Many times, team members are excellent at taking care of clients and patients but forget the "small stuff" that must be completed to keep the practice running smoothly. This small stuff is known as indirect production, which affects direct production (occurs when clients and patients are present). If supplies are missing from the exam room drawer, and a doctor or technician must leave the room to obtain the supply, efficiency is decreased and direct production is affected. Ear cones must be cleaned and disinfected between patients, and paper towel dispensers must be refilled. If these tasks are not completed, again, efficiency is decreased. Task lists can help ensure these and other tasks are completed.

Teams should try to maximize team members, schedules, and equipment. Maximizing the client schedule can help increase the profits of the practice (see Chapter 13). Nail trims and suture removal appointments can be made for technicians, and yearly exams or ear infection appointments can be made for a veterinarian. An example of maximizing equipment comes in the form of dental machines. Routine dental prophylaxis (grade 1 and 2) can be scheduled for veterinary technicians throughout the day, allowing the veterinarian to see more patients. If a technician needs the assistance of a veterinarian, one can help as needed. The dental machine will not produce profits sitting alone and should be used to its maximum potential.

Time Management of Leaders

It is essential to work efficiently, especially in a veterinary practice. There is never enough time in the day or week to complete all tasks needed. Leaders need to know how to perform a task, how to prioritize tasks, and how long each task will take. Understanding the relation of time to production is essential. Planning and scheduling of work decrease wasted time.

The behaviors that result in wasted time include failure to plan and budget time, interruptions, failure to follow through and complete tasks, slowness in making decisions, unnecessary work, and failure to delegate. Other time wasters include lack of privacy and desk clutter. When items are needed and cannot be found, time is wasted looking for them. Efficient time management requires that staff organize tasks, maintain a daily schedule, establish deadlines, and organize work flow.

To help maintain a daily work flow, a manager may create a to-do list and determine priorities that need to be accomplished. Many people make a list when tasks become overwhelming but do not create a list for everyday tasks. A to-do list helps managers prioritize tasks and can ensure they are completed on a daily basis. If a task does not get completed on the day stated, it can roll over to the following day, especially if the priorities of the listed tasks change. Long-term lists can also be developed to keep long-range goals in mind. Often, managers become overwhelmed with short-term goals and lose sight of long-term tasks.

Leaders must set standards high and set an example for other team members. If a manager cannot complete tasks early or on time, the rest of the team cannot be expected to complete their tasks on time either. A calendar or planner can also help keep personal and work appointments organized. Each person responds to organization differently, and different methods should be tried as long as the ultimate goal is reached: completion of all tasks created and assigned.

Decreasing Loss

An essential task of a manager is to develop practices and policies to increase profits and decrease loss. Loss can come in a variety of avenues. Missed charges top the list, followed by employee theft, excess use of products and supplies in the hospital, and undercharging for services provided.

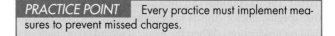

PRACTICE POINT   Every practice must implement measures to prevent missed charges.

BOX 3-9 | Methods to Decrease Loss

- Implement internal controls to prevent employee theft
- Use travel sheets to decrease missed charges
- Implement electronic medical records
- Team members should be accountable for all supplies used
- Set appropriate fees
- Manage inventory appropriately

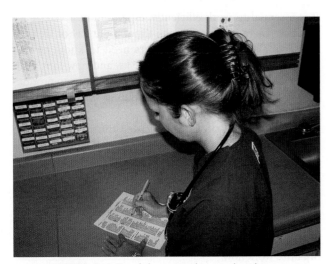

FIGURE 3-6 Travel sheets can decrease lost charges.

It is unfortunate to think that the great team that has been developed is at risk for employee theft. However, employee theft can account for a high percentage of loss each year (see Chapter 20). Internal controls must be implemented to prevent the temptation. The cost adds up if each employee takes one box of heartworm preventive medication home (Box 3-9).

Missed charges account for a majority of lost money. Fecal smears, heartworm tests, and nail trims are often forgotten. Practices should audit a minimum of 20 records per day and review for lost charges. Almost every record will have at least one item that was not charged. It is imperative to implement procedures to help control loss through missed charges (review Chapter 14 and Chapter 20 for additional details). Unfortunately, many practices do not implement measures to track missed charges, and the amount of money lost is never known.

Travel Sheet

Many paper medical record practices have found that travel sheets are an excellent way to decrease lost charges (Figure 3-6). A travel sheet lists the most common procedures provided and products carried in the practice. The travel sheet is attached to the medical record and travels with it throughout the day. When a service is performed, the procedure is then circled or highlighted on the sheet (Figure 3-7). In multiple-doctor practices, it is advised to use a specific colored highlighter for each veterinarian. The receptionist can then be sure to add charges under that specific doctor (this is imperative when veterinarians are paid on production). When the medical record is complete, the receptionist can enter the charges and double-check the record against the travel sheet, looking for any missed charges.

For those who wish to save paper, travel sheets can be laminated and reused. Simply place them in a pile and clean them at the end of the day.

Inpatient charges are missed more often than outpatient charges. Team members may only miss one charge for an outpatient; that number is at least doubled, if not tripled, for hospitalized patients. Outpatients are considered those that do not remain in the hospital. Exams, vaccines, fecal checks, and so forth are all outpatient services. Inpatient services include hospitalization, IV fluids, injections administered, and laboratory diagnostics that are completed while the patient is hospitalized. It may be useful for practices to develop a specific travel sheet for hospitalized patients. Each time a test or treatment is completed, it should be circled on the sheet with the specific colored highlighter of the veterinarian who ordered the treatment or test.

Each hospital may create individualized hospital travel sheets that can include the most common hospitalized procedures performed in that particular practice. Each patient will have one hospital travel sheet per day, allowing charges to be entered as soon as the opportunity presents. Team members are less likely to forget charges for patients when the case is fresh in their mind versus later, just before patient discharge (Figure 3-8).

Electronic medical records (EMRs) eliminate many missed charges, because the system is set up to invoice clients when a particular service or product is selected.

Accountability

Team members should be held accountable for the amount of materials used in clinic to provide services for clients. For example, a sloppy surgeon who drops suture material on a daily basis can cost the practice a significant amount. Technicians who use a wad of gauze to clean a wound (instead of two to three pieces per scrub) increase costs. Not every employee contributes to loss, but if each is held accountable, the lost dollars will decrease. Meetings are a great place to discuss loss and brainstorm ideas to reduce it as well as bring awareness to product loss.

Inventory Management

It is important to realize that inventory control is a large factor in controlling loss within the practice. A good inventory system ensures that product will be available for use while inventory is maintained at a cost-effective level. Reorder points and reorder quantities are vital to a successful inventory system. Inventory levels should be decreased to help reduce shrinkage. Excess products can be kept in a central supply location, allowing the inventory manager to monitor supply use closely. See Chapter 15 for details of effective inventory management.

Appropriate Fee Setting

Many practices do not charge appropriately for the services provided. Veterinarians often believe the costs are too high

Client Number _____ Client Name _____ Pet _____ Doctor _____

DISCOUNTS
0107 Monthly Special
0108 Senior Wellness
Senior Citizen

OFFICE CALL
0214 Brief Office Call
0216 Regular Office Call
0219 Well K-9/Fe Exam
0222 Exotics Exam-Reg
0220 Exotics Exam-Brief
226 Exam w/ vaccines
0228 Pre-Op Exam
0232 Recheck N/C
0234 Recheck
0109 Health Certificate
0106 Int'l Health Certificate
0104 Duplicate Rabies Tag

FELINE VACCINES
0608 FVRCP Booster
0612 FVRCP 1 year
0609 FVRCP 3 year
0613 FELV Booster
0610 FELV 1 year
0611 FVRCP/FELV
0607 Rabies Only Fe -1 yr
0618 Rabies Feline 1 year
0605 Feline Yearly Exam
0621 Feline Sr Wellness

PET WEIGHT_____

CANINE VACCINES
0603 Parvo
0615 Bordetella
0616 DHPP Booster
0602 DHPP 1 year
0617 DHPP 3 year
0604 Rabies Canine 1 year
0601 Rabies 3 year
0690 Canine Yearly Exam
0620 Canine Sr Wellness
0606 Rattlesnake Vaccine
0619 Lepto

ANESTHESIA
0302 Anesthesia
0304 Extended
0306 Short
0308 Local
0310 Tranquilization
0316 Geriatric Anesthesia

GROOMING
0506 Beak Trim- Small
0508 Beak Trim- Large
0510 Nail Trim
0512 Nail Trim- Exotic
0514 Wing Trim- Small
0516 Wing Trim- Large
0520 Trim Teeth
0518 Pluck ears
0502 Medicated Bath
0501 Shave Cat

DENTAL
0702 Sm Normal Prophy
0704 Lg Normal Prophy
0701 Feline Normal Prophy
0706 Severe Periodontal Dz
0710 Follow-Up
0714 Tooth Ext. Minimum
0716 Tooth Ext. Moderate
0718 Tooth Ext. Extensive
0712 Dental Sutures

HOSPITALIZATION
0902 Board-Canine
0904 Board-Feline
0903 Overnight Board, Sx
0906 Day Board/Obsvtn
907 Hospital Day
0908 Hospital Overnight
909 Hospital Day w/ IV
0910 Hospital Weekend
0912 Hospital Exotic
911 O2 Therepy Half Day
0914 O2 Therepy Full Day
0916 IV Care Daily
0918 IV Care Intensive
0920 IV Catheter
0922 IV Catheter, 2nd
0924 IV Fluids per Liter
0926 IV Fluids One time
0928 Fluid Additives
0925 IV Fluids Hetastarch
0930 SQ Fluids Once
0932 SQ Fluids Per Day
0934 SQ Fluids Exotic
0936 SQ Fluids Disp.
938 SQ Fluids No Tech/Dr.

RADIOLOGY
4125 Radiographs
4126 Radiographs-dental

LAB SERVICES
3505 ACTH Stim
3515 Autoimmune Profile
3520 Avian Comp Profile
3526 Avian Post Purchase
3535 Bile Acids
3611 BIPS
3621 Blood Pressure
3560 CBC/Diff
3580 Coagulation Profile
3770 Chemistry #1
3775 Chemistry >2
3590 Culture and Sensitivity
3605 Cytology In house
3593 Cytology-Lab
3610 DTM
3615 Ear Mite Check
3620 Ear Smear
3631 Electrolytes
3603 EKG
3626 EKG >1 per day
3628 EKG Senior Wellness
3630 EKG Repeat
3641 Ehrlichia Canis PCR
3655 Fecal-Direct
3660 Fecal Flotation/Smear
3665 Fecal- Recheck
3675 FELV Snap Test
3685 FELV/FIV Snap Test
4081 Fine Needle Aspirate
3695 Fungal Serology
3815 General Health Profile
3710 Heartworm SNAP
3715 Heartworm Difil
3705 HCT/TP
3720 Histopath
3725 Histopath Additional
3730 Histopath Derm
3731 Histopath-Bone Decal
3527 Mammalian Comp Prof
0438 Necropsy In house
0436 Necropsy NMDL
0441 Necropsy Avian-NMDL
3745 Parvovirus Snap Test
3750 Phenobarb Levels
3749 Platelet Count
3601 Pre-Op EKG
3755 Pre-Op Profile
3785 Reptile Std. Profile
3786 Reptile Comp Profile
3795 Schirmer Tear Test
3805 Skin Scrape

LAB SERVICES
3821 T-4 Equilibrum Dialysis
3820 T-4 Dogs
3822 T-4 Cats
3830 Tick Born Dz Panel
4141 Tonopen
3850 Urinalysis- In house
3855 Urinalysis-Lab
3880 Urinalysis-SG
3854 Urinalysis Sediment
3853 Urinalysis-Stick
3852 Urinalysis- Yearly Exam
3860 Vaginal Smear

CLINICAL PROCEDURES
4005 Abdominocentesis
4010 Anal Sac Expression
4015 Anal Sac recheck
4020 Artifical Insemination
4025 Bandage Wound Sm
4030 Bandage Wound Med
4035 Bandage Wound Lg
3085 Cast
4050 Clean Ears
4055 Clip/Clean Wound Sm
4060 Clip/Clean Wound Med
4065 Clip/Clean Wound Lg
4070 Corneal Stain (1)
4071 Corneal Stain (2)
4080 Enema
4083 Flush Anal Glands
4085 Flush ears (1)
4090 Flush ears (2)
4095 Flush Nasal Duct
4105 Home Again Implant
4110 Pass Stomach Tube
4130 Semen Collection/Eval
7002 Splint-Small
5126 Re-Splint Small
7001 Splint-Medium
5131 Re-Splint Medium
7000 Splint-Large
5136 Re-Splint-Large
4140 Thoracocentesis
4145 Transtracheal Wash
4150 Urinary Catheter

EUTHANASIA
WT_____
Dog _____ Cat _____
Mass Cremation
Private Cremation
402 Exotic

FIGURE 3-7 Sample travel sheet.

Continued

and that clients cannot afford to pay those fees. In reality, the veterinary practice has a large overhead cost that is, for the most part, hidden. Payroll taxes, team member benefits, and credit card fees are just a few of the hidden costs veterinary practices encounter. Obvious costs include product purchases, utilities, and mortgages (or rent) that must be paid monthly regardless of the profit the practice produces. See Chapter 20 for more information on budgeting and financial planning in a veterinary hospital.

> **PRACTICE POINT** Review service fees and implement an appropriate fee structure to help reduce loss.

If clients complain of the fees they are charged, they may not fully understand the value associated with those fees. Client education techniques should be reviewed to ensure clients are being fully educated by the team when they (the client) visit the practice. Clients value honesty, compassion, and timeliness. They want to understand the information being presented to them. Without this knowledge, they will not accept the recommendations (Chapters 2, 10, and 20 include more information regarding methods to increase the value for clients).

When developing a pricing structure, fees should be divided into two categories: shopped and nonshopped services. Shopped services include vaccinations, heartworm tests, and routine procedures. These fees can be competitively priced with other practices in the community. The fees should cover the cost of the product, the cost of the inventory needed to complete that service, the time of the technician and/or veterinarian to complete the service, and overhead associated with the practice. For example, a heartworm test should include the cost of the test itself, the syringe and needle

SURGICAL PROCEDURES	4405 Feline Neuter	CONSULTS	INJECTIONS
4205 Abcess Debride	4410 Feline Neuter/Declaw	202 Cardiology	
4210 Amputate Limb Sm	4420 Feline OVH	213 Repeat EKG	# of ML _____
4215 Amputate Limb Lg	4425 Feline OVH In heat	204 Internal Medicine	
4220 Amputate Digit	4430 Feline OVH Pregnant	206 Miscellaneous	1220 Amiglyde #1
4225 Amputate Tail	4435 Feline OVH Declaw	208 OFA 1225 Amiglyde >1	
4235 Ant. Cruc. Repair	4441 FHO Feline	210 Radiology	1256 Baytril 100mg/ml
4240 Aural Hematoma-K-9	4442 FHO Canine	212 Shipping	1255 Baytril 22.7mg/ml
4341 Aural Hematome-Fe	4455 Growth Removal SM		1265 Cephazolin
4245 Biopsy - Wedge	4460 Growth Removal MED	**HEARTWORM MEDICATION**	1270 Cephazolin >1
4250 Biopsy - Punch	4465 Growth Removal LG	HG Small # _____	1281 Cortrosyn
4246 Biopsy - Bone	4470 Growth Removal >1	HG Medium # _____	1289 Dexameth 2mg/ml
4260 C-Section	4480 Hernia Repair Inguinal	HG Large # _____	1290 Dexameth 4mg/ml
4265 C-Section w/ OVH	4485 Hernia Repair Abdom	HG Feline 0-5# #6	1305 Diphenhydramine
4270 Canine Neuter <50	4490 Hernia Repair Diaphm.	HG Feline 5-15# #6	Ivomec
4275 Canine Neuter >50	4495 Hernia Repair Umbil.		1335 Immiticide
4285 Canine OVH <50	4505 Patellar Luxation #1	Revolution Feline	1390 Methyl Pred Acetate
4290 Canine OVH 50-99	4510 Patellar Luxation #2	Revolution Canine	1410 Pred Acetate
4272 Canine OVH >100	4511 Prostatic Wash		1417 Solu-delta Cortef 100mg
4295 Canine OVH/Heat	4515 Puppy Dewclaws Each	Frontline Feline	1418 Solu-delta Cortef 500mg
4305 Canine OVH/Preg	4520 Puppy Tail Docks Each	Frontline Canine	1430 Torbugesic
4236 Cranial Cruc. SM (1)	4525 Pyometra w/ OVH	Frontline In Hosp Use	
4238 Cranial Cruc. LG (1)	4530 Rabbit Neuter		**E-COLLAR**
4237 Cranial Cruc. SM (2)	4535 Rabbit OVH	**POST OP PAIN MEDS**	
4239 Cranial Cruc. LG (2)	4540 Staple Wound per staple	Rimadyl 25mg	**N/C ITEMS**
4315 Cherry Eye Repair 1	4545 Stenotic Nares Repair	Rimadyl 75mg	818 HG SM
4320 Cherry Eye Repair 2	4550 Suture Wound SM	Rimadyl 100mg	822 HG M
4325 Cryptorchid Fe-Flank	4555 Suture Wound MED	Metacam	826 HG LG
4330 Cryptorchid Fe-Abdm	4560 Suture Wound LG	Buprinex	2790 Strongid
4345 Cryptorchid K-9 Abdm	4575 Third Eyelid Flap	Tramadol	510 Nail Trim
4340 Cryptorchid K-9 Flank			
4350 Cystotomy			
4355 Debride wound			
4360 Declaw/Tendonectomy			
4365 Dewclaw Unjointed #1			
4370 Declaw Jointed #1			
4375 Drain Placement			
4385 Entropion per lid			
4390 Exploratory			
4395 Eye Enucleation			

FIGURE 3-7, cont'd

needed to draw the blood for the test, and the technician's time to draw the blood and run the test. A percentage needs to be added on top to contribute to the hidden overhead costs of the practice. Many times, practices forget to add the cost of the supplies needed to complete the service as well as the staff and overhead costs.

Once shopped service fees have been set, nonshopped fees can be determined. Review Chapter 20 for more information on appropriate fee setting. Pharmaceuticals must also be charged appropriately and include the cost for the label, the pill vial, and the time to count the pills to be dispensed. Review Chapter 15 for appropriate inventory pricing structures. Outside laboratory fees are generally doubled, adding $5 to $10 to cover the cost of supplies used to obtain the sample, plus labeling, packaging, and filling out the form.

Motivating and Retaining Team Members

Chapter 5 covers the selection of employees and retaining current team members. The selection process of team members is important. It is critical to choose the best employee possible, not just fill a position with anyone available.

People who work well together understand the importance of positive reinforcement. It is essential for maintaining the team's enthusiasm and motivation. The simplest form of positive reinforcement comes in words and phrases that recognize an individual's hard work and dedication to the practice. Positive reinforcement is a tremendous incentive for strengthening teams. Lack of recognition and appreciation is a top reason for employee dissatisfaction. Seize the moment to show each team member the recognition he or she deserves (Box 3-10).

Positive reinforcement should be given on an individual basis. A team member who has gone above and beyond expectations should be rewarded immediately with something that is useful for that particular person. For example, if an employee has just purchased a new home and has previously discussed the need to buy new kitchen utensils, then a simple reward of new pots and pans may be warranted. If a team member is remodeling a home, a gift certificate to a local hardware store may be appropriate. However, a gift certificate to the local roller rink for a team member who is 50 years old would devalue the positive reinforcement. Take the time to reward appropriately, and the positive reinforcement will double in value.

Job enrichment is also important for retaining team members. For example, the main job of kennel attendants is to clean the kennels on a daily basis; however, by allowing them to assist technicians, the job can be enriched (Figure 3-9). They can hold animals for treatments or help position patients for radiographs. Individuals can get bored with their daily duties. By allowing them to do something other than clean kennels, their job can be exciting and interesting and

CLIENT'S LAST NAME				WORKING DIAGNOSIS										
PET'S NAME					PRIMARY DOCTOR									

DATE:	8AM	9	10	11	12	1	2	3	4	5	6	7	8
FEED													
WATER													
WALK/LITTER													
TEMPERATURE													
WEIGHT													
APPETITE?													
ATTITUDE?													
URINE?													
BM OR DIARRHEA													
VOMIT?													

OFFICE CALL	HOSPITALIZATION	LAB SERVICES	LAB SERVICES
0214 Brief Office Call	0902 Board-Canine	3611 BIPS	0000 Urinalysis
0216 Regular Office Call	0904 Board-Feline	3621 Blood Pressure	3860 Vaginal Smear
0222 Exotics Exam-Reg	0903 Overnight Board, Sx	3560 CBC/Diff	**CLINICAL PROCEDURES**
0220 Exotics Exam-Brief	0906 Day Board/Obsvtn	3770 Chemistry #1	4005 Abdominocentesis
0232 Recheck N/C	907 Hospital Day	3775 Chemistry >2	4010 Anal Sac Expression
0234 Recheck	0908 Hospital Overnight	3590 Culture and Sensitivity	0000 Bandage Wound
FELINE VACCINES	909 Hospital Day w/ IV	3605 Cytology In house	3085 Cast
0608 FVRCP Booster	0910 Hospital Weekend	3610 DTM	4050 Clean Ears
0612 FVRCP 1 year	0912 Hospital Exotic	3615 Ear Mite Check	4055 Clip/Clean Wound Sm
0609 FVRCP 3 year	911 Oxygen Therepy Half Day	3620 Ear Smear	4060 Clip/Clean Wound Med
0613 FELV Booster	0914 Oxygen Therepy Full Day	3631 Electrolytes	4065 Clip/Clean Wound Lg
0610 FELV 1 year	0916 IV Care Daily	3603 EKG	4070 Corneal Stain (1)
0611 FVRCP/FELV	0918 IV Care Intensive	3626 EKG >1 per day	4071 Corneal Stain (2)
0618 Rabies Feline 1 year	0920 IV Catheter	3655 Fecal-Direct	4080 Enema
0605 Feline Yearly Exam	0922 IV Catheter, 2nd	3660 Fecal Flotation/Smear	4083 Flush Anal Glands
0621 Feline Sr Wellness	0924 IV Fluids per Liter	3675 FELV Snap Test	4085 Flush ears (1)
CANINE VACCINES	0926 IV Fluids One time	3685 FELV/FIV Snap Test	4090 Flush ears (2)
0603 Parvo	0928 Fluid Additives	4081 Fine Needle Aspirate	4110 Pass Stomach Tube
0615 Bordetella	0925 IV Fluids Hetastarch	3815 General Health Profile	7002 Splint-Small
0616 DHPP Booster	0930 SQ Fluids Once	3710 Heartworm SNAP	5126 Re-Splint Small
0602 DHPP 1 year	0932 SQ Fluids Per Day	3705 HCT/TP	7001 Splint-Medium
0617 DHPP 3 year	0934 SQ Fluids Exotic	3745 Parvovirus Snap Test	5131 Re-Splint Medium
0604 Rabies Canine 1 year	0936 SQ Fluids Disp.	3750 Phenobarb Levels	7000 Splint-Large
0601 Rabies 3 year	**RADIOLOGY**	3601 Pre-Op EKG	5136 Re-Splint-Large
0690 Canine Yearly Exam	4125 Radiographs	3755 Pre-Op Profile	4140 Thoracocentesis
0620 Canine Sr Wellness	**CONSULTS**	3795 Schirmer Tear Test	4145 Transtracheal Wash
0606 Rattlesnake Vaccine	202 Cardiology	3805 Skin Scrape	4150 Urinary Catheter
0619 Lepto	213 Repeat EKG	0000 T-4	**E-COLLAR**
	204 Internal Medicine		
	210 Radiology		

FIGURE 3-8 Sample hospital travel sheet.

BOX 3-10 | Ideas for Motivating Team Members

- Setting goals together
- Thinking "career"
- Humor
- Benefits packages
- Lifelong learning (CE)
- Paid time off
- Generational preferences
- Praise
- Coupons or gift cards to local restaurants
- Celebrating victories
- "Firing" bad clients

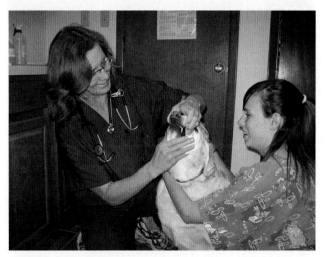

FIGURE 3-9 Encouraging team members to assist outside of their regular responsibilities keeps them motivated.

give them incentive to take the next step up the ladder within the veterinary hospital.

Do team members have pride in the workplace? Is there a waiting list to be hired, or does the practice hire the first person that comes along? Do team members understand how the business is run? Consider factors that contribute to pride in the workplace, starting with the mission, visions, and values.

If team members know what direction they are going and the goals they need to achieve, they will have pride; without knowing these things, they will not have pride. Share goals, income and expenses with everyone. Create an open books management system, keeping *everyone in the loop*.

Is each employee used to the fullest potential? This was discussed previously with staff leveraging. Each team member must be able to use all of the skills they have been taught. Capitalize on each person's strengths to overcome the weaknesses of others. This creates empowerment, thus resulting in accountability and productivity of each person.

> **PRACTICE POINT**   Motivate team members by using them to their fullest potential.

What opportunities are available for career development? Previous sections of this chapter have highlighted how continuing education is beneficial to every team member. Allow the team to become inspired, champion new ideas, and problem solve issues as they arise.

What opportunities do team members have to express their opinion? Listen to employees and integrate their thoughts into everyday solutions.

National Association of Veterinary Technicians in America: 2011 Demographics Survey

In 2011, the National Association of Veterinary Technicians in America (NAVTA) completed a demographics survey and released some amazing data. For a full review of the survey, visit www.navta.net. High points of the survey include issues facing veterinary technicians (Box 3-11) as well as the most fulfilling aspects of a veterinary technician's job (Box 3-12). Every one of these issues has been described earlier, and it is

---

BOX 3-11	Issues Facing Veterinary Technicians

- Lack of professional recognition
- Job burnout
- Underutilization
- Lack of resources to complete tasks efficiently
- Lack of raises/pensions
- Undermanaged
- Understaffed
- Relationship with management
- Long hours

BOX 3-12	Most Fulfilling Aspects of a Veterinary Technician's Job

- Caring for animals in the best way possible
- Making a difference in a pet's life
- Client education
- Assisting in diagnosis
- Staying current with CE
- Developing client relationships

---

up to the leader to effectively implement tools to prevent the *issues veterinary technicians face* and capitalize on the *most fulfilling aspects*.

⚖️ VETERINARY PRACTICE and the LAW

Creating a positive culture for the team is an essential element to a successful practice. Positive cultures have high client retention and compliance rates, low employee turnover, and most important, team accountability and buy-in. Without this positive culture, many scenarios can develop, placing the practice in hot water. Negative cultures breed internal theft, employee burnout, and potential claims of psychological assessment. If team members do not know the vision and mission of the practice, they simply show up to work each day, completing duties as needed. The tasks may not be completed to expectation, creating lapses in patient care and safety violations resulting in injury to either patients or team members. When team members are terminated, they are often terminated for unknown reasons, with expectations and corrective actions never being recorded. Prevent these legal issues from arising by creating a positive team culture, starting with leadership.

REVIEW QUESTIONS

1. What are some characteristics of effective leaders?
2. What are four steps of management?
3. Why are these four steps critical to the management of a veterinary practice?
4. What are two theories of effective management? Define each.
5. How can you become a better leader?
6. Why are respect and rapport imperative when managing a team?
7. What are some methods that can be used to empower team members?
8. How long should a meeting last?
9. What is a consensus?
10. Why should conflicts be resolved immediately?
11. What are the 4 *R*'s of team management?
    a. Rights, responsibilities, reliability, reality
    b. Responsibility, respect, rapport, recognition
    c. Reasons, retention, resources, responsibility
    d. None of the above
12. Which of the following characteristics should a team leader possess?
    a. Selfishness
    b. Enthusiasm
    c. Sincerity
    d. Dishonesty
    e. All of the above
    f. Both B and C
13. Which of the following is the correct definition of emotional intelligence?
    a. The ability to become emotionally attached/detached as needed

b. The ability to stay emotionally stable in a professional environment
c. The ability to identify, assess, and control one's emotions
d. The ability to be relate to other people on an emotional level

14. Which of the following examples would be the best way to delegate tasks?
a. Rely on one responsible individual to delegate all needed tasks to.
b. Only give easier, time-consuming tasks to others on the team.
c. Delegate tasks as needed to different individuals on the team to prevent overloading one person.
d. None of the above

15. Which of the following are issues involving veterinary technicians?
a. Lack of professional recognition
b. Long hours
c. Job burnout
d. Lack of raises/pensions
e. All of the above

Recommended Reading

Ackerman L, Stowe JD: *Blackwell's five minute veterinary practice management consult*, Ames, IA, 2007, Blackwell.

Belaso JA, Stayer RC: *Flight of the buffalo: soaring to excellence, learning to let employees lead*, New York, 1994, Grand Central Publishing.

Hersey P, Blanchard K: *Management of organized behavior*, ed 10, Upper Saddle River, NJ, 2012, Prentice Hall.

NAVTA demographics survey; *The NAVTA Journal*, Sept/October 2012.

Nelson R: *1501 ways to reward employees*, New York, 2012, Workman Publishing Company.

Tropman J: *Making meetings work: achieving high quality group decisions*, ed 2, Thousand Oaks, CA, 2003, Sage Press.

Veterinary Ethics and Legal Issues

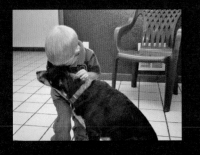

OUTLINE

Code of Ethics, *73*
    Veterinary Ethics, *77*
Legal Issues, *78*
    Veterinary Practice Act, *78*
    Definitions of Law, *78*
    Consent, *79*
    Emergency Care, *79*

Malpractice, *81*
Abandoned Animals, *82*
Impending Laws, *82*
Medical Records, *82*
**Most Common Complaints to the Board
of Veterinary Medicine,** *83*

KEY TERMS

Administrative Ethics
Civil Law
Code of Ethics
Consent
Contract Law
Criminal Law
Informed Consent
Law
Malpractice
Negligence
Normative Ethics
Personal Ethics
Professional Ethics
Social Ethics
Standard of Care
Tort
Veterinary Ethics
Veterinary Practice Act

LEARNING OBJECTIVES

When you have completed this chapter, you should be able to:

1. Differentiate ethics and law.
2. Define the branches of ethics.
3. Identify a veterinary practice act.
4. Differentiate criminal and civil law.
5. Describe informed consent.
6. Develop an informed consent form.
7. Clarify methods used to prevent malpractice and negligence.
8. Manage abandoned animals.
9. List the most common complaints in veterinary medicine.

CRITICAL COMPETENCIES

1. **Analytical Skills** - the ability to analyze information and use logic to address problems; the ability to quickly and accurately grasp complex information and concepts and to make correct inferences.
2. **Critical and Strategic Thinking** - the ability to think critically about situations and to understand the relevance of information for different problems; use critical reasoning to generate and evaluate alternative courses of action or points of view relevant to an issue.
3. **Decision Making** - the ability to make good decisions, solve problems, and decide on important matters; the ability to gather and analyze relevant data and choose decisively between alternatives.
4. **Integrity** - honesty, trustworthiness, and adherence to high standards of ethical conduct.
5. **Resourcefulness** - the ability to understand what it takes to complete the job; apply knowledge, skills, and expertise to perform tasks quickly and efficiently.
6. **Writing and Verbal Skills** - the ability to comprehend written material easily and accurately; ability to express thoughts clearly and succinctly in writing.

In the law and ethics domain, practice managers monitor procedures and policies of the practice to determine whether events or processes comply with laws, regulations, and standards.

Knowledge Requirements

The tasks related to legal and ethical standards require knowledge of state/provincial and federal laws, legal codes, government regulations, professional standards, and agency rules.

Three areas of ethics exist and affect each team member on every level. Social, personal, and professional ethics are interrelated, yet they affect each person differently. Social ethics are the consensus principles adopted or accepted by society at large and codified into laws and regulations. Laws include those against murder, rape, and stealing along with ordinances such as those that regulate pets on leashes. Personal ethics define what is right or wrong on an individual basis. This can include religious beliefs and values as they relate to relationships and marriages. Professional ethics, as stated, are developed by the professionals of a particular discipline, developing rules, codes, and conduct for the profession to follow.

Code of Ethics

Ethics is a branch of philosophy and a systematic, intellectual approach to the standards of behavior. The purpose of a professional code of ethics is to help members of a profession achieve high levels of behavior through moral consciousness, decision making, and practice. A sense of ethics in daily practice challenges veterinarians to determine right from wrong. Each organization within the profession also has a code of ethics for its members and is based on moral principles that reflect concern and care for the client and patient.

Historically, ethics relate to standards of conduct promoted by and demanded of members of veterinary associations. The American Veterinary Medical Association (AVMA) *Principles of Veterinary Medical Ethics* is a document on ethical issues in veterinary practice focusing more on the relationships one has with colleagues than on the broader range of moral and ethical issues relating to animals (Box 4-1).

The Veterinary Hospital Managers Association (VHMA) holds a strong code of ethics for the profession, practice, and patient. Practice and hospital managers must protect the interest and integrity of the practice itself while providing a professional image for the profession (Figure 4-1).

BOX 4-1 | **AVMA Principles of Veterinary Medical Ethics**

Introduction

Veterinarians are members of a scholarly profession who have earned academic degrees from comprehensive universities or similar educational institutions. Veterinarians practice the profession of veterinary medicine in a variety of situations and circumstances.

Exemplary professional conduct upholds the dignity of the veterinary profession. All veterinarians are expected to adhere to a progressive code of ethical conduct known as the Principles of Veterinary Medical Ethics (the Principles). The basis of the Principles is the Golden Rule. Veterinarians should accept this rule as a guide to their general conduct, and abide by the Principles. They should conduct their professional and personal affairs in an ethical manner. Professional veterinary associations should adopt the Principles or a similar code as a guide for their activities.

Professional organizations may establish ethics, grievance, or peer review committees to address ethical issues. Local and state veterinary associations should also include discussions of ethical issues in their continuing education programs.

Complaints about behavior that may violate the Principles should be addressed in an appropriate and timely manner. Such questions should be considered initially by ethics, grievance, or peer review committees of local or state veterinary associations, when they exist, and/or when appropriate, state veterinary medical boards. Members of local and state committees are familiar with local customs and circumstances, and those committees are in the best position to confer with all parties involved.

The Judicial Council may address complaints, prior to, concurrent with, or subsequent to review at the state or local level, as it deems appropriate.

All veterinarians in local or state associations and jurisdictions have a responsibility to regulate and guide the professional conduct of their members.

Colleges of veterinary medicine should stress the teaching of ethical and value issues as part of the professional veterinary curriculum for all veterinary students.

The National Board of Veterinary Medical Examiners is encouraged to prepare and include questions regarding professional ethics in the National Board Examination.

The AVMA Judicial Council is charged to advise on all questions relating to interpretation of the Bylaws, all questions of veterinary medical ethics, and other rules of the Association. The Judicial Council should review the Principles periodically to ensure that they remain complete and up to date.

Professional Behavior

Veterinarians should first consider the needs of the patient: to relieve disease, suffering, or disability while minimizing pain or fear.

Veterinarians should obey all laws of the jurisdictions in which they reside and practice veterinary medicine. Veterinarians should be honest and fair in their relations with others, and they should not engage in fraud, misrepresentation, or deceit.

Veterinarians should report illegal practices and activities to the proper authorities.

The AVMA Judicial Council may choose to report alleged infractions by nonmembers of the AVMA to the appropriate agencies.

Veterinarians should use only the title of the professional degree that was awarded by the school of veterinary medicine where the degree was earned. All veterinarians may use the courtesy titles *Doctor* or *Veterinarian*. Veterinarians who were awarded a degree other than DVM or VMD should refer to the *AVMA Directory* for information on the appropriate titles and degrees.

It is unethical for veterinarians to identify themselves as members of an AVMA recognized specialty organization if such certification has not been awarded.

Continued

BOX 4-1 | AVMA Principles of Veterinary Medical Ethics—cont'd

It is unethical to place professional knowledge, credentials, or services at the disposal of any nonprofessional organization, group, or individual to promote or lend credibility to the illegal practice of veterinary medicine.

Veterinarians may choose whom they will serve. Both the veterinarians and the client have the right to establish or decline a Veterinarian-Client-Patient Relationship (see Section III) and to decide on treatment. The decision to accept or decline treatment and related cost should be based on adequate discussion of clinical findings, diagnostic techniques, treatment, likely outcome, estimated cost, and reasonable assurance of payment. Once the veterinarians and the client have agreed, and the veterinarians have begun patient care, they may not neglect their patient and must continue to provide professional services related to that injury or illness within the previously agreed limits. As subsequent needs and costs for patient care are identified, the veterinarians and client must confer and reach agreement on the continued care and responsibility for fees. If the informed client declines further care or declines to assume responsibility for the fees, the VCPR may be terminated by either party.

In emergencies, veterinarians have an ethical responsibility to provide essential services for animals when necessary to save life or relieve suffering, subsequent to client agreement. Such emergency care may be limited to euthanasia to relieve suffering, or to stabilization of the patient for transport to another source of animal care.

When veterinarians cannot be available to provide services, they should arrange with their colleagues to assure that emergency services are available, consistent with the needs of the locality.

Veterinarians who believe that they haven't the experience or equipment to manage and treat certain emergencies in the best manner, should advise the client that more qualified or specialized services are available elsewhere and offer to expedite referral to those services.

Regardless of practice ownership, the interests of the patient, client, and public require that all decisions that affect diagnosis, care, and treatment of patients are made by veterinarians.

Veterinarians should strive to enhance their image with respect to their colleagues, clients, other health professionals, and the general public. Veterinarians should be honest, fair, courteous, considerate, and compassionate. Veterinarians should present a professional appearance and follow acceptable professional procedures using current professional and scientific knowledge.

Veterinarians should not slander, or injure the professional standing or reputation of other veterinarians in a false or misleading manner.

Veterinarians should strive to improve their veterinary knowledge and skills, and they are encouraged to collaborate with other professionals in the quest for knowledge and professional development.

The responsibilities of the veterinary profession extend beyond individual patients and clients to society in general. Veterinarians are encouraged to make their knowledge available to their communities and to provide their services for activities that protect public health.

Veterinarians and their associates should protect the personal privacy of patients and clients. Veterinarians should not reveal confidences unless required to by law or unless it becomes necessary to protect the health and welfare of other individuals or animals.

Veterinarians who are impaired by alcohol or other substances should seek assistance from qualified organizations or individuals. Colleagues of impaired veterinarians should encourage those individuals to seek assistance and to overcome their disabilities.

The Veterinarian-Client-Patient Relationship

The veterinarian-client-patient relationship (VCPR) is the basis for interaction among veterinarians, their clients, and their patients. A VCPR exists when all of the following conditions have been met:

- The veterinarian has assumed responsibility for making clinical judgments regarding the health of the animal(s) and the need for medical treatment, and the client has agreed to follow the veterinarian's instructions.
- The veterinarian has sufficient knowledge of the animal(s) to initiate at least a general or preliminary diagnosis of the medical condition of the animal(s). This means that the veterinarian has recently seen and is personally acquainted with the keeping and care of the animal(s) by virtue of an examination of the animal(s), or by medically appropriate and timely visits to the premises where the animal(s) are kept.
- The veterinarian is readily available, or has arranged for emergency coverage, for follow-up evaluation in the event of adverse reactions or the failure of the treatment regimen.

When a VCPR exists, veterinarians must maintain medical records (see Section VII).

Dispensing or prescribing a prescription product requires a VCPR.

Veterinarians should honor a client's request for a prescription in lieu of dispensing.

Without a VCPR, veterinarians merchandising or use of veterinary prescription drugs or their extra-label use of any pharmaceutical is unethical and is illegal under federal law.

Veterinarians may terminate a VCPR under certain conditions, and they have an ethical obligation to use courtesy and tact in doing so.

If there is no ongoing medical condition, veterinarians may terminate a VCPR by notifying the client that they no longer wish to serve that patient and client.

If there is an ongoing medical or surgical condition, the patient should be referred to another veterinarian for diagnosis, care, and treatment. The former attending veterinarian should continue to provide care, as needed, during the transition.

Clients may terminate the VCPR at any time.

Attending, Consulting, and Referring

An *attending veterinarian* is a veterinarian (or a group of veterinarians) who assumes responsibility for primary care of a patient. A VCPR is established.

Attending veterinarians are entitled to charge a fee for their professional services.

When appropriate, attending veterinarians are encouraged to seek assistance in the form of consultations and referrals. A decision to consult or refer is made jointly by the attending veterinarian and the client.

BOX 4-1 | AVMA Principles of Veterinary Medical Ethics—cont'd

When a consultation occurs, the attending veterinarian continues to be primarily responsible for the case.

A *consulting veterinarian* is a veterinarian (or group of veterinarians) who agrees to advise an attending veterinarian on the care and management of a case.

The VCPR remains the responsibility of the attending veterinarian.

Consulting veterinarians may or may not charge fees for service.

Consulting veterinarians should communicate their findings and opinions directly to the attending veterinarians.

Consulting veterinarians should revisit the patients or communicate with the clients in collaboration with the attending veterinarians.

Consultations usually involve the exchange of information or interpretation of test results. However, it may be appropriate or necessary for consultants to examine patients. When advanced or invasive techniques are required to gather information or substantiate diagnoses, attending veterinarians may refer the patients. A new VCPR is established with the veterinarian to whom a case is referred.

The *referral veterinarian or receiving veterinarian* is a veterinarian (or group of veterinarians) who agrees to provide requested veterinary services. A new VCPR is established. The referring and referral veterinarians must communicate.

Attending veterinarians should honor clients' requests for referral.

Referral veterinarians may choose to accept or decline clients and patients from attending veterinarians.

Patients are usually referred because of specific medical problems or services. Referral veterinarians should provide services or treatments relative to the referred conditions, and they should communicate with the referring veterinarians and clients if other services or treatments are required.

When a client seeks professional services or opinions from a different veterinarian without a referral, a new VCPR is established with the new attending veterinarian. When contacted, the veterinarian who was formerly involved in the diagnosis, care, and treatment of the patient should communicate with the new attending veterinarian as if the patient and client had been referred.

With the client's consent, the new attending veterinarian should contact the former veterinarian to learn the original diagnosis, care, and treatment and clarify any issues before proceeding with a new treatment plan.

If there is evidence that the actions of the former attending veterinarian have clearly and significantly endangered the health or safety of the patient, the new attending veterinarian has a responsibility to report the matter to the appropriate authorities of the local and state association or professional regulatory agency.

Influences on Judgment

The choice of treatments or animal care should not be influenced by considerations other than the needs of the patient, the welfare of the client, and the safety of the public.

Veterinarians should not allow their medical judgment to be influenced by agreements by which they stand to profit through referring clients to other providers of services or products.

The medical judgments of veterinarians should not be influenced by contracts or agreements made by their associations or societies.

When conferences, meetings, or lectures are sponsored by outside entities, the organization that presents the program, not the funding sponsor, shall have control of the contents and speakers.

Therapies

Attending veterinarians are responsible for choosing the treatment regimens for their patients. It is the attending veterinarian's responsibility to inform the client of the expected results and costs, and the related risks of each treatment regimen.

It is unethical for veterinarians to prescribe or dispense prescription products in the absence of a VCPR.

It is unethical for veterinarians to promote, sell, prescribe, dispense, or use secret remedies or any other product for which they do not know the ingredient formula.

It is unethical for veterinarians to use or permit the use of their names, signatures, or professional status in connection with the resale of ethical products in a manner which violates those directions or conditions specified by the manufacturer to ensure the safe and efficacious use of the product.

Genetic Defects

Performance of surgical or other procedures in all species for the purpose of concealing genetic defects in animals to be shown, raced, bred, or sold, as breeding animals is unethical. However, should the health or welfare of the individual patient require correction of such genetic defects, it is recommended that the patient be rendered incapable of reproduction.

Medical Records

Veterinary medical records are an integral part of veterinary care. The records must comply with the standards established by state and federal law.

Medical records are the property of the practice and the practice owner. The original records must be retained by the practice for the period required by statute.

Ethically, the information within veterinary medical records is considered privileged and confidential. It must not be released except by court order or consent of the owner of the patient.

Veterinarians are obligated to provide copies or summaries of medical records when requested by the client. Veterinarians should secure a written release to document that request.

Without the express permission of the practice owner, it is unethical for a veterinarian to remove, copy, or use the medical records or any part of any record.

Fees and Remuneration

Veterinarians are entitled to charge fees for their professional services.

In connection with consultations or referrals, it is unethical for veterinarians to enter into financial arrangements, such as fee splitting, which involve payment of a portion of a fee to a recommending veterinarian who has not rendered the professional services for which the fee was paid by the client.

Continued

BOX 4-1 | AVMA Principles of Veterinary Medical Ethics—cont'd

Regardless of the fees that are charged or received, the quality of service must be maintained at the usual professional standard.

It is unethical for a group or association of veterinarians to take any action which coerces, pressures, or achieves agreement among veterinarians to conform to a fee schedule or fixed fees.

Advertising

Without written permission from the AVMA Executive Board, no member or employee of the American Veterinary Medical Association (AVMA) shall use the AVMA name or logo in connection with the promotion or advertising of any commercial product or service.

Advertising by veterinarians is ethical when there are no false, deceptive, or misleading statements or claims. A false, deceptive, or misleading statement or claim is one which communicates false information or is intended, through a material omission, to leave a false impression.

Testimonials or endorsements are advertising, and they should comply with the guidelines for advertising. In addition, testimonials and endorsements of professional products or services by veterinarians are considered unethical unless they comply with the following:

- The endorser must be a bona fide user of the product or service.
- There must be adequate substantiation that the results obtained by the endorser are representative of what veterinarians may expect in actual conditions of use.
- Any financial, business, or other relationship between the endorser and the seller of a product or service must be fully disclosed.
- When reprints of scientific articles are used with advertising, the reprints must remain unchanged, and be presented in their entirety.
- The principles that apply to advertising, testimonials, and endorsements also apply to veterinarians' communications with their clients.
- Veterinarians may permit the use of their names by commercial enterprises (e.g., pet shops, kennels, farms, feedlots) so that the enterprises can advertise under veterinary supervision, only if they provide such supervision.

Euthanasia

Humane euthanasia of animals is an ethical veterinary procedure.

Glossary
Pharmaceutical Products

Several of the following terms are used to describe veterinary pharmaceutical products. Some have legal status, others do not. Although not all of the terms are used in the Principles, we have listed them here for clarification of meaning and to avoid confusion.

Ethical Product: A product for which the manufacturer has voluntarily limited the sale to veterinarians as a marketing decision. Such products are often given a different product name and are packaged differently than products that are sold directly to consumers. "Ethical products" are sold only to veterinarians as a condition of sale that is specified in a sales agreement or on the product label.

Legend Drug: A synonymous term for a veterinary prescription drug. The name refers to the statement (legend) that is required on the label (see *veterinary prescription drug* later).

Over-the-Counter (OTC) Drug: Any drug that can be labeled with adequate direction to enable it to be used safely and properly by a consumer who is not a medical professional.

Prescription Drug: A drug that cannot be labeled with adequate direction to enable its safe and proper use by non-professionals.

Veterinary Prescription Drug: A drug that is restricted by federal law to use by or on the order of a licensed veterinarian, according to section 503(f) of the federal Food, Drug, and Cosmetic Act. The law requires that such drugs be labeled with the statement: "Caution, federal law restricts this drug to use by or on the order of a licensed veterinarian."

Dispensing, Prescribing, Marketing, and Merchandising
Dispensing is the direct distribution of products by veterinarians to clients for use on their animals.

Prescribing is the transmitting of an order authorizing a licensed pharmacist or equivalent to prepare and dispense specified pharmaceuticals to be used in or on animals in the dosage and in the manner directed by a veterinarian.

Marketing is promoting and encouraging animal owners to improve animal health and welfare by using veterinary care, services, and products.

Merchandising is the buying and selling of products or services.

Advertising and Testimonials
Advertising is defined as communication that is designed to inform the public about the availability, nature, or price of products or services or to influence clients to use certain products or services.

Testimonials or endorsements are statements that are intended to influence attitudes regarding the purchase or use of products or services.

Fee Splitting
The dividing of a professional fee for veterinary services with the recommending veterinarian (see Section VIII B).

Bold print states the principles, and standard print explains or clarifies the principle to which it applies. Revised by the Council in October 2006. Approved by the Ethics Board in November 2006.
Courtesy American Veterinary Medical Association, Schaumburg, Ill.

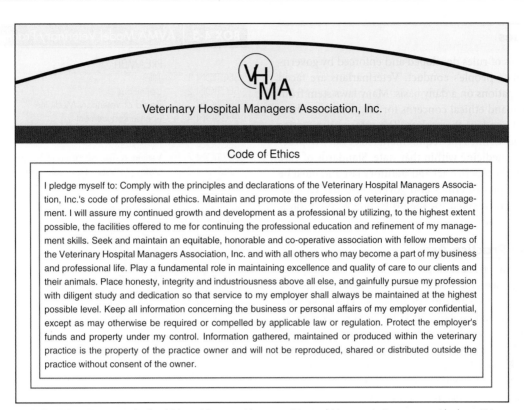

FIGURE 4-1 VHMA Code of Ethics. (Courtesy Veterinary Hospital Manager's Association, Alachua, FL.)

Veterinary practice managers understand the ethical requirements of veterinary practice, as outlined by the AVMA and CVPM code of ethics, and ensure that professional and support staff fulfil their ethical responsibilities.

The National Association of Veterinary Technicians in America (NAVTA) code of ethics for veterinary technicians is a combination of professional ethics that focus both on practicing medicine and protecting the profession as a whole (Box 4-2). NAVTA strives to provide excellent guidelines for its members as well as the public.

Veterinary Ethics

Four branches of veterinary ethics exist: descriptive, official, administrative, and normative. *Descriptive ethics* refers to the study of ethical views of veterinarians and veterinary professionals regarding their behavior and attitudes. This relates to what members of the profession think is right and wrong and does not involve making value judgments about what is moral or immoral in a professional's behavior. Official veterinary ethics involve the creation of the official ethical standards adopted by organizations of professionals and imposed on their members. Administrative veterinary ethics involve actions by administrative government bodies that regulate veterinary practice and activities in which veterinarians engage. Many organizations incorporate the AVMA's principles of ethics into their statutes or regulations. License revocation can result if any civil or criminal

| BOX 4-2 | NAVTA Code of Ethics |

1. Aid society and animals through providing excellent care and service for animals.
2. Prevent and relieve the suffering of animals.
3. Promote public health by assisting with the control of zoonotic disease and informing the public about these diseases.
4. Assume accountability for individual professional actions and judgments.
5. Protect confidential information provided by clients.
6. Safeguard the public and profession against individuals deficient in professional competencies or ethics.
7. Assist with efforts to ensure conditions of employment are consistent with the excellent care for animals.
8. Remain competent in veterinary technology through commitment and lifelong learning.
9. Collaborate with members of the veterinary medical profession in efforts to ensure quality health care services for all animals.

Courtesy National Association of Veterinary Technicians in America, www.navta.net.

violation of these regulations occurs. Normative ethics refer to the search for correct principles of good and bad, right and wrong, and justice or injustice. The difference between ethics and law lies in enforcement; the government enforces laws, whereas the professional associations that developed the ethics enforce ethics.

Legal Issues

Laws are bodies of rules developed and enforced by government to regulate people's conduct. Veterinarians are faced with legal obligations on a daily basis. Many laws stem from society's moral and ethical concerns for life, death, and how people should conduct themselves. The veterinary practice act of each state defines the requirements necessary to practice veterinary medicine within that state. Standards of care rise from both the practice act and statutory law and must be followed. Principles of ethics also govern veterinary medicine and are implemented for the protection of the profession and society itself.

Veterinary Practice Act

The veterinary practice act emphasizes that the right to practice veterinary medicine is a privilege granted by state law and is thus subject to regulation to protect and promote public health, safety, and welfare. This statute is enacted as an exercise of the powers of the state to promote public health, safety, and welfare by ensuring the delivery of competent veterinary medical care. Therefore veterinary medicine must be practiced by individuals who possess the personal and professional qualifications specified in this act.

AVMA has created a model practice act that most states have followed while developing their state veterinary practice acts. Laws and regulations vary among the states; therefore each practice should be familiar with its own state's veterinary practice act (Box 4-3).

Because veterinary practice acts are umbrella laws that govern the practice of veterinary medicine, changes cannot be made easily. Changes must be submitted to the House and Senate, and then ultimately signed into law by the governor. State associations and boards can circulate proposed changes among members of the veterinary and veterinary technician communities, soliciting opinions and changes that members may recommend. Once the board and associations agree, a lobbyist may be hired to find state senators and representatives to support the bill. It may be introduced into the legislative process, amended, and updated various times before the final product is presented to the governor for acceptance. The governor can then accept or deny the bill, but cannot make changes.

Practice acts are then regulated and enforced by the state veterinary medical board, which oversees both veterinarians and veterinary technicians. This group is responsible for testing and licensure, collection of renewal fees, and the evaluation of complaints presented by the public. With adequate evidence of wrongdoing, boards can revoke any professional veterinary license. The most common complaints are listed later in this chapter.

Definitions of Law

A law generally consists of established rules, statutes, and administrative agency rules that can be enforced to establish limits of conduct for governments and individuals in society. Law is divided into two categories: civil and criminal.

BOX 4-3	AVMA Model Veterinary Practice Act

	PREAMBLE
SECTION 1	Title
SECTION 2	Definitions
SECTION 3	Board of Veterinary Medicine
SECTION 4	License Requirement
SECTION 5	Veterinarian-Client-Patient Relationship Requirement
SECTION 6	Exemptions
SECTION 7	Veterinary Technicians and Technologists
SECTION 8	Status of Persons Previously Licensed
SECTION 9	Application for License: Qualifications
SECTION 10	Examinations
SECTION 11	License by Endorsement
SECTION 12	Temporary Permit
SECTION 13	License Renewal
SECTION 14	Discipline of Licensees
SECTION 15	Impaired Veterinarian
SECTION 16	Hearing Procedure
SECTION 17	Appeal
SECTION 18	Reinstatement
SECTION 19	Veterinarian-Client Confidentiality
SECTION 20	Immunity from Liability
SECTION 21	Cruelty to Animals—Immunity for Reporting
SECTION 22	Abandoned Animals
SECTION 23	Enforcement
SECTION 24	Severability
SECTION 25	Effective Date

Courtesy American Veterinary Medical Association, Schaumburg, Ill.

Civil law relates to the duties between people and the government. A contract dispute between a veterinarian and an employee is an example of a case that falls under civil law. Criminal law prosecutes crimes committed against the public as a whole. Most criminal laws focus on acts that injure people or pets or offend public morality. Violation of civil law generally results in fines paid to the opposing party, whereas violation of criminal law results in jail time and/or fines.

> **PRACTICE POINT** A noncompete agreement falls under the division of civil law.

Civil law can be further broken down into tort and contract law. A tort is a civil offense to an opposing party in which harm has occurred. Standards of care exist for the protection of one's body, business interests, personal property, and reputation. Tort law permits people to sue for relief of an injury that occurred as a result of damages inflicted on their bodies, to their families, or to their property. Furthermore, tort law can be determined to be intentional or unintentional and must be proved to the court. An *intentional tort* is defined as just that: an intentional action that has taken place in which harm has occurred to another member of society. Examples of intentional torts include assault and battery, defamation of character, invasion of privacy, immoral conduct, and fraud. An example of an unintentional tort claim would be the failure to practice the standard of care. If a veterinarian did not

practice the standard of care that has been developed by veterinary professionals and an animal suffered injury because of neglect, the veterinarian could be guilty of an unintentional tort of negligence. Torts are generally resolved with a civil trial and a monetary settlement is made.

Contract law deals with duties established by individuals as a result of contractual agreement. This area of law was developed to ensure that promises made by people would be fulfilled; if they are not fulfilled, a breach of duty is established.

Veterinary practice managers understand and ensure compliance of contract law as it pertains to associates, staff, and clients.

A crime is an unlawful activity against a member of the public and is prosecuted by a public official, normally the district attorney or the attorney general's office. A crime is further classified as a misdemeanor or a felony. A misdemeanor charge is less serious than that of a felony and generally results in less jail time.

> **PRACTICE POINT** Animal abuse cases fall into the division of criminal law.

Negligence is the performance of an act that a reasonable person under the same circumstances would not perform. Malpractice can be considered a form of negligence and can be considered intentional or unintentional. Overall, malpractice can refer to any unprofessional, illegal, or immoral conduct. Malpractice is the dereliction of duty, resulting in injury to the patient. Box 4-4 lists the most common errors in veterinary practice that can result in malpractice claims.

Consent

By definition, consent is the voluntary acceptance or agreement to what is planned or is done by another person. Informed consent is when a veterinary practice has given information to a client regarding the proposed treatment, allowing the client to make an informed decision regarding whether to proceed with a treatment. Courts have established several elements that must be fully addressed to have complete informed consent. The consent must be given freely, and the treatment and diagnosis must be given in understandable terms. The risks, benefits, and prognosis of the defined procedure must be stated as well as the prognosis if no treatment is elected. The practice must provide a statement of alternative treatments or procedures along with the risks, benefits, and cost of each. The client must be given the right to ask questions and have them answered. See Figure 2-10, *A* to *K*, for a variety of sample consent forms. Figure 4-2 is an example of an informed consent form; the pet owner and technician sign each section together after the risks and benefits have been discussed and understood by the owner.

BOX 4-4 | Acts of Malpractice

- Incorrect drug administration
- Incorrect strength of drug administration
- Failure to clean animals that have defecated and/or urinated on themselves
- Abandonment
- Leaving foreign objects in a patient after surgery
- Failure to exercise good judgment
- Failure to communicate
- Loss or damage to patients personal property
- Disease transmission
- A patient attacking another while in the veterinary practice
- Use of defective equipment or medication

If an informed consent is challenged in a court of law and these conditions have not been met, the court may conclude that the client did not consent to the procedure and the veterinarian may be held liable. Documentation of the discussion must be in the record. If a record does not indicate that risks were discussed, the court can assume the discussion did not occur. A signed consent form does not indicate that an informed consent occurred, because many people sign consent forms without reading them. Therefore a verbal discussion **must** occur. Practices should never rely on clients who state "do what is best" because this is not informed consent; they have not been educated on the risks and benefits of the procedure. The average client does not possess the skill or knowledge to make informed decisions without all of the available information.

Information should be given to clients in a manner that they can understand. Each client should be evaluated for the level of education, skill, and knowledge that he or she possesses with which to comprehend the information. It may be questioned of minors or those who's reasoning or judgment is impaired (by mental illness, intoxication, etc.) whether their understanding of the information is valid; acceptance of consent should be made with caution in these cases.

The best consent form available is one that is tailored to specific clients and the procedure being recommended. If anesthesia is advised to complete a procedure, the consent form should clearly indicate that death is a risk. A blank should be placed next to that statement for both the client and the team member reviewing the consent form to sign. All risks, benefits, and prognoses should be listed as such and initialed by both individuals. This will help the court determine whether each topic was fully addressed and whether the client was fully informed before signing the form.

Emergency Care

Veterinary practices often face a dilemma when a Good Samaritan brings in a pet that has been hit by a car. Can the practice treat this emergency? Who is the owner? Can the owner be contacted? Is the Good Samaritan going to be responsible for the bill? The first thought that most practices

---

ABC Veterinary Clinic
Surgery, Anesthesia, and Treatment Consent Form

Client Name _____ Patient Name _____

Date _____ Procedure _____ Male/Female

Your pet has been scheduled for a procedure requiring sedation or anesthesia. By signing this form, you authorize ABC Veterinary Clinic and its agents to administer tranquilizers, anesthetics, and analgesics that are deemed appropriate. Please be aware that all drugs have a potential for adverse side effects in any particular animal. The chances of such occurrence are extremely low; however, death can result in any anesthetized patient.

Owner initials _____ Tech initials_____

In an effort to ensure your pet's safety and to anticipate any problems before they occur, we advise pre-anesthetic blood work and electrocardiogram prior to anesthesia. Blood work will determine the kidney and liver functions, which participate in the metabolism of anesthesia. An electrocardiogram can detect abnormal arrhythmias, heart rate, and conductivity.

I accept/decline blood work   I accept/decline an electrocardiogram

Owner initials _____ Tech initials_____

IV fluids are advised for all patients undergoing anesthesia. IV fluids help maintain blood pressure of the patient while offering support for the kidneys to metabolize the medications. Pets may take longer to recover without IV fluids.

I accept/decline IV fluids

Owner initials _____ Tech initials_____

Heartworm tests are recommended for dogs over 6 months of age. Heartworm disease can cause anesthetic complications. We advise FeLV/FIV testing for cats. FeLV or FIV infection can delay healing of any surgical site.

I accept/decline heartworm test   I accept/decline FeLV/FIV test

Owner initials _____ Tech initials_____

Vaccinations are important for disease prevention in your pet. We advise that pets be current on vaccines. Rabies vaccination is required by law; every pet must receive a rabies vaccine.

Vaccines due (booster?): DHPP FVRCP FeLV   Rabies

Owner Initials _____ Tech Initials_____

FIGURE 4-2 Consent form.

experience is that there is no consent to treat the animal. However, if the owners are found, they may hold the practice liable for not performing lifesaving techniques.

Veterinary practice managers understand and ensure compliance with the legal and ethical guidelines surrounding confidentiality of staff, clients, and patients.

The *law of unjust enrichment* allows protection for the practice if critical factors are met. If there is value to the pet, the courts may allow a recovery of cost. The more valuable the pet appears, the greater the chance of recovery. Value can be based on either economic or emotional attachment with

respect to the human-animal bond. The severity of the injuries must be proven. Photographs documenting injuries and supportive treatment will help assure the client and the court that unnecessary procedures were not completed. Attempts to reach the owner must be documented in the record with the name of the person trying to make contact, phone numbers, time of the calls, as well as the number of attempts made. Once the patient is stable, only supportive care should be rendered. Plating a fracture would not be considered supportive care of a trauma patient unless it was a lifesaving technique.

Many times, the only way for a practice to recover the costs associated with emergency care is to take the client to court (if the owner was identified). This has led to many

Did pet eat this morning?	Yes	No
Has pet had any allergies or vaccine reactions in the past?	Yes	No
Are we declawing the pet?	Yes	No
Are we removing dewclaws?	Yes	No
Does the pet have 2 testicles?	Yes	No
If the pet is pregnant, can we continue with surgery?	Yes	No
Does the pet have an umbilical hernia?	Yes	No
May we repair?	Yes	No
Does the pet have retained teeth?	Yes	No
May we remove?	Yes	No
Does the pet need an Elizabethan collar?	Yes	No
Dental: OK to extract teeth?	Yes	No
OK to take dental radiographs if indicated?	Yes	No
OK to apply Doxirobe gel if indicated?	Yes	No
Is pet currently on antibiotics?	Yes	No
When was last dose? _____		
How many pills are left? _____		
Growth Removal: Histopath?	Yes	No
Location of growths: _____		

You may contact me **today** at: _____

Alternative contact phone number: _____

I understand that anesthesia is a risk and authorize the above procedures. I understand that I will be contacted first if any changes in the discussed protocol occur.

Client signature _____ Date _____

FIGURE 4-2, cont'd

practices refusing to treat animals without owners. There is no law that states that practices must treat; in fact, duty to treat is only initiated once a valid client-patient relationship has been established. Once a valid client-patient relationship has been established, a practice must continue the treatment until the animal recovers, the veterinarian has completed all the treatments agreed upon, the patient dies, or the client terminates the client-patient relationship. However, according to the AVMA Code of Ethics, *veterinarians have an ethical responsibility to provide essential services for animals when necessary to save life or relieve suffering, subsequent to client agreement. Such emergency care may be limited to euthanasia to relieve suffering, or to stabilization of the patient for transport to another source of animal care.*

Treatment can be declined by the practice because of the client's inability to pay; however, once treatment has begun,

it is extremely difficult to terminate treatment if the result would be neglect or harm to the animal. If treatment by the veterinarian must be terminated for any reason, including nonpayment of services, the veterinarian should make a good faith effort to find a veterinarian that will continue the treatment.

Veterinary practices are ethically obligated to provide emergency services to their clients after hours (as stated in the AVMA Code of Ethics); if they do not provide services themselves, they must refer their clients to a location that accepts emergencies after hours.

Malpractice

Lawsuits against veterinarians and veterinary technicians are almost always based on neglect versus breach of contract, defamation, or breach of warranty. *Negligence* is

defined as performing an act that a person of ordinary prudence would not have done under similar circumstances (or failure to perform an act that a person of ordinary prudence would have done). If a veterinarian or technician is sued for negligence, four basic elements must be proven in the court of law. The first is the establishment of a valid client-patient relationship. This is rarely an issue because most client-patient relationships were established when the patient was presented to the practice by the owner. Second, breach of duty must be proven. *Breach of duty* is the failure of the veterinarian or technician to act in accordance with the standard of care. This breach can occur by either performing an act that should not have been performed or not performing an act that should have been performed. Third, *proximate cause* must be established. Proximate cause is the connection between the negligent act of the veterinarian and/or technician and the harm to the patient caused by the act. Fourth, damages or harm incurred by the patient as a result of the negligent act must be displayed.

> **PRACTICE POINT** Veterinary technicians who fail to complete treatments on the weekend can be held liable for negligence.

The *standard of care* can be defined as the duty to exercise the care and diligence that is ordinarily exercised by a reasonably competent veterinarian under normal circumstances. With the availability of specialists in many metropolitan and suburban areas around the United States, the standard of care will be held to the specialist level. This means that veterinarians should refer or recommend referrals to a specialty center when a case is complex and requires the intervention of a specialist. Veterinarians may be held liable if they do not make the recommendation and/or not document the referral recommendation in the record. If the client declines the referral, the declined treatment should be documented clearly.

To help avoid a malpractice lawsuit against a veterinarian or practice, several topics can be addressed with team members. Medical records must be complete, with every detail of the case. "If it is not in the record, it did not happen," is a common statement in the court of law. Every treatment and recommendation must be clearly documented along with any refusals the client has made. Clients must be informed when making decisions, and proof of informed consent must be included in the record. If a patient is in need of a higher level of care, the veterinarian must advise referral of the case. Should the client decline, it should be clearly documented in the record.

Most veterinarians purchase liability insurance through AVMA, which is supported by Professional Liability Insurance Trust (PLIT). This insurance provides coverage for veterinarians, veterinary technicians, and support staff that are engaged in activities involved in the practice. Each veterinarian in the practice must carry his or her own liability insurance.

Abandoned Animals

Many animals are left at practices unclaimed, especially puppies with parvovirus or other incurable or expensive ailments. Practices may make repeated attempts to contact the owner, to which no replies are made. Because a valid client-patient relationship was developed when the owner dropped off the pet, the practice is responsible for providing treatment that will prevent harm or neglect to the patient. The practice is not required to perform lifesaving techniques; however, the pet cannot receive injury by withholding treatment. After repeated attempts to contact the owner, a certified letter should be sent to the owner indicating the confirmation of abandonment of the pet. Local and state laws should be reviewed indicating the length of time the practice is required to hold the pet to confirm abandonment. A second certified letter may be required by some localities. If there is no response from the owner within the stated time, the pet can be considered abandoned and the practice can make the pet available for adoption or euthanize it, whichever provides the best outcome for the practice.

Impending Laws

Local laws have been amended in several cities that animals may no longer be considered to be owned, but rather to be cared for by guardians. This can affect the veterinarian-client relationship in many ways. In human cases, a guardian is generally given that authority or designation to care for a person who is a minor, incapacitated, or disabled. A *guardian ad litem* is a person appointed to protect the interests of a minor or legally incompetent person in a lawsuit or, in this case, an animal.

Change in the status of owner to guardian can present many issues. Who will determine what is best for the animal—the guardian or veterinarian? Could the veterinarian be sued for wrongful death on behalf of the pet? Other questions will certainly be raised as well as concerns for animal abuse or neglect by veterinarians. If a veterinarian does not immediately provide pain relief for an animal or send home postoperative pain medication, the practice may be held liable for neglect.

Medical Records

The laws concerning the legal ownership of records vary from state to state; however, in general, medical records are owned by the practice, not the pet owner. The owner can request a copy of the medical record at anytime. In fact, most clients request copies of records when they are changing veterinary hospitals.

> **PRACTICE POINT** The veterinary practice, not the pet owner, owns the medical record.

Clients should sign a medical record release for medical records to be copied and released to someone other than the client. This includes faxing records to other hospitals, boarding facilities, or new owners. The only time medical records should be released without consent is if the patient has a reportable disease that must be reported to the state or U.S. Department of Agriculture.

It should be kept in mind that medical records are legal documents. Therefore they must be legible at all times. Medical records are generated to ensure consistent and accurate care as well as protect the veterinarian in the event of a malpractice suit. Inaccurate, illegible medical records could be interpreted as professional incompetence with substandard care. It must also be remembered: if it was not written down, it did not occur.

If mistakes are written in a record, a single line should be drawn through the mistake, initialed, and corrected. Correction fluid or scratch-outs should not be permitted because this could be interpreted as altering of records, rendering them inadmissible in the court of law (see Chapter 14 for more information on medical records).

Most Common Complaints to the Board of Veterinary Medicine

A complaint is a formal action noting dissatisfaction with the services of a licensed veterinarian or credentialed veterinary technician. A complaint is filed with the state veterinary board office, which then sends a letter to the veterinarian and/or technician. An investigator is assigned to the case and completes all needed interviews and record reviews. The complaint is reviewed by the review committee, who then submits it to the board. The board takes ultimate action against the veterinarian or technician and can dismiss the case or settle the case without a hearing (continuing education and fines may be imposed). If the complaint is found to be severe, a Notice of Contemplated Action is sent requesting a hearing. The result of the hearing may impose continuing education, fines, license suspension, or revocation. All decisions can be appealed.

Patient owners tend to file complaints because of dissatisfaction resulting from experiences at the practice. Dissatisfaction may come from service that displeased them or did not fulfill their expectations. Many times, clients are unsatisfied with the side effect a treatment may have produced. For example, a cast or splint may have been too tight, resulting in cast or bandaging sores. A common complaint is that a pet chewed a cast off and removed the sutures or staples without the veterinary team having warned the owner to keep the pet from chewing. Other times, the wrong medication was dispensed, infuriating owners.

Occasionally, a patient incurs severe trauma, necessitating the team to become dedicated to taking care of the patient's immediate needs. The aftercare and prognosis of the pet are the last items communicated to the owner and are often forgotten. Many clients become upset that they spent so much money saving a pet. They feel that if they had only known the prognosis and the amount of aftercare required, they may have chosen to euthanize the pet instead. The entire treatment process, from the immediate care to the year after the trauma, must be communicated to the owner and documented in the record to prevent this complaint from arising.

Clients are often unhappy with the results of a surgery or treatment. Many fractures do not heal properly, and the client believes the veterinarian is responsible. The team must recommend the best procedure available to repair fractures, regardless of whether the practice provides that procedure. If possible, the patient should be referred to a practice that is able to provide the best possible procedure. If the client declines the referral and opts for the lesser treatment, it must be noted in the record. The recommendation should also be written on a release sheet that the owner signs when the patient is discharged; this provides proof that the owner was made aware of the recommendation.

The unexpected death of a patient is also a common complaint. If a client brings a pet to the practice for treatment, regardless of the use of anesthesia, the owner must sign a treatment authorization form. As stated earlier, an informed consent **must** be discussed with the owner, listing the risks and benefits of treatments or procedures. The client must be fully informed that death may result. A simple blood draw on an unhealthy cat can induce a sudden, unexpected death. It is imperative that risks be discussed with the owner.

Team members treating clients disrespectfully loses clients for the practice and can result in formal complaints. Disrespect may include being rude to a client, not listening to client wishes, or not returning a client's phone calls.

Many clients are unsatisfied with the invoice at the end of the procedure. Estimates must be provided to owners at all times, regardless of whether the information is given over the phone or in the examination room. The estimate copy must remain in the medical record for future referencing. If the estimate should change in any way, the client must be notified immediately of the impending change. If the owner did not approve services, a formal complaint may be filed.

Poor communication is the top complaint. Communication is integral to most aspects of the veterinary practice, from the receptionist to the veterinarian. Many times, veterinary technicians relay too much information and overstep their professional boundaries. Veterinary technicians cannot diagnose a disease; only veterinarians are permitted to do so. In the process of providing information to the client before the veterinarian has seen the case, the technician may give incorrect or invalid information. The different information provided by the veterinarian and veterinary technician can confuse the client, resulting in a complaint.

When patients are discharged from the hospital, a signed copy of the information provided must remain with the record; this covers the practice if clients state they did not receive the information. When the patient is discharged, the team member must ensure that the client fully understands the instructions and can medicate the patient as advised.

Conduct, record keeping, premises, and pharmaceutical citations are four common violations given in veterinary medicine. Correct conduct is defined in the following:

> Veterinarians shall exercise the same degree of care, skill, and diligence in treating patients as are ordinarily used in the same or similar circumstances by reasonably prudent members of the veterinary medical profession in good standing. A veterinarian shall not use or participate in any form of representation or advertising or solicitation which contains false, deceptive, or misleading statement or claims.

Record keeping is a difficult challenge for many practices; however, records must be fully completed to prevent a violation (see Chapter 14).

WHAT WOULD YOU DO/NOT DO?

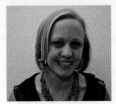

Fluffy was admitted to the hospital for lab work because she just "was not feeling right." Teresa, the technician admitting the case was advised to perform a CBC/chemistry, radiographs, and a urinalysis by Dr. Mortinger. Teresa reviewed the medical record as she placed the lab work results in the folder. She did not see an estimate for the services that were recommended and asked Dr. Mortinger if an estimate had been provided, as it is practice policy. Dr. Mortinger said the clients advised her that they did not need an estimate; "do whatever is needed" was their reply. Since the blood work returned normal results, with slight changes in the radiographs and urinalysis, the veterinarian advised an ultrasound of the abdomen. The owners agreed; "do whatever is needed," they replied again. The ultrasound revealed a tumor in the bladder, with high suspicions of a transitional cell carcinoma. The veterinarian called the owners to deliver the news, who were devastated that their dog had cancer. "She was just in to see you last month for her yearly exam! How could you have missed this on her exam, Dr. Mortinger?" The owners were on their way to practice to pick up Fluffy.

Once the owners arrived, Lori, the receptionist reviewed the invoice with the owners before the pet was released. The owners were enraged at the price of the invoice and refused to pay for the services. "We did not authorize those services! You just wait," exclaimed Mrs. Smith. "Not only did Dr. Mortinger miss cancer in my dog last month, she ran tests I did not know about! I WILL file a complaint, and I am going to sue her!"

What Should the Team Members Have Done?

First, since it was practice policy, an estimate should have initially been created, regardless of whether the owners felt they needed one. An estimate lists all of the advised services, along with a cost. Second, when Teresa noticed that an estimate not provided, she should have made one and called with owner with an updated estimate when the ultrasound was approved. Third, if Lori could have placed the owner in a room, other clients would not have heard the outburst of Mrs. Smith.

An estimate may have prevented the shock in price, and would have clearly listed the services. The owners may have responded differently had communication been clearer. At this point in the conversation, it would be wise to place the Smith family into a room, and have a veterinarian explain the history of bladder tumors and provide written information regarding treatment options. Providing communication may reduce the anger, allowing the client to understand that this type of tumor is not usually diagnosed on a yearly exam.

Ensure the medical records are complete, including an explanation of the scenario that had just occurred. Should the client want to file a complaint with the state board of veterinary medicine and continue with a suit of malpractice or negligence, then the professional liability company must be contacted for further information. The case should no longer be discussed with the client.

The most common premises violation is that a surgery room must be a room separate and distinct from all other rooms that is reserved for aseptic surgical procedures requiring aseptic preparation. Only items used for surgical procedures may be kept in the surgical room. Dental machines cannot be stored in the surgical room because they are not part of an aseptic procedure.

Veterinarians should honor a client's request to dispense or provide a written prescription for a drug that has been determined by the veterinarian to be appropriate for the patient. Therefore clients who wish to purchase medication on the Internet must be provided with a prescription (at their request). Practices who do not fulfill the request are in violation.

Many other complaints arise in veterinary medicine for malpractice and negligence; however, the examples previously listed are the most common ones that can be easily prevented by the veterinary health care team. Every team member must provide courteous customer service with valid, factual information. Communication must be the priority of the entire team, specifically regarding any changes to estimates, treatment plans, or increased wait times to clients.

VETERINARY PRACTICE and the LAW

Veterinary assistants are not licensed, and in most states their role is not clearly defined. Veterinary practice acts may allow veterinarians to delegate clinical tasks to qualified veterinary assistants to be performed under direct supervision. Some states do define the roles and regulations of veterinary assistants; therefore the legal status should be determined in the practicing state.

Credentialed veterinary technicians are licensed in most states; however, the state veterinary practice act may not clearly define the roles or procedures that technicians are allowed to perform. Just as with assistants, practice acts state that the veterinarian(s) can delegate duties to qualified technicians, provided that they are under the direct supervision of the veterinarian.

Licensed technicians are responsible for maintaining a professional image and must renew their license annually or biannually. Licenses can be revoked for lack of continuing education, misconduct, or drug abuse.

REVIEW QUESTIONS

1. Define civil law.
2. Define contract law.
3. Define negligence.
4. Define malpractice.
5. Why are ethics important to the veterinary profession?
6. Why is an informed consent imperative?
7. Why would a consent form be upheld in court?
8. What branch of law does animal abuse fall under?
9. What is PLIT? Whom does it cover?
10. Why is medical record legibility important?
11. Which association created the Principles of Veterinary Medical Ethics?
    a. AVMA
    b. NAVTA
    c. VHMA
    d. PLIT
12. What does the acronym VCPR stand for?
    a. Veterinary-client public records
    b. Veterinarian-client-patient relationship
    c. Veterinary cardiac pulmonary resuscitation
    d. Veterinary conduct and professional responsibilities
13. Which of the following are considered a branch of veterinary ethics?
    a. Normative
    b. Descriptive
    c. Administrative
    d. Official
    e. All of the above
14. What two categories are law divided into?
    a. Civil and federal
    b. Criminal and common
    c. Criminal and civil
    d. Federal and criminal
15. What is the correct definition of an *intentional tort*?
    a. An intentional action that has taken place in which harm has occurred to another member of society
    b. Crimes committed against the public as a whole
    c. A civil offense to an opposing party in which harm has occurred
    d. An injury occurring to a member of society due to negligence

Recommended Reading

Wilson JF: *Laws and ethics for the veterinary profession*, Yardley, PA, 1990, Priority Press.

Wilson JF, Fishman AJ, Nemder JD: *Contracts, benefits, and practice management for the veterinary profession*, Yardley, PA, 2009, Priority Press.

Wilson JF: *Legal consents for veterinary practices*, ed 4, Yardley, PA, 2006, Priority Press.

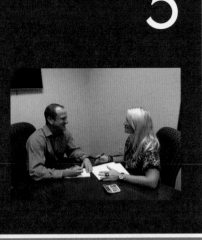

CHAPTER 5

Human Resources

OUTLINE

Organizational Behavior, 88
Laws That Require Familiarity, 88
Fair Labor and Standards Act, 89
Family and Medical Leave Act, 89
Uniformed Services Employment and Reemployment Rights Act, 89
Immigration Reform and Control Act, 89
Employee Polygraph Protection Act, 93
Equal Employment Opportunity, 93
Occupational Safety and Health Administration, 93
Pregnancy and Maternity Leave, 93
Required Posters, 93
Employee Manual, 93
Developing an Employee Manual, 100
Laws of Importance, 106
Social Media Policy, 107
Job Descriptions and Duties, 107
Hiring the Perfect Team, 109
When to Hire, 109
Reviewing Resumes, 110
Reviewing Letters of Reference, 110
References, 110
Using Social Media to Review Candidates, 110
Asking the Right Questions, 110
Questions Not to Ask, 111
Pre-employment Screening, 111
The First Day for a New Hire, 111

Employee Procedure Manual, 112
Developing an Employee Procedure Manual, 113
Implementing an Employee Procedure Manual, 113
Updating the Employee Procedure Manual, 114
Standards of Care, 115
Team Training, 115
Developing a Training Protocol, 116
Providing All Levels of Continuing Education, 121
Role-Playing, 122
Methods to Retain Employees, 122
Termination, 123
Payroll, 124
Determining Staff Wages, 125
Veterinarians, 125
Technicians, 126
Assistants, Receptionists, and Kennel Attendants, 127
Groomers, 127
Determining Raises, 127
Managing Payroll, 127
Records, 128
Payroll Taxes, 128
Forms W-2 and W-4, 129
Workers' Compensation Insurance, 129
Personnel Files, 129
Contract Employee Versus Employee, 131
Theft and Embezzlement, 135

KEY TERMS

401(k)
1099-MISC
Benefits
COBRA
Contract Employee
Direct Deposit
Employee Manual
Employee Polygraph Protection Act
Employee Procedure Manual
Equal Employment Opportunity
ERISA
Fair Credit Reporting Act
FLSA1
FMLA
FUTA
IRCA
Noncompete Agreement
Organizational Behavior
OSHA
References
Resume
SEPs
sIRA
USERRA
W-2
W-4
Workers' Compensation Insurance

LEARNING OBJECTIVES

When you have completed this chapter, you should be able to:

1. Compare and review resumes.
2. Discuss methods used to interview candidates effectively.
3. Describe questions that can legally be asked of candidates.
4. Clarify specific laws associated with human resources.
5. Identify required posters.
6. Develop an employee personnel manual.
7. Develop an employee procedure manual.
8. Calculate staff wages when hiring new employees.
9. Calculate raises.
10. Efficiently manage payroll and calculate taxes.
11. Explain how to maintain payroll files.
12. Develop team training protocols.
13. List methods used to effectively terminate team members.

1. **Adaptability** - being open to change and flexible work methods; the ability to adapt behavior to changing conditions or new information.
2. **Analytical Skills** - the ability to analyze information and use logic to address problems; the ability to quickly and accurately grasp complex information and concepts and to make correct inferences.
3. **Compliance** - being reliable, thorough, and conscientious in carrying out work assignments; have an appreciation for the importance of organizational rules and policies.
4. **Continuous Learning** - have a curiosity for learning; actively seek out new information, technologies, and methods; keep skills updated and apply new knowledge to the job.
5. **Creativity** - the ability to think creatively about situations, to see things in new and different ways; use imagination and creativity to develop innovative solutions to problems.
6. **Critical and Strategic Thinking** - the ability to think critically about situations and to understand the relevance of information for different problems; use critical reasoning to generate and evaluate alternative courses of action or points of view relevant to an issue.
7. **Decision Making** - the ability to make good decisions, solve problems, and decide on important matters; the ability to gather and analyze relevant data and choose decisively between alternatives.
8. **Integrity** - honesty, trustworthiness, and adherence to high standards of ethical conduct.
9. **Leadership** - a willingness to lead and take charge; the ability to motivate others and mobilize group effort toward common goals.
10. **Oral Communication and Comprehension** - the ability to express one's thoughts verbally in a clear and understandable manner, and the ability to actively listen and attend to what others are saying; must have good group presentation skills.
11. **Persuasion** - the ability to change the attitudes and opinions of others and to persuade them to accept recommendations and change behavior.
12. **Planning and Prioritizing** - the ability to effectively manage time and workload to meet deadlines; the ability to organize work, set priorities, and establish plans for achieving goals.
13. **Relationship Building** - the ability to develop constructive and cooperative working relationships with others and maintain them over time; must also be able to settle disputes, resolve grievances and conflicts, and negotiate with others.
14. **Resilience** - the ability to cope effectively with pressure and setbacks; the ability to handle crisis situations effectively and remain undeterred by obstacles or failure.
15. **Resourcefulness** - the ability to understand what it takes to complete the job; apply knowledge, skills, and expertise to perform tasks quickly and efficiently.
16. **Writing and Verbal Skills** - ability to comprehend written material easily and accurately; ability to express thoughts clearly and succinctly in writing.

In the human resources domain, the veterinary practice manager plans, directs, and coordinates the human resource management activities of the organization. Work activities include recruiting and hiring staff, providing guidance and direction to subordinates, setting performance standards and monitoring performance, and scheduling the work of others.

Knowledge Requirements

These human resource tasks require knowledge of (1) principles and procedures for recruitment, selection, training, and evaluation of personnel; (2) management principles involved in strategic planning, leadership, compensation, and scheduling; and (3) methods of writing job descriptions and manuals.

Organizational Behavior

Basic management of a veterinary practice includes organizational development and employee development. Organizational development is the development, improvement, and effectiveness of an organization and includes the culture, values, system, and behaviors of such practice. Employee development helps improve the vision, empowerment, learning, and problem-solving abilities of team members.

The vision of such a practice is built by the owner and shared by the team. All team members should know what the vision of the practice is and live it on a daily basis. With vision comes structure, practice culture, norms, codes of conduct, and core values. The culture created should be positive and provide an open communication policy for all employees. A code of conduct can be established and written in the employee manual, allowing all employees to know what is expected of them. Review Chapter 3 for more information on the formation and implementation of a mission, visions and values of a practice.

Team development is essential to the success of a practice. Creating the perfect team takes time and begins before team members are hired. It then continues with correct hiring procedures. Job descriptions must be detailed and job duties should be clear, allowing potential and current employees to know what is expected of them. Retaining the perfect team is of utmost importance and must be a top priority for the practice. Encouraging teamwork and motivation will help ensure high employee retention rate, as do positive feedback, daily coaching, and evaluations. Effective organizations have teams, not individuals.

> **PRACTICE POINT**   Creating the perfect team takes time and begins before team members are hired.

Team members are required to communicate with practice management, clients, and other team members. Team meetings can help facilitate communication among employees and allow discussion of protocols and procedures. Meetings should run on time and be as effective as possible in the short time allotted. Communication with clients is essential because this is where most client dissatisfaction occurs. Exceptional client communication increases client compliance because they can accept the recommendations made by the team more easily.

Development of employee and procedure manuals may take time, but they greatly increase the efficiency and communication of a practice. By allowing the team to help create the manuals, fewer duties and descriptions are forgotten and more ideas are included. Manuals can help hold the team together and allow greater leadership in all areas of the practice. When a team creates manuals together, implementing and using them is achieved with greater success.

WHAT WOULD YOU DO/NOT DO?

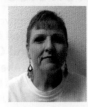

It has been brought to the attention of a practice manager that inappropriate behavior may have occurred between team members at a recent continuing education seminar held out of town. Rumor has it that a male veterinarian and a female veterinary technician had a couple of alcohol beverages and shared a room together. Other team members that attended the seminar with the pair felt that this gave the technician benefits over themselves and that favoritism may occur from this point on.

What Should a Practice Manager Do?

First, the employee manual must be consulted to see if any reference is made to employee relations. If no reference is made, nothing can be done. If reference is made, then both team members should be interviewed individually, verifying the rumor. The interview may reveal false information; if the rumor is true, both team members must be sanctioned as outlined in the employee manual. Third, a team meeting should be held outlining the employee manual, communicating the expectations of all team members. Open communication must be a top priority to prevent events such as this from occurring.

Laws That Require Familiarity

Before the employee manual can be developed, managers should have a clear understanding of laws and how they affect the veterinary practice. Laws and regulations change on a regular basis at both the federal and state levels. Every practice manager and office manager should be familiar with changes that occur, update the team with changes, and add to or modify the employee manual as needed (Box 5-1). The Society for Human Resource Management (www.shrm.org) is an excellent organization to become a member of, helping managers to stay abreast of current federal and state changes.

 Veterinary practice managers understand and comply with employment and labor laws.

> **BOX 5-1 | Laws to be Familiar With**
>
> - Family and Medical Leave Act
> - Uniformed Services Employment and Reemployment Rights Act
> - Fair Labor and Standards Act
> - Equal Employment Opportunity
> - Occupational Safety and Health Administration
> - Immigration Reform and Control Act
> - Employee Polygraph Protection Act

Fair Labor and Standards Act

The Fair Labor and Standards Act (FLSA) was created to establish minimum wage and overtime pay standards as well as regulate the employment of minors (see Figure 5-2). State minimum wage may be more or less than the federal minimum wage; whichever is higher supersedes the other. Minimum wage changes periodically and managers should be aware of changes. Any employee working more than a 40-hour workweek must be paid overtime at 1.5 times the regular rate of pay. The FLSA makes reference to a workweek as 7 consecutive, regularly recurring, 24-hour periods totaling 168 hours. For the first 40 hours worked in any given workweek, each employee must be paid at least minimum wage. Overtime pay must be paid for any hours worked above 40 in a given week at the stated hourly wage. Some states have rules that supersede these federal guidelines, requiring overtime to be paid when work exceeds 8 hours in 1 day. *(At the time of publication, this law is undergoing evaluation and may change; visit the Web site of the Department of Labor for updated regulations).*

PRACTICE POINT	FLSA applies to every practice.

An exemption to overtime pay applies to any individual involved in executive, administrative, or professional duties. In the case of a professional employee, at least 80% of the duties must require knowledge of an advanced type of science or learning, artistic work, or teaching. Veterinarians and most practice managers qualify as exempt.

It is imperative to monitor team member hours because staff members in veterinary medicine often work long and hard hours. Excess hours lead to burnout (see Chapter 6). Prevention of burnout is imperative or the employee retention rate will drop dramatically. Veterinary technicians do not qualify as exempt, therefore, any hours accumulated after 40 hours must be paid as overtime. Practices can receive large fines from the Department of Labor for not paying team members overtime.

Another exemption to FLSA is full-time students (who may be paid at 85% of minimum wage), apprentices, or handicapped workers. The Wage and Hour Division of the U.S. Department of Labor issues certificates of exemptions, which must be applied for by the employer, to pay wages less than minimum wage.

Employees must be at least 16 years of age to work in non–farm-related jobs; youths who are 14 or 15 years old may be allowed to work outside school hours with a work permit. They are allowed to work only 3 hours per day during school days and 8 hours per day on non-school days. Work cannot begin before 7 AM and cannot end after 7 PM. During the summer, hours are extended until 9 PM. Work permits can generally be obtained from the school district that the child is enrolled in. Again, state regulations may supersede this federal law; checking with the state department of labor is advised.

According to federal guidelines, employers are required to keep records on wages and hours for a minimum of 3 years after the termination of the employee; some states require longer record retention.

Family and Medical Leave Act

The Family and Medical Leave Act (FMLA) was established in 1993 to protect and preserve the integrity of the family. It was designed to benefit employees without adversely affecting employers (see Figure 5-3). It allows employees to take up to 12 weeks of unpaid leave for the following reasons:

- Incapacity due to pregnancy, prenatal medical care, or childbirth
- To care for the employee's child after birth, or placement for adoption or foster care
- To care for the employee's spouse, son, daughter, or parent who has a serious health condition
- A serious health condition that makes the employee unable to perform the employee's job.

Military Family Leave Entitlements

Eligible employees whose spouse, son, daughter, or parent is on covered active duty or call to covered active duty status may use their 12-week leave entitlement to address certain qualifying exigencies. Qualifying exigencies may include attending certain military events, arranging for alternative childcare, addressing certain financial and legal arrangements, attending certain counseling sessions, and attending post-deployment reintegration briefings.

The employee is guaranteed his or her job, or an equivalent one, upon return to work. Employees must have worked for the organization for at least 12 months, with at least 1250 hours acquired during those 12 months. The employee must give the employer at least 30 days notice before leaving regarding when the period will begin and end. If these requirements are not met, the employer can deny the leave. FMLA applies to organizations with more than 50 employees; an organization with fewer employees is exempt from the act.

Uniformed Services Employment and Reemployment Rights Act

The Uniformed Services Employment and Reemployment Rights Act (USERRA) was created to protect individuals who are enrolled in any branch of the military service. USERRA protects the rights of employees who voluntarily or involuntarily leave an employment position to undertake any military service. Employers cannot discriminate against past, present, and potential employees who are uniformed service members. Employees have the right to return to the employment position they had before leaving as well as any benefits that are or were available at that time.

Immigration Reform and Control Act

The Immigration Reform and Control Act (IRCA) prohibits employer discrimination against any employee or potential employee because of national origin. Form I-9 should be filled out by new hires to confirm that they can legally work in the United States. Form I-9 is required to be completed by employers and states that the employer has examined the required documents verifying employment eligibility (Figure 5-1) (see the Evolve site accompanying this text for the complete form). Documents to verify include a birth

Employment Eligibility Verification

Department of Homeland Security
U.S. Citizenship and Immigration Services

USCIS
Form I-9
OMB No. 1615-0047
Expires 03/31/2016

►**START HERE.** Read instructions carefully before completing this form. The instructions must be available during completion of this form.
ANTI-DISCRIMINATION NOTICE: It is illegal to discriminate against work-authorized individuals. Employers **CANNOT** specify which document(s) they will accept from an employee. The refusal to hire an individual because the documentation presented has a future expiration date may also constitute illegal discrimination.

Section 1. Employee Information and Attestation *(Employees must complete and sign Section 1 of Form I-9 no later than the **first day of employment**, but not before accepting a job offer.)*

Last Name *(Family Name)*	First Name *(Given Name)*	Middle Initial	Other Names Used *(if any)*

Address *(Street Number and Name)*	Apt. Number	City or Town	State	Zip Code

Date of Birth *(mm/dd/yyyy)*	U.S. Social Security Number	E-mail Address	Telephone Number
	☐☐☐-☐☐-☐☐☐☐		

I am aware that federal law provides for imprisonment and/or fines for false statements or use of false documents in connection with the completion of this form.

I attest, under penalty of perjury, that I am (check one of the following):

☐ A citizen of the United States

☐ A noncitizen national of the United States *(See instructions)*

☐ A lawful permanent resident (Alien Registration Number/USCIS Number): _____

☐ An alien authorized to work until (expiration date, if applicable, mm/dd/yyyy) _____ . Some aliens may write "N/A" in this field.
(See instructions)

For aliens authorized to work, provide your Alien Registration Number/USCIS Number **OR** Form I-94 Admission Number:

1. Alien Registration Number/USCIS Number:_____

OR

2. Form I-94 Admission Number: _____

If you obtained your admission number from CBP in connection with your arrival in the United States, include the following:

Foreign Passport Number: _____

Country of Issuance: _____

Some aliens may write "N/A" on the Foreign Passport Number and Country of Issuance fields. (*See instructions*)

3-D Barcode
Do Not Write in This Space

Signature of Employee:	Date *(mm/dd/yyyy)*:

Preparer and/or Translator Certification *(To be completed and signed if Section 1 is prepared by a person other than the employee.)*

I attest, under penalty of perjury, that I have assisted in the completion of this form and that to the best of my knowledge the information is true and correct.

Signature of Preparer or Translator:	Date *(mm/dd/yyyy)*:

Last Name *(Family Name)*	First Name *(Given Name)*

Address *(Street Number and Name)*	City or Town	State	Zip Code

🛑 *Employer Completes Next Page* 🛑

FIGURE 5-1 Form I-9.

Section 2. Employer or Authorized Representative Review and Verification

(Employers or their authorized representative must complete and sign Section 2 within 3 business days of the employee's first day of employment. You must physically examine one document from List A OR examine a combination of one document from List B and one document from List C as listed on the "Lists of Acceptable Documents" on the next page of this form. For each document you review, record the following information: document title, issuing authority, document number, and expiration date, if any.)

Employee Last Name, First Name and Middle Initial from Section 1:

List A Identity and Employment Authorization	OR	**List B** Identity	AND	**List C** Employment Authorization
Document Title:		Document Title:		Document Title:
Issuing Authority:		Issuing Authority:		Issuing Authority:
Document Number:		Document Number:		Document Number:
Expiration Date *(if any)(mm/dd/yyyy)*:		Expiration Date *(if any)(mm/dd/yyyy)*:		Expiration Date *(if any)(mm/dd/yyyy)*:
Document Title:				
Issuing Authority:				
Document Number:				
Expiration Date *(if any)(mm/dd/yyyy)*:				
Document Title:				
Issuing Authority:				**3-D Barcode** **Do Not Write in This Space**
Document Number:				
Expiration Date *(if any)(mm/dd/yyyy)*:				

Certification

I attest, under penalty of perjury, that (1) I have examined the document(s) presented by the above-named employee, (2) the above-listed document(s) appear to be genuine and to relate to the employee named, and (3) to the best of my knowledge the employee is authorized to work in the United States.

The employee's first day of employment *(mm/dd/yyyy)*: _____ **(*See instructions for exemptions*.)**

Signature of Employer or Authorized Representative	Date *(mm/dd/yyyy)*	Title of Employer or Authorized Representative		
Last Name *(Family Name)*	First Name *(Given Name)*	Employer's Business or Organization Name		
Employer's Business or Organization Address *(Street Number and Name)*	City or Town		State	Zip Code

Section 3. Reverification and Rehires *(To be completed and signed by employer or authorized representative.)*

A. New Name *(if applicable)* Last Name *(Family Name)* First Name *(Given Name)*	Middle Initial	**B.** Date of Rehire *(if applicable) (mm/dd/yyyy)*:

C. If employee's previous grant of employment authorization has expired, provide the information for the document from List A or List C the employee presented that establishes current employment authorization in the space provided below.

Document Title:	Document Number:	Expiration Date *(if any)(mm/dd/yyyy)*:

I attest, under penalty of perjury, that to the best of my knowledge, this employee is authorized to work in the United States, and if the employee presented document(s), the document(s) I have examined appear to be genuine and to relate to the individual.

Signature of Employer or Authorized Representative:	Date *(mm/dd/yyyy)*:	Print Name of Employer or Authorized Representative:

Form I-9   03/08/13 N

FIGURE 5-1, cont'd

Continued

LISTS OF ACCEPTABLE DOCUMENTS
All documents must be UNEXPIRED

Employees may present one selection from List A
or a combination of one selection from List B and one selection from List C.

LIST A Documents that Establish Both Identity and Employment Authorization	LIST B Documents that Establish Identity	LIST C Documents that Establish Employment Authorization
OR		AND
1. U.S. Passport or U.S. Passport Card	1. Driver's license or ID card issued by a State or outlying possession of the United States provided it contains a photograph or information such as name, date of birth, gender, height, eye color, and address	1. A Social Security Account Number card, unless the card includes one of the following restrictions: (1) NOT VALID FOR EMPLOYMENT (2) VALID FOR WORK ONLY WITH INS AUTHORIZATION (3) VALID FOR WORK ONLY WITH DHS AUTHORIZATION
2. Permanent Resident Card or Alien Registration Receipt Card (Form I-551)		
3. Foreign passport that contains a temporary I-551 stamp or temporary I-551 printed notation on a machine-readable immigrant visa	2. ID card issued by federal, state or local government agencies or entities, provided it contains a photograph or information such as name, date of birth, gender, height, eye color, and address	2. Certification of Birth Abroad issued by the Department of State (Form FS-545)
4. Employment Authorization Document that contains a photograph (Form I-766)	3. School ID card with a photograph	3. Certification of Report of Birth issued by the Department of State (Form DS-1350)
	4. Voter's registration card	
5. For a nonimmigrant alien authorized to work for a specific employer because of his or her status: a. Foreign passport; and b. Form I-94 or Form I-94A that has the following: (1) The same name as the passport; and (2) An endorsement of the alien's nonimmigrant status as long as that period of endorsement has not yet expired and the proposed employment is not in conflict with any restrictions or limitations identified on the form.	5. U.S. Military card or draft record	4. Original or certified copy of birth certificate issued by a State, county, municipal authority, or territory of the United States bearing an official seal
	6. Military dependent's ID card	
	7. U.S. Coast Guard Merchant Mariner Card	5. Native American tribal document
	8. Native American tribal document	6. U.S. Citizen ID Card (Form I-197)
	9. Driver's license issued by a Canadian government authority	7. Identification Card for Use of Resident Citizen in the United States (Form I-179)
	For persons under age 18 who are unable to present a document listed above:	8. Employment authorization document issued by the Department of Homeland Security
6. Passport from the Federated States of Micronesia (FSM) or the Republic of the Marshall Islands (RMI) with Form I-94 or Form I-94A indicating nonimmigrant admission under the Compact of Free Association Between the United States and the FSM or RMI	10. School record or report card	
	11. Clinic, doctor, or hospital record	
	12. Day-care or nursery school record	

Illustrations of many of these documents appear in Part 8 of the Handbook for Employers (M-274).

Refer to Section 2 of the instructions, titled "Employer or Authorized Representative Review and Verification," for more information about acceptable receipts.

FIGURE 5-1, cont'd

or naturalization certificate, a U.S. passport, a valid foreign exchange passport authorizing employment in the United States, a resident alien card (green card), Social Security card, and driver's license or state identification card.

Form I-9 should not be filled out until the first day of employment, and verification documents do not have to be copied; however, all employee records must be treated the same. Either all employee verification documents must be copied, or none at all. Managers must ensure the document is filled out entirely and correctly. Form I-9 can be inspected at any time, and violations for incomplete or incorrect forms can add up. Form I-9 must be kept for 3 years from the date of hire, or 1 year after termination, whichever is longer.

> **PRACTICE POINT**   Form I-9 should be filled out on the first day of employment (not before).

Employee Polygraph Protection Act

The Employee Polygraph Protection Act prohibits most employers from using lie detector tests for either pre-employment screening or during the course of employment. Employers cannot discriminate against employees who refuse to take a lie detector test. An exemption does apply to a practice that prescribes and dispenses controlled substances. It is advised to review this law further for additional information as it applies to veterinary medicine (see Figure 5-4).

Equal Employment Opportunity

An Equal Employment Opportunity policy prohibits discrimination against employees on the basis of race, color, sex, religion, or national origin. Employers cannot deny a promotion, terminate, or not hire a potential employee for any of those reasons. Equal Employment Opportunity also prevents discrimination of those with disabilities who can perform the job as described in the job duties. The law also requires that organizations provide to qualified applicants and employees with disabilities reasonable accommodation that does not impose undue hardship on the employer. The Age Discrimination in Employment Act of 1967 protects applicants and current employees over the age of 40 years from discrimination on the basis of age in hiring, promotion, discharge, and compensation. Title VII of the Civil Rights Act of 1964 prohibits sex discrimination in payment of wages to men and women performing substantially equal work in the same establishment.

Occupational Safety and Health Administration

The Occupational Safety and Health Administration (OSHA) has set safety standards to protect employees. Employers must provide a safe work environment and comply with safety standards set forth by OSHA (see Chapter 21 for more information). OSHA has the authority to inspect workplace environments without advance notice to the employer. Safety hazard plans should be in place to help protect employees

| BOX 5-2 | Posters That Must be Displayed in a Highly Visible Area |

- Occupational Safety and Health Administration
- Equal Employment Opportunity
- Family and Medical Leave Act
- Employee Polygraph Protection Act
- Immigration Reform and Control Act
- Uniformed Services Employment and Reemployment Rights Act
- Fair Labor and Standards Act

from dangers, and they must be enforced by the employer on a daily basis (see Figure 5-6).

Pregnancy and Maternity Leave

State labor boards or commissions should be contacted to determine the most recent regulations regarding the required length of pregnancy and maternity leave. Employers cannot prohibit pregnant employees from working once risks associated with their position have been discussed. It is unlawful to exclude employees from job duties unless the claim is supported by objective, scientific evidence. If employees insist on continuing to work in a potentially harmful environment, they should sign a statement releasing the employer from liability.

Required Posters

Posters informing employees of their rights are required and must be posted in a location visible by all employees. Posters can be picked up at any local or state labor department free of charge and do not have to be purchased from solicitors. Federal posters required include OSHA: It's the Law, Equal Employment Opportunity, Family and Medical Leave Act of 1993, Employee Polygraph Protection Act, Immigration Reform and Control Act, the Uniformed Services Employment and Reemployment Rights Act, and the Fair Labor Act (Box 5-2; Figures 5-2 to 5-6). Some states require more than these federally mandates posters. Visit the state department of labor for updated requirements.

> **PRACTICE POINT**   Visit your state labor board to determine if your state requires more than the federal posters to be posed in your clinic.

Employee Manual

Before hiring can begin, a successful plan must be implemented. An employee manual, job descriptions, and expectations must be developed; otherwise the hiring process will have potholes in it. Many practices are quick to hire and slow to fire, thereby creating a negative work environment. Managers often choose not to deal with issues that should be addressed immediately, because there is no structure in place to support the managers decision. Creating an employee manual, job descriptions, and

Text continued on p. 99

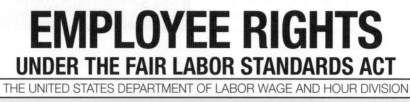

EMPLOYEE RIGHTS
UNDER THE FAIR LABOR STANDARDS ACT

THE UNITED STATES DEPARTMENT OF LABOR WAGE AND HOUR DIVISION

FEDERAL MINIMUM WAGE
$7.25 PER HOUR
BEGINNING JULY 24, 2009

OVERTIME PAY　At least 1½ times your regular rate of pay for all hours worked over 40 in a workweek.

CHILD LABOR　An employee must be at least **16** years old to work in most non-farm jobs and at least 18 to work in non-farm jobs declared hazardous by the Secretary of Labor.

Youths **14** and **15** years old may work outside school hours in various non-manufacturing, non-mining, non-hazardous jobs under the following conditions:

No more than
- **3** hours on a school day or **18** hours in a school week;
- **8** hours on a non-school day or **40** hours in a non-school week.

Also, work may not begin before **7 a.m.** or end after **7 p.m.**, except from June 1 through Labor Day, when evening hours are extended to **9 p.m.** Different rules apply in agricultural employment.

TIP CREDIT　Employers of "tipped employees" must pay a cash wage of at least $2.13 per hour if they claim a tip credit against their minimum wage obligation. If an employee's tips combined with the employer's cash wage of at least $2.13 per hour do not equal the minimum hourly wage, the employer must make up the difference. Certain other conditions must also be met.

ENFORCEMENT　The Department of Labor may recover back wages either administratively or through court action, for the employees that have been underpaid in violation of the law. Violations may result in civil or criminal action.

Employers may be assessed civil money penalties of up to $1,100 for each willful or repeated violation of the minimum wage or overtime pay provisions of the law and up to $11,000 for each employee who is the subject of a violation of the Act's child labor provisions. In addition, a civil money penalty of up to $50,000 may be assessed for each child labor violation that causes the death or serious injury of any minor employee, and such assessments may be doubled, up to $100,000, when the violations are determined to be willful or repeated. The law also prohibits discriminating against or discharging workers who file a complaint or participate in any proceeding under the Act.

ADDITIONAL INFORMATION
- Certain occupations and establishments are exempt from the minimum wage and/or overtime pay provisions.
- Special provisions apply to workers in American Samoa and the Commonwealth of the Northern Mariana Islands.
- Some state laws provide greater employee protections; employers must comply with both.
- The law requires employers to display this poster where employees can readily see it.
- Employees under 20 years of age may be paid $4.25 per hour during their first 90 consecutive calendar days of employment with an employer.
- Certain full-time students, student learners, apprentices, and workers with disabilities may be paid less than the minimum wage under special certificates issued by the Department of Labor.

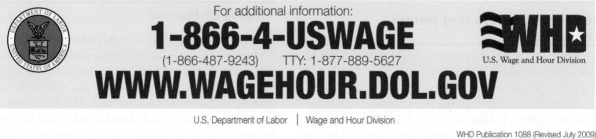

For additional information:
1-866-4-USWAGE
(1-866-487-9243)　　TTY: 1-877-889-5627

WHD
U.S. Wage and Hour Division

WWW.WAGEHOUR.DOL.GOV

U.S. Department of Labor　|　Wage and Hour Division

WHD Publication 1088 (Revised July 2009)

FIGURE 5-2 Minimum wage.

EMPLOYEE RIGHTS AND RESPONSIBILITIES
UNDER THE FAMILY AND MEDICAL LEAVE ACT

Basic Leave Entitlement

FMLA requires covered employers to provide up to 12 weeks of unpaid, job-protected leave to eligible employees for the following reasons:

- for incapacity due to pregnancy, prenatal medical care or child birth;
- to care for the employee's child after birth, or placement for adoption or foster care;
- to care for the employee's spouse, son, daughter or parent, who has a serious health condition; or
- for a serious health condition that makes the employee unable to perform the employee's job.

Military Family Leave Entitlements

Eligible employees whose spouse, son, daughter or parent is on covered active duty or call to covered active duty status may use their 12-week leave entitlement to address certain qualifying exigencies. Qualifying exigencies may include attending certain military events, arranging for alternative childcare, addressing certain financial and legal arrangements, attending certain counseling sessions, and attending post-deployment reintegration briefings.

FMLA also includes a special leave entitlement that permits eligible employees to take up to 26 weeks of leave to care for a covered service-member during a single 12-month period. A covered servicemember is: (1) a current member of the Armed Forces, including a member of the National Guard or Reserves, who is undergoing medical treatment, recuperation or therapy, is otherwise in outpatient status, or is otherwise on the temporary disability retired list, for a serious injury or illness*; or (2) a veteran who was discharged or released under conditions other than dishonorable at any time during the five-year period prior to the first date the eligible employee takes FMLA leave to care for the covered veteran, and who is undergoing medical treatment, recuperation, or therapy for a serious injury or illness.*

*The FMLA definitions of "serious injury or illness" for current servicemembers and veterans are distinct from the FMLA definition of "serious health condition".

Benefits and Protections

During FMLA leave, the employer must maintain the employee's health coverage under any "group health plan" on the same terms as if the employee had continued to work. Upon return from FMLA leave, most employees must be restored to their original or equivalent positions with equivalent pay, benefits, and other employment terms.

Use of FMLA leave cannot result in the loss of any employment benefit that accrued prior to the start of an employee's leave.

Eligibility Requirements

Employees are eligible if they have worked for a covered employer for at least 12 months, have 1,250 hours of service in the previous 12 months*, and if at least 50 employees are employed by the employer within 75 miles.

*Special hours of service eligibility requirements apply to airline flight crew employees.

Definition of Serious Health Condition

A serious health condition is an illness, injury, impairment, or physical or mental condition that involves either an overnight stay in a medical care facility, or continuing treatment by a health care provider for a condition that either prevents the employee from performing the functions of the employee's job, or prevents the qualified family member from participating in school or other daily activities.

Subject to certain conditions, the continuing treatment requirement may be met by a period of incapacity of more than 3 consecutive calendar days combined with at least two visits to a health care provider or one visit and a regimen of continuing treatment, or incapacity due to pregnancy, or incapacity due to a chronic condition. Other conditions may meet the definition of continuing treatment.

Use of Leave

An employee does not need to use this leave entitlement in one block. Leave can be taken intermittently or on a reduced leave schedule when medically necessary. Employees must make reasonable efforts to schedule leave for planned medical treatment so as not to unduly disrupt the employer's operations. Leave due to qualifying exigencies may also be taken on an intermittent basis.

Substitution of Paid Leave for Unpaid Leave

Employees may choose or employers may require use of accrued paid leave while taking FMLA leave. In order to use paid leave for FMLA leave, employees must comply with the employer's normal paid leave policies.

Employee Responsibilities

Employees must provide 30 days advance notice of the need to take FMLA leave when the need is foreseeable. When 30 days notice is not possible, the employee must provide notice as soon as practicable and generally must comply with an employer's normal call-in procedures.

Employees must provide sufficient information for the employer to determine if the leave may qualify for FMLA protection and the anticipated timing and duration of the leave. Sufficient information may include that the employee is unable to perform job functions, the family member is unable to perform daily activities, the need for hospitalization or continuing treatment by a health care provider, or circumstances supporting the need for military family leave. Employees also must inform the employer if the requested leave is for a reason for which FMLA leave was previously taken or certified. Employees also may be required to provide a certification and periodic recertification supporting the need for leave.

Employer Responsibilities

Covered employers must inform employees requesting leave whether they are eligible under FMLA. If they are, the notice must specify any additional information required as well as the employees' rights and responsibilities. If they are not eligible, the employer must provide a reason for the ineligibility.

Covered employers must inform employees if leave will be designated as FMLA-protected and the amount of leave counted against the employee's leave entitlement. If the employer determines that the leave is not FMLA-protected, the employer must notify the employee.

Unlawful Acts by Employers

FMLA makes it unlawful for any employer to:

- interfere with, restrain, or deny the exercise of any right provided under FMLA; and
- discharge or discriminate against any person for opposing any practice made unlawful by FMLA or for involvement in any proceeding under or relating to FMLA.

Enforcement

An employee may file a complaint with the U.S. Department of Labor or may bring a private lawsuit against an employer.

FMLA does not affect any Federal or State law prohibiting discrimination, or supersede any State or local law or collective bargaining agreement which provides greater family or medical leave rights.

FMLA section 109 (29 U.S.C. § 2619) requires FMLA covered employers to post the text of this notice. Regulation 29 C.F.R. § 825.300(a) may require additional disclosures.

For additional information:
1-866-4US-WAGE (1-866-487-9243) TTY: 1-877-889-5627
WWW.WAGEHOUR.DOL.GOV

U.S. Department of Labor | Wage and Hour Division

WHD Publication 1420 · Revised February 2013

FIGURE 5-3 FMLA.

EMPLOYEE RIGHTS

EMPLOYEE POLYGRAPH PROTECTION ACT

THE UNITED STATES DEPARTMENT OF LABOR WAGE AND HOUR DIVISION

The Employee Polygraph Protection Act prohibits most private employers from using lie detector tests either for pre-employment screening or during the course of employment.

PROHIBITIONS
Employers are generally prohibited from requiring or requesting any employee or job applicant to take a lie detector test, and from discharging, disciplining, or discriminating against an employee or prospective employee for refusing to take a test or for exercising other rights under the Act.

EXEMPTIONS
Federal, State and local governments are not affected by the law. Also, the law does not apply to tests given by the Federal Government to certain private individuals engaged in national security-related activities.

The Act permits polygraph (a kind of lie detector) tests to be administered in the private sector, subject to restrictions, to certain prospective employees of security service firms (armored car, alarm, and guard), and of pharmaceutical manufacturers, distributors and dispensers.

The Act also permits polygraph testing, subject to restrictions, of certain employees of private firms who are reasonably suspected of involvement in a workplace incident (theft, embezzlement, etc.) that resulted in economic loss to the employer.

The law does not preempt any provision of any State or local law or any collective bargaining agreement which is more restrictive with respect to lie detector tests.

EXAMINEE RIGHTS
Where polygraph tests are permitted, they are subject to numerous strict standards concerning the conduct and length of the test. Examinees have a number of specific rights, including the right to a written notice before testing, the right to refuse or discontinue a test, and the right not to have test results disclosed to unauthorized persons.

ENFORCEMENT
The Secretary of Labor may bring court actions to restrain violations and assess civil penalties up to $10,000 against violators. Employees or job applicants may also bring their own court actions.

THE LAW REQUIRES EMPLOYERS TO DISPLAY THIS POSTER WHERE EMPLOYEES AND JOB APPLICANTS CAN READILY SEE IT.

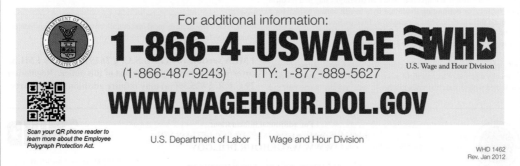

For additional information:

1-866-4-USWAGE ≋WHD
(1-866-487-9243)   TTY: 1-877-889-5627   U.S. Wage and Hour Division

WWW.WAGEHOUR.DOL.GOV

Scan your QR phone reader to learn more about the Employee Polygraph Protection Act.

U.S. Department of Labor | Wage and Hour Division

WHD 1462
Rev. Jan 2012

FIGURE 5-4 EPPA.

Equal Employment Opportunity is

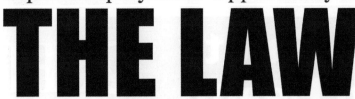

THE LAW

Private Employers, State and Local Governments, Educational Institutions, Employment Agencies and Labor Organizations

Applicants to and employees of most private employers, state and local governments, educational institutions,
employment agencies and labor organizations are protected under Federal law from discrimination on the following bases:

RACE, COLOR, RELIGION, SEX, NATIONAL ORIGIN
Title VII of the Civil Rights Act of 1964, as amended, protects applicants and employees from discrimination in hiring, promotion, discharge, pay, fringe benefits, job training, classification, referral, and other aspects of employment, on the basis of race, color, religion, sex (including pregnancy), or national origin. Religious discrimination includes failing to reasonably accommodate an employee's religious practices where the accommodation does not impose undue hardship.

DISABILITY
Title I and Title V of the Americans with Disabilities Act of 1990, as amended, protect qualified individuals from discrimination on the basis of disability in hiring, promotion, discharge, pay, fringe benefits, job training, classification, referral, and other aspects of employment. Disability discrimination includes not making reasonable accommodation to the known physical or mental limitations of an otherwise qualified individual with a disability who is an applicant or employee, barring undue hardship.

AGE
The Age Discrimination in Employment Act of 1967, as amended, protects applicants and employees 40 years of age or older from discrimination based on age in hiring, promotion, discharge, pay, fringe benefits, job training, classification, referral, and other aspects of employment.

SEX (WAGES)
In addition to sex discrimination prohibited by Title VII of the Civil Rights Act, as amended, the Equal Pay Act of 1963, as amended, prohibits sex discrimination in the payment of wages to women and men performing substantially equal work, in jobs that require equal skill, effort, and responsibility, under similar working conditions, in the same establishment.

GENETICS
Title II of the Genetic Information Nondiscrimination Act of 2008 protects applicants and employees from discrimination based on genetic information in hiring, promotion, discharge, pay, fringe benefits, job training, classification, referral, and other aspects of employment. GINA also restricts employers' acquisition of genetic information and strictly limits disclosure of genetic information. Genetic information includes information about genetic tests of applicants, employees, or their family members; the manifestation of diseases or disorders in family members (family medical history); and requests for or receipt of genetic services by applicants, employees, or their family members.

RETALIATION
All of these Federal laws prohibit covered entities from retaliating against a person who files a charge of discrimination, participates in a discrimination proceeding, or otherwise opposes an unlawful employment practice.

WHAT TO DO IF YOU BELIEVE DISCRIMINATION HAS OCCURRED
There are strict time limits for filing charges of employment discrimination. To preserve the ability of EEOC to act on your behalf and to protect your right to file a private lawsuit, should you ultimately need to, you should contact EEOC promptly when discrimination is suspected:
The U.S. Equal Employment Opportunity Commission (EEOC), 1-800-669-4000 (toll-free) or 1-800-669-6820 (toll-free TTY number for individuals with hearing impairments). EEOC field office information is available at www.eeoc.gov or in most telephone directories in the U.S. Government or Federal Government section. Additional information about EEOC, including information about charge filing, is available at www.eeoc.gov.

Employers Holding Federal Contracts or Subcontracts

Applicants to and employees of companies with a Federal government contract or subcontract
are protected under Federal law from discrimination on the following bases:

RACE, COLOR, RELIGION, SEX, NATIONAL ORIGIN
Executive Order 11246, as amended, prohibits job discrimination on the basis of race, color, religion, sex or national origin, and requires affirmative action to ensure equality of opportunity in all aspects of employment.

INDIVIDUALS WITH DISABILITIES
Section 503 of the Rehabilitation Act of 1973, as amended, protects qualified individuals from discrimination on the basis of disability in hiring, promotion, discharge, pay, fringe benefits, job training, classification, referral, and other aspects of employment. Disability discrimination includes not making reasonable accommodation to the known physical or mental limitations of an otherwise qualified individual with a disability who is an applicant or employee, barring undue hardship. Section 503 also requires that Federal contractors take affirmative action to employ and advance in employment qualified individuals with disabilities at all levels of employment, including the executive level.

DISABLED, RECENTLY SEPARATED, OTHER PROTECTED, AND ARMED FORCES SERVICE MEDAL VETERANS
The Vietnam Era Veterans' Readjustment Assistance Act of 1974, as amended, 38 U.S.C. 4212, prohibits job discrimination and requires affirmative action to employ and advance in employment disabled veterans, recently separated veterans (within

three years of discharge or release from active duty), other protected veterans (veterans who served during a war or in a campaign or expedition for which a campaign badge has been authorized), and Armed Forces service medal veterans (veterans who, while on active duty, participated in a U.S. military operation for which an Armed Forces service medal was awarded).

RETALIATION
Retaliation is prohibited against a person who files a complaint of discrimination, participates in an OFCCP proceeding, or otherwise opposes discrimination under these Federal laws.

Any person who believes a contractor has violated its nondiscrimination or affirmative action obligations under the authorities above should contact immediately:

The Office of Federal Contract Compliance Programs (OFCCP), U.S. Department of Labor, 200 Constitution Avenue, N.W., Washington, D.C. 20210, 1-800-397-6251 (toll-free) or (202) 693-1337 (TTY). OFCCP may also be contacted by e-mail at OFCCP-Public@dol.gov, or by calling an OFCCP regional or district office, listed in most telephone directories under U.S. Government, Department of Labor.

Programs or Activities Receiving Federal Financial Assistance

RACE, COLOR, NATIONAL ORIGIN, SEX
In addition to the protections of Title VII of the Civil Rights Act of 1964, as amended, Title VI of the Civil Rights Act of 1964, as amended, prohibits discrimination on the basis of race, color or national origin in programs or activities receiving Federal financial assistance. Employment discrimination is covered by Title VI if the primary objective of the financial assistance is provision of employment, or where employment discrimination causes or may cause discrimination in providing services under such programs. Title IX of the Education Amendments of 1972 prohibits employment discrimination on the basis of sex in educational programs or activities which receive Federal financial assistance.

INDIVIDUALS WITH DISABILITIES
Section 504 of the Rehabilitation Act of 1973, as amended, prohibits employment discrimination on the basis of disability in any program or activity which receives Federal financial assistance. Discrimination is prohibited in all aspects of employment against persons with disabilities who, with or without reasonable accommodation, can perform the essential functions of the job.

If you believe you have been discriminated against in a program of any institution which receives Federal financial assistance, you should immediately contact the Federal agency providing such assistance.

EEOC 9/02 and OFCCP 8/08 Versions Useable With 11/09 Supplement

EEOC-P/E-1 (Revised 11/09)

FIGURE 5-5 EEO.

FIGURE 5-6 OSHA. It's the law.

performance expectations before hiring will create a structure that every veterinary practice needs.

An employee manual provides a guide for team members and acts as a quick resource when a personnel issue arises (Figure 5-7). (See the Evolve site accompanying this text for the complete document.) A manual can solve workplace problems quickly and fairly because topics and policies have already been determined. Employee manuals also hold managers and leaders accountable. If it is stated in the manual, then the procedure must be followed (harassment, coaching, termination, etc.). If managers do not follow the guidelines that have been established, potential lawsuits from previous or disgruntled employees could result. In addition, a negative workplace culture is being developed (if managers don't follow the rules, why should employees?).

If an employee manual has not been developed, it is important to take the time to establish one. It may be a good idea to have the practice attorney review the manual before distribution to ensure the practice is legally protected in every way possible (in addition, state laws differ regarding employment laws). Violations of the terms of the manual can be seen as a breach of contract; therefore it is important to state in the front of the manual that it is not a contract, and that the manual can be changed and updated at any time. New employees should read the manual, sign a document stating that they have received it, and understand that it is not a contract—simply a guide to employee policy. If any changes have been made, employees should read them and sign a document indicating that they have received the update.

Courtesy of Patterson Veterinary University

EQUAL EMPLOYMENT OPPORTUNITY POLICY STATEMENT

Equal Employment Opportunity has been, and will continue to be, a fundamental principle at ABC, where employment is based upon personal capabilities and qualifications without discrimination because of race, color, religion, sex, age, national origin, disability, or any other protected characteristic as established by law.

This policy of Equal Employment Opportunity applies to all policies and procedures relating to recruitment and hiring, compensation, benefits, termination and all other terms and conditions of employment.

The Manager has overall responsibility for this policy and maintains reporting and monitoring procedures. Employees' questions or concerns should be referred to the Manager.

Appropriate disciplinary action may be taken against any employee willfully violating this policy.

NON-DISCRIMINATION AND ANTI-HARASSMENT POLICY

The ABC Company is committed to a work environment in which all individuals are treated with respect and dignity. Each individual has the right to work in a professional atmosphere that promotes equal employment opportunities and prohibits discriminatory practices, including harassment. Therefore, ABC expects that all relationships among persons in the workplace will be business-like and free of bias, prejudice and harassment.

Equal Employment Opportunity

It is the policy of ABC to ensure equal employment opportunity without discrimination or harassment on the basis of race, color, national origin, religion, sex (with or without sexual conduct), age, disability, [alienage or citizenship status, marital status, creed, genetic predisposition or carrier status, sexual orientation] or any other characteristic protected by law. ABC prohibits and will not tolerate any such discrimination or harassment.

Definitions of Harassment

a. **Sexual harassment** constitutes discrimination and is illegal under federal, state and local laws. For the purposes of this policy, sexual harassment is defined, as in the Equal Employment Opportunity Commission Guidelines, as unwelcome sexual advances, requests for sexual favors and other verbal or physical conduct of a sexual nature when, for example: (i) submission to such conduct is made either explicitly or implicitly a term or condition of an individual's employment; (ii) submission to or rejection of such conduct by an individual is used as the basis for employment decisions affecting such individual; or (iii) such conduct

FIGURE 5-7 Example of two pages of employee manual. Full document is on the Evolve site. (Courtesy Patterson Veterinary Supply, Inc.)

Continued

Courtesy of Patterson Veterinary University

has the purpose or effect of unreasonably interfering with an individual's work performance or creating an intimidating, hostile or offensive working environment.

Sexual harassment may include a range of subtle and not so subtle behaviors and may involve individuals of the same or different gender. Depending on the circumstances, these behaviors may include, but are not limited to: unwanted sexual advances or requests for sexual favors; sexual jokes and innuendo; verbal abuse of a sexual nature; commentary about an individual's body, sexual prowess or sexual deficiencies; leering, catcalls or touching; insulting or obscene comments or gestures; display or circulation in the workplace of sexually suggestive objects or pictures (including through e-mail); and other physical, verbal or visual conduct of a sexual nature. Sex-based harassment that is, harassment not involving sexual activity or language (e.g., male manager yells only at female employees and not males) may also constitute discrimination if it is severe or pervasive and directed at employees because of their sex.

b. Harassment on the basis of any other protected characteristic is also strictly prohibited. Under this policy, harassment is verbal or physical conduct that denigrates or shows hostility or aversion toward an individual because of his/her race, color, religion, national origin, age, disability, [alienage or citizenship status, marital status, creed, genetic predisposition or carrier status, sexual orientation] or any other characteristic protected by law or that of his/her relatives, friends or associates, and that: (i) has the purpose or effect of creating an intimidating, hostile or offensive work environment; (ii) has the purpose or effect of unreasonably interfering with an individual's work performance; or (iii) otherwise adversely affects an individual's employment opportunities.

Harassing conduct includes, but is not limited to: epithets, slurs or negative stereotyping; threatening, intimidating or hostile acts; denigrating jokes and display or circulation in the workplace of written or graphic material that denigrates or shows hostility or aversion toward an individual or group (including through e-mail or other internet communication sites).

Individuals and Conduct Covered

These policies apply to all applicants and employees, and prohibit harassment, discrimination and retaliation whether engaged in by fellow employees, by a supervisor or manager or by someone not directly connected to ABC (e.g., an outside vendor, consultant or client).

Conduct prohibited by these policies is unacceptable in the workplace and in any work-related setting outside the workplace, such as during business trips, business meetings and business-related social events.

Retaliation Is Prohibited

FIGURE 5-7, cont'd

Employment and labor laws change frequently, and policies and manuals must be updated to reflect these changes. Practices should reserve the right to update and modify employee manuals at any time. It is important to remain flexible, and employees should be made aware of changes as they occur; once again, it is important that they sign a form acknowledging any updates. When changes are implemented, save the file under a new name on the computer (indicating the date the changes were made). Keep all copies of all documents in case dates of when the changes were made ever have to be proven.

| PRACTICE POINT | Employee manuals keep both the employer and employee accountable to one another. |

Developing an Employee Manual

Employee manuals should maintain a positive tone, avoiding any authoritarian manner. Their purpose is to create a positive work environment, prevent problems before they arise, and allow communication to occur freely. Creating an atmosphere of open communication between team members and management can minimize problems related to human resources.

 Veterinary practice managers create, review, and update job descriptions/manuals.

Many topics are addressed in employee manuals, including the philosophy or mission of the practice. Benefits are generally offered by all practices; however, the extent of the benefits can vary from practice to practice. Benefits packages

| BOX 5-3 | Sample Table of Contents for Employee Personnel Manual |

Statement or purpose of manual
Philosophy and/or mission statement
Laws of importance
    Americans with Disabilities Act
    Confidentiality
    Equal employment opportunity
    Family Medical Leave Act
    Pregnancy safety
    Sexual harassment policy
Employment policies
    Appearance, dress code, uniforms
    Attendance, work schedule policy
    Code of Conduct
    Drug and alcohol abuse policy
    Drug-free work place
    Employment on an at-will basis
    Employment statuses
    Hours of operation
    Probationary period
    Punctuality
    Romantic relationships
    Social media policy
    Violence in the workplace
Compensation
    Compensation schedule
    Overtime
    Personnel records
Benefits
    Continuing education
    Disability

Dues and license fees
Holiday's recognized/holiday pay
Insurance
    Disability, health, liability
Retirement
Sick leave
Vacation
Veterinary services
Workers' compensation benefits
Noncompete agreement
Jury duty
Training procedures
    Probationary period
Safety
    OSHA/SDS
    Reporting an accident
    Security
Termination procedures
    Resignation
    Dismissals
        Immediate dismissals
Signature page
    Each state has different laws regarding employee manuals and laws that must be covered. It is advised to contact an attorney for review. Employment and labor laws change frequently, and policies and manuals must be updated to reflect the changes. Practices should reserve the right to update and modify employee manuals at any time. It is important to remain flexible, and employees should be made aware of changes as they occur and sign a form acknowledging the update.

OSHA, Occupational Safety and Health Administration; *SDS*, Safety Data Sheet.

can play a large role in attracting and retaining employees. Each benefit that is offered should be defined, and there should be clear statements about which employees qualify for them. If seasonal team members are employed, length of employment and benefits should be stated. Noncompete agreements must be addressed in employee manuals, as well as work schedule policies, codes of conduct, social media policies, and safety procedures (Box 5-3).

The following topics are covered in summary; review Box 5-3 for a complete listing of topics.

Philosophy and Mission Statements

Employee manuals should cover a variety of topics, including an overview of the practice mission, visions, and values. The practice mission may be the same as a purpose statement: the fundamental reason for the organization to exist. What is the purpose? What services are provided? Why are they important? These are just a few questions that can be answered when developing the practice mission. A vision may include goals the practice wishes to achieve and how they will be achieved. A positive and achievable goal must be established. The statement should be measurable and simple, and all team members should be able to participate in achieving the mission and vision of the practice (review Chapter 3).

Full-Time and Part-Time Employment

Full-time and part-time employment must be defined. Each practice can determine the number of hours per week required for a full-time position. Some practices may choose 40 hours per week, others may only require 34 hours. Overtime must be paid for any employee who works more than 40 hours per week (or as stated by state law). Those in violation can be penalized severely. *(Authors note: At time of publication, this law is being revised, which may change the number of hours required to be a full-time employee. Monitor state labor boards for continuously updated information.)*

Seasonal Employees

Some practices are extremely busy during specific months and must hire seasonal employees to survive the busy time. Job descriptions, duties, and dates of employment should be established, preventing any miscommunication. Seasonal employees should also sign that they have received, read, and understand the employee manual. Benefits are generally not offered to seasonal employees; however, this is at the discretion of the practice.

Benefits

Once full-time and part-time employees have been established, the benefits each position receives should be defined.

BOX 5-4 | Examples of Employee Benefits

- Health insurance
- Dental/vision insurance
- Continuing education
- Vacation
- Sick leave
- Holiday pay
- Professional liability insurance
- Disability insurance
- Life insurance
- Retirement plans
- Dues and licenses
- Veterinary care

Many benefit plans are included in full-time employment; however, it is up to the practice to decide what to offer. No governing agency requires benefits to be offered, but they certainly help in recruiting and retaining employees. It is highly recommended to offer as many benefits as possible to all employees (Box 5-4).

PRACTICE POINT   Benefits are not required by law, but they help attract and retain team members.

Employee salary and benefits statements should be provided to employees on an annual basis. Employees generally only see the monetary compensation they have received, as shown on their year-end Form W-2. Annual statements provide the overall picture because many employees do not know the value of the benefits they receive, and employers need to know that they are compensating their employees fairly.

Statements can be developed by each practice and basic information should be included in each statement. Statements should run for the entire fiscal year, giving a clear picture to the employee of how much the employer has paid in the previous year. Pretax compensation should be listed, along with Medicare and Social Security contributions made by the employer (team members do not realize the practice contributes to these funds). Insurance, vacation, continuing education, uniforms, sick days, holidays, pet health care, and any other benefits should be listed individually because each employee's benefit summary will be different. It should not take an excessive amount of time to prepare the statements, as all of the information should be easily retrievable through the accounting software (QuickBooks).

It is advised to discuss the statements with employees instead of handing them out without comment so that the employees will comprehend the full compensation and benefits plan. Historically, employees only consider their paycheck as compensation and forget that benefits are a real cost to the employer (Box 5-5).

Vacation

The amount of vacation that may be taken is determined by the practice and is generally built up over time. Vacation pay

---

BOX 5-5 | Example of Benefits Statement

Name of employee:	D. J. Stover
Period covered:	January 1, 2013, to December 31, 2013
Date of hire:	April 15, 1993
Salary or hourly wage:	$45,768.98 = $22/hour
Emergency compensation:	$0
Bonus:	$2500
Social Security and Medicare contribution:	$2837.68 + $663.63 = $3501.31
Health insurance:	$309.87/month (pay 100%) = $3718.44
Liability insurance:	$1200
Disability insurance:	$102/month = $1224
Holiday pay:	8 paid days; $22/hour × 8 hours/day = $176 × 8 days = $1408
Vacation:	3 weeks, 40 hours/week; $22 × 40 = $880/week × 3 = $2640
Sick time:	1 week (40 hours) = $22 × 40 = $880
Retirement:	3% of matching contribution = $3042/year
Uniforms:	New uniforms twice yearly = $180
Continuing education:	$1500 to be used at your discretion
Dues:	City and state veterinary medical associations, American Veterinary Medical Association = $350
Licenses:	State, controlled substances = $325
Pet medical care:	Total discounted services this year = $1650.89
Miscellaneous:	Lunches, ice cream breaks = $67.89/employee
Total benefits:	$20,187.53
Total salary and benefits:	$65,956.51
Benefits as a percentage of salary:	31%

---

should be offered and employees should be encouraged to take it. Without a vacation, stress, fatigue, irritability, and decreased production will result, which are all detrimental to the practice.

Factors to consider when determining vacation for the practice include length of employment time required before vacation can be used, time allotment, eligibility, accrual, schedule approval, and whether unused vacation is paid at the time of termination or resignation. As a general guideline, practices may allow 1 week per year for the first year, then increase 1 week per year to a maximum of 3 weeks. Practices often state that vacation should be used up within the fiscal year and should not be allowed to roll over to the following year (this is the choice of a practice). No law states how vacation should be determined or used. Team members should be asked to give sufficient notice to use vacation time, allowing schedules to be adjusted accordingly. Overtime is not paid when vacation is used within the week.

Another method of vacation determination is to base the time accrued by the number of hours worked per week. A long-term employee may receive 8 hours of vacation for every 100 hours of work.

PRACTICE POINT Practices are highly encouraged to offer vacation as a benefit; it is an important time that allows the employee to rest, relax, and rejuvenate, which helps prevent burnout in the long run.

Sick Leave

Just as with vacation, the amount of sick leave is generally built up with the time of service, and its use should be encouraged. Allowing one person time off when they are sick is better than having four people sick at once. Trying to prevent the spread of a virus is more economically advantageous!

Factors to account for when determining the rules for sick leave include how long a person must be employed before receiving paid sick leave, accrual, whether the practice will allow it to accrue year to year, and whether it is paid on termination or resignation. Overtime is not paid when using sick leave.

Insurance

Liability insurance is available in a variety of forms. Veterinarians must carry liability insurance, which is generally paid for by the practice. It is imperative that the liability insurance be high enough to cover any accident that may occur within the practice. This includes any animal-related injury, client injury, or accusation of malpractice. Managers must ensure these premiums are paid annually.

Health insurance can and should be available for full-time team members. It is generally cheaper for a business to offer health insurance than for individuals to buy health insurance. Practices may offer to pay 100% of the monthly payment, or less if they so choose. The employee is then responsible for the remaining percentage if the employer does not cover the entire premium.

Health insurance policies should be reviewed on an annual basis because premiums and coverage change frequently. When deciding which insurance plan to choose, team members should review both health maintenance organization (HMO) and preferred provider organization (PPO) plans because they can differ greatly in the doctors and laboratories covered as well as in co-payments and annual deductibles. HMOs are usually well managed and generally cover all medical expenses if patients use the doctors and laboratories within the approved network. PPOs offer a network of physicians and laboratories and encourage patients to use them; this is not required, but subscribers receive a lower amount of coverage if they choose a doctor that is out of network.

PRACTICE POINT Health insurance availability in a practice is a critical factor when potential employees are considering employment.

The Patient Protection and Affordable Care Act applies to businesses with 50 full-time employees or more; at the time of publication, practices with less than 50 employees are not required to provide health insurance. Visit www.shrm.org for the latest up-to-date information. It is important to consider that even if the practice does not offer health insurance as a benefit, every team member must have insurance, or will be fined by the government. Practices must keep this in mind, paying employees enough to cover their cost of healthcare.

Disability insurance is a benefit that some employers offer. Disability insurance is maintained to protect the employee against injury that results in the inability to perform tasks needed to complete the job. Back injuries, bite wounds that result in permanent damage, and carpal tunnel syndrome are just a few conditions that may prevent a team member from working to their full capacity. Three forms of disability insurance are available. *Own occupation* disability insurance covers any disability that does not allow a team member to return to that particular line of work. For example, if a veterinarian could no longer perform surgery because of a permanent hand injury but could see patients in a limited way, he would receive a small disability pension. *Any occupation* disability insurance covers any disability that does not allow the team member to return to any occupation. *Residual coverage* is important to professionals who become partially disabled and incur a loss of income from reduced duties. Residual benefits are based on the percentage of income lost. Team members need coverage in case they are permanently injured, especially if they are the main income producer of the family.

Workers' compensation insurance is not required in all states, but it is recommended. The Workers' Compensation Act was developed to protect the employer against any accident or injury that occurs on the job site. This type of compensation is detailed later in this chapter.

Insurance agents are excellent at helping small businesses find the right insurance plan at all levels. Ask clients and other local practices for referrals of reputable and reliable agents who provide courteous service. They can maximize the benefits for both the employer and employee while finding the most economically feasible policy.

Retirement Funds

A great benefit to offer employees is a retirement fund. Retirement funds are a growing trend in veterinary medicine and complement the benefits package well. The most common form of a retirement fund in general veterinary practice is a SIMPLE IRA (sIRA). SIMPLE is the abbreviation for Savings Incentive Match Plan for Employees, and IRA is short for Individual Retirement Account. sIRA plans are established by employers who want to allow eligible employees to set aside part of their pretax compensation as a part of their retirement savings plan. The employer must contribute either dollar for dollar or a percentage to all eligible employees. The employee can either contribute a set dollar amount per pay period or a percentage of the total pretax compensation. 401(k) plans are another common form of retirement fund in which employers are not required to contribute to the employee's account but can do so if they wish. Employees determine how much they wish to contribute on a monthly basis to their 401(k) plan.

Practices may also create a profit-sharing plan for employees in which they receive an annual share of the practice's profits. Profit-sharing gives employees a sense of ownership

in the company. This plan generally requires a plan administrator, and the percentage of profits is determined by management. Simplified Employee Pension plans (SEPs) are similar to profit-sharing plans and are appropriate for small organizations. They are funded by tax-deductible employer contributions, and employees are not allowed to contribute.

Retirement funds are highly regulated by the government through the Employee Retirement Income Security Act (ERISA) because of past negligence and abuse in the management of pension plans. Professional guidance from a broker is advised to determine which plan is best for the practice.

Retirement funds encourage team members to stay with the practice for the long term and reward employees for their dedication and hard work. The employer's match is tax deductible, making contributions a benefit for the practice.

Continuing Education

Continuing education (CE) should be a benefit available to all team members required to hold a license as well as those expected to continue to improve their job description and duties and those wanting to better themselves and the practice. Hospitals may determine a specific amount and give that dollar amount to each individual on a yearly basis, allowing team members to attend whichever form of CE they prefer. The set amount should include travel expenses, hotel, CE registration fees, and money to cover the cost of meals. If the practice chooses to cover those costs individually, team members should bring receipts back to the practice for reimbursement. These receipts should be kept for year-end taxes.

> **PRACTICE POINT** Every team member deserves continuing education. Create a budget for CE and use it!

Allowing a set dollar amount per team member can prevent overspending and holds team members accountable for their spending. They may choose CE on a local or state level, which ultimately saves money for the practice. CE can average $895 to $1850 per person for national or regional conferences (includes airfare, hotel, registration, and food).

Many local and state veterinary medical associations, along with manufacturers, hold continuing education events throughout the year, covering a variety of topics. Lunches or dinners are often offered at these free lectures, defraying some costs of attending. Technicians and veterinarians alike are normally invited to attend.

Holiday Pay

Practices may elect whether to pay employees for certain holidays. Holidays include New Year's Eve; New Year's Day; Martin Luther King, Jr. Day; Presidents' Day; Easter; Memorial Day; Independence Day; Labor Day; Veterans Day; Thanksgiving; Christmas Eve; and Christmas Day. Some practices only observe the major holidays; others prefer to observe a day that is meaningful to the practice. Holiday pay is usually paid to an employee who would normally work those hours on days when the practice has chosen to close.

Holiday pay is generally only 8 hours of pay, and overtime is not paid when holiday pay has been accumulated.

Uniforms

If team members are required to wear scrubs, the practice should provide them or compensate individuals for their purchase. The benefit to the practice in providing scrubs is the ability to control the clothing appearance of team members. If scrubs do not appear professional, they can be replaced without harassment. Employees should be held accountable for maintaining their uniforms in the best condition possible. Requiring all team members to wear the same color uniform on specific days adds to the professional appearance of the staff. Ask the team to pick the best colors and assign days to those colors. When having input, the team will comply much easier with the request. Many companies offer discounts when large orders are placed. Inquire with several companies to find the best price that fits the budget of the practice.

Membership Fees

Both veterinarians and credentialed technicians pay a variety of membership fees each year. State veterinary medical associations, national organizations, and specialty boards are just a few. Practices may offer to cover the dues, especially if the organization or association helps the practice in some way. Many state and national organizations have a voice in government affairs, and political action committees watch out for and defend veterinary interests. Practices should analyze all potential dues and set a guideline to follow when choosing to cover such expenses.

Licenses

Licenses held by veterinarians and technicians are renewed each year or biannually with a fee. Practices may wish to cover this expense, including the controlled substance license, state license, and any other license required to practice veterinary medicine.

The total cost of licensure fees and dues to organizations for one veterinarian averages $1200 per year. Practices should remember that these fees could be considered a write-off at the end of the year when taxes are being completed.

Employee Discounts

The practice has the discretion to determine employee discounts and how much they should be. Many practices allow team members to purchase items at a reduced cost. Internal Revenue Service (IRS) guidelines must be taken into consideration when providing discounts to team members. Employee discounts on *services* (greater than a 20% discount) are reported as fringe benefits and must be reported as pay. Visit www.irs.gov/pub/irs-pdf/p15b.pdf every January for the most current update of fringe benefits. Practices not reporting fringe benefits risk paying back taxes and fines. In lieu of employee discounts, hospitals may wish to extend pet health insurance to employees and cover the premium associated with this benefit.

PRACTICE POINT Be aware of the IRS guidelines on employee discounts: lack of compliance brings fines to both the employee and employee.

Code of Conduct

Employees are expected to maintain professionalism while on the premises. The code of conduct section of the employee manual should define each area in which there are specific expectations of team members. Appearance, confidentiality, quality of patient care, equipment care, and accountability for supplies and equipment are some topics that should be addressed.

Appearance is more than just looks. Clients respect and trust team members who appear professional. Body piercings, hair color, and tattoos should be addressed. Cleanliness, body odor, and wrinkle-free uniforms may be discussed as well as the appropriate application of makeup.

Although it seems impossible that team members will misunderstand that client and patient confidentiality is of utmost importance, it must be addressed in the employee manual. Team members must also understand that employee information and phone numbers are confidential and must never be given out. Information can never be given out without employee or client consent.

If a pet is lost and an unknown person calls the practice indicating that he or she has found a pet, the phone number and information should be written down, informing the unknown person that the client will be calling. The client should then be called and the information passed on to him or her. Never give the client's name and phone number to an unknown person. The practice does not know if the unknown person really has the pet, or if the person has criminal intentions. The practice can be held liable for giving out confidential information if this scenario ever occurs.

Work Schedule Policy

All team members need to be aware of the work schedule policy. Veterinarians are expected to be available during set appointment hours, and vacation or personal time must be scheduled in advance to accommodate the request. All other team members are expected to cover the shifts that have been assigned to them and must schedule vacation time in advance. Most practices will grant time off to team members as long as their shifts have been covered. The practice must establish a policy, include it in the employee manual, and enforce it. Team members who do not follow policy should be given a written warning. See the section on termination procedures in this chapter for guidance on documenting and enforcing procedures.

Team members should be made aware of the issues that arise when the practice is short staffed. Members must be held accountable for their shifts, and any absence (unless for an emergency or illness) is unacceptable. Team shortages contribute to increased stress levels, decreased team efficiency, and a decline in patient and client care. Shortages also produce individual resentment, again leading to decreased team morale.

Jury Duty

When team members are summoned for jury duty, they are obligated by law to attend. School, work, or any other excuse is not allowed. Team members should be encouraged to have their shift covered before jury duty, and management should help with this coverage. Jury duty is a public service and should be served with pride.

Training Procedures

Training procedures should be clearly defined in the employee manual. New team members should be advised of the training schedule (if one is available) and when they are expected to master those skills (more information on developing a training program is provided later in this chapter). The manual should indicate whether there is a probationary period (generally 30 days) and the step that follows the probation. If the new employee does not succeed during the probationary period, the manual should indicate that the employee would be terminated. If the employee does succeed, the manual should indicate whether the team member would receive an evaluation and/or a raise. Some practices have a 30-day probationary period, give an evaluation at 30 days, re-evaluate again at 90 days with a raise at that time. Manuals should also indicate how often evaluations will occur thereafter. It is recommended to provide (at minimum) yearly written evaluations for each team member, keeping copies in each team member's personnel file. See Chapter 3 for evaluation recommendations. In addition, coaching should occur on a daily basis. Employees cannot be expected to improve without daily feedback and negative criticism that happens once a year.

PRACTICE POINT Phase training programs are much more successful than simply *throwing the employee in* to learn the policies and procedures of the hospital.

Noncompete Agreements

Veterinarians, groomers, or other team members who are paid on a production basis or who are significant income producers for the practice may be asked to sign a noncompete or restrictive covenant agreement (NCA). An NCA is a contract that protects the business and employer by preventing the employee from opening a business or taking employment at a location within a certain number of miles of the practice. The purpose is to safeguard the veterinary practice when protectable interests are at risk. Owners have the right to protect tangible and intangible property.

An example of intangible property is practice goodwill. Practice goodwill is the reputation within the community, with colleagues and staff, and in doctor and client/patient relationships. Intangible property, also known as *incorporeal property,* describes something that a person or corporation can have ownership of and can transfer ownership to another person or corporation, but has no physical substance.

Tangible property is anything that can be touched and includes both real and personal property. Examples of tangible property are equipment, buildings and vehicles.

State laws vary regarding covenants, and they must be reasonable. The scope of activity is generally restricted and includes a time limitation and a geographic restraint. Historically, courts would not enforce covenants, and some are still reluctant to do so. If an NCA restricts a professional's ability to earn a living or restricts the public from having the benefit of the competition, courts may not enforce the NCA. Courts are slowly changing and will critically analyze the previous factors, including the restricted geographic location.

Safety and Security Procedures

Employees should receive safety training during the first few days of employment; team safety should be of utmost importance. Chapter 21 covers the development and implementation of a safety program if one is not already in use. OSHA recognizes and enforces employee safety, and rules and regulations have been implemented that employers must enforce (see Chapter 22).

Security in and around the practice 24 hours a day is very important. The outside premises should be well lit and secure for team members who are walking pets. Security cameras may be needed depending on the location of the practice.

Employee entrance doors should be locked at all times, preventing the entry of clients or criminals. The door should only be locked from the outside, allowing access out the door in the event of an emergency and quick escape from the building is needed.

The nature of the practice occasionally requires that staff members have access to the facility after hours. Consequently, security becomes an individual matter. Each team member has the responsibility to see that the practice is secured if he or she is the last person to leave. Keys should be issued to employees at the discretion of the practice manager and returned at the end of employment or at the request of the practice manager or owner. The practice may also wish to install key pads, allowing codes to be engaged/disengaged accordingly.

Reporting Accidents

Each accident should be reported to the owner and/or practice manager. Injuries can be serious and should not be hidden from management. When injuries occur, management should investigate and implement protocols to prevent the injury from reoccurring to another person. Proper forms must be completed when an injury has occurred, and the practice manager is responsible for ensuring that the forms are forwarded to the proper authorities when warranted (see Chapter 21 for OSHA Forms 300, 301, and 301A).

Probationary Period

Many practices use a probationary period when hiring new employees. This trial period allows new team members to try the position and see if they are a match for the practice. The practice reserves the right to terminate the new employees at the end of the trial period if they do not appear to be fulfilling the job requirements. The probationary period should be clearly stated in the offer of employment letter and employee manual, including the length of the period, and that the practice reserves the right to end employment without cause. Review state laws regarding lengths of probationary periods; states may require practices to pay unemployment if the length of time exceeded state requirements.

> **PRACTICE POINT**   Probationary periods must be clearly stated in the employee manual, along with the stage that follows (further training, promotion, or termination).

It can be detrimental to maintain employees who do not fit into the practice. Poor work ethic, poor performance, and negative attitudes are contagious, and if employees with these habits are kept for long-term employment, they can begin to affect the top notch team members.

Termination Procedures

Termination procedures are discussed in detail later in this chapter. However, the procedure should be discussed and clearly defined in the employee manual. Team members must be advised what to expect if the situation arises. Defined termination procedures also offer some protection to the practice if an unemployment claim or lawsuit ever arises.

Laws of Importance

Several legal topics need to be addressed and covered in the employee manual. These and other laws were discussed in detail earlier in this chapter.

Equal Employment Opportunity

A practice must follow Equal Employment Opportunity (EEO) guidelines. The practice cannot discriminate on the basis of race, color, sex, religion, or national origin and must state this to employees and potential employees.

Pregnancy

A practice cannot discriminate against pregnant team members. It is advised to state in the manual that team members are requested to inform management as soon as they are aware of the pregnancy so that all precautions can be addressed. A pregnant team member must decide what she can and cannot do. Safety issues can be addressed, such as radiation exposure, anesthesia, and heavy lifting; however, the team member must decide her own safety level. She cannot be changed from technician status to reception status unless she requests to do so.

> **PRACTICE POINT**   Pregnant women cannot be discriminated against in their job duties.

Sexual Harassment

Every team member must be protected from sexual harassment from both management and other team members. Sexual harassment occurs whenever unwelcomed sexual conduct is made a term or a condition of employment. It can occur when unwelcomed sexual conduct has the purpose or effect

of interfering with an individual's work performance or creating an offensive work environment. It can also occur when a supervisor conditions the granting of an employment benefit upon the receipt of sexual favors. Unwelcomed sexual conduct can be in the form of jokes, suggestive comments, insults, threats, suggestive noises, whistles, cat calls, touching, pinching, brushing against someone, assault, or coerced sexual intercourse. Policies must be developed, stated, and followed to protect the practice from a potential lawsuit. Promotion, demotion, or pay based on sexual innuendo cannot be allowed and must be clearly stated. The manual should also indicate with whom the employee should discuss possible sexual harassment violations, and that the discussion will occur without the possibility of retaliation. Practices must have a zero tolerance policy when it comes to sexual harassment.

Psychological Harassment

Psychological harassment is just as important as sexual harassment. Psychological harassment is characterized by bullying, gossiping, and creating a hostile work environment through behaviors that are not sexually related. Psychological harassment can come from managers, leaders, or other co-workers. However, if a manager does not stop or prevent psychological harassment from a co-worker, the manager can be charged with negligence. A zero tolerance policy for both sexual and psychological harassment must be included in the employee manual.

Managers must handle any harassment claims immediately. The longer the claim waits to be dealt with, the higher the risk of being held liable.

Social Media Policy

Social media is a broad term for Facebook, Twitter, Linked In, blogs, or Web pages. It has become an increasing popular way for communication among clients, friends and colleagues. However, it can affect the practice in a negative manner. Social media rules must be established, including who the social media manager is for the practice. The social media manager must review any information, pictures, or links before posting. Clients must authorize the use of patient photos before they can be used.

Team members must understand they are ambassadors for the practice, and anything posted (even if just to friends) will be disseminated to the world. Employees should be reminded to think twice before posting, and should withhold comments they would not want their spouse, mother, or grandmother to read. They must be held accountable for what they have posted, and reminded that the social media policy applies to not only those responsible for managing the practices social media pages, but all team members employed. Consider the following statement to be a part of a social media policy: *Ultimately, you are solely responsible for what you post online. Before creating online content, consider the risks and benefits that are involved. Keep in mind that any of your conduct that adversely affects your job performance, the performance of fellow team members, clients,*

patients, and distributor/manufacture representatives may result in disciplinary action up to and including termination. Inappropriate postings may include (but are not limited to) discriminatory remarks, harassment, threats of violence, or unprofessional comments. In addition, a manager may also include: refrain from using social media while on work time, unless it is work related and has been approved by management. Do not use the practice's email address to sign up for any social media networks, blogs, or tools for personal use.

Codes of conduct (in conjunction with their social media habits), zero tolerance of harassment, and release of confidential information must also be outlined, and rules can be applied just as stated in the employee manual (if termination can occur as stated in the employee manual for the previously discussed topics, it can also occur in regard to social media policy violations). Laws and regulations affecting social media are changing on a regular basis, and managers must remain vigilant when developing and maintaining policies. Visit the Society for Human Resource Management at www.shrm.org for the most up-to-date regulations and acceptable social media policies. Because social media laws change, remind employees the social media policy can be updated at anytime.

Job Descriptions and Duties

Now that the employee manual has been developed, job descriptions can be focused on. Job descriptions must be detailed and include every aspect and expectation of that job. Team members cannot be held to expectations if the duty was not listed in the job description; with that being said, the phrase "and any other task assigned by a supervisor" can be added to most job descriptions. If the practice is large and has several departments, a description may include a statement such as "Every employee works for ABC Veterinary Hospital as a whole, not for a particular supervisor or department." It is clearly defined that each team member is to help anyone who needs help, not just those within his or her own department.

Examples of summarized job duties and descriptions in Box 5-6 are in no way complete (also review the job duties in Chapter 1, Boxes 1-2 to 1-4, 1-6, 1-8 to 1-10, and 1-12). They can be added to or deleted. Each practice varies, and duties and descriptions should be developed for each hospital.

Hard skills are competencies that are required of the position or could be learned through training. Examples of hard skills for veterinary technicians would include placing a catheter, giving vaccinations, or administrating tablets to a dog. Soft skills are competencies that cannot be taught and are generally developed in individuals as they mature. Soft skills competencies include a strong work ethic, promptness, attentiveness, or leadership abilities. Both sets of skills are critical to evaluate when creating job descriptions and searching for the right candidate. Because hard skills can be trained and soft skills cannot, oftentimes it is advantageous to hire an employee based on a strong set of soft skills.

BOX 5-6	Sample of Summarized Job Descriptions

Kennel Assistant

A kennel assistant will be expected to assist a veterinarian, veterinary technician, or assistant in the care of animals. This may include restraining, cleaning, and walking the patients. The kennel assistant will maintain the constant cleanliness of the kennels, cages, and ward area, including the care and feeding of all animals. Kennel assistants are expected to have knowledge of cleaning and disinfecting methods and use proper chemicals and equipment to complete the task safely and efficiently. The assistant should be able to patiently treat sick and debilitated patients as well as understand and carry out written and oral instructions. Kennel assistants must be able to lift and carry patients up to 50 lb as needed and required by team members. If any problems arise, kennel assistants should report them to the practice manager immediately.

Veterinary Assistant

A veterinary assistant will be expected to assist the veterinarian and veterinary technician in the care of animals. This may include restraining, cleaning, and walking the patients; providing medical care assigned by the veterinarian; as well as offering any communication to the client as specified by the veterinarian. The assistant will also perform laboratory analysis, take and develop radiographs, and assist the receptionist with answering the phone and providing customer service as needed. An assistant is expected to be pleasant, patient, courteous, and polite to clients and team members at all times and contribute to keeping the office flowing in an organized, efficient manner. Assistants must have knowledge of vaccination protocols, pharmacology, nutrition, animal husbandry and care and must be able to lift and carry patients up to 50 lb as needed and required by team members. If any problems arise, assistants should report them to the practice manager immediately.

Veterinary Technician

A veterinary technician will be expected to assist the veterinarian in the care of animals. This may include restraining, cleaning, and walking the patients; providing medical care assigned by the veterinarian; as well as offering any communication to the client as specified by the veterinarian. The technician will also perform laboratory analysis, take and develop radiographs, and assist the receptionist with answering the phone and providing customer service as needed. The technician may oversee the kennel and veterinary assistants and provide continuing education for these staff members. The veterinary technician is held to the highest standard of care and must ensure all patients receive the appropriate treatments and nutrition and be kept in a safe and clean environment. A technician must be able to educate clients on the care and condition of their pets. Veterinary technicians are expected to be pleasant, patient, courteous, and polite to clients and team members at all times and contribute to keeping the office flowing in an organized, efficient manner. Technicians must have knowledge of vaccination protocols, pharmacology, nutrition, and animal husbandry and care. Veterinary technicians must be able to lift and carry patients up to 50 lb as needed by team members. If any problems arise, veterinary technicians should report them to the practice manager immediately.

Receptionist

A receptionist is expected to provide the highest level of customer service and care. This is to be done by answering phones, scheduling appointments, answering client questions, pulling patient charts, checking clients in and out, and accepting payments. A receptionist will maintain a professional appearance and behave in a professional manner at all times, speak clearly and slowly for clients to understand, and relay reliable information to clients as directed by the veterinarian and/or veterinary technicians. If any problems arise, the receptionist should report them to the office manager immediately.

Office Manager

An office manager is expected to provide the highest level of customer service and care. This is to be done by answering phones, scheduling appointments, answering client questions, pulling patient charts, checking clients in and out, and accepting payments. Office managers will maintain a professional appearance and behave in a professional manner at all times, speak clearly and slowly for clients to understand, and relay reliable information to clients as directed by the veterinarian and/or veterinary technician. Managers are responsible for the training of receptionists and for overseeing all duties that are expected of them. The office manager is held to the highest standard and should ensure that all customers are satisfied and have received the value of service they have paid for. If any problems arise, office managers should report them to the practice manager immediately for guidance.

Practice Manager

The practice manager oversees the kennel assistant, veterinary assistant, veterinary technician, reception, and office management teams. The practice manager ensures that all team members receive proper training and that all standards of care are being met. The practice manager may oversee inventory management, scheduling, and maintenance of equipment. If problems arise, the practice manager should report them to the hospital administrator or owner for guidance.

Veterinarian

A veterinarian will see patients to diagnose and treat disease, perform surgery, and prescribe medications. A veterinarian will delegate duties of laboratory analysis and animal care to technicians and assistants, allowing more client/veterinarian interaction and education. Veterinarians are held to the highest standard of care; they are ultimately responsible for the care and treatment of patients and must advise clients of the best options available for their patients. Problems with training or with team members not completing their duties correctly should be discussed with the practice manager and hospital administrator.

Hospital Administrator

A hospital administrator oversees the entire function of the veterinary hospital. The administrator is responsible for creating and maintaining budgets, finances, hospital protocols, and procedures. This position requires the use of accounting and financial tools, which must be used for the practice to be successful.

PRACTICE POINT Ensure that job descriptions are lengthy and detailed; then use these descriptions in the performance evaluations.

Each description should have the following fundamentals addressed:

- *A position title.* This helps give form to the position and may help create a hierarchy in larger hospitals.
- *A summary.*
- *Duties and responsibilities.* Skilled, specialized, and basic duties must all be listed. Essential skills, such as lifting a 50-lb dog or providing client education, cannot be left out.
- *Description of required skills and qualifications.*
- *Accountability.* State the person to whom this person or position will report.

Job descriptions and duties should be given to each applicant during the interview process. Applicants must fully understand the entire job of a veterinary hospital. This will allow the interviewer and candidate to compare skills and abilities and determine whether the applicant is a match for the position.

Although job descriptions are not required by law, they can certainly protect a practice against potential lawsuits, unemployment, and discrimination suits. Job descriptions also add clarity and consistency for team members (everyone knows what everyone else's job duties and expectations include). Job descriptions must be tied to performance expectations, and reviewed with employees during annual or semiannual evaluations (see Chapter 3 for more details). These descriptions and job duties must be evaluated annually to check for any changes that may have occurred. Has the practice purchased new equipment? Have protocols changed? If yes, then job descriptions could also be changed or added to.

Hiring the Perfect Team

Now that the employee manual and job descriptions are complete, a plan can be created for hiring a team member. But how do you know "who" you need to hire? What position will benefit the practice the most (veterinary assistant, veterinary technician, or veterinarian)? Having a plan in place will prevent a quick-to-hire mentality that practices often have. Managers must know who they want to hire and what qualifications and skills they are looking for. Having a plan prevents "emotional hiring" (hiring someone simply because you like them, but they lack the skills or qualifications needed).

Veterinary practice managers recruit, interview, and hire new employees.

When to Hire

Knowing which position to hire for can be difficult without a true evaluation of the hospital practices. Managers must be diligent about this investigation, as it can have a positive or negative effect on the practice's finances and on the team's morale. There are five key factors that managers should evaluate: veterinary/staff ratio, veterinary production, team member's production, hospital flow, and staff payroll percentages.

Benchmarks show that the average number of full-time staff members to one full-time equivalent veterinarian is 4.8 (AAHA, 2013). It is critical for veterinarians to have the ability to leverage duties to team members. If leveraging cannot occur (because of low staff numbers), veterinarians are doing the duties of technicians (versus only their duties of prescribing medications, diagnosing, and performing surgery). Teams must be strong in numbers to generate income. Veterinary production numbers are then evaluated as well. As stated previously, if the team is not leveraged, the veterinarian cannot produce money. In the average general practice, the team's efforts will bring in approximately 50% of the income (passive income) and the veterinarian(s) will generate the remaining 50% (active income). If practices are not producing these numbers, staffing, leveraging, and training must be investigated.

PRACTICE POINT Be cognizant of the active and passive income patterns when determining who and when to hire.

Team member production is also critical. Perhaps a team is strong and assumes all of the responsibilities it should, allowing the veterinarian to complete their three duties diligently. However, if the team is overworked and understaffed, they may not be able to support the 50% passive income that every practice should strive for. In addition, overworked team members get home from work and do not have any energy left to have a life outside of their job. Diligent managers will investigate and ensure employees are not spread too thin and have a balance between work and life; without this balance, burnout is inevitable (see Chapter 6).

Hospital flow is just as critical to evaluate as the veterinary/staff ratio and veterinary/team member productions. The following questions should be asked:

- How many times does the phone ring before it is answered? Once answered, how long do clients have to wait on hold?
- How long does it take for a client to get an appointment? (is the wait time 1 week, 2 weeks, etc.?)
- How long are clients waiting before they enter the exam room?
- How long are clients waiting before they are seen by the veterinarian?
- Are patient care standards being met?
- Are client service standards being met?

Being able to answer these questions can help determine what positions should be hired for. If there is a backlog of appointments, is it because the veterinarian is overbooked (or is the team too busy, therefore eliminating appointments?) Can training and increased team accountability and/or responsibility alleviate some of this backlog?

Phones should ring no more than two times (see Chapter 2), and chaos at the front desk can create a negative perception of the practice by clients. Can hiring a receptionist alleviate this issue?

Patient care and customer service must be the number one priority of every practice. If either of these areas is ever compromised, an investigation into what, where, why, and how it occurred must ensue. Did the patient not receive treatments because the team is short staffed? Was the wrong treatment administered because of a lack of training? Did the customer not receive the service expected because the team was rushed?

> **PRACTICE POINT** Great customer service is provided when team members are not short staffed, rushed or under educated. Make sure your team meets these standards to provide the best possible care.

Payroll percentages should always be monitored, especially for overtime. Overtime will definitely hurt the practice financially; however, it will also hurt the employee because working long hours (and being underpaid) results in burnout. Employees that are burned out are less motivated, bring in less money, do not work together as a "team," and eventually leave the practice. Managers must not rely only on percentages; all of the previous factors must be evaluated. Most often, when payroll budgets are cut, so is the customer service provided to clients (decreased customer service yields lost clients, referrals, and compliance).

Having a team of highly motivated, positive team members with a strong work ethic can make a practice successful and take it to the next level; one employee who lacks motivation and enthusiasm can break the entire team. Sometimes, practices need to hire for personality and work ethic, and then train for the skill that is needed. One cannot hire for skill and train personality or work ethic. Team members either have it or they do not, and it is useless to hire an unmotivated person. Unmotivated and irritable staff members affect all team members and create a negative environment. This can be detrimental to a practice and should be prevented at all costs.

Reviewing Resumes

Applicants may provide a resume for review when applying for a position within the hospital. Resumes should be short and to the point, with applicants clearly stating what they are looking for in a position. Do not make notes on resumes because they remain part of the personnel file if the applicant is hired. Notes should be made on a separate piece of paper. Also remember that the threat involving claims of discrimination in the hiring process is real, so good defensive tactics must be practiced throughout the entire hiring process (treat all prospects the same; ask the same interview questions and check all references).

Reviewing Letters of Reference

It is important to follow up on any letter of reference. Some letters are written to ease a difficult termination; others may have been unwilling to express any reservations that were held at the time of the employee resignation or termination. Therefore, an outstanding letter of reference is not always a true reflection of the applicant's abilities. Phone calls are advised on all applicants; one candidate cannot be treated differently from another.

References

It is imperative to call all references listed. If a candidate has not provided a list of references with the resume and/or application, one should be asked for at the time of the interview. It can be difficult to obtain useful information when calling references. Because of the increase in defamation lawsuits, past employers are reluctant to provide any information, either positive or negative. Information that is permissible must be factual and documented in written evidence. All references on all candidates should be checked, and the same questions should be asked. One applicant cannot be treated differently from another. Calling references can also reveal discrepancies with the applicant's resume and/or interview.

Using Social Media to Review Candidates

Employers looking to hire candidates must use caution; searching social media sites may reveal information about an individual's protected status under federal or state law. This information may include a person's age, race, political affiliation, national origin, or disabilities. At the time of publication, 28 states have laws that protect applicants from employers that may discriminate against them for engaging in lawful activities such as smoking (which may be revealed in social media photos). If an applicant feels that they did not get hired because of content on their social media page, they can bring a case of discrimination before the National Labor Relations Board.

Asking the Right Questions

With the *best team* in mind, it is essential to ask the right questions when interviewing potential candidates (Figure 5-8). Questions such as "Tell me about yourself," "What do you know about our practice?" and "What is your single greatest achievement?" stimulate discussion instead of eliciting a yes or no answer. "Describe a typical day in your last job" promotes

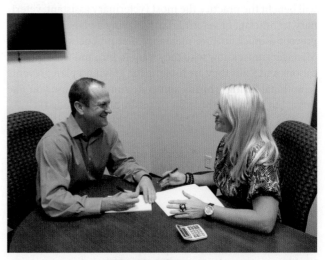

FIGURE 5-8 Interview.

discussion regarding work ethic. Questions should prompt the candidate to show his or her skill and potential. Open-ended questions allow the applicant to discuss the question asked. *What, when, where, why,* and *how* are excellent words to use when asking an open-ended question. Every person believes he or she has an excellent work ethic and a great personality; the interviewer must be able to distinguish whether this is true. Closed-ended questions allow only a yes or no answer (Box 5-7).

One may also ask candidates if previous employers can be called; answers may provide a clue to the past employment history. Once employers are called, an important question to ask is, "Would you rehire this person?" The response can provide valuable information regarding the candidate.

If a potential employee's original interview goes well, a working interview may be considered to help determine an individual's work ethic and skill. Many applicants may state they are qualified for the position, and a working interview will help determine whether certain skills are met. This also allows team members to weigh in and give their opinion of the potential hire. It is important to remind all team members what questions cannot be asked during this working interview.

Questions Not to Ask

The hiring process is highly regulated by federal and state laws, which exist for the protection of potential employees. Many questions cannot be asked in an interview. Any questions related to marriage, age, gender, religion, and military status are strictly prohibited. The interviewer cannot ask female applicants different questions than male applicants and cannot ask if they have any children. See Box 5-8 for a list of questions that cannot be asked.

Pre-employment Screening

The Fair Credit Reporting Act is a federal law that regulates prescreening reports issued to employers by outside agencies called *credit reporting agencies.* Employers may use these consumer reports to help screen employees. These can also be referred to as part of a background check. State regulations vary regarding the amount of credit information that can be obtained from these reports. Please review state regulations

when considering this information. Background checks are a matter of public record; however, employers must have the consent of the applicant before any reports are obtained. Managers should consider hiring a payroll firm in order to obtain the most complete background checks. Local companies may only complete a local search; however, potential employees can have a history in any other state!

Practices can also administer a grammar and/or spelling test, perhaps including some medical terminology. A typing test may also be appropriate if the position includes a large amount of typing or transcription services.

The First Day for a New Hire

A new team member's first day can be intimidating, overwhelming, and daunting. The employee should be introduced to the rest of the staff, given a tour of the practice, and then taken to a quiet area to review practice policy and procedures. The new employee should fill out new hire forms, including Form W-4 (federal income tax withholding form), state tax forms (if required), Form I-9 (employment eligibility verification form), forms for accepting or declining any employee benefit plans, and emergency contact information. Copies of any credentials should be made at this time. The employee should receive his or her own copy of the employee personnel manual, review it verbally with a manager, and sign a document stating he or she has received, read, and understands the manual.

> *PRACTICE POINT*   Do you remember what it was like the first day you started in the practice? Most responses include feeling scared, intimidated, and overwhelmed. Find ways to prevent your new hire from experiencing these feelings.

The new team member should be given a copy of the procedure manual and reassured that he or she is not expected to know all the information within the manual on the first day. The phase training program that the hospital has implemented should be explained, along with the expected dates of completion. The new employee should be allowed to observe

BOX 5-7	Asking the Right Questions

- Are you currently employed? Why or why not?
- How long have you been employed at your current job?
- Why would you want to leave your current position?
- Describe a typical day at your last job.
- What did you enjoy about your past job?
- What position do you expect to fill?
- If you joined our team, what abilities would you bring?
- Describe your summer employment.
- What do you feel are your outstanding qualities?
- What was the least enjoyable aspect of your last job?
- What are some areas you feel you need improvement on?
- Are you able to work a weekend schedule?
- When would you be available to begin work?
- What is your salary requirement?

BOX 5-8	Questions NOT to Ask

- Do you have any children?
- What is your national origin?
- Where are your parents from?
- What is your maiden name?
- Have you ever been arrested?
- Do you have any physical disabilities?
- Have your wages ever been garnished?
- What type of military service have you been involved with?
- What is your native language?
- What clubs and societies do you belong to?
- Have you ever filed for workers' compensation?
- What is your religion?
- What holidays do you observe?
- Do you prefer to be addressed as Ms., Miss, or Mrs.?
- When did you graduate from high school?

the whole team for the rest of the day and encouraged to ask questions. Hands-on training can begin the following day. Taking the new employee to lunch adds a personal touch to the day. Team members can ask questions and learn about each other out of the office. Overwhelming the new employee during the first week sets him or her up for failure, and it is ultimately a management issue.

Employee Procedure Manual

An employee procedure manual not only helps train new employees, it also provides a guide to look up procedures as needed. Procedure manuals take time to develop and must be updated frequently to provide consistency with all team members (Box 5-9).

BOX 5-9 Sample Table of Contents for Employee Procedure Manual

Animal bites
Artificial insemination
Bandages/splints/casts
    Pressure bandages
    Wound management
        Dry bandages
        Wet-to-dry bandages
    Splints/casts
Blood transfusions
    Fresh frozen plasma
    Whole blood
        Equipment needed
Catheters
    Butterfly
    Foley catheters
    IV catheters
    Jugular catheters
    Polypropylene catheters
    Red rubber catheters
    Tom cat catheters
Common diseases
    Dog
    Cat
Common emergencies
    CPR
    Anaphylactic reaction
    Blocked cat
    Dyspneic animal
    Dystocia
    Gastric torsion
    Seizures
    Toxicities
Declaws
    Equipment
    Procedure
    Paper strips
Dentals
    Machine
    Gum disease
    Anatomy of the mouth
Determining age of cats and dogs
Diets
    Dogs
    Cats
    Ferrets
    Rabbits
    Reptiles
    Snakes
    Birds
    Special diets (Hills, Waltham, Purina)

Fluids
    Types
    Additives
    Catheter types and sizes
    Catheter use and maintenance
    Heparin bags and prep
    Administration of fluids
    Drip rate calculation
Heartworm disease
    Life cycle of the heartworm
    Treatment
    Prevention
Instruments
    Care and handling
    Autoclaving
    General pack
    Cold sterilization
    General cold pack
Kennel care
    Duties
    Cleaning procedures
    Blankets
Laboratory equipment and procedures
    Centrifuges
    Microscopes
    IDEXX ProCyte Dx Hematology Analyzer
    Hemocytometer
    Refractometer
    Tonometer
    Diagnostic tests and lab work
        Blood work abbreviations
        Heartworm test
        SNAP
        Parvo
        FELV
        FELV/FIV/HWT
        WBC
        HCT or PCV
        TP
        UA
        Fecal
        DTM
        Ear smear
        Ear mite check
        Skin scrape
        Staining slides
    Protocols for common blood work
        ACTH stimulation
        Bile acids
        Phenobarbital
        Thyroid

Logs
  Lab log
  Surgery log
  Controlled drug log
  Radiology log
Medications
  Abbreviations
  Weight conversions
  Labels
  Administration
Neutering pets; see spaying/neutering pets
Pregnancy
  Care of female
  Care of puppies and kittens
  Problems with pregnancy
  Cesarean section
  Gestation/reproductive maturity
Radiology
  Machine function
  Radiology chart
  Radiology log
  Filing
  Radiation safety
  Aprons and care of
  Dark room/processor
Reproductive disorders
  Cryptorchidism
  Incontinence
  Mastitis
  Metritis
  Prostate
    Cystic hyperplasia
    Prostate tumors
  Pyometra
Restraint (for exam and venipuncture)
  Dog
  Cat
  Ferret
  Rabbits
  Iguana
  Birds

Room
  Room prep
  Supplies
Safety data sheets
  Location
  How to read
Safety plan and hazards communication (OSHA)
Spaying/neutering pets
  Age
  Benefits
  Risks associated with surgery
  Postoperative care
Surgery
  NPO
  Autoclave
    Care and maintenance
  Packs
    Instrument packs
    Cold pack
    Gown and towel pack
    Towel pack
    Drapes
  Needles and suture material
  Surgery prep
  Biopsy prep
  Anesthesia
    Drugs
    Endotracheal tubes
    Monitoring
  Anesthetic machines and maintenance
  Isoflurane refill
  Oxygen
Syringes
  Varieties and gauges of needles
Vaccines and protocols
  Dog
  Cat
  Ferret

ACTH stim, Adrenocorticotropic hormone stimulation; *CPR,* cardiopulmonary resuscitation; *DTM,* dermatophyte test medium; *FELV,* feline leukemia; *FIV,* feline immunodeficiency virus; *HCT,* hematocrit; *NPO,* nothing by mouth; *PCV,* packed cell volume; *TP,* total protein; *UA,* urinalysis; *WBC,* white blood cell count.

Developing an Employee Procedure Manual

Every procedure that is used in the practice should be listed. To start, team members may be asked to write up different procedures that are used on a daily basis. An outline can be useful to help organize procedures by department or technique, which then can be developed into a table of contents. The procedure manual can be organized in alphabetical order for easy and quick retrieval. Information included in each section should define the procedure, list the steps to accomplish the procedure, and include an explanation as to why the procedure is completed in that fashion. This allows team members to completely understand and be able to explain procedures to clients when

needed. Figure 5-9 lists several topics that can be included in a manual.

Implementing an Employee Procedure Manual

When team members participate in creating an employee procedure manual, they are more likely to help implement it and make use of it. Once it has been completed, each team member should receive a copy, and a hard copy should be kept within the practice. It should be placed in a central location and be easy to find. Paperless practices can upload the employee procedure manual onto the computer system, allowing team members to access it from any computer in the clinic.

Animal Bites:

Any bite is BAD! If you are bitten under any circumstances, you need to report it to Nancy and go to your doctor. Cats are the worst. They have the most bacteria and the worst bacteria. You must receive antibiotics from your doctor. If you do not, call Nancy. Be sure the doctor does not suture the wound closed.

Artificial Insemination:

In both dogs and cats, breeding can occur naturally between a male and a female, or by *artificial insemination (AI):* To breed by AI, semen must be collected from the male and then either inserted directly into the female or deep-frozen for later use. The female must be in the proper stage of the estrous cycle. Once the semen is collected, it must be inserted into the female as soon as possible. If it is frozen it needs to warm to room temperature, be evaluated, and inserted into the female.

Equipment needed for AI:
- Rubber vulva
- Collection vial
- Slides to evaluate semen (place on microscope to warm slides)
- AI tube
- 12-mL syringe
- KY Jelly

Bandages/Splints/Casts:

Bandages: Bandages are used to protect an area (an incision), apply pressure to a specific area, or cover a wound. Bandages used to protect an area (e.g., after a dewclaw surgery) generally have a Telfa pad over the area, with some absorbent gauze and vet wrap. A bandage used to apply pressure (e.g., after a declaw surgery) requires absorbent gauze and vet wrap. If it is to apply pressure to the abdominal area, we may use an Ace bandage. For wound management, various types of bandages can be used. A **wet to dry bandage** is used when a wound cannot be sutured closed. A Kotex pad soaked with saline is applied to the wound, which is normally wrapped lightly with an Ace bandage. These bandages need to be changed at least twice daily. **A dry bandage** normally consists of a Telfa pad on the wound, which is wrapped with cotton bandage material, brown Kling gauze, then vet wrap. These bandages need to be changed frequently depending on the case and the doctor. A bandage must have "stirrups" (tape on the leg itself and wrapped around the bandage material). This helps stabilize the bandage to prevent it from slipping.

Splints/Casts: These are used to stabilize a broken bone. A splint may be used in place of a cast if there is an underlying wound dressing that needs to be changed frequently. Both splints and casts require a lot of padding to prevent pressure sores. First apply stirrups to both sides of the leg. Wrap the leg with cotton gauze high enough to protect the leg from the top of the cast or splint (always wrap from the toes toward the shoulder). Next, wrap the leg with brown Kling gauze, being sure not to wrap the leg too tight. If you are applying a splint, one stirrup should be taped onto the bandage and the other onto the splint. Secure the splint with additional tape as needed. Wrap the splint with brown Kling gauze and vet wrap. Be sure to check the toes daily for swelling. If

FIGURE 5-9 Example of employee procedure manual.

> **PRACTICE POINT**   Ask all team members to help in the creation of an employee procedures manual. This will help improve accountability of team members and improve implementation procedures.

When new employees are hired, they must also receive their own copy. Each section can then be covered and explained over the course of several weeks. Covering all information within a short period of time will overwhelm new team members and they will be unlikely to remember what is covered in the manual. The procedure manual can be used to develop a training guide and schedule, covered later in this chapter. When team members question a protocol, they can reference the employee procedure manual. In many cases, certain techniques are used so infrequently that their protocols are forgotten.

Updating the Employee Procedure Manual

Each time a vaccine protocol, laboratory procedure, or surgical prep technique changes, the employee manual must be updated. Team members should receive a single sheet indicating the change, and employees should sign a form indicating they have received the update (similar to the employee manual protocol).

Changes can be hard for some team members to implement, especially when a routine with a particular procedure has been established. They may become resistant to the change, even though it has been formally established and they have signed the form indicating they are aware of the change. Some employees resist change because of their discomfort level with the change or new procedure. Training these employees with a different approach may improve compliance; these team members should also be

there is any swelling, the splint needs to be redone. If you are applying a cast, soak the cast material in warm water for 1 minute. (Be sure to use gloves so that you do not get adhesive on your hands.) Apply the cast material and allow it to dry (approximately 3 to 5 minutes). Tape the stirrups onto the cast and wrap with vet wrap. ALWAYS leave space at the toes to check for swelling.

DO NOT ALLOW CASTS OR SPLINTS TO GET WET. If the animal must be outside, the foot can be wrapped in a plastic bag to protect the cast or splint. If the pet comes inside, remove the bag because sweaty paw pads will also get the splint or cast wet.

Blood Transfusions:

We have several different options when administering a transfusion. Once the method has been chosen, make sure all the products needed are available. If this is the first transfusion for the pet, the blood does not have to be cross-matched. If the pet has had prior transfusions, the blood must be matched to the donor. Reactions can occur in any animal. All patients must be monitored during and after the administration of the transfusion.

- *Plasma transfusion:* Fresh frozen plasma is used to treat animals with low protein or clotting factors. It must be ordered from the Animal Blood Bank. It is shipped overnight on ice and must be frozen until ready to use. Once you are ready to use it, thaw it to room temperature and use it within 24 hours. It is administered with a standard 15 d/mL IV infusion set.
- *Whole blood:* Whole blood is used to replace all blood components. It is generally donated from a staff member's pet. The doctor must determine that the donating pet is healthy, has not donated in the past 12 weeks, is parasite free, and is large enough to donate the amount of blood needed. The donor is placed on a table, and either the jugular vein or cephalic vein is clipped as for a catheter. A blood collection set is used. One end is inserted into the appropriate sized ACD bottle (a hemostat clip is placed on the line to prevent vacuum loss in the bottle). The 14-g needle is inserted into the vein (and secured as with an IV catheter and line). Once the blood flashes back, remove the hemostat and gently agitate the bottle while it is filling. Once the bottle is full, apply the hemostat onto the line again and remove the collection set from the donor pet. Apply a tight bandage to the site to prevent a hematoma if a cephalic vein is used. The donor pet should be fed a great meal after the donation. This donated blood is good for 3 weeks. It should be discarded after that. When administering the transfusion, a blood transfusion set is used. Prep the cephalic vein as you would for a general IV catheter. Insert the transfusion set into the collection bottle and allow the chamber to fill. Insert a catheter and flush with a heparin solution. Attach the transfusion set and administer at the recommended dose. Observe for any reaction.

The following supplies are needed for whole blood transfusions:
  - Blood collection set
  - Blood administration set
  - ACD bottle
  - Catheter
  - Tape
  - Vet wrap
  - Treats for the blood donor

FIGURE 5-9, cont'd

Continued

asked why they oppose the change. They may have valuable insight that management has forgotten, and taking the new approach may help other employees implement the change as well.

Standards of Care

Standards of care (SOCs) are simply that: guidelines and treatment protocols that have been established allowing the highest quality of medical care to be recommended for every patient. SOCs are developed by the veterinarians for the most common cases that a practice sees. These guidelines include diagnostics and treatment of such diseases as heartworm, parvovirus, and ear infections. When SOCs are established, every team member is on the same page recommending the same treatment protocol to clients. This enhances client compliance and communication. See Chapter 11 for more information on SOCs.

Employee procedure manuals and SOCs are excellent training protocols for all the team members, new and experienced.

Team Training

There cannot be enough emphasis placed on the importance of team training. The success of a practice depends on the *quality* and *quantity* of training. New employees without any training should start with the basics, preventing them from becoming overwhelmed with new information. New team members with experience should still follow a training protocol, taking care not to skip procedures and protocols. New employees with experience can breeze through training but are likely to miss critical practice protocols when a phase training program is not followed. Training should be fun and creative. ***Telling is not training,*** and it will reduce the amount of information that is retained.

Catheters:

Butterfly: These catheters come with 25-g and 28-g needles. They are commonly used for subcutaneous fluids in exotic animals, ferrets, birds, and very small dogs and cats. We also use them to administer IV drugs to exotic pets. They are great for subcutaneous fluids when an animal is extremely wiggly; it allows movement without injuring the animal.

Foley catheters: These are generally used to do a cystogram (injecting dye into the bladder of a pet). Foley catheters have 2 ports: one to inject medication into and the other to inflate the balloon.

IV catheters: Selection of types of catheters and gauge depends on species and size, fragility of veins, length of time the catheter will be in place, and type of fluids administered.   A 24-g catheter is commonly used for cats, a 22-g catheter for a small to medium dog, and a 20-g catheter for a large dog. A larger dog should also have a longer (2-inch catheter) versus the normal 1-inch catheter for medium and small dogs.

Jugular catheters: These are used to do transtracheal washes on pets. We commonly use 16-g and 18-g catheters.

Polypropylene catheters: We commonly use these catheters for blocked dogs. These catheters come in a variety of sizes in a large white tube. They are sterile in the tube, so be sure not to empty them or touch them when you remove one.

Red rubber catheters: These can be used for either tube feeding an animal or to insert into a blocked cat. They are individually packaged and come in sizes from 3 French to 14 French.

"Tom cat" catheters: These are used for blocked cats and come in one size. They are also packaged individually and are sterile in each package.

FIGURE 5-9, cont'd

Veterinary practice managers create and manage personnel training and development programs (including safety training).

> **PRACTICE POINT** Ask all team members to help in the creation of an employee procedures manual; this will help improve accountability of team members and improve implementation procedures.

An excellent attitude is the No. 1 skill that is often forgotten. Practices overlook training and development of positive attitudes. A great attitude starts at the top and trickles down to the rest of the team. Owners, associates, and management must have a positive attitude every day; this encourages the rest of the team to follow. Positive attitudes are contagious and can lift the spirits of those around them; bad attitudes foster failure.

Developing a Training Protocol

The creation of a phase training list that must be completed will help ensure that team members are trained properly. Each practice is different; development of these modules can be done on an individual basis. Some protocols may work well in one practice but not in another. Tweaks and changes should be made to protocols to continue to produce the best quality of training. Training takes time and must be done in phases. Too much information will overload the new employee, who may not return to work the following day.

An excellent protocol has different levels of training and allows team members a reasonable amount of time to master the skills within each phase. It is important that inexperienced team members understand why protocols are completed in such a manner, and that the protocols give examples of possible consequences of misinterpreted instructions. Skills should be detailed to ensure complete understanding of each skill. For example, customer service has a variety of skills under its umbrella: answering the phone courteously, greeting clients as they enter the practice, and answering questions a client may have (Box 5-10).

Training should occur during open hours. Hands-on training is much more effective than talking or reading, and when team members have to practice the skill over and over, and under the supervision of another team member, they are more likely to retain the information.

Basic modules for kennel assistants should include kennel duties and tasks. Included in a basic module would be cleaning techniques, chemicals, and the knowledge of diseases and their transmission. Animal handling, restraint, exercise, and basic nutrition may be addressed in modules to follow.

Veterinary assistants should be expected to know all the material for kennel assistants, a perfect example for module 1. The following modules can then cover surgery, laboratory, radiology, and pharmacology. Credentialed veterinary technicians are expected to know all the modules, allowing tasks to be added as the practice members become comfortable with the new team members' abilities.

Phase training should be tailored to each new team member depending on experience. Modules contain a tremendous amount of information, and team members are expected to learn most of it and in a short time frame. Time should be taken to fully explain procedures and protocols to

BOX 5-10 | Phase Training

Kennel Assistant Module 1
- Policies and paperwork
  - Employee personnel manual
  - Employee procedures manual
  - Employee expectations
  - Professional ethics
  - W-4, I-9, and benefits forms
  - Time clock
  - Mailbox
  - Dress code
- Cleaning
  - Prevent transmission of disease
    - What diseases are transmitted and how
  - Isolation
    - Keep all isolation cleaning items in isolation
  - Chemicals to clean with
    - Chlorhexidine
    - Vindicator
    - A-33
    - Clorox
  - Chemicals not to clean with
    - Lysol
    - Ammonia
  - Equipment
    - Scrub brushes
    - Mops and buckets
    - Brooms
  - Technique
    - Scrubbing
    - Contact time
    - Rinsing and drying
  - Laundry
    - Hot water
    - Detergent and bleach
  - Towels and blankets
    - Safety of blankets for patients
      - No holes or shredded blankets
  - Proper disposal of sharps
    - Biohazard containers
  - Proper disposal of bodies
    - Private burial
    - Mass or private cremation

Kennel Assistant Module 2
- Nutrition
  - Knowledge of different types of food
    - Puppy, maintenance, and senior formulas; prescription formulas
  - Amount to feed each animal
    - Measure
  - NPO
  - PO
- Hospital sheets
  - Following treatments required
- Walking patients safely
  - Removing patients from cages/kennels safely
  - Slip leash
  - At least 3 times daily, more if indicated
  - With IV fluids

- With bandaging material, casts, or other
- Cats
  - Clay litter
  - Nonabsorbable litter
  - Paper litter

Kennel Assistant Module 3
- Hospital maintenance
  - Trash
  - Sweeping/mopping
  - Cleanliness
    - Vents, fans, display shelving
  - Light fixtures
    - Working light bulbs and ballasts
  - Outside: weeds, animal waste and front porch appearance

Kennel Assistant Module 4
- Restraint techniques
  - Dogs and cats
  - Psychological restraint
  - Lifting appropriately
  - Handling the fractious patient
  - Lateral recumbency
  - Sternal recumbency
- Restraint for venipuncture (blood draw)
  - Jugular
  - Cephalic
  - Saphenous
  - Femoral
- Use precautions when necessary
  - Muzzles
  - Slip leash
  - Know when to hold tighter or use less restraint
- Understand client concerns when restraining animals
- E-collars
- Normal vital signs
  - Temperature
  - Pulse
  - Respiratory rate
- Grooming
  - Combing and brushing
  - Ear cleaning
  - Nail trimming
  - Anal sac expression
  - Bathing

Veterinary Assistant Module 1
- Kennel Assistant Modules 1 to 4

Veterinary Assistant Module 2
- Interaction with clients and patients
  - Treat animals as if they were your own
  - Make clients feel comfortable at all times
  - Offer coffee or water to those that must wait extended periods of time
  - Listen to what they say
  - Show you care
  - Offer to carry items and patients for clients
  - Always provide an answer. If you don't have the answer, find the correct answer ASAP

Continued

BOX 5-10	Phase Training—cont'd

- Cleaning between patients
  - Prevent transmission of disease
  - Wash hands after each patient
  - Clean table and exam room between each patient
  - Clean any instruments used between patients
- Animal care protocol
  - Hospital sheets
  - Proper food and proper feeding times for each patient
  - Provide fresh water at all times, unless otherwise indicated
  - Provide a clean blanket or towel at all times unless otherwise indicated
  - Prevention of nosocomial infections
  - Patient monitoring
    - Observe patient for any BM, urination, vomit, or abnormal condition. Indicate on hospital sheet and alert a veterinarian.
    - Patients should be monitored at all times while in the hospital
- Performing medicated baths
  - Be familiar with product and procedure for bathing
  - Dermazole shampoo
  - Pyoben shampoo
  - Flea/tick dip
  - Lime/sulfur dip
- Medical records
  - Reading and understanding medical records
  - SOAP Format
  - Writing a complete medical record
  - Abbreviations
    - Vomit, diarrhea, client, decline, patient, other common abbreviations used in practice
  - Initials
  - Filing of records
  - Updating records
- Exam room
  - History taking
  - Recording observations
  - TPR
  - Preparing room for veterinarian
  - Cleanliness
  - Stocking of
  - Sexing of animals
  - Aging dogs and cats
  - Mixing vaccines
  - Filling syringes
- Customer service
  - Greeting clients with a smile
  - Listening to what the client wants
  - Satisfying customer needs
  - Ensuring the customer perceives the value in the service they received
- Computer software
  - Client information
  - Patient history
  - Invoicing
  - Circle sheet or tracking sheet
- Protocol and procedures
  - Flow of patient appointments
  - Exam room

- Surgical
- Vaccinations
- Dental care
- Laboratory testing
- Patient treatments
- Common questions and concerns
  - Heartworm disease and products carries
  - Fleas and ticks; products carried
  - Dietary nutritional needs and products carried
  - Shampoos and conditioners; products carried

Veterinary Assistant Module 3
- Surgeries performed in practice
  - Routine OVH/castrations
  - Declaw
  - Dewclaw
  - Dental prophylaxis
  - Orthopedic procedures
  - Exploratory laparotomies
- Surgical protocol
  - Scheduling of
  - Surgery logs
  - NPO
  - Pre-anesthetic
  - Anesthesia
    - Anesthetic planes
  - Intubation
    - Selection of appropriate tube
    - Inflation of cuff
  - Eye lubrication
    - Why
    - How
    - What lubricant to use
  - IV fluids
    - Prepping site with aseptic technique
      - Clip
      - Clean
      - Betadine, alcohol, chlorhexidine
    - IV catheters
      - 18 g, 20 g, 22 g
      - Length
    - IV fluids
      - Normosol
      - NaCl
      - Dextrose
    - Securing of
  - Procedures
    - Sterile field
    - Opening packs
    - Suture material
      - Types of suture
      - Opening suture pack
    - Needles
      - Types of needles
      - Sterilizing of
      - Opening of
    - Gowning the surgeon
    - Monitoring the recovering patient
      - TPR

BOX 5-10 | Phase Training—cont'd

- Removal of ET
- Release instructions
- Equipment
  - Surgical table
    - Tilting, raising, and lowering
  - Monitors
    - Surgical monitor
    - Blood pressure machine
    - ECG
    - SPO_2
  - Anesthetic machine
    - Proper use of
    - Proper administration of gases
    - Selecting appropriate anesthetic hoses
    - Refilling gas compartment
  - Surgical instruments and packs
    - Names and uses of individual instruments
- Maintenance of equipment
  - Change soda lime
  - Change/maintain scavenger system
  - Clean daily and check for leaks:
    - Machine, including valves and bags
    - Anesthetic hoses
    - Masks
  - Surgical laundry
  - Cleaning of surgical suite
    - Table and lights
    - Counters
- Autoclave protocol
  - Use of
  - Pack preparation
    - Cleaning, lubricating, and maintaining instruments
  - Preparation of individual instruments
  - Proper labeling and taping
  - Length of time autoclave is good for
  - Maintenance of
  - Distilled water

Veterinary Assistant Module 4
- X-ray
  - Introduction
  - Safety
  - Equipment
    - Thyroid collar
    - Lead gloves
    - X-ray gown
    - Eye protection
    - Radiation badge
      - Proper use and placement of
  - Log
  - Film
    - Maintenance and use of cassettes
    - Storage of
    - Filing of radiographs
    - Identification of
  - Technique
    - Use of calipers
    - Understanding and determining kVp and mAs
    - Collimation

- Anatomy of positions
  - D/V, V/D, A/P, lateral
  - Abdominal, thoracic
- Developer
  - Manual vs. automatic vs. digital
  - Maintenance of
  - Chemicals
    - Developing solution
    - Fix solution
  - Cleaning
  - Disposing of chemicals
- Ultrasound
- Endoscopy
- Laboratory
  - Common external parasites
    - Prepping for
      - Ear smear
      - Skin scrape
      - Cytology
  - Common internal parasites
    - Collecting fecal samples
    - Prepping fecal
    - Reading fecal
  - Equipment
    - HCT/PCV Machine
      - Determining HCT
    - Chemistry machine
      - BUN, CREA, SGPT, ALT, BILI, GLU, CHOL, AMYL, PHOS, Ca, etc.
    - CBC machine
      - WBC, RBC, PLT, HCT
    - Electrolyte machine
      - Na, CL, K
    - Microscope
      - How to use and clean
      - Different levels of power
      - Oil immersion
        - Cytology
    - Refractometer
      - How to use and clean
      - Determining urine specific gravity and TP
    - Centrifuge
      - HCT, small and large
    - Tonometer
      - How to use, calibrate, and clean
    - Blood pressure machine
      - How to use
      - Measuring for correct cuff size
      - Doppler versus surgical monitor
    - ECG machine
      - Location of clips
      - Alcohol on clips for better conduction
    - Blood tubes
      - SST
        - Serum separator tubes
        - Tests that cannot be drawn with SST
      - RTT
        - Serum used for

Continued

BOX 5-10	Phase Training—cont'd

- PTT
  - EDTA anticoagulant
  - Plasma used for
- BTT
  - Citrate anticoagulant
  - Plasma used for
- GTT
  - Lithium heparin anticoagulant
  - Plasma used for
- Using aseptic technique to obtain blood samples
- Testing available in house
  - CBC/chemistry/electrolytes/blood gases
  - Urinalysis
  - Heartworm 4DX (heartworm, *Ehrlichia canis*, Lyme disease, and anaplasmosis)
  - FeLV/FIV/HWT
  - Parvo
  - Spec CPL
- Testing available outside
  - Laboratory forms
  - Bile acids
  - Phenobarbital levels
  - ACTH stimulation
  - T-4
    - Total T-4
    - Equilibrium dialysis
    - Thyroid panels
- Maintenance of equipment
  - Daily
  - Weekly
  - Monthly
- Stains
  - Wright stain
  - Diff-Quick
  - New methylene blue
  - Urinalysis stain
- Urinalysis
  - Collection of sample
    - Free catch
    - Cystocentesis
    - Catheterization
  - Evaluation of sample
    - Microscopic
    - Stick
    - Specific gravity
  - Urine culture and sensitivity
    - Collection of
    - Sample submission
- Necropsy
  - Material needed
  - Sample submission

Veterinary Assistant Module 5
- Patient discharge
  - Discharge instructions
  - Medications
  - Pet's personal items: collars, blankets and toys
- Pharmacology
  - Handling controlled substances
  - Most common drugs used

- Antibiotics
- Anti-inflammatory
- Antihistamines
- Cardiac
- Ophthalmic
- Otic
- Gastrointestinal
- Shampoos/conditioners
- Skin care
- Injectable medications
- Tranquilizers
- Thyroid
- Miscellaneous
- Drug location
- Drug storage
  - Amber bottle versus clear bottle
- Drug use
- Potential drug interactions
- Normal dosing
- Normal instructions
- Labeling
- Counting
- Reading a prescription label
- Direction abbreviations
  - SID
  - BID
  - TID
  - QID
  - PRN
  - EOD
  - PO
  - IV
  - IM
  - SQ
- Reading the instructions to the owner
- Administering medications to the patient
  - Oral solution
  - Pills or capsules
  - Aural medication
  - Ocular medication
  - Topical medication

Veterinary Assistant Module 6
- Patient treatments
  - Injections
    - SQ
    - IV
    - IM
  - Administering other medications
    - PO
    - AU/AD/AS
    - OU/OD/OS
    - Topically
- Monitoring IV fluids and catheters
- Developing patient hospitalization sheets
- Developing patient release sheets

Veterinary Technician Module 1
- Kennel Assistant Modules 1 to 4

BOX 5-10 | Phase Training—cont'd

Veterinary Technician Module 2
- Veterinary Assistant Modules 1 and 2

Veterinary Technician Module 3
- Veterinary Assistant Module 3
- Place IV catheter
- Determine drip rate
- Induce and maintain anesthesia
- Monitor recovering surgical patients
- Perform dental prophylaxis

Veterinary Technician Module 4
- Veterinary Assistant Modules 4 and 5
- Obtain lab samples with aseptic technique
- Perform cystotomy
- Problem solve x-ray techniques when needed

Veterinary Technician Module 5
- Veterinary Assistant Module 6

Veterinary Technician Module 6
- Develop leadership skills
- Provide CE for kennel and veterinary assistants
- Provide assistance with inventory control
- Provide accountability for products and supplies used
- Help develop protocols and procedures for practice
- Provide an excellent attitude that is contagious to the rest of the team

Receptionist Training Module 1
- Policies and paperwork
  - Employee personnel manual
  - Employee procedures manual
  - Forms W-4 and I-9, and benefits forms
  - Time clock
  - Mailbox
  - Dress code
- Cleanliness of reception area
- Greeting clients
  - Responding to client questions and concerns
- Client service
- Telephone calls
  - Customer service
  - Friendly, positive tone
  - Length of time on hold

Receptionist Training Module 2
- Procedures and protocols
  - Examinations
  - Vaccinations
  - Surgery
- Invoicing
  - Entering invoice
  - Reviewing invoice with client
  - Accepting payment
  - Change
  - Documenting transaction
- Appointments
  - Making
  - Accepting
  - Canceling/moving

Receptionist Training Module 3
- Medical records
  - Creating new medical records
  - Updating patient records
  - Making entries in medical records
  - Filing
  - Retrieving
  - Reviewing for complete records
- Morning procedure
  - Checking clients in
  - Checking clients out
- Afternoon procedure
  - End of day procedures
- Computer software
  - Searching for history and past transactions
- Common questions and concerns
  - Heartworm disease; products carried
  - Fleas and ticks; products carried
  - Dietary nutritional needs; products carried
  - Shampoos and conditioners; products carried

Receptionist Training Module 4
- Prescriptions
  - Medications
  - Abbreviations
  - Labeling
  - Reviewing instructions with clients

---

ensure the new employee fully understands them. It may be wise to explain the procedures and protocols multiple times, using a variety of methods for explanation.

New team members should be encouraged to read the employee procedures manual and the training modules. Once these are read, they can observe team members completing the skills, complete the skills themselves, and then be tested on the concept. Once a new team member has completed the first module with satisfaction, the second module can be started, with an estimated date of completion in mind.

It takes a *team* to train a *team*—and using *all* team members to train new employees improves efficiency greatly. Ten

people training an individual produces much more knowledge than just one person doing training. However, one supervisor should be in charge of overseeing the testing procedure to ensure the employee can complete the procedures and techniques as expected. If any area needs improvement, it can be addressed at that time.

Providing All Levels of Continuing Education

New employees are not the only team members who need training. Long-term and advanced assistants and technicians may not need the basic training that new employees do, but disease knowledge, treatments, and protocols may change

frequently. If team members are not encouraged to attend outside continuing education seminars, then continuing education should be brought to the practice. Practices can incorporate manufacturers' representatives into the meeting schedule. Sales consultants have a variety of topics available and often allow the practice to pick topics they want to educate the staff about.

> **PRACTICE POINT** Recall the mission and vision set by the hospital, and set continuing education goals for team members to help attain those goals.

Continuing education inspires and encourages team members to improve the quality and quantity of care they provide to both clients and patients. When team members receive quality education, they can educate the clients at a much higher level.

Continuing education also contributes to the prevention of team member burnout. Keeping employees engaged and excited is critical to practice success.

Role-Playing

A technique that yields a high success rate is role-playing. If a receptionist's or technician's job is to educate a client about heartworm disease, then team members should be able to recite the information to any other employee. Once they have mastered the words and the ability to convey the information to team members, then they can educate any client. Team members are more nervous when having to role-play in front of their peers; this is an excellent test of their knowledge and confidence. They will come across as much more professional and educated in front of clients when they have confidence in the information they are conveying.

Role-playing should be included in any training protocol. Receptionists will find it beneficial while making appointments or confronting upset clients. Assistants and technicians will find it beneficial when educating clients about diseases, and kennel assistants will become aware of potential problems in the kennel and how to fix them before they arise.

Methods to Retain Employees

Employee turnover rates not only affect the clinic financially, but also decrease the team morale and efficiency as well. It takes a large amount of time and dedication to train employees. Training an employee reduces the amount of time spent with patients and clients, decreases the quality of care patients receive, and increases staff wages during the training period. A program to promote team spirit and satisfaction can decrease these negative side effects. Job satisfaction includes respect for one another, recognition, achievement, and challenges.

> **PRACTICE POINT** Team member loyalty does not just happen. Leaders must implement measures to retain and motivate team members.

Providing an environment that is open, friendly, and promotes communication is important. People spend the majority of their time at work. They should not have to be upset about coming to work, hate their jobs, or avoid team members because of an unfriendly work environment. Team members should be encouraged to talk with management about personnel issues without the fear of retaliation. Supervisors and practice owners should listen to team members and discuss issues with teams before they become a problem. Ask team members to complete an employee survey. Find out how they feel and what their concerns are, and address them. They will feel that their opinion counts, and more than likely, if one employee has a problem with a topic, another does as well. Management may never know of the problem unless the team members are asked.

Each manager has his or her own techniques for conflict resolution. The ultimate goal should be to prevent and solve problems, not react and discipline. Creation of an enjoyable environment comes from the practice owners, associates, and managers. If harmony is nonexistent among these key individuals, the rest of the team cannot be expected to get along and enjoy their jobs. When team members are happy, the quality and quantity of patient and client care increase as well as the efficiency among the team members.

Salary is important to team members and should be kept within a reasonable range for the area. Team members cannot be expected to complete highly skilled tasks and procedures for minimum wage. However, if job satisfaction is high, salary may be less important.

Continuing education for team members is very important to increasing staff retention. Employees should be constantly fed new information to keep them motivated. Motivated employees seek new information on a daily basis, yearning for a challenge. Satisfying this craving for knowledge is a benefit for both the practice and the employer.

> Veterinary practice managers oversee continuing education and licensure/certification of staff.

Team member involvement helps retain employees as well. If team members are involved in decision making and helping to create and implement protocols and procedures, they are likely to feel needed. Team members take pride in tasks they had a role in developing and will ensure the success of those tasks. The practice benefits from team involvement as well; the ideas of the entire staff are better than the ideas of just one or two. Sometimes, a new or improved idea can be created from ideas taken from several points of view, making for excellent problem prevention and solving.

Maintaining the same team also helps put clients at ease when they arrive at the practice. Clients know they will receive the same quality of care when they see the same team members each time. Receptionists know the client when they walk in the door, technicians know their pets' history, and

they can leave their pets, if needed, knowing they will receive exceptional care. Client satisfaction of this magnitude will help increase the average client transaction, client retention, and client compliance.

Many ideas can be implemented to increase staff retention. As stated earlier, it must start with the management. Team appreciation is important and can be done several ways. Birthday cakes and cards are special; the entire team benefits from the joy and smiles singing "Happy Birthday" brings. Christmas holiday parties are expected and come at a stressful time of the year. Find other days to show employee appreciation. Inexpensive hiking trips can be planned; consider a night at the movies or special ice cream breaks in the middle of the day. Cruise deals can be found online for relatively inexpensive amounts. Trips taken together promote friendship and harmony outside the work environment. Trips can be more productive than a bonus given yearly and can include continuing education for the staff. The memories made from a trip far outweigh the money given in bonus form. Celebrate small victories frequently. Celebrating large victories places less emphasis on the "small stuff." Small stuff is important, too, and often is what keeps the practice rolling smoothly.

One of the most satisfying ideas for teams is to compliment an individual for a job well done as soon as it is accomplished. Many people only receive criticism, never a compliment. When team members receive compliments throughout the day, the spirit of the entire team is lifted a notch. Other team members will see the compliments and strive to achieve a compliment as well. Rarely do individuals become competitive at this stage because they know they are appreciated as well. It takes a team to be complete! Review Chapter 3 for great leadership ideas.

Termination

Termination procedures must be clearly stated *and followed* to protect the practice against unemployment claims, or worse, discrimination. In general, an employee is given a verbal warning and a method to correct the mistake, accident, or violation. The warning is documented in the personnel file, along with the date and the signature of the manager correcting the action (Figure 5-10). Two or three written warnings are then allowed (practice decides), again each documented in the personnel file. Each written warning should be dated, along with the employee's and manager's signatures. The last warning should also state that the next step is termination.

 Veterinary practice managers discipline and discharge employees.

Termination must take place when a team member has been verbally warned and written up for unsatisfactory performance of duties, excessive tardiness, or absenteeism. Dishonesty and unethical behavior, criminal activity within the hospital (stealing or embezzlement) or outside the hospital (drug use), and improper use of personal protective equipment (PPE) should be grounds for immediate termination (no warnings are needed). Immediate dismissal guidelines must be stated in the employee manual, just as the steps to proper termination are.

When guidelines are placed in the employee manual, managers must follow through. Allowing team members to slide and not discipline them as needed decreases employee accountability (they know they can get away with bad behavior), and decreases team morale (other team members become upset because corrective action has not been taken). Further, if all employees are not treated exactly the same way regarding discipline procedures, the threat of discrimination is high. For example, if one employee is terminated for excessive tardiness whereas another is not, the terminated employee can claim discrimination. The threat of discrimination is real, and managers must take every action to prevent such accusations.

> **PRACTICE POINT** A plan must be created for terminating employees; otherwise anger, emotion, and foul words will contaminate the conversation.

The following guidelines should be used when the decision to terminate is final:

- Ensure that the employee was verbally corrected, all written warnings are documented, and that the employee understood the correction and signed each entry.
- Do not fire employees while upset, angry, or in the midst of an argument. When emotions are high, incorrect words, phrases, and actions will be said or will take place. Wait until the emotions subside, and ensure correct termination procedures are followed. This will help protect the practice against wrongful dismissal complaints.
- If the employee has insurance through the practice, the Consolidated Omnibus Budget Reconciliation Act (COBRA) requires the practice to continue coverage for a specified time. COBRA also requires employers to continue coverage for former employees who have a medical condition that would prevent them from obtaining immediate coverage from a new employer.

Once a termination has been found to be warranted, time and procedure are of essence. The termination should occur at the end of the day, so that if any negative interaction occurs, it is less disruptive to clients and staff. Return of the door key should be requested at that time. The employee should sign termination papers, indicating the reason for termination. The entire procedure should be documented by the manager immediately, before any facts are forgotten. All documentation and paperwork should be placed in the employee's file and locked in a file cabinet. It is imperative to remember that all information regarding the termination should be kept confidential and not shared with other team members.

If an employee resigns, the practice should ask the employee to write a letter of resignation. If possible, the

ABC Veterinary Hospital

Employee Warning Notice

Employee Information	
Employee Name:	Date:
Employee ID:	Job Title:
Manager:	Department:

Type of Warning

☐ First Warning   ☐ Second Warning   ☐ Final Warning

Type of Offense

☐ Tardiness/Leaving Early   ☐ Absenteeism   ☐ Violation of Company Policies
☐ Substandard Work   ☐ Violation of Safety Rules   ☐ Rudeness to Customers/Coworkers
☐ Other: _____

Details

Description of Infraction:

Plan for Improvement:

Consequences of Further Infractions:

Acknowledgement of Receipt of Warning

By signing this form, you confirm that you understand the information in this warning. You also confirm that you and your manager have discussed the warning and a plan for improvement. Signing this form does not necessarily indicate that you agree with this warning.

_____   _____
Employee signature   Date

_____   _____
Manager signature   Date

_____   _____
Witness signature (if employee understands warning but refuses to sign)   Date

FIGURE 5-10 Sample discipline form.

reason for leaving should be indicated as well as the final date of employment. An exit interview can be completed the last day of employment. Exit interviews can give the practice needed information: why the employee is resigning, his or her thoughts of items or ideas in the practice that need improvement, and ways the person might recommend or institute changes. These are just some ideas of how a practice can benefit from losing an employee.

Hospitals can develop their own termination procedures with more or fewer verbal and written warnings. Whatever method is chosen must be reasonable for both the employer and employee, defined in the employee personnel manual, and documented in the personnel file.

Payroll

It is important for a manager to understand the entire payroll process. Becoming as organized as possible in its management will ensure a successful system. Payroll can be time-consuming and tedious and must be maintained by a motivated, intelligent team member. That team member must be held accountable for correct payroll procedures and must ensure that all tax payments are submitted on time. The person who signs and prepares the payroll tax form is held accountable by the IRS; if any mistakes occur or payments are received late, that individual will be responsible for the late fees and corrections.

Pay periods are defined as the length of time covered by each payroll period and generally cover weekly, biweekly, or semimonthly periods. An example of 1 week would be Monday morning through Sunday night. A practice can determine what pay period works best as well as days of the week to start and stop the period.

Weekly pay periods pay employees once a week, generating 52 paychecks per year. The disadvantage to weekly pay periods is the administrative costs associated with processing payroll on a weekly basis. Biweekly payroll decreases administrative costs by processing payroll every other week,

producing only 26 checks per year. Employees must learn how to balance their budgets to accommodate biweekly checks. Because there are not a balanced number of weeks in every month, there will be 2 months out of the year when payroll occurs three times within the month. This can make reports appear incorrect, as these months will appear less profitable, and should not be used in comparison with previous year-to-month analysis. If the months are analyzed, the increased payroll period should be noted. Semimonthly payroll eliminates this appearance in the analysis because payroll occurs evenly on the first and the fifteenth of each month and produces 24 pay periods per year.

> **PRACTICE POINT** The disadvantage to weekly payroll is the increase in human resources costs associated with processing payroll.

When determining payday, the day that team members receive their checks, it is important to allow sufficient time between the end of the pay period and payday for payroll preparation. Generally, 3 days is sufficient. If a bookkeeper or accountant is used, he or she may ask for less time.

Determining Staff Wages

Determining wages for different levels of staff can be a challenge, because a balance must be made between budgeting and maintaining an educated and dedicated staff. Team members must be compensated for their skill while creating and maintaining an environment that is enjoyable. When considering wages, the benefits package that is available to the staff must be remembered (team members should be reminded of the benefits received during their annual review). The location of the practice within the United States also plays a factor in wage determination, as the cost of living in some areas is higher than in others. Practices in large cities, referral practices, and specialty centers will also have higher compensation rates than those in smaller cities and general practice.

 Veterinary practice managers manage employee benefit programs.

To help a new practice determine a pay scale or an existing practice update its scale, a chart can be developed to show minimum, maximum, and average ranges for each position, as well as to determine any discrepancies a current practice may have in its pay scale system. It is critical to have consistent procedures for setting pay levels for each position. The first step is to list all the jobs in the practice and to rank them according to importance. This allows the most important jobs to be ranked highest, providing the highest compensation. For new practices, this is ideal; for existing practices, it may reveal less important jobs receiving higher pay because the employee was recently hired. In general, wages have risen, but salaries of long-term employees have not.

The second step is to chart what current employees are being paid. The third step is to insert the benchmark pay scales available from the American Animal Hospital Association (AAHA), Veterinary Hospital Managers Association (VHMA), or National Commission on Veterinary Economic Issues (NCVEI) to determine where the practice sits in the national average. As previously stated, the location of the practice in the United States is a factor in pay scales, but a practice should at least be at or above the 75th percentile. This will help recruit and retain excellent team members.

> **PRACTICE POINT** Visit www.vhma.org for up-to-date compensation and benefits for each position in the hospital.

Veterinarians

Hiring a veterinarian for a practice is very important; not only should the person be able to fit into the practice, he or she has to be able to fit into the budget of the practice. To determine whether a practice can support another veterinarian, reports should be generated looking at the average number of clients seen on a yearly basis. To support a full-time–equivalent veterinarian, 800 to 1200 active clients are needed per year. Therefore the practice needs to see at least an additional 800 clients per year to justify a new veterinarian.

Once it has been determined that another veterinarian is needed and can be fairly compensated, then the practice must decide before hiring how it will compensate the veterinarian and how much he or she will be compensated.

Pro-sal, a combination of production and salary is one form of compensation; salary only and production only are the other two forms commonly used in veterinary medicine. If the practice commonly accepts after-hours emergencies, doctors may be paid additional money to compensate for their time. Under professional liability, veterinarians have a legal duty to accept emergencies or refer them to an emergency practice after hours.

Pro-Sal Formula

The most common form of compensation is a pro-sal formula, also referred to as the *production reconciliation hybrid*. This allows veterinarians to receive a base salary and a production bonus once a predetermined dollar amount has been reached. If this formula is chosen, the base salary must first be determined and is normally based on the veterinarian's experience. The production bonus then needs to be set; the practice must determine how much the veterinarian must produce before receiving the bonus. The practice should also decide what percentage of the production will be paid as a bonus and whether the bonus is paid on a monthly or quarterly basis. When calculating the pro-sal rate, the salary is guaranteed, regardless of the production. The production total is then subtracted from the salary, and the veterinarian receives the remainder.

An example of pro-sal is as follows:

A veterinarian is paid $60,000 base salary per year, with a 10% production bonus once production has reached $10,000 per month. Bonuses are paid monthly for the previous month's production. Payday is on the first and the fifteenth of each month.

To figure salary pay:

- **$60,000 ÷ 24 (24 pay periods per year) = $2500 per check.**
- The veterinarian produced $33,000 for the previous month:
- **$33,000 × 10% = $3300**
- **$3300 (production) − $2500 (guaranteed salary) = $800**
- The gross pay for the first of the month is **$2500 + $800 = $3300.**
- The gross pay for the fifteenth of the month is **$2500.**

The definition of gross pay is the total amount earned before any taxes or other withholdings.

Salary

In brief, salary-compensated veterinarians receive a set amount, regardless of the amount of dollars produced. Some practices prefer to pay veterinarians a set salary as opposed to any other form of pay, because it seems to decrease the competition among veterinarians in the practice. It promotes a team environment, and all doctors and staff help each other accomplish all tasks, diagnoses, and treatments needed. A practice needs to determine a set salary for a veterinarian; again, this is generally based on his or her experience. As previously stated, veterinarians are exempt from overtime under FLSA. Hours should be monitored to prevent burnout.

An example of salary pay is similar to the previous example:

- **The veterinarian receives $60,000 in salary per year.**
- **Payday occurs on the first and the fifteenth of each month:**
- **$60,000 ÷ 24 = $2500 per pay period.**

Production

Production compensation pays a veterinarian a percentage of the amount of dollars produced. The practice must determine the percentage before hiring a veterinarian; average amounts are 18% to 25% in small-animal practice and 25% to 30% in large-animal practice.

It is also necessary to determine what is paid as production. Inventory and procedures should all be evaluated (there is no set standard; it is up to the practice to determine what products or services qualify).

In general, veterinarians are paid just as the rest of the staff, either biweekly or on the first and the fifteenth of each month. A report is generated for each veterinarian indicating the dollar amount produced for that specific period. The dollar amount produced is then multiplied by the percentage determined and paid as gross salary.

A production-only salary can be easy to figure as well:

- A veterinarian is paid **20%** of production of all services and products.
- Payday occurs on the first and the fifteenth of each month.

- The payroll manager should pull a report of that specific veterinarian's production from the first to the fourteenth of the month. If the veterinarian produced $15,000 during that period, **$15,000 × 20% = $3000 gross pay.**
- The second pay period report would run from the fifteenth to the thirtieth or thirty-first of the month. If the veterinarian produced $16,236 for that period, then **$16,236 × 20% = $3247.20 gross pay.**

Production as the basis for salary can decrease the overall team spirit and can promote competition among veterinarians. Some veterinarians will perform diagnostic procedures that may not be necessary to increase their production numbers. This can lead to claims of gouging.

It also promotes competition between veterinarians in choosing wealthy clients and big cases over yearly exams, vaccines, and small procedures. It can also discourage veterinarians from participating in any procedures that do not produce an income or that only produce a small amount of income. If the practice offers healthy shelter-pet checks for a reduced cost, production-only veterinarians may choose not to see them. In healthy practices that have a positive culture, all of the issues just discussed can be prevented, producing a win-win for everyone involved.

The practice must determine which formula is going to work best for the practice. Some practices may find that competition is not a problem within the hospital and that either a pro-sal or production-only formula yields the best results. Others may find the salary formula to be the easiest and least time-consuming formula to use. The advantage to percentage-based compensation is that it can motivate veterinarians to work hard and produce more income. It emphasizes the medical and business aspect of veterinary medicine and compensates veterinarians for their successful efforts and the skills involved in practicing high-quality medicine. It can also eliminate opportunities for claims of discrimination, because pay is based on production, not determined by management.

Practices must be well staffed and trained for a pro-sal or production formula to work efficiently. Veterinarians must be able to effectively delegate duties, treatments, and diagnostics to technicians while they continue seeing patients. If they cannot delegate duties, they may become upset with management over the lack of staff training.

Emergency Pay

If emergencies are accepted after hours, veterinarians may be paid salary plus emergency pay. Some practices pay the set emergency fee per animal seen: an average of $35 to $50 per case before 11 PM and $50 to $75 after 11 PM. Other practices may pay 30% to 50% of the exam cost, plus a percentage of the diagnostics performed before the office opens. Yet another option may be to pay 10% of the exam fee and 18% to 22% of the total client transaction.

Technicians

Credentialed technicians are usually compensated based on experience and should be paid on an hourly basis.

Technicians are generally dedicated and will work hours in excess of 40 hours per week to ensure that the necessary duties, tasks, and treatments are completed for every patient. FLSA of 1938 states that all employees who work over 40 hours within a 1-week period must be paid overtime.

Practices may set an average start rate with a set number of years of experience to create consistency when hiring team members. Industry benchmarks are available from AAHA, VHMA, and NCVEI to help practices determine wage levels for technicians in each area of the United States.

Assistants, Receptionists, and Kennel Attendants

Many practices start team members without any experience at a minimum wage, allowing for raises as tasks and duties are mastered. Assistants without a certificate, receptionists, and kennel attendants generally do not have any veterinary experience, which is gained through the workplace environment. Some receptionists may be hired who have previous customer service experience, which should be considered when determining wages. Customer service skills are an invaluable resource to a practice and should not be overlooked.

Groomers

Some groomers are paid on a production percentage, just as veterinarians may be paid, whereas others may be paid hourly. Independent groomers may simply be paid a fee for each animal that is groomed; others may only rent the space within the veterinary practice.

Independent groomers must have their own tax identification numbers; therefore taxes are not taken out of the groomers' paychecks. They are responsible for paying their own federal and state taxes. At the end of the year, independent groomers receiving pay over $600 within the fiscal year must be issued Form 1099-MISC (when others are issued Form W-2) for taxation purposes. Form 1099-MISC cites all monies paid to the contractor on an untaxed basis. The groomer submits Form 1099-MISC with his or her taxes (Figure 5-11).

Determining Raises

Employees may receive raises on a scheduled basis. The practice should establish a policy as to when raises will be considered for all team members. Some practices may give raises after 3 months of employment, then on a yearly basis. Some practices give raises based on merit, whereas others give raises with the completion and mastering of skills. Cost-of-living raises must also be considered for those not receiving a raise based on merit or skill.

> **PRACTICE POINT** Employees should be given raises based on performance, not length of time employed by the practice.

Raises should not be given at the same time employee evaluations are given; they tend to decrease the value of the evaluation. Evaluations should be completed first, and then raises can follow within a few months.

A budget should be developed that includes raises for employees. When a set dollar amount has been budgeted for raises, the amount can be distributed among team members. Lists can be developed rating team members, allowing a specific percentage or dollar amount increase. Those team members that go above and beyond the call of duty must be placed at the top of the list for the largest raises. Those with less skill and lower quality of work ethic can be placed at the end of the list. Veterinarians may be compensated based on production or receive a percentage increase, whichever the budget allows.

If the clinic's budget does not allow a set raise for employees, yet team members need to be rewarded for excellent work, then a one-time bonus can be given. A bonus allows team members to know they are appreciated, but it affects the bottom line less than employee raises do. A bonus is a one-time payout, as opposed to a raise, which permanently increases expenditures. With that said, raises should not be overlooked because employees may seek employment at other practices offering higher pay.

Managing Payroll

Payroll has many different aspects, and organization is the key to managing it successfully. Some practices have a bookkeeper or accountant manage payroll; others use internal office managers to complete the tasks.

> **PRACTICE POINT** Outsourcing payroll can save the practice money in terms of human resource dollars.

Intuit QuickBooks is an excellent source for payroll software. Frequent tax updates are sent as well as tips for organizing payroll records. QuickBooks calculates the taxes that are withheld from the employee and those contributed by the employer. If direct deposit is used, a link is available to complete the deposit. When extra money is withheld from employees for insurance or retirement plans, QuickBooks establishes a sheet indicating what and how much should be withheld. Payroll sheets are developed for each employee, and taxes to be paid are calculated. Team members must take the time to enter the information initially, and QuickBooks does all the rest.

Calculating Payroll

Examples are used to help explain a payroll calculation if a manual method is used instead of software.

Regular rate calculations:

Example A: Wanda is paid $10 per hour and works 34 hours per week. Payroll is paid every other Monday; therefore the work week is Monday, 12:00 AM through Sunday, 12:59 PM.

- 34 hours per week × 2 = 68 hours per 2-week period
- 68 hours × $10.00 = $680.00 before taxes

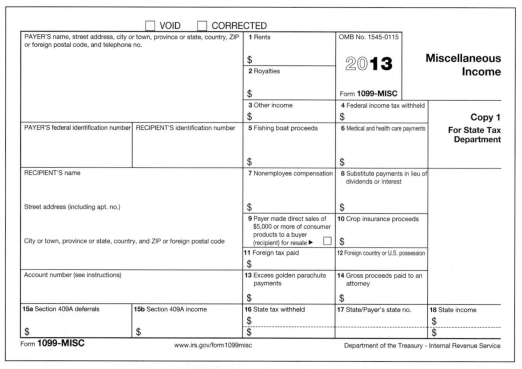

FIGURE 5-11 Form 1099-MISC.

Overtime rate calculations:

Example B: This period, Ann has worked 44 hours during week 1 and 32 hours during week 2. She is paid $10 per hour; overtime is paid at $15 per hour (1½ times the regular rate).

- **Week 1:** 40 hours × $10.00 = $400.00; 4 hours × $15.00 = $60.00
- **Week 2:** 32 hours × $10.00 = $320.00
- $400.00 + $60.00 + $320.00 = $780.00 before taxes

Example C: This period, Alex accrues 44 hours in week 1 and 52 hours during week 2.

- **Week 1:** 40 hours × $10.00 = $400.00; 4 hours × $15.00 = $60.00
- **Week 2:** 40 hours × $10.00 = $400.00; 12 hours × $15.00 = $180.00
- $400.00 + $60.00 + $400.00 + $180.00 = $1040.00 before taxes

More examples of calculations are available in Chapter 24.

Records

States have different requirements regarding the length of time to keep employee payroll records; check with the state department of labor. All records should be kept in a locked cabinet for confidentiality purposes.

Employees should receive a payroll check stub with each paycheck (those with direct deposit should receive a stub on the day of payroll). Payroll stubs should indicate the employee's name, wage, and gross income (income before taxes and other withholdings), along with Social Security and Medicare withholdings. Contributions to a sIRA or 401(k) program should also be stated, along with any withholdings for insurance. Payroll stubs for full-time employees may also state the vacation and sick hours available. A summary sheet for all employees should be kept on file for each payroll period.

Direct Deposit

With the technology available today, many practices and employees prefer to use direct deposit for payroll checks. The check is deposited directly into the employee's checking account on the date of payroll; the employee does not need to go to the bank to deposit the check.

Practices may contact their bank for direct deposit procedures. Normally, an authorization form is submitted from each employee to the practice's bank. The form includes the employee's name, address, current bank, and checking account number. The employee authorizing the direct deposit should also sign it. The bank may also request a voided check to ensure the correct routing number is entered when the initial deposit is set up. Paycheck amounts are usually due at the bank 2 to 3 business days before payday. This ensures that the funds will be transferred on payday.

The advantages of direct deposit are numerous. Less paper is used, and it takes less time for the staff to write checks and place them in secured envelopes. Team members who do not have checking accounts may continue to request regular payroll checks; this should not be a problem because those checks can be written as they previously were.

Payroll Taxes

Several taxes are withheld from employees, and the employer is responsible for paying those as well as additional taxes. The practice bookkeeper, accountant, or team member responsible for payroll will determine this amount and must ensure that the taxes are paid on time. State revenue departments

dislike late payments and often penalize heavily for those that are late.

> PRACTICE POINT   All taxes should be automatically deducted from the practice checking account, ensuring no late payment occurs.

Social Security and Medicare

Taxes withheld from an employee payroll checks include income tax, Social Security, and Medicare. Social Security and Medicare fall under the Federal Insurance Contribution Act (FICA), wherein 6.2% of the gross pay is withheld for Social Security and 1.45% is withheld for Medicare. The employer is responsible for contributing the same amount to FICA. The total employee income taxes, as well as the employee and employer portions of FICA, are paid to the IRS through a federal tax deposit (FTD) system.

FTDs are required and must be paid on either a monthly basis or a semiweekly basis. The amount of tax due within a select period determines whether practices must pay monthly or semiweekly. Form 8109 must be filled out with the deposit and can be submitted electronically or at the practice's banking institution (Figure 5-12).

Federal Unemployment Tax Act

In addition to reporting FICA contributions on Form 941, employers are also responsible for taxes under FUTA, which are reported on Form 940. These taxes are paid solely by the employer, not withheld or deducted from the employee. FUTA only taxes the first $7000 paid to an employee in 1 year; the rate is 0.06%. A few states do not have an unemployment program; therefore tax in these states may be slightly higher.

Unemployment tax is generally paid quarterly; the amount of tax due depends on the schedule of payments. Just as with Form 941, payments are made electronically or at the practice's banking institution (Figures 5-13 and 5-14).

Forms W-2 and W-4

Employees are required to fill out Form W-4 (Figures 5-15) once they are hired for employment. The form asks questions to determine how many deductions should be withheld from the payroll check, along with requiring the employee's Social Security number, address, and signature. This form should be kept in the employee's personnel file in case it is ever needed again, or if the employee wishes to change the number of deductions on the form.

At the end of the year, as taxes are prepared, the accountant or bookkeeper will produce a Form W-2 for each employee, summarizing his or her earnings for the year (Figure 5-16). These forms include gross earnings and Social Security and Medicare, insurance, and retirement withholdings. These forms are due to employees no later than January 31 of each year.

> PRACTICE POINT   Employees must receive their Form W-2 by January 31st of each year.

Workers' Compensation Insurance

As stated earlier, workers' compensation insurance protects the employer from injuries individuals might receive while on the job. Injuries include falls, animal bites, accidents, or exposure to harmful substances. Workers' compensation insurance is regulated by individual states, not the federal government; therefore not all states require coverage. Depending on the state, a business may be able to contribute to a state fund, a private insurance fund, or a combination of both. Some states also allow practices to be self-insured. It is advised to check with the state to ensure the practice is in compliance.

If an employee is bitten, falls, or injures himself or herself in any way on the job site, workers' compensation insurance pays for physician visits, medications, and hospitalization that may be required. Insurance will also pay the team member's wages if more than 5 days of work are lost because of the injury. Many practices do not require team members to visit a doctor when an accident has occurred because they are afraid that the cost of insurance will increase with each claim filed. However, if an injury worsens, and the team member does not seek medical attention, then the employer can be liable to pay for all medical costs. Workers' compensation may deny a claim if it is not filed within a specific number of days after the injury. All serious injuries, including dog and cat bites, should, at minimum, be examined by a physician to protect the employer against future liabilities.

If an employee becomes injured, a "first report of injury" form should be filled out. If medical attention is needed, the employee should be sent with the form provided by the company providing the insurance. The form should have the practice name, the policy number, and a place to input employee information. This paper can be presented to the medical office, which can then file the claim.

Once the medical visit has been completed, the practice can submit the first report of injury and the insurance form to the state division of labor as well as the insurance carrier. Workers' compensation should follow up with the rest of the documentation. If claims are not filed, the employee is responsible for the bill received from the medical office.

If the practice chooses not to carry workers' compensation insurance, the practice owner is exposed to liability. If a team member sustains an extensive injury on the job, the practice will be responsible for paying for the medical bills of the team member. Surgery can become costly, along with follow-up visits and physical therapy. Careful consideration should be taken if the practice chooses not to carry workers' compensation insurance.

Personnel Files

There should be a file of confidential information on each employee. These files can be kept in a locking file cabinet that only the owner and practice manager can access. All information regarding an employee should be kept together and be well organized for easy retrieval.

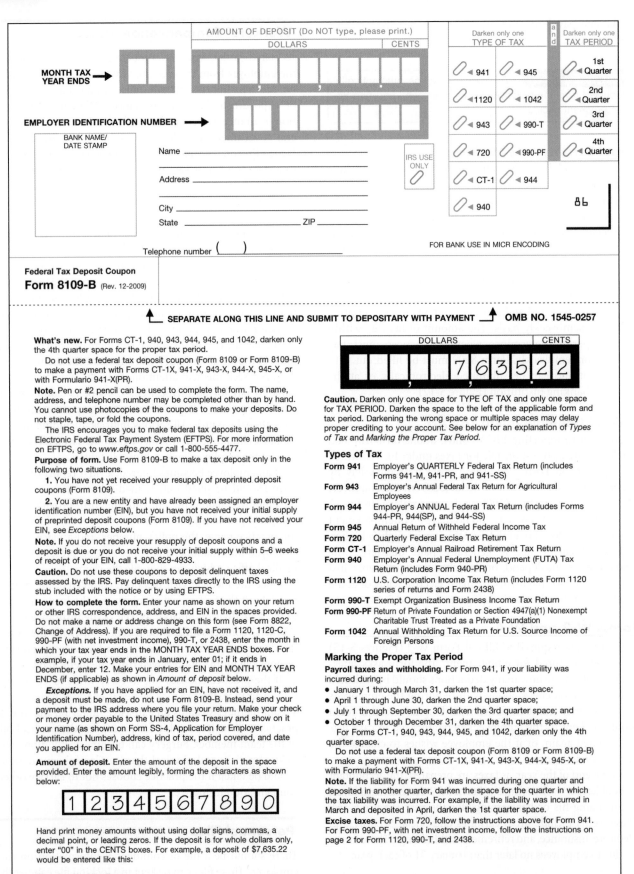

FIGURE 5-12 FICA Form 8109.

Form 940-V, Payment Voucher

Purpose of Form

Complete Form 940-V, Payment Voucher, if you are making a payment with Form 940, Employer's Annual Federal Unemployment (FUTA) Tax Return. We will use the completed voucher to credit your payment more promptly and accurately, and to improve our service to you.

Making Payments With Form 940

To avoid a penalty, make your payment with your 2012 Form 940 **only if** your FUTA tax for the fourth quarter (plus any undeposited amounts from earlier quarters) is $500 or less. If your total FUTA tax after adjustments (Form 940, line 12) is more than $500, you must make deposits by electronic funds transfer. See *When Must You Deposit Your FUTA Tax?* in the Instructions for Form 940. Also see sections 11 and 14 of Pub. 15 (Circular E), Employer's Tax Guide, for more information about deposits.

Caution. *Use Form 940-V when making any payment with Form 940. However, if you pay an amount with Form 940 that should have been deposited, you may be subject to a penalty. See* Deposit Penalties *in section 11 of Pub. 15 (Circular E).*

Specific Instructions

Box 1—Employer Identification Number (EIN). If you do not have an EIN, you may apply for one online. Go to IRS.gov and click on the *Apply for an EIN Online* link under *Tools*. You may also apply for an EIN by calling 1-800-829-4933, or you can fax or mail Form SS-4, Application for Employer Identification Number. If you have not received your EIN by the due date of Form 940, write "Applied For" and the date you applied in this entry space.

Box 2—Amount paid. Enter the amount paid with Form 940.

Box 3—Name and address. Enter your name and address as shown on Form 940.

• Enclose your check or money order made payable to the "United States Treasury." Be sure to enter your EIN, "Form 940," and "2012" on your check or money order. Do not send cash. Do not staple Form 940-V or your payment to Form 940 (or to each other).

• Detach Form 940-V and send it with your payment and Form 940 to the address provided in the Instructions for Form 940.

Note. You must also complete the entity information above Part 1 on Form 940.

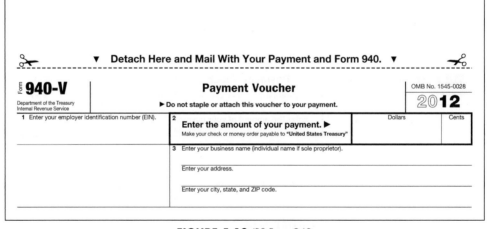

FIGURE 5-13 IRS Form 940.

 Veterinary practice managers maintain confidential employee records.

The team member's resume may be located at the front of the file, followed by the Form W-4, the employee benefits form, and an emergency contact form. Raises, evaluations, reprimands, and any disciplinary history can be included next, followed by copies of any credentials the team member may have. Other documents may include job descriptions, interview reports, background verification reports, offer of employment letters, and training records. Garnishment orders, credit reports, and medical records should be stored in a separate file, again in a locked cabinet. It is recommended that these records be kept for a minimum of 7 years after an employee has left the practice in case employment verification should be needed by another employer, or in case of tax or payroll audits or job-related illnesses or injuries. State and local laws may vary regarding the length of years records must be kept; whichever period is longer should supersede the other.

Contract Employee Versus Employee

Some veterinarians prefer to be contract employees instead of staff members. This is especially true for relief veterinarians. Contract employees, as stated previously for groomers, are responsible for their own taxes. Therefore contract employees are paid a straight fee; taxes are not withheld from their paychecks.

Form 941-V, Payment Voucher

Purpose of Form

Complete Form 941-V, Payment Voucher, if you are making a payment with Form 941, Employer's QUARTERLY Federal Tax Return. We will use the completed voucher to credit your payment more promptly and accurately, and to improve our service to you.

Making Payments With Form 941

To avoid a penalty, make your payment with Form 941 **only if:**

• Your total taxes after adjustments for either the current quarter or the preceding quarter (Form 941, line 10) are less than $2,500, you did not incur a $100,000 next-day deposit obligation during the current quarter, and you are paying in full with a timely filed return, or

• You are a monthly schedule depositor making a payment in accordance with the Accuracy of Deposits Rule. See section 11 of Pub. 15 (Circular E), Employer's Tax Guide, for details. In this case, the amount of your payment may be $2,500 or more.

Otherwise, you must make deposits by electronic funds transfer. See section 11 of Pub. 15 (Circular E) for deposit instructions. Do not use Form 941-V to make federal tax deposits.

Caution. *Use Form 941-V when making any payment with Form 941. However, if you pay an amount with Form 941 that should have been deposited, you may be subject to a penalty. See* Deposit Penalties *in section 11 of Pub. 15 (Circular E).*

Specific Instructions

Box 1—Employer identification number (EIN). If you do not have an EIN, you may apply for one online. Go to IRS.gov and click on the *Apply for an EIN Online* link under "Tools." You may also apply for an EIN by calling 1-800-829-4933, or you can fax or mail Form SS-4, Application for Employer Identification Number, to the IRS. If you have not received your EIN by the due date of Form 941, write "Applied For" and the date you applied in this entry space.

Box 2—Amount paid. Enter the amount paid with Form 941.

Box 3—Tax period. Darken the circle identifying the quarter for which the payment is made. Darken only one circle.

Box 4—Name and address. Enter your name and address as shown on Form 941.

• Enclose your check or money order made payable to the "United States Treasury." Be sure to enter your EIN, "Form 941," and the tax period on your check or money order. Do not send cash. Do not staple Form 941-V or your payment to Form 941 (or to each other).

• Detach Form 941-V and send it with your payment and Form 941 to the address in the Instructions for Form 941.

Note. You must also complete the entity information above Part 1 on Form 941.

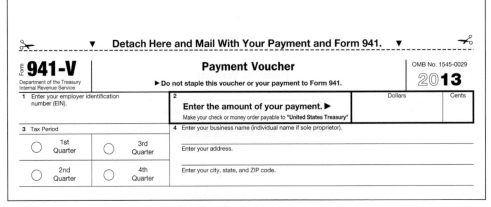

FIGURE 5-14 IRS Form 941.

PRACTICE POINT Verify the status of contract employees to prevent severe penalties from the IRS.

The IRS is strict regarding the classification of contract employment versus employee. IRS code states that independent contractors are not required to follow instructions as to how to perform a task, duty, or job. The work must be performed at irregular intervals and cannot be full time. Contractors control their own hours and have the right to pursue other jobs. They must work without supervision and are paid by the job, not the hour. They are responsible for their own dues and licenses, which should be made available when contracted.

An example of an independent contractor would be a specialist who comes into a practice, performs surgery, and leaves. These doctors do not develop a client/patient relationship, are paid for the job performed, and generally bring their own technicians to assist. A relief veterinarian who covers for a short time, filling in for an absent veterinarian, is also an independent contractor. Veterinarians who work shifts for an emergency clinic must use caution if they choose to use the term *independent contractor*. They cannot continually work the same shift and cannot be considered to work full time.

Veterinarians who work as contract employees should have copies of all credentials, including state and controlled substance licenses and U.S. Department of Agriculture accreditation, on file. Verification of contract licenses should also be checked with the state board of veterinary medicine. It is the practice's responsibility to ensure that proper documentation is verified when hiring relief and contract veterinarians.

Form W-4 (2013)

Purpose. Complete Form W-4 so that your employer can withhold the correct federal income tax from your pay. Consider completing a new Form W-4 each year and when your personal or financial situation changes.

Exemption from withholding. If you are exempt, complete **only** lines 1, 2, 3, 4, and 7 and sign the form to validate it. Your exemption for 2013 expires February 17, 2014. See Pub. 505, Tax Withholding and Estimated Tax.

Note. If another person can claim you as a dependent on his or her tax return, you cannot claim exemption from withholding if your income exceeds $1,000 and includes more than $350 of unearned income (for example, interest and dividends).

Basic instructions. If you are not exempt, complete the **Personal Allowances Worksheet** below. The worksheets on page 2 further adjust your withholding allowances based on itemized deductions, certain credits, adjustments to income, or two-earners/multiple jobs situations.

Complete all worksheets that apply. However, you may claim fewer (or zero) allowances. For regular wages, withholding must be based on allowances you claimed and may not be a flat amount or percentage of wages.

Head of household. Generally, you can claim head of household filing status on your tax return only if you are unmarried and pay more than 50% of the costs of keeping up a home for yourself and your dependent(s) or other qualifying individuals. See Pub. 501, Exemptions, Standard Deduction, and Filing Information, for information.

Tax credits. You can take projected tax credits into account in figuring your allowable number of withholding allowances. Credits for child or dependent care expenses and the child tax credit may be claimed using the **Personal Allowances Worksheet** below. See Pub. 505 for information on converting your other credits into withholding allowances.

Nonwage income. If you have a large amount of nonwage income, such as interest or dividends, consider making estimated tax payments using Form 1040-ES, Estimated Tax for Individuals. Otherwise, you may owe additional tax. If you have pension or annuity

income, see Pub. 505 to find out if you should adjust your withholding on Form W-4 or W-4P.

Two earners or multiple jobs. If you have a working spouse or more than one job, figure the total number of allowances you are entitled to claim on all jobs using worksheets from only one Form W-4. Your withholding usually will be most accurate when all allowances are claimed on the Form W-4 for the highest paying job and zero allowances are claimed on the others. See Pub. 505 for details.

Nonresident alien. If you are a nonresident alien, see Notice 1392, Supplemental Form W-4 Instructions for Nonresident Aliens, before completing this form.

Check your withholding. After your Form W-4 takes effect, use Pub. 505 to see how the amount you are having withheld compares to your projected total tax for 2013. See Pub. 505, especially if your earnings exceed $130,000 (Single) or $180,000 (Married).

Future developments. Information about any future developments affecting Form W-4 (such as legislation enacted after we release it) will be posted at *www.irs.gov/w4*.

Personal Allowances Worksheet (Keep for your records.)

A Enter "1" for **yourself** if no one else can claim you as a dependent . . . . **A** _____

B Enter "1" if:
- You are single and have only one job; or
- You are married, have only one job, and your spouse does not work; or
- Your wages from a second job or your spouse's wages (or the total of both) are $1,500 or less.

. . . **B** _____

C Enter "1" for your **spouse.** But, you may choose to enter "-0-" if you are married and have either a working spouse or more than one job. (Entering "-0-" may help you avoid having too little tax withheld.) . . . . **C** _____

D Enter number of **dependents** (other than your spouse or yourself) you will claim on your tax return . . . **D** _____

E Enter "1" if you will file as **head of household** on your tax return (see conditions under **Head of household** above) . . **E** _____

F Enter "1" if you have at least $1,900 of **child or dependent care expenses** for which you plan to claim a credit . . . **F** _____

(**Note.** Do **not** include child support payments. See Pub. 503, Child and Dependent Care Expenses, for details.)

G **Child Tax Credit** (including additional child tax credit). See Pub. 972, Child Tax Credit, for more information.
- If your total income will be less than $65,000 ($95,000 if married), enter "2" for each eligible child; then **less** "1" if you have three to six eligible children or **less** "2" if you have seven or more eligible children.
- If your total income will be between $65,000 and $84,000 ($95,000 and $119,000 if married), enter "1" for each eligible child . . . **G** _____

H Add lines A through G and enter total here. (**Note.** This may be different from the number of exemptions you claim on your tax return.) ▶ **H** _____

For accuracy, complete all worksheets that apply.
- If you plan to **itemize** or **claim adjustments to income** and want to reduce your withholding, see the **Deductions and Adjustments Worksheet** on page 2.
- If you are **single** and have **more than one job** or are **married and you and your spouse both work** and the combined earnings from all jobs exceed $40,000 ($10,000 if married), see the **Two-Earners/Multiple Jobs Worksheet** on page 2 to avoid having too little tax withheld.
- If **neither** of the above situations applies, **stop here** and enter the number from line H on line 5 of Form W-4 below.

--------------------------------- Separate here and give Form W-4 to your employer. Keep the top part for your records. ---------------------------------

Form **W-4**
Department of the Treasury
Internal Revenue Service

Employee's Withholding Allowance Certificate

▶ Whether you are entitled to claim a certain number of allowances or exemption from withholding is subject to review by the IRS. Your employer may be required to send a copy of this form to the IRS.

OMB No. 1545-0074

2013

1 Your first name and middle initial	Last name	2 Your social security number

Home address (number and street or rural route)

3 ☐ Single ☐ Married ☐ Married, but withhold at higher Single rate.
Note. If married, but legally separated, or spouse is a nonresident alien, check the "Single" box.

City or town, state, and ZIP code

4 If your last name differs from that shown on your social security card, check here. You must call 1-800-772-1213 for a replacement card. ▶ ☐

5 Total number of allowances you are claiming (from line **H** above **or** from the applicable worksheet on page 2) **5** _____

6 Additional amount, if any, you want withheld from each paycheck . . . . **6** $ _____

7 I claim exemption from withholding for 2013, and I certify that I meet **both** of the following conditions for exemption.
- Last year I had a right to a refund of **all** federal income tax withheld because I had **no** tax liability, **and**
- This year I expect a refund of **all** federal income tax withheld because I expect to have **no** tax liability.

If you meet both conditions, write "Exempt" here . . . . ▶ **7** _____

Under penalties of perjury, I declare that I have examined this certificate and, to the best of my knowledge and belief, it is true, correct, and complete.

Employee's signature
(This form is not valid unless you sign it.) ▶

Date ▶

8 Employer's name and address (Employer: Complete lines 8 and 10 only if sending to the IRS.)	9 Office code (optional)	10 Employer identification number (EIN)

For Privacy Act and Paperwork Reduction Act Notice, see page 2.   Cat. No. 10220Q   Form **W-4** (2013)

FIGURE 5-15 IRS Form W-4.

Form W-4 (2013)

Deductions and Adjustments Worksheet

Note. Use this worksheet *only* if you plan to itemize deductions or claim certain credits or adjustments to income.

1 Enter an estimate of your 2013 itemized deductions. These include qualifying home mortgage interest, charitable contributions, state and local taxes, medical expenses in excess of 10% (7.5% if either you or your spouse was born before January 2, 1949) of your income, and miscellaneous deductions. For 2013, you may have to reduce your itemized deductions if your income is over $300,000 and you are married filing jointly or are a qualifying widow(er); $275,000 if you are head of household; $250,000 if you are single and not head of household or a qualifying widow(er); or $150,000 if you are married filing separately. See Pub. 505 for details . . .   **1** $ _____

2 Enter: { $12,200 if married filing jointly or qualifying widow(er) / $8,950 if head of household / $6,100 if single or married filing separately }   **2** $ _____

3 **Subtract** line 2 from line 1. If zero or less, enter "-0-" . . . .   **3** $ _____

4 Enter an estimate of your 2013 adjustments to income and any additional standard deduction (see Pub. 505)   **4** $ _____

5 **Add** lines 3 and 4 and enter the total. (Include any amount for credits from the *Converting Credits to Withholding Allowances for 2013 Form W-4* worksheet in Pub. 505.) . . . .   **5** $ _____

6 Enter an estimate of your 2013 nonwage income (such as dividends or interest) . . . .   **6** $ _____

7 **Subtract** line 6 from line 5. If zero or less, enter "-0-" . . . .   **7** $ _____

8 **Divide** the amount on line 7 by $3,900 and enter the result here. Drop any fraction . . . .   **8** _____

9 Enter the number from the **Personal Allowances Worksheet,** line H, page 1 . . . .   **9** _____

10 **Add** lines 8 and 9 and enter the total here. If you plan to use the **Two-Earners/Multiple Jobs Worksheet,** also enter this total on line 1 below. Otherwise, **stop here** and enter this total on Form W-4, line 5, page 1   **10** _____

Two-Earners/Multiple Jobs Worksheet (See *Two earners or multiple jobs* on page 1.)

Note. Use this worksheet *only* if the instructions under line H on page 1 direct you here.

1 Enter the number from line H, page 1 (or from line 10 above if you used the **Deductions and Adjustments Worksheet**)   **1** _____

2 Find the number in **Table 1** below that applies to the **LOWEST** paying job and enter it here. **However,** if you are married filing jointly and wages from the highest paying job are $65,000 or less, do not enter more than "3" . . . .   **2** _____

3 If line 1 is **more than or equal to** line 2, subtract line 2 from line 1. Enter the result here (if zero, enter "-0-") and on Form W-4, line 5, page 1. **Do not** use the rest of this worksheet . . . . . .   **3** _____

Note. If line 1 is **less than** line 2, enter "-0-" on Form W-4, line 5, page 1. Complete lines 4 through 9 below to figure the additional withholding amount necessary to avoid a year-end tax bill.

4 Enter the number from line 2 of this worksheet . . . .   **4** _____

5 Enter the number from line 1 of this worksheet . . . .   **5** _____

6 **Subtract** line 5 from line 4 . . . .   **6** _____

7 Find the amount in **Table 2** below that applies to the **HIGHEST** paying job and enter it here . . . .   **7** $ _____

8 **Multiply** line 7 by line 6 and enter the result here. This is the additional annual withholding needed . .   **8** $ _____

9 Divide line 8 by the number of pay periods remaining in 2013. For example, divide by 25 if you are paid every two weeks and you complete this form on a date in January when there are 25 pay periods remaining in 2013. Enter the result here and on Form W-4, line 6, page 1. This is the additional amount to be withheld from each paycheck   **9** $ _____

Table 1

Married Filing Jointly		All Others	
If wages from **LOWEST** paying job are—	Enter on line 2 above	If wages from **LOWEST** paying job are—	Enter on line 2 above
$0 - $5,000	0	$0 - $8,000	0
5,001 - 13,000	1	8,001 - 16,000	1
13,001 - 24,000	2	16,001 - 25,000	2
24,001 - 26,000	3	25,001 - 30,000	3
26,001 - 30,000	4	30,001 - 40,000	4
30,001 - 42,000	5	40,001 - 50,000	5
42,001 - 48,000	6	50,001 - 70,000	6
48,001 - 55,000	7	70,001 - 80,000	7
55,001 - 65,000	8	80,001 - 95,000	8
65,001 - 75,000	9	95,001 - 120,000	9
75,001 - 85,000	10	120,001 and over	10
85,001 - 97,000	11		
97,001 - 110,000	12		
110,001 - 120,000	13		
120,001 - 135,000	14		
135,001 and over	15		

Table 2

Married Filing Jointly		All Others	
If wages from **HIGHEST** paying job are—	Enter on line 7 above	If wages from **HIGHEST** paying job are—	Enter on line 7 above
$0 - $72,000	590	$0 - $37,000	590
72,001 - 130,000	980	37,001 - 80,000	980
130,001 - 200,000	1,090	80,001 - 175,000	1,090
200,001 - 345,000	1,290	175,001 - 385,000	1,290
345,001 - 385,000	1,370	385,001 and over	1,540
385,001 and over	1,540		

Privacy Act and Paperwork Reduction Act Notice. We ask for the information on this form to carry out the Internal Revenue laws of the United States. Internal Revenue Code sections 3402(f)(2) and 6109 and their regulations require you to provide this information; your employer uses it to determine your federal income tax withholding. Failure to provide a properly completed form will result in your being treated as a single person who claims no withholding allowances; providing fraudulent information may subject you to penalties. Routine uses of this information include giving it to the Department of Justice for civil and criminal litigation; to cities, states, the District of Columbia, and U.S. commonwealths and possessions for use in administering their tax laws; and to the Department of Health and Human Services for use in the National Directory of New Hires. We may also disclose this information to other countries under a tax treaty, to federal and state agencies to enforce federal nontax criminal laws, or to federal law enforcement and intelligence agencies to combat terrorism.

You are not required to provide the information requested on a form that is subject to the Paperwork Reduction Act unless the form displays a valid OMB control number. Books or records relating to a form or its instructions must be retained as long as their contents may become material in the administration of any Internal Revenue law. Generally, tax returns and return information are confidential, as required by Code section 6103.

The average time and expenses required to complete and file this form will vary depending on individual circumstances. For estimated averages, see the instructions for your income tax return.

If you have suggestions for making this form simpler, we would be happy to hear from you. See the instructions for your income tax return.

FIGURE 5-15, cont'd

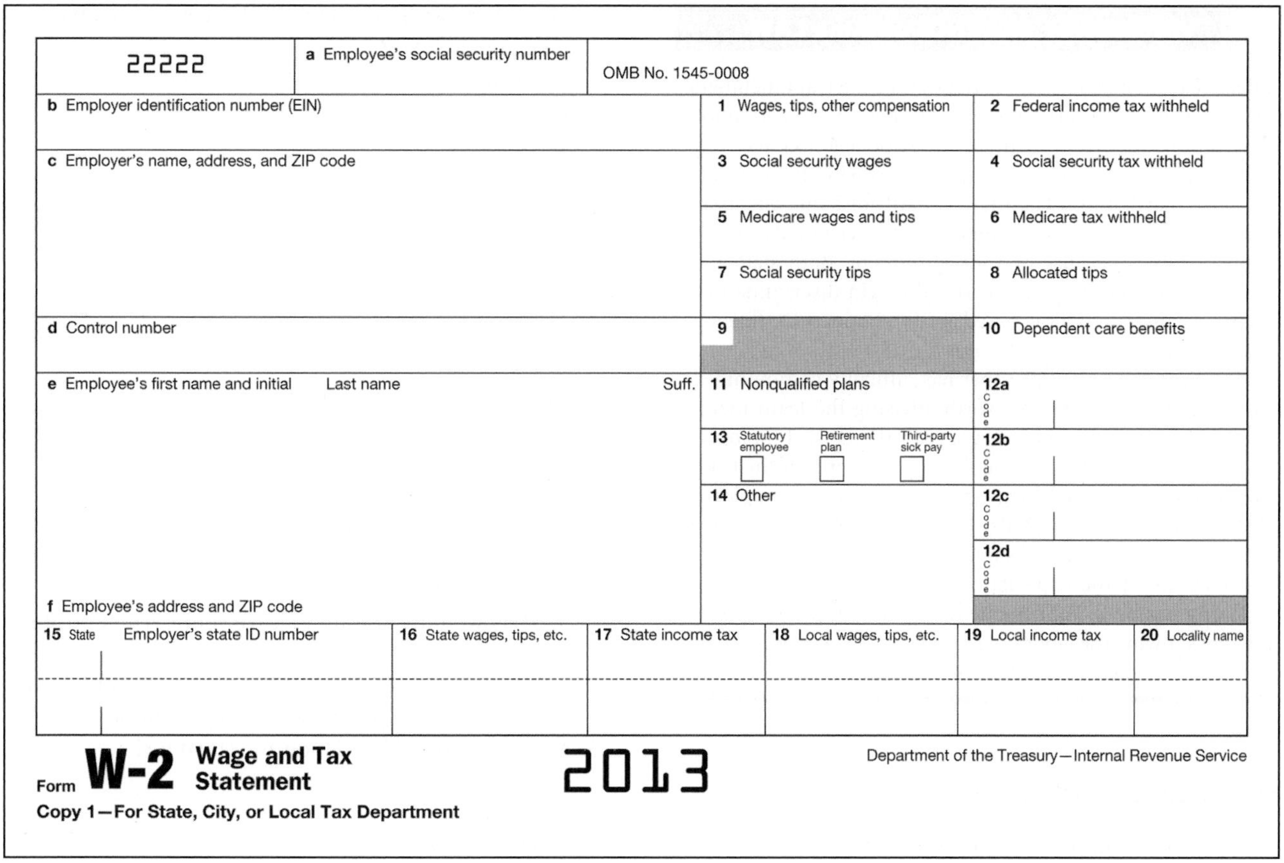

22222	**a** Employee's social security number		

b Employer identification number (EIN)

c Employer's name, address, and ZIP code

d Control number

e Employee's first name and initial   Last name   Suff.

f Employee's address and ZIP code

OMB No. 1545-0008

1 Wages, tips, other compensation | 2 Federal income tax withheld
3 Social security wages | 4 Social security tax withheld
5 Medicare wages and tips | 6 Medicare tax withheld
7 Social security tips | 8 Allocated tips
9 | 10 Dependent care benefits
11 Nonqualified plans | 12a Code
13 Statutory employee / Retirement plan / Third-party sick pay | 12b Code
14 Other | 12c Code
| 12d Code

| 15 State | Employer's state ID number | 16 State wages, tips, etc. | 17 State income tax | 18 Local wages, tips, etc. | 19 Local income tax | 20 Locality name |

Form **W-2** Wage and Tax Statement **2013**
Copy 1—For State, City, or Local Tax Department
Department of the Treasury—Internal Revenue Service

FIGURE 5-16 IRS Form W-2.

At the end of the year, any contract veterinarian receiving pay over $600 within the fiscal year must be issued Form 1099-MISC for taxation purposes (others are issued Form W-2). Form 1099-MISC cites all monies paid to the contractor on an untaxed basis. The veterinarian submits Form 1099-MISC with his or her taxes. (See Figure 5-11 for an example of Form 1099-MISC).

If an independent contractor fails to file and pay his or her own taxes, and a practice used the contractor's services for over $600 and did not issue Form 1099-MISC at the end of the year, the practice can be held responsible for all back taxes, interest, and penalty charges. It is imperative to contact a certified public accountant regarding the state and federal regulations that may apply to a practice when using a relief or contracted veterinarian.

It is also becoming popular for credentialed veterinary technicians to contract out their services. Technicians may provide relief services at hospitals that need coverage or provide consulting services. These are also considered contract employees who must also follow the aforementioned procedures.

Theft and Embezzlement

Employee theft and embezzlement are the leading causes of unexplained inventory reduction and cash flow. Having excess inventory supplies available on the floor unfortunately invites employee theft. Team members see the extra supplies and think taking one box of Heartgard is not going to hurt the practice. However, if each employee took one box of heartworm preventative for each pet, the cost would be considerable. Theft normally does not stop with one box. Soon it becomes dog food or medication and, if the team member is not caught, can move to bigger, more expensive items. When employees purchase items, one team member should be responsible for entering charges for all employees. This can ensure correct charges for products and that all products are being charged for.

Team members can be crafty at embezzling cash. More than one person should be responsible for handling cash and balancing the cash drawer at the end of the night. Additionally, another person should be responsible for the deposits, and the office manager must balance the printed deposit slip to the daily total.

If employee theft or embezzlement is suspected, the practice attorney should be contacted for further advice. Some practices may install cameras to try to catch employees in the act. Proof of theft should be required. Once the practice has proof of the theft, the employee can be terminated. Practices must use caution when suspecting employee theft; a lawsuit can be initiated by the terminated employee if there is a lack of evidence. See Chapter 20 for more information on theft and embezzlement.

⚖ VETERINARY PRACTICE and the LAW

Effective team management includes training team members in proper oral communication. It is imperative to add to job descriptions that team members must be able to effectively communicate with clients. Team members with thick accents or those that talk too fast may be hard for some clients to understand; however, employers cannot discriminate against team members because of a foreign accent. Both state and federal laws protect against national origin discrimination, including discrimination based on foreign accent, fluency, and cultural traits (e.g., clothing).

If an excellent team member has difficulty communicating with clients, it may be worth advising the team member to seek the assistance of a speech therapist. Employers may want to contribute to the therapy assistance if the team member is a potential long-term and dedicated employee that has heightened soft skills. This assistance can be deemed continuing education, and should be tied to the performance expectations. If the expectations are not met (and proper coaching has been implemented), the employee can be dismissed; showing the labor board every action had been taken to improve the team members' performance.

REVIEW QUESTIONS

1. Give two examples of questions that cannot be asked during an interview.
2. What is the FLSA?
3. What is USERRA?
4. What is OSHA?
5. What posters are required to be posted in a practice?
6. Where should the required posters be posted?
7. What is the benefit of developing an employee manual?
8. What payroll taxes are employers responsible for?
9. What is a contract employee?
10. Why provide training in phases?
11. How many weeks does the FMLA cover an employee to take unpaid leave?
    a. 14 weeks
    b. 6 weeks
    c. 12 weeks
    d. 8 weeks
12. Which act requires employers to pay minimum wage and overtime pay?
    a. FMLA
    b. EPPA
    c. EEO
    d. FLSA
13. What does NCA stand for?
    a. National Contract-Employees Association
    b. Noncompete Agreement
    c. No Contract Act
    d. Nonimmigrant Control Act
14. Which of the following is a question you should *not* ask during an interview?
    a. Why would you want to leave your current position?
    b. What is your salary requirement?
    c. What was the least enjoyable aspect of your last job?
    d. When did you graduate from high school?
15. What does the abbreviation AD stand for?
    a. Right ear
    b. Right eye
    c. Once daily
    d. Adrenal disease

Recommended Reading

AAHA: *Financial & productivity pulse points*, ed 7, Lakewood, CO, 2013, AAHA Press.

Donnelly AL: *AAHA guide to creating an employee handbook*, ed 3, Lakewood, CO, 2009, AAHA Press.

Employment Law Guide: Laws, Regulations and Technical Assistance Service (Web site): www.dol.gov/compliance/guide/. Accessed August 4, 2013.

Stress, Burnout, and Compassion Fatigue

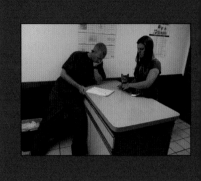

OUTLINE

Stress Identification, *138*
  Positive and Negative Stress, *138*
  Choice, Control, and Consequences, *138*
  Stages of Stress, *139*
  Role of Neurotransmitters, *139*
  Personalities and Stress, *139*
  Identifying Stressors, *139*
Coping with Stress, *140*
Substance Abuse and Dependence, *141*
  Factors Affecting Substance Abuse, *141*
  Recognizing Substance Abuse, *141*

Intervention, *141*
  Steps of Drug Intervention, *142*
Preventing Career Burnout, *142*
Compassion Fatigue, *143*
  Signs and Symptoms of Compassion
    Fatigue, *144*
  Impact of Compassion Fatigue on
    Individuals, *144*
  Impact of Compassion Fatigue on
    the Practice, *144*
  Managing Compassion Fatigue, *144*

KEY TERMS

Dependence
Intervention
Neurotransmitters
Stress
Stressors
Substance Abuse

LEARNING OBJECTIVES

When you have completed this chapter, you should be able to:

1. Identify stress.
2. Explain the stages associated with stress.
3. Identify common stressors.
4. List methods used to control stress.
5. Describe substance abuse.
6. List methods of intervention.
7. Identify characteristics associated with burnout.

CRITICAL COMPETENCIES

1. **Compliance** - being reliable, thorough, and conscientious in carrying out work assignments; having an appreciation for the importance of organizational rules and policies.
2. **Integrity** - honesty, trustworthiness, and adherence to high standards of ethical conduct.
3. **Leadership** - a willingness to lead and take charge; the ability to motivate others and mobilize group effort toward common goals.
4. **Planning and Prioritizing** - the ability to effectively manage time and workload to meet deadlines; the ability to organize work, set priorities, and establish plans for achieving goals.
5. **Relationship Building** - the ability to develop constructive and cooperative working relationships with others and maintain them over time; must also be able to settle disputes, resolve grievances and conflicts, and negotiate with others.

Stress is responsible for a variety of effects in human beings, including physical illness, mental illness, and death. Stress has become accepted in today's society, and at times appears to be unavoidable. Many factors, such as irritable clients, complex cases, and a high volume of patients, can produce a high level of stress in veterinary medicine.

People choose to handle stress in different ways, either positively or negatively, such as with exercise (positive) or with drugs and alcohol (negative). Unfortunately, many choose to cope with stress through drugs and alcohol. Drugs and alcohol may relieve the emotional and physical effects of stress; however, the use of these substances generally creates more problems than they are worth. It is important to identify the source(s) associated with stress and attempt to control the situation. This will allow lower levels of stress, positively affecting physical and mental health.

Stress in the veterinary profession also contributes to burnout and compassion fatigue. Burnout is defined as physical and/or emotional exhaustion that is related to the effects of long-term stress. Compassion fatigue is the effects and characteristics that result from the long-term caring (emotionally and physically) for pets and clients. All team members should make an effort to prevent either from occurring.

Stress Identification

Stress can be defined as the state produced when the body responds to any demand for adaptation or adjustment (Figure 6-1). Stress produces stressors that can be identified as internal, external, or environmentally related. Internal stressors include a person's emotions and sensitivities. A person may be more sensitive to words or phrases said to them and may respond with more emotion than typical. External stressors may include limited time schedules and large workloads. Many people take on too many projects, filling their schedule and workloads to capacity, causing

unusual stress and reactions. Environmental stressors many be as simple as hot or cold weather and complex noises. Too many alarms on a surgery monitor can cause a person to respond differently than what is considered normal.

Positive and Negative Stress

Stress comes in two forms: positive (good) stress and negative (bad) stress. Positive stress is the body's natural ability to learn how to cope with stress; it may energize a person to cope with the challenges presented. Good stress produces satisfaction and relief once the action or actions causing the stress are over. However, if positive stress continues for an unreasonable amount of time, it can turn into a negative stressor and affect the person negatively (Box 6-1). Good stress can result in an overly energized person who eventually becomes overworked, leading to exhaustion. A person who is exhausted ultimately becomes an overwhelmed individual.

Bad stress can inadvertently affect a person physically, emotionally, and mentally. Bad stress affects blood pressure and heart rate and can make individuals respond in an unusual manner to normal situations. The normal situation of running out of milk may trigger a person's temper. Bad stress must be taken control of to prevent conflict between family and co-workers.

Choice, Control, and Consequences

Three factors affect good and bad stress: choice, control, and consequences. *Choice* is determined by the individual. An individual chooses to be involved in a project and chooses to have good stress associated with the project. For example, a technician chooses to remodel an exam room by applying new colors of paint, adding a border around the perimeter of the room, and staining the baseboards. The good stress provides satisfaction once the project is completed.

> **PRACTICE POINT**   Three factors affect how team members respond to stress: choice, control, and consequence.

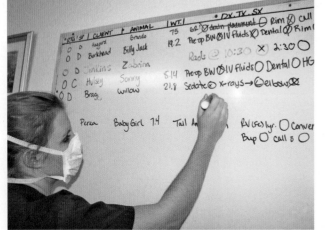

FIGURE 6-1 High patient load and insufficient staff can produce stress in veterinary team members.

BOX 6-1	Physical Ailments That May be Triggered by Stress
• Allergies	• Heart attack
• Anxiety	• Heartburn
• Asthma	• Hypertension
• Backaches	• Hyperventilation
• Chest pains	• Insomnia
• Chronic fatigue	• Muscle aches
• Colitis	• Nausea
• Depression	• Nosebleeds
• Dermatitis	• Perspiration
• Dizziness	• Sexual dysfunction
• Dry mouth	• Temporomandibular joint
• Erratic breathing	disorders
• Facial tics	• Ulcers
• Headaches	

Control is how a person wishes to respond to and master stress. Clients and emergencies determine the schedule of a practice. The practice may set up the daily schedule, but walk-ins and emergencies ultimately change the schedule on a daily basis. The increased business and complex cases add stress to each team member's daily routine; however, if team members can have a quick powwow, then each member's stress level will decrease because a plan has been discussed and implemented. The team has taken control, ultimately reducing stress.

Consequence is the result of an action. For example, once cancer has been diagnosed, death is a likely outcome at some point in the patient's future. Therefore death is the consequence of the diagnosis. If the anticipated result is expected, the stress produced is a good stress (resulting in little effect on the heart rate and blood pressure). However, if an unexpected death results from anesthesia, bad stress results. Death is not a normal consequence of anesthesia and produces a large amount of stress on the staff.

Stages of Stress

The body automatically responds to stress mentally and physically. The body's fight-or-flight response occurs automatically and is necessary for survival. Several stages exist in the fight-or-flight response: alarm, adaptation, exhaustion, and death. Stage 1, alarm, is the initial response to fight or flight. The body releases increased endorphins and hormones and the blood flow within the body is increased. This affects and increases the breathing rate, blood sugar levels, adrenal gland secretion, cortisone production, and perspiration. Adrenal gland secretion of epinephrine increases the individual's heart and respiratory rate. A prolonged increase in heart rate increases blood pressure, which ultimately has negative effects on the cardiac system. The adrenal glands' activity, over a prolonged period, may cause muscle tension and digestive tract disorders. Diarrhea, nausea, ulcers, and constipation can result from oversecretion of the adrenal glands. If stage 1 continues, the body learns to adapt to the conditions and tries to compensate for the abnormalities, resulting in stage 2, adaptation. After a prolonged period, the body adapts and becomes exhausted (stage 3), resulting in burnout, fatigue, and eventually death (stage 4).

Role of Neurotransmitters

During stressful situations, neurotransmitters in the brain are called on and can be oversecreted in a manner similar to hormone release and adrenal gland response during stage 1. Overproduction of neurotransmitters can cause anxiety, anger, and depression. After prolonged release, a person is no longer able to cope with normal stressors. This is when many turn to drugs or alcohol to try to eliminate the stress. Drugs and alcohol distort or eliminate the exchange of information in the brain, releasing the stress felt by these individuals.

Personalities and Stress

Personalities predispose people to experience stress differently. It is not known how personality affects stress, whether it is learned or genetic; however, personalities are grouped into types. The stress-prone personality is generally a type A personality. These individuals are perfectionists, often multitask, expect a high level of performance from themselves as well as their co-workers, and tend to be successful. Stress-prone individuals are at a higher risk for heart disease and hypertension. Stress-hardy personalities are less prone to stress, are in control of their lives, and do not have to be the best in all they do. They often control and compartmentalize the stress and deal with it later. Type B personalities manage stress well, rarely letting others know they are suffering from any type of stress.

Identifying Stressors

Identifying stressors can help one cope with stress in a successful manner. Individuals in the veterinary field generally experience life-event, environmental, personal, client, and career stressors. Life-event stressors can include death, divorce, retirement, pregnancy, financial difficulties, and holidays. The list of life-event stressors that can affect an individual is endless, and each person will respond to each situation differently. For example, the holiday season can be extremely stressful for a person with financial difficulty or a large, overbearing family. Holidays may be peaceful and enjoyable for an individual with financial success and a small, close-knit family. How the person deals with the stress is individualized, as is whether they choose to control the situation or not.

> **PRACTICE POINT**   Identifying stressors will help team members cope with stress.

Environmental stressors include climate, weather, pollution, crime, and traffic. In veterinary medicine, environmental stressors include noise levels, alarms, equipment, and inventory. Several noises and alarms may occur at once, including the ringing phones, barking dogs, and surgical monitor warnings. Equipment maintenance and breaks can be a huge stressor, especially for the technician who is in charge of maintaining and repairing equipment. Inventory shortages can be a stress to doctors, who may feel that supplies are always limited, preventing them from practicing the medicine they want.

Personal stressors may include lack of self-confidence and self-esteem. Team members who lack both self-confidence and self-esteem may have a harder time educating and taking care of clients as well as being successful in their personal lives.

Client stressors include clients who are angry or grieving. Dealing with a know-it-all and the elderly can also be stressful. Angry clients make every team member's day miserable and are able to invoke every stressor. Grieving clients experience several emotions, including denial, anger, and eventually acceptance. Many times the team must cater to every stage and emotion of grief. This can add stress to each team member's daily routine, again invoking several other stressors. Know-it-all clients generally think they know more

than the veterinarians themselves, although they have not attended veterinary school. These clients may choose to treat the patient themselves, regardless of the recommendations that have been made by the team. Teams should understand that they cannot control this type of client or their actions and should simply document the recommendations in the record. Some elderly clients want to talk about every animal they have owned, share every encounter the current pet has ever experienced, and want the best treatment available. Unfortunately, many cannot afford the best care available. The team may feel guilty and will sometimes make concessions to help this type of client. Stress can be eliminated with this type of client, knowing that this client will take time and patience; preplanning would be of benefit to the staff. Satisfaction can be obtained from this type of stress when it is managed in the correct fashion.

Career stressors may include long hours, low pay, and unappreciated work ethic. Many technicians and veterinarians enter the profession with the understanding of low pay and long hours, but years of unappreciated work eventually have a compounding effect. Team members can take actions to minimize career stressors by controlling the situation. Leaders of the practice and team members must work together to eliminate long hours; each member should be responsible for capping his or her own hours. An individual can only put forth so many productive hours within a week's period. Balancing work and life is essential when managing career stress. Pay scales can be evaluated and potentially increased by enhancing the skill set, knowledge, and value of each employee. Team members should consistently strive for higher levels of education, higher levels of care, and excellent levels of client education. An invaluable employee may receive higher compensation and be rewarded for the excellent work ethic put forth. Job satisfaction and dedication can decrease stress; again, long hours must be capped to prevent burnout.

Coping with Stress

Once stressors have been identified, they must be analyzed as to which ones can be dealt with, coped with, and/or eliminated. Changes in lifestyle, mental and physical activities, and relaxation methods can be instituted to help eliminate, or at least reduce, stress. Nutrition, sleep, and exercise (Figure 6-2) play a vital role in reducing stress and should be taken into consideration when making lifestyle changes.

> **PRACTICE POINT** Cope with stress by eating healthy, exercising regularly, and sleeping well.

Regular healthy eating habits are one of the best protectors against stress. Protein is especially helpful in counteracting the effects of stress on the body. Micronutrients from fruits and vegetables help improve the

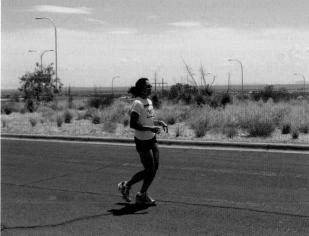

FIGURE 6-2 Exercise can alleviate stress and prevent a person from becoming burnt out in his or her profession.

immune system, which is impaired as a side effect of stress. Since the blood glucose level is altered, individuals tend to overeat sugars, fats, and carbohydrates during stressful periods. These nutrients, although essential in small and limited amounts, are counterproductive in alleviating stress.

Sleep is imperative to reducing stress. Sleep needs vary from person to person and may change throughout one's life cycle. Most adults need 7 to 8 hours of sleep per night; each must learn the amount required to function properly, produce work at an acceptable level, and rise in the morning feeling refreshed. The REM (rapid eye movement) phase of sleep is also essential. Dreams occur during REM sleep, and it has been determined that this type of sleep is necessary to rest the body. Those who consume alcohol and use drugs do not experience a normal REM phase and therefore experience sleep deprivation.

Exercise reduces stress by reducing and releasing tension, restoring normal chemical balances, relieving mild depression, and decreasing the risk of cardiac disease. Exercise should be part of a normal daily routine and should include activities that are enjoyable. Each person enjoys activities on different levels; therefore finding one that satisfies both the mind and body is imperative. Many people enjoy running and the endorphins it produces, allowing the mind to solve problems and relieve stress as the body exerts energy. Others enjoy hiking, kayaking, weightlifting, or riding bikes. Any exercise program must be enjoyable to be beneficial. Each person must experiment and find the right activity.

Mental changes and activities can be initiated to reduce the effects of stress. Laughter, the best medicine, should be part of every person's day. Hobbies may be adopted, taking the mind away from stressors and allowing increased concentration on other topics. Music, reading, and art can also be forms of stress relief depending on the individual.

Expressing feelings is an excellent outlet for stress. Friends, family, and co-workers can be exceptional listeners for someone who needs to vent. Once feelings are released,

the stress level decreases. Talking with co-workers may not only alleviate stress, but also produce solutions to reduce the stress as well. Many times if one co-worker is experiencing stress associated with the practice, others are as well.

It is known that chronic and/or uninterrupted stress is very harmful. It is important therefore to take breaks and decompress. Walks can be taken instead of coffee breaks. Team members should use weekends to relax and avoid scheduling so many events that Monday mornings seem like a relief. Creating a predictable schedule at work and home provides structure and routine in one's life. Thinking and planning ahead allow various scenarios to be considered, good and bad, which may become realities at work or home. One cannot prevent the unexpected from happening; however, visualizing what is possible can provide a comfortable framework from which to respond. With this kind of preparation, stress can be turned into a positive force. Individuals can learn signals associated with stress and take measures to reduce them before they become a problem.

Various mental health care providers offer stress-management counseling in the form of individual or group therapy. Stress counseling and group discussion therapy has been shown to reduce stress symptoms and improve overall health and attitude.

Substance Abuse and Dependence

Not every person who uses drugs or alcohol to deal with stress is an abuser or becomes dependent on the product. However, the likelihood of dependence on the product is high. Substance abusers may use the drug or alcohol intermittently or on a regular basis. Either type of user may develop substance dependence. Stress has long been recognized as one of the most powerful triggers for drug or alcohol cravings and abuse.

Substance dependence is indicated by symptoms of tolerance to the effects of a drug and symptoms of withdrawal without the drug. The user eventually requires more of the substance to obtain the desired effects. When the individual is not using the substance, he or she may have symptoms such as cravings, anxiety, and/or depression. Once a user becomes dependent on a substance, he or she continues to use it regardless of the consequences. This is when individuals lose their families and jobs. The use of the substance has now become an addiction.

Factors Affecting Substance Abuse

Some risk factors for addiction have been determined; these include genes, chronic pain, sociocultural factors, and environment. Individuals who have families with a history of addictions must exercise caution at all times because the risk of addiction to alcohol or drugs is high. Individuals who suffer chronic pain have a higher chance of developing an addiction because it begins to take more of the substance to decrease the pain associated with chronic conditions. Sociocultural factors include age, occupation, ethnicity, and social class (including friends and acquaintances). Environmental factors include stresses associated with an occupation or family as well as the ability to access drugs. Individuals in the health care industry have a higher percent chance of becoming dependent on substances because of the availability and ease of access.

Recognizing Substance Abuse

It can be hard to recognize drug abuse or determine the correct time to intervene. Users hide the secret, keep it confidential, and eventually become isolated. These actions eventually lead to a feeling of helplessness; however, users justify the use of drugs because of the high levels of stress they may be enduring or the increased workload and fatigue that they experience.

Many substance abusers experience a change in behavior, practice poor personal hygiene, and dress in a sloppy, wrinkled, and unprofessional manner. They begin to withdraw from family, friends, and co-workers. They neglect their duties and cases, are disorganized, and exhibit poor judgment. Many start to write prescriptions for themselves, steal controlled substances from the practice, experience financial problems, and begin to have unexplained absences from work. This results in conflict and career instability.

It is important to intervene to protect clients and other team members. The practice may be at risk for malpractice suits because the impaired team member will make poor judgments. Those convicted of drug abuse can have their licenses revoked, which can prevent the license from ever being renewed.

Intervention

A drug intervention is a process that helps a drug addict recognize the extent of his or her problem. Individuals who are addicted to drugs or alcohol usually do not know their addiction is out of control. They tend to look at those around them as a measure of how right or wrong their actions are. Those who surround themselves with individuals who are caught up in the grasp of drug addiction are not able to see the drastic effects of their own dependence.

> **PRACTICE POINT** Intervention, although risky, can save a person's career, *and life.*

These individuals need objective feedback on their behavior. It is through a nonjudgmental, noncritical, systematic drug intervention process that the individuals are able to see their own lifestyle choices. When they truly understand the impact that their alcohol dependence or drug addiction has on others, they may begin to see that they are hurting those around them.

The individual who is suspected of having a substance abuse problem may try to minimize his or her use, change the topic, joke about use, or say phrases such as "my substance use is no worse than anyone else's." Even if the individual begins to share some life problems that he or she has been experiencing, know that those problems will not get better unless the individual stops the use of alcohol or substances.

The goal of an intervention is for the addict to accept the reality of his or her addiction and to seek help. The process of conducting an intervention is a difficult and delicate matter.

It is important that it is done correctly; otherwise the individual may feel cornered and become defensive. Advice from a trained professional is useful in determining the proper strategy and timing of a specific intervention.

If team members suspect that an individual has a problem with drugs or alcohol, they should get involved. It is the active involvement by concerned others that begins the process of lifestyle change. Intervention is the first step. Professional treatment is the second. Both are necessary steps for addicts to become free of their dependencies.

Steps of Drug Intervention

1. Time the drug abuse intervention. If possible, plan to talk with the addict when he or she is unimpaired. Choose a time when both the addict and the intervener are in a calm frame of mind and when a discussion can be done privately.
2. Be specific. Tell the co-worker that you are concerned about his or her drug or alcohol abuse and want to be supportive in getting help. Back up concerns with examples of the ways in which the drug abuse has caused problems for patients, clients, and co-workers, including any recent incidents.
3. State the consequences. The basic intent is to make the abuser's life more uncomfortable if he or she continues using drugs or alcohol. Let the abuser know that all measures will be taken to protect the staff, clients, and patients, and that he or she will no longer be able to practice veterinary medicine or perform technician duties while under the influence.
4. Listen. If, during an intervention, the abuser begins asking questions such as, "Where would I have to go?" or "For how long?" it is a sign that he or she is reaching out for help. Do not directly answer these questions. Instead, have the abuser call and talk with a professional. Offer support and do not delay. Once an agreement to seek professional help has been accomplished, seek admittance immediately.

Intervention is imperative; if a veterinarian or credentialed veterinary technician chooses not to accept help, then assistance must be obtained from the state board of veterinary medicine to remove the license. If a team member who is not licensed is the addict, he or she must be terminated to protect the integrity of the practice and the safety of fellow team members and patients.

Preventing Career Burnout

One of the most common causes of career change in veterinary medicine is burnout. Burnout can be defined as physical or emotional exhaustion, especially as a result of long-term stress. It is also an expression used to describe what might be better defined as depression or extreme exhaustion. Veterinarians and veterinary technicians are generally a very dedicated group and will work until the bitter end to ensure patients and clients are taken care of.

PRACTICE POINT Take care of yourself! Prevent burnout!

Negative attitudes are often a result of burnout, and are more contagious than positive attitudes. Clients will perceive the negativity, resulting in decreased compliance. The end result may be lost clients, lost revenue, and, ultimately, loss of valuable team members. Physical symptoms of burnout include ulcers, fatigue, overeating, gastroenteritis, cardiac abnormalities, backaches, and nausea. Behavioral issues associated with burnout include withdrawal, increased alcohol intake, agitation, depression, distraction, and increased spending.

Burnout victims hate to go to work; they have lost the enthusiasm and passion that drove them into the veterinary profession. Often the one suffering from burnout is the last person to identify and admit that burnout has occurred. Team workers, family, and friends can identify burnout much earlier; however, the victim cannot change until acceptance of the condition has occurred.

Breaks and vacations are a necessity to reinvigorate the team, individuals, and practice owners. They should be looked at as an investment, not a loss, because the invigoration brings new ideas, motivation, and enthusiasm back to the business. Continuing education can be stimulating, rejuvenating, and exciting for the entire team and is considered an investment as well as prevention for burnout (Figure 6-3).

Boundaries must be set for work and personal items. A team worker's personal life cannot be sacrificed for the sake of the practice. Time must be taken to enjoy activities outside the practice; family, health, and fun must be listed as priorities. Creating a balanced life may prevent burnout in the long run.

Exercise programs may be instituted for the entire team. It can take a lot of motivation to invigorate team members who have not exercised regularly, but the benefits that each team member will receive will be extremely rewarding. The exercise team leader may save a life by instituting an exercise program and save a valuable employee from leaving the profession. "A body in motion stays in motion" is a true statement and a mantra to live by.

Assistants may look into schools to receive credentials. This may allow an increase in salary, responsibilities, and knowledge. Education never devalues a person; it increases the value

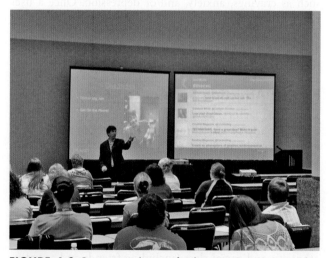

FIGURE 6-3 Continuing education for the entire team is essential to preventing burnout.

to the team and to the individual and allows the continuous challenge of climbing the ladder within a career. Credentialed technicians may look toward specialty boards, community-involved events, and continuing education for challenges and rewards. Since many practices lack an experienced practice manager, a technician may take the management challenge and develop methods to improve the practice financially. The possibilities are endless; it is up to the individual to seek challenges, prevent burnout, and continue to motivate others to succeed in a potentially rewarding career.

WHAT WOULD YOU DO/NOT DO?

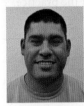 Alex, a longtime employee, is scheduled to work 34 hours per week, but he has been accumulating over 44 hours a week by covering other employees shifts. Although it is great that he is helping to prevent the practice from being understaffed, it is beginning to take a toll on Alex's personality. Generally, Alex is very friendly and provides excellent customer service. The clients usually rave about his service, until recently. The office manager has received client complaints about Alex's rude tone of voice and condescending attitude; one comment from a client stated he didn't have time to explain a procedure. Another client stated that he made her feel stupid because she didn't understand the vaccination schedule when she asked for clarification.

What Should the Practice Manager Do?

The practice manager must address the negative attitude that has overcome Alex and ask him what has happened recently that has affected him so much. Alex may be having personal issues that have shortened his temper, but he may be unaware how he has affected others around him. After asking what has happened, the office manager may ask him how a change can improve the situation. Alex may penalize himself enough and change his behavior without any penalty from the practice. Should Alex become defensive about his attitude, he may be encouraged to take some vacation time to relax and unwind. If he does not wish to take time off for himself, he may be advised to decrease his hours until things can work out for him, leaving him under less stress. Good managers protect their employees from burning out by asking questions and learning about the problem or problems and finding methods to prevent such problems. Many times, ineffective managers are quick to blame and criticize, which creates resentment and unhappiness in a work environment.

Knowing the goals of the practice can also help prevent employee burnout. Employees that "show up to get the job done and leave" are at a higher risk for burnout than those that want to help the practice grow. However, team members must know how to help the practice reach its goal. Having successful team meetings, brainstorming sessions, and open communication are an exceptional way to create a positive team culture, where every team member is on board. Review Chapter 3 for more information on leadership and team management.

Compassion Fatigue

The difference between burnout and compassion fatigue is that burnout vanishes when a team member leaves the practice and enters another (Figure 6-4). The excitement and drive for the profession returns. With compassion fatigue, one must leave the profession to be cured.

Compassion fatigue (CF) is a term that gained prevalence in human health care fields, particularly in nursing. It can be described as *the cost of caring for others in emotional need* (Figley, 2006). Veterinary professionals are known for their love and passion for pets and animals. This passion, coupled with positive and negative outcomes of the cases seen on a daily basis, puts team members in a position to face compassion fatigue in their lives. There is also some evidence that many team members have suffered some form of abuse in their past, be it mental, emotional, physical, or sexual. Many individuals turn to animals as a form of comfort and support. The animals provide the support, love, and security needed to face and overcome these special situations. Team members become attached to these patients, and if a negative outcome occurs, the team member is highly affected.

Not all team members have been exposed to abuse, but the common factor is the desire to help animals that cannot help themselves. Team members will give their all to their patients, their jobs, and the work, putting the cause ahead of themselves. It is this exact dedication that can subject them to the onset of compassion fatigue.

Practice managers are encouraged to define and understand compassion fatigue, identify signs and symptoms of CF in themselves and others, and lay groundwork for skills to help manage and prevent CF from setting in.

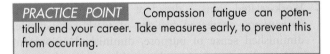 *PRACTICE POINT* Compassion fatigue can potentially end your career. Take measures early, to prevent this from occurring.

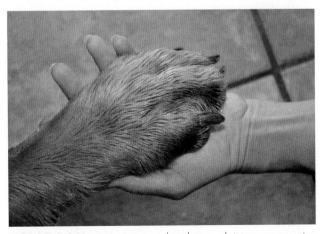

FIGURE 6-4 Veterinary team members have such intense compassion for their patients, inevitably leading to compassion fatigue at some point during their career.

Signs and Symptoms of Compassion Fatigue

The signs and symptoms of compassion fatigue can be very apparent, yet often those individuals experiencing them are unaware. These signs can display differently in every individual.*

- Cognitive signs – decreased concentration and/or ability to concentrate, apathy, rigidity, preoccupation with trauma, confusion, disorientation, difficulty making decisions, loss of meaning, decreased self-esteem, thoughts of self-harm, perfectionism
- Emotional signs – powerlessness, anxiety, guilt, numbness, fear, helplessness, sadness, depression, feeling depleted, shock, blunted or enhanced effects/responses, experiencing troubling dreams, sudden recall of a frightening or highly emotional experience while working with a pet/patient, cynicism, hypersensitivity to emotional material, insensitivity to emotional material, emotional roller coaster
- Behavioral signs – irritable, withdrawn, moody, clingy, appetite changes, losing things, hypervigilance over patients and co-workers, isolating oneself, poor sleep, substance abuse, nightmares, accident-prone, lower tolerance for frustration
- Spiritual signs – questioning life's meaning, pervasive hopelessness, loss of purpose (in job and/or in life), questioning religious beliefs, loss of faith, skepticism
- Somatic signs – sweating, rapid heartbeat, difficulty breathing, aches and pains, dizziness, impaired immune system, headaches, difficulty falling or staying asleep, stomachaches
- Interpersonal signs – failure to develop non–work-related aspects of life, voicing excessive complaints, difficulty separating personal and professional life, poor self-care, projection of anger or blame, mistrust, decreased interest in intimacy or sex, loneliness, impact on parenting (protectiveness), isolation from friends
- Work-related signs – dread of working with certain co-workers, decreased feelings of work competence, diminished sense of purpose, diminished enjoyment with career, dread of working with certain clients or situations

Impact of Compassion Fatigue on Individuals

CF can have a myriad of effects on the individual, starting with job dissatisfaction. Interactions with co-workers can become difficult as communication breaks down. Individuals no longer enjoy work or working with their team members. Anxiety and depression can also begin to creep in, further affecting relationships both at work and on the home front. The individual can begin to feel demoralized and begin experiencing sleep disturbances and traumatic memories of past cases and pets. Oftentimes someone suffering from CF will be less resilient to physical ailments and

*Adapted from Figley, 1995.

can become irritable very easily. Outside of the workplace, CF can also take a toll on personal relationships, affect family dynamics, and further an individual's state of anxiety or depression.

Impact of Compassion Fatigue on the Practice

CF can debilitate not only individuals, but also the veterinary team (Figure 6-5). CF sufferers will begin calling in and coming to work late. That absenteeism and tardiness gives rise to overtime hours for other employees. The individuals working those overtime hours are now potentially getting pushed into their "red zone" and the cycle begins. This cycle will directly affect the finances of the practice.

Managing Compassion Fatigue

There are four easy steps to help manage CF:
- *Recognize* triggers and stressors of CF.
- *Reduce* the triggers and stressors once they have been identified. Working excessive overtime is often a trigger; practice managers and team members must be able to determine when these triggers arise and implement methods to reduce them.
- *Restore* – Practice balancing life and work. Once the triggers are identified and reduced, restore the balance in life. Implement activity, a great nutrition plan, and a good night's sleep, each and every day.
- *Repeat* – Curing CF is not an option; however, managing it with the *R*'s just listed and repeating the cycle can greatly decrease the effects.

When feeling out of control, overwhelmed, depressed, or hopeless, seek professional help from someone experienced in compassion fatigue. There is no shame in seeking help with these emotional situations that team members are expected to deal with on a daily basis.

Entire courses are available to help team members and practice managers to become familiar with and successfully

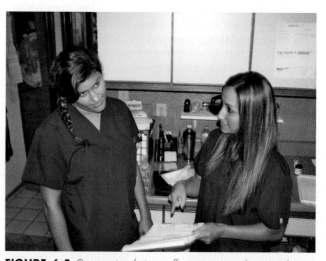

FIGURE 6-5 Compassion fatigue affects team member attitudes not only toward patients, but also toward each other, often creating a hostile work environment.

manage CF. The previous summary is provided as an informational resource only, and the author encourages further research for the development and implementation of a CF program within the practice.

⚖ VETERINARY PRACTICE and the LAW

Team members that work excess hours and get burned out on the profession do not take the time to discuss procedures, disease, and conditions with clients. Exhausted team members have short tempers with clients and do not provide clients with information to give informed consent. Short tempers and poor nonverbal communication prevent clients from asking questions, and these behaviors may prevent clients from returning to the practice in the future. Veterinarians and team members that do not clearly communicate with clients are at a higher risk of having a complaint filed with the state veterinary board. Complaints must be fully investigated and may result in license revocation.

Team members experiencing stress, burnout, or compassion fatigue can be at a higher risk for turning to drugs or alcohol to alleviate the symptoms associated with each. Managers and owners must be diligent about preventing burnout from occurring, and must learn to recognize symptoms when it does occur. Controlled substances in the practice must be closely monitored, and random drugs tests may be implemented. Impaired team members are at a higher risk for injury, job abandonment, and decreased employee accountability. Veterinarians can have their licenses revoked for controlled substance abuse, and if an injury occurs while a team member is impaired, applications for workers' compensation may be denied.

REVIEW QUESTIONS

1. What symptoms physically occur in someone under undue stress?
2. How does good stress differ from bad stress?
3. What factors affect stress?
4. What three methods can reduce stress?
5. What stressors may affect someone in the veterinary profession?
6. What is substance abuse?
7. What factors have been determined to increase the likelihood of substance abuse?

8. By what evidence does an individual reveal that he or she is a substance abuser?
9. Why should one intervene if substance abuse is suspected?
10. What can happen to a professional convicted of drug use?
11. What can too much *positive stress* lead to?
    a. Satisfaction
    b. Exhaustion
    c. Energy
    d. Relief
12. How many stages of stress are there?
    a. 6
    b. 4
    c. 3
    d. 2
13. Which of the following describes *somatic signs* of compassion fatigue?
    a. Decreased concentration
    b. Impaired immune system
    c. Irritability
    d. Anxiety
14. What are the four steps of managing compassion fatigue?
    a. Restore, repeat, reduce, recognize
    b. Respect, relax, resign, restore
    c. Rest, resolve, restore, resume
    d. None of the above
15. Which of the following are considered to be risk factors for addiction?
    a. Genetics
    b. Sociocultural factors
    c. Environment
    d. Chronic pain
    e. All of the above

Recommended Reading

Figley CR: *Compassion fatigue: coping with secondary traumatic stress disorder in those who treat the traumatized*, New York, 1995, Psychology Press.

Figley CR, Roop RG: *Compassion fatigue in the animal-care community*, Washington, DC, 2006, Humane Society Press.

HelpGuide: Stress symptoms, signs, and causes, (Web site): www.helpguide.org/mental/stress_signs.htm. Accessed November 22, 2013.

Mayo Clinic (2006). Stress Management: Know your triggers. (Web site): mayoclinic.com/health/stress-management/SR00031. Accessed November 22, 2013.

Practice Design

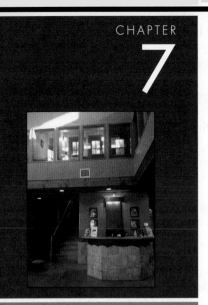

KEY TERMS

Ergonomics
Maintenance Diets
Motion Economy
Therapeutic Diets
Time and Motion

OUTLINE

Principles of Time and Motion, *147*
Body Positioning, *147*
Ergonomics, *148*
Miscellaneous Factors to Consider, *148*
Health and Safety of Reception Team
   Members, *149*
Design and Function of Effective
   Practices, *149*

Creating Comfortable Reception
   Areas, *149*
Creating Comfortable Exam Rooms, *150*
Consultation Rooms, *152*
Retail Area, *152*
Middle Area, *152*
Treatment Area, *152*

LEARNING OBJECTIVES

When you have completed this chapter, you should be able to:

1. Discuss motion economy.
2. Clarify how to complete tasks more efficiently.
3. Distinguish proper body position.
4. Define ergonomics.
5. Describe the design and function of effective practices.
6. Develop comfortable reception areas.
7. Develop comfortable consultation rooms.
8. Develop an effective retail area.

CRITICAL COMPETENCIES

1. **Adaptability** - being open to change and flexible work methods; the ability to adapt behavior to changing conditions or new information.
2. **Analytical Skills** - the ability to analyze information and use logic to address problems; the ability to quickly and accurately grasp complex information and concepts and to make correct inferences.
3. **Continuous Learning** - a curiosity for learning; actively seek out new information, technologies, and methods; keep skills updated and apply new knowledge to the job.
4. **Creativity** - the ability to think creatively about situations, to see things in new and different ways; use imagination and creativity to develop innovative solutions to problems.
5. **Critical and Strategic Thinking** - the ability to think critically about situations and to understand the relevance of information for different problems; use critical reasoning to generate and evaluate alternative courses of action or points of view relevant to an issue.
6. **Decision Making** - the ability to make good decisions, solve problems, and decide on important matters; the

ability to gather and analyze relevant data and choose decisively between alternatives.
7. **Leadership** - a willingness to lead and take charge; the ability to motivate others and mobilize group effort toward common goals.
8. **Planning and Prioritizing** - the ability to effectively manage time and work load to meet deadlines; the ability to organize work, set priorities, and establish plans for achieving goals.
9. **Relationship Building** - the ability to develop constructive and cooperative working relationships with others and maintain them over time; must also be able to settle disputes, resolve grievances and conflicts, and negotiate with others.
10. **Resilience** - the ability to cope effectively with pressure and setbacks; the ability to handle crisis situations effectively and remain undeterred by obstacles or failure.
11. **Resourcefulness** - the ability to understand what it takes to complete the job; apply knowledge, skills, and expertise to perform tasks quickly and efficiently.

Many veterinary practices are located in older buildings and are beginning to look at remodeling, upgrading, or moving into a new building. Many things must be taken into consideration when moving to a new building. Selecting a location that is easy to find for both new and existing clients will increase the growth of the practice. The building should look clean and professional from the outside (Figure 7-1). The hospital or practice sign should be easy to see and read from the street (Figure 7-2). Team members will be responsible for the input of ideas to increase efficiency at the new or updated location; this demands an understanding of the principles of motion economy and the placement of equipment

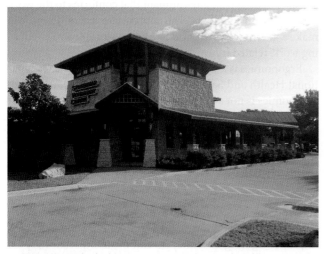

FIGURE 7-1 The building must appear clean and professional on the outside. (Photo courtesy Stanton Foster, Stonebriar Veterinary Centre, and Dr. Jennifer Wilcox.)

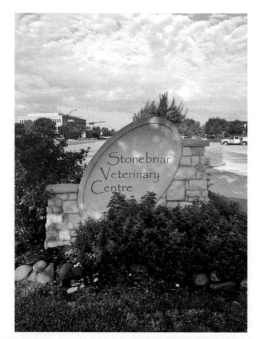

FIGURE 7-2 Hospital signs should be professional and clearly visible from the street. (Photo courtesy Stanton Foster, Stonebriar Veterinary Centre, and Dr. Jennifer Wilcox.)

to create an environment that helps the team work in a smarter way and more comfortably. The goal of motion economy is to be more efficient, not to work harder and more strenuously.

Principles of Time and Motion

When determining the placement of office equipment and supplies, the principles of time and motion should be considered. Time and motion refer to the amount of time and degree of motion required to perform a given task. This is important in the receptionist's office and exam rooms of a general practice. Many studies have been completed to understand how to minimize the amount of time and motion it takes to perform basic tasks. To improve motion economy, it is necessary to eliminate unnecessary steps or tasks, rearrange equipment, organize procedures, and simplify tasks. The principles of motion economy can aid in accomplishing these goals, thereby reducing stress and increasing productivity within the practice (Box 7-1).

Body Positioning

Receptionists should consider sitting whenever possible to eliminate undue stress on the back, neck, and legs. Improper posture while standing can lead to fatigue, which can decrease productivity. While seated in a chair, a person should have the thighs parallel to the floor, the lower legs vertical, and the feet firmly on the floor (Figure 7-3). While using the keyboard, the arms should be positioned so that the forearms and wrists are as close to horizontal as possible. The back and neck should be erect, with the upper arms perpendicular to the floor. It should be remembered that the receptionist should always face clients; a team member's back can appear rude and unapproachable.

> **PRACTICE POINT** The building must appear clean and professional on the outside.

BOX 7-1	Applying the Principle of Motion Economy in the Business Office

- Position objects as close to the point of use as possible.
- Use motions that require the least amount of movement.
- Minimize the number of materials used for a given procedure.
- Use smooth, continuous movements, not zigzag motions.
- Organize materials in a logical sequence.
- Use ergonomically designed chairs to provide good body posture.
- Provide lighting that eliminates shadows.
- Provide work areas that are at elbow level.
- Computer screens should be positioned within 10 to 40 degrees of horizontal.

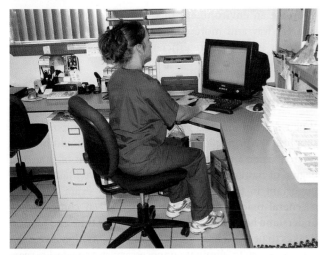

FIGURE 7-3 Receptionists should maintain proper posture by keeping their feet flat on the floor, legs perpendicular, and back straight.

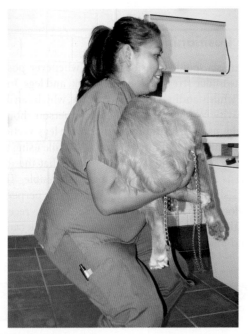

FIGURE 7-4 Always lift with the legs, not the back, to prevent debilitating injuries.

Technicians working on the floor all day must have a correct body posture to reduce future back problems. Body posture should be straight, with no slumping. Team competitions can be held to correct each others' body posture on a daily basis. Team members must also remember to lift *with their legs,* not their backs, to prevent back injuries. This is especially true when lifting bags of dog food for clients. Most back problems are due to continual, long-term, incorrect lifting procedures; therefore injuries may not be felt for years. Management must initiate and enforce correct lifting procedures to protect the team from future painful and potentially debilitating conditions (Figure 7-4).

Ensure that counters are high enough that team members and clients are not hunched over to write on documents or perform treatments. In the reception area, this includes counters for both the clients and the reception team. For the technical team, this includes the pharmacy, laboratory, and treatment counters.

Ergonomics

Ergonomics is the science that studies the relationship between people and their work environments. Interrelated physical and psychological factors are involved in the creation of a stress-free work environment. By understanding the abilities that people have and their work patterns, it is possible to design an environment that conforms to the work needs of team members. The appropriate use of design can make a job much more productive and efficient while reducing work-related injuries and discomforts.

Ergonomics is a safety concern and relates to the Occupational Health and Safety Administration (OSHA). Although ergonomics is not a standard OSHA policy, it does fall under the general duty clause, in that employers are responsible for providing a safe working environment.

Miscellaneous Factors to Consider

Physiologic factors include color, lighting, acoustics, heating and cooling, space, furniture, and equipment. Poor lighting can play a large factor in team member inefficiencies; improper lighting causes eyestrain, misinterpreted hospital sheets and records, or missed parasites on a pet. Consider placing skylights in every room of the practice; natural lighting enhances moods, while at the same time decreasing utility bills. Windows may be placed in offices, reception areas, and treatment rooms.

Acoustics can play a vital role in kennel assistants' duties because they spend most of their time within the kennel ward. Barking dogs with a piercing tone can wear down even the best attitude, decreasing the efficiency of the team member (let alone a recovering patient!). When working in noisy areas for extended periods of time, personal hearing protectors can be worn (Figure 7-5). Refer to Chapter 21 for more information on OSHA regulations that pertain to hearing protection.

Heating and cooling have an effect on clients and team members as well as patients. Clients may become irritated easier when the facilities are hot; team members may not work as efficiently when it is either too hot or too cold. Patients will not recover as well in cold environments and may need additional blankets to maintain body temperature, thus decreasing the efficiency of the team. Consider individual thermostats for the surgery room (keeping it cooler) and recovery (keeping it warmer).

Smaller spaces always decrease the efficiency of a team, as does too large a space with wasted room. When designing a practice, whether remodeling an old or new building, space efficiency matters. However, it is important to

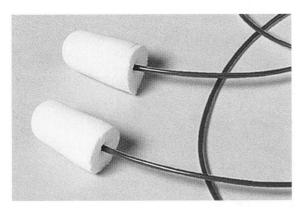

FIGURE 7-5 Hearing protectors should always be used in noisy kennels. (From Bassert JM, McCurnin DM: *McCurnin's clinical textbook for veterinary technicians*, ed 7, St Louis, 2010, Saunders Elsevier.)

keep in mind where the practice will be in 10 years. Some practices may need to grow into a larger space with time (but having the space available is much easier than not having space at all).

Color plays a large role in how a client perceives the practice and the team. An attractive, cheerful, and efficient reception area confirms the confidence the practice has conveyed to the client. A dark, dirty, and cluttered reception area can bring doubts or mistrust to the client. Light colors with warm hues can create a cheerful setting, whereas cool colors, such as light green and blue, can produce a tranquil setting. Tranquil settings can benefit both the team and the client during difficult and stressful situations.

Physical factors include the use of proper equipment to help prevent injury. Office chairs should have a broad base with four to five casters for proper balance. They should also have a well-padded seat with lumbar back support. Computer monitors should be placed at the appropriate height and distance from the receptionist to prevent straining the eyes and neck. Computer keyboards should have an ergonomic design and should also be placed at the proper height to prevent bursitis or tendonitis. Technicians should always use proper restraint equipment when indicated and get help when lifting or transporting large and heavy animals or equipment.

Don't forget pet elimination areas! If space allows, two areas may be developed: one for the clients and another for hospitalized patients. Creating an elimination area reminds clients to walk their pet before entering the hospital, and is also an ideal area when urine samples need to be collected on outpatients. Relief areas for hospitalized animals should be fenced in, preventing the escape of patients, and creating a safe environment for team members.

> **PRACTICE POINT**   Pet elimination areas for hospitalized patients should be fenced in, for safety reasons.

Health and Safety of Reception Team Members

A variety of factors can affect the health and safety of receptionists. For example, spending hours a day looking at a computer screen can result in eyestrain and fatigue. Repetitive keyboarding can lead to wrist discomfort and possible bursitis or tendonitis. Inappropriate body posture can lead to back discomfort. To help relieve eyestrain, computer monitors should have appropriate lighting and be placed at an angle to decrease glare on the screen. The use of an ergonomically designed mouse and keyboard can decrease fatigue in the wrist, and an ergonomically designed chair can help facilitate correct body posture while seated at a desk (Figure 7-6).

Design and Function of Effective Practices

The size, type of practice, and services offered are three main factors that affect the design and efficiency of a hospital. The primary goal is to develop a solution that optimizes the efficiency of the team while providing clients and patients with a high standard of care.

Most practices are divided into three parts: the front, middle, and back. The front generally consists of the reception area and exam room. The middle refers to the laboratory, pharmacy, and treatment area, and the back refers to kennel wards and storage area.

Creating Comfortable Reception Areas

The reception area is the gateway to the practice and provides the clients with the first impression of the hospital (Figure 7-7). Overcrowding and congestion always occur in the reception area, especially as clients arrive for appointments and to pick up patients or medications. Congestion doubles as clients check out with their pets. This congestion can lead to undesirable pet interaction and client dissatisfaction.

It can be advisable to develop separate waiting areas for dog and cat patients, reducing the stress on both the owners and pets. A practice may also have separate check-in and checkout areas, reducing the congestion associated with both procedures. If a practice boards or grooms patients, a separate entrance may benefit both clients and team members.

> **PRACTICE POINT**   Consider the clients expectations while sitting in the reception area. Then consider designing the area to exceed those expectations.

A warm atmosphere can be created with comfortable chairs, nice artwork on the walls, and plants. Chairs should be made of a material that is easy to clean, does not stain, and is durable. Seats should have some space between them. Clients do not like to sit right next to each other, especially those with large dogs. Plants should be hung from the ceiling or on the wall to prevent dogs from urinating on them. A restroom should be provided off the reception area for the convenience of clients.

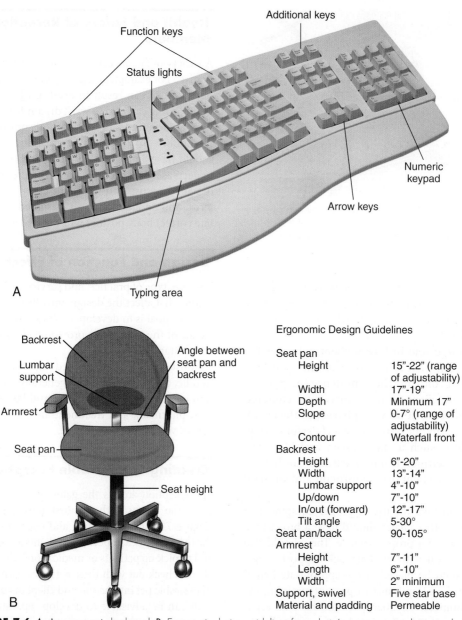

FIGURE 7-6 A, An ergonomic keyboard. **B,** Ergonomic design guidelines for a chair (measurements relative to chair seat). (**A** From Finkbeiner B, Finkbeiner C: *Practice management for the dental team,* ed 6, St Louis, 2006, Mosby Elsevier; **B** from Jacobs K: *Ergonomics for therapists,* ed 3, St Louis, 2008, Mosby Elsevier.)

Portrait photos of team members can be placed on the wall in the lobby (Figure 7-8). Photos may be a professional portrait or a spontaneous photo, showing activities team members participate in with their pets outside the office.

Photo albums can be created of clients and their pets (clients should be asked for permission to place photos in the album). A hospital photo album can also be created, showing different rooms of the practice, activities that occur in those rooms, and team members performing activities. Many clients wonder what it looks like behind the scenes and what occurs once their pet leaves the exam room; this is a wonderful creation to appease their minds. Picture collages also warm up rooms, giving clients something to look at while they wait.

Creating Comfortable Exam Rooms

Exam rooms are frequently white, dirty, and smell of the previous patient. Cleanliness is imperative to owners and should be to the entire team as well. Rooms should be swept and mopped after each patient to decrease the chance of transmitting disease. Cleanliness also prevents the transmission of odors. Warm, neutral tones calm clients. Practices may add nicely framed pictures or client education posters. Thumbtacks should not be used to hang posters; holes in the wall and torn posters devalue the practice. Wall borders also add a nice touch to rooms, along with comfortable chairs that allow clients to sit near patients on the examination table. Rooms should not be cluttered with models, treats, or diagnostic equipment (Figure 7-9). Countertops and sinks should be clean at all times.

WHAT WOULD YOU DO/NOT DO?

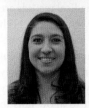

Lori, a veterinary technician, recently attended continuing education and learned about the benefits of adding colors to exam and treatment rooms. The rooms in her practice are white and always appear dirty. She envisions a colorful exam room with border of puppies and kittens. To her, the color should be a soft, calming color. She learned that calming colors will help ease client tensions when they are in the rooms. Lori is afraid to approach the practice manager with her idea for fear of rejection.

What Should Lori Do?

Lori should put a proposal together that lists all of the elements she learned in continuing education. She could research the best possible colors and find a border that would match the color combination that she has in mind. Second, she could put an estimate together of the total cost of painting the room, including her labor, paint, and materials. Once all of this information is together, she can propose her plan to the practice manager and owner, who may be excited and have ideas to add as well. Team members should always feel that their ideas and contributions are important and not be afraid to present them. Practice managers love to have team members who are independently motivated and willing to put forth an extra step to add a personal touch to the practice.

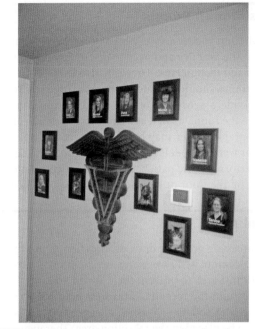

FIGURE 7-8 Professional portraits can be placed on the wall in the lobby. (Courtesy Ben Wilson and Star of Texas Veterinary Hospital.)

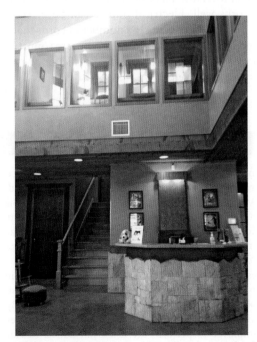

FIGURE 7-7 A reception area should give a warm, comfortable feeling to clients and staff. (Courtesy Stanton Foster, Stonebriar Veterinary Centre, and Dr. Jennifer Wilcox.)

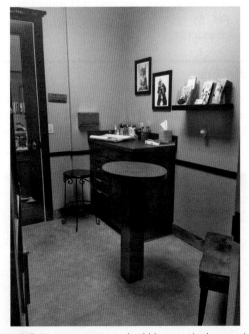

FIGURE 7-9 Examination rooms should be warmly decorated, clean, and in excellent condition. This room is decorated and designed especially for feline patients. (Courtesy Stanton Foster, Stonebriar Veterinary Centre, and Dr. Jennifer Wilcox.)

Consultation Rooms

Consultation rooms are very nice to have for clients who arrive at the practice and need to discuss patient care with doctors and technicians. They can also be used for euthanasia. Rooms should be quiet, away from high traffic areas, and provide a sense of comfort. Nicely framed pictures may line the room, as well as a comfortable couch or chair. A radiograph viewer may be added for consultation purposes, as well as models for client education. If a euthanasia is performed, the patient may have a nice, comfortable blanket on the floor or be held in the arms of the client.

Retail Area

Retail areas are great for drawing attention to products the practice promotes; however, extra attention needs to be given to this area to prevent theft. Retail areas that can be placed behind the reception area may hold more valuable items such as collars or leashes; cheaper toys and smaller items can be placed in the reception area. Therapeutic diets should be placed behind the counter, allowing maintenance diets to remain in the reception area. Many practices have limited space to carry excess products, so care must be taken when choosing what products will be carried. It should be determined what and how the practice will benefit if it chooses to carry a product. However, clients look to veterinary practices for recommendations of products to purchase, food to feed, and toys that should be allowed for their pet. An appropriate balance must be determined within each practice.

Middle Area

The middle area of a veterinary practice generally includes the pharmacy and laboratory areas, which must also function in an efficient manner (Figures 7-10 and 7-11). If the pharmacy and laboratory share the same space, there must be enough room for computers, laboratory equipment, prescription filling, and a location to write on records. If electronic medical records are used, enough computers must be available, enhancing both the speed of service to the client, and team member satisfaction. Equipment should be placed in ergonomically efficient locations, reducing the workload of team members as they complete tasks associated with the laboratory area. Laboratory equipment must be placed far enough apart to allow fans to efficiently cool the equipment. Electrical outlets should not be overloaded, which can cause a fire hazard.

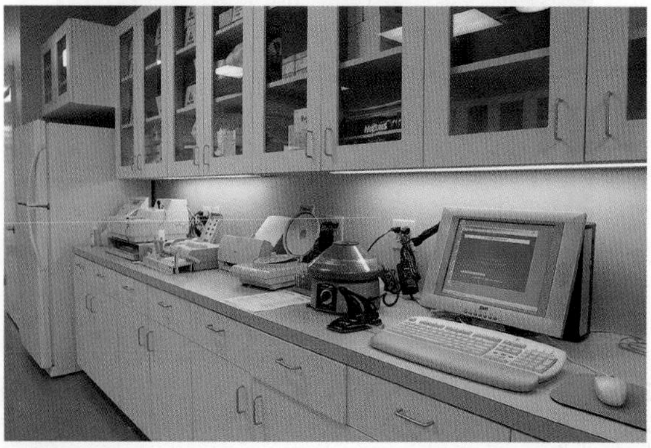

> **PRACTICE POINT**   The middle area must be the most efficient area of the hospital, taking into consideration time, motion, and ergonomics.

Treatment Area

The treatment area may also encompass radiology (Figure 7-12), surgery (Figure 7-13), and the treatment area (Figure 7-14), whereas the back may be considered the kennel, isolation wards, and storage areas. Floors should have an anti-slip surface, reducing accidental slipping on wet floors. The treatment area should be set up to allow traffic to flow freely and uncongested. Treatment tables should be positioned to allow team members to work from any angle; therefore placement of tables in the center of a room works well. Electrical outlets can be placed in the ceiling if needed, reducing the number of cords that a team member might trip on. The treatment area must remain clutter free, allowing the team to work efficiently, especially when space is limited.

FIGURE 7-10 The laboratory is located just beyond the examination rooms. (From Bassert JM, McCurnin DM: *McCurnin's clinical textbook for veterinary technicians,* ed 7, St Louis, 2010, Saunders Elsevier.)

⚖ VETERINARY PRACTICE and the LAW

When developing, designing, or remodeling a practice, the Americans with Disabilities Act (ADA) must be considered. The ADA is a federal law that protects those with disabilities, and it includes team members and clients. Clients must be able to have full access to the facility; this includes parking lot ramps, bathroom access (wide doors and handrails), and wide doors for wheelchair access to all rooms.

Team members with disabilities cannot be discriminated against if they can complete the job requirements as listed in the job description section of the employee manual. By law, employers must make reasonable accommodation to enable the employee to perform the listed job duties. Reasonable accommodation may include making existing facilities used by employees readily accessible and usable by individuals with disabilities.

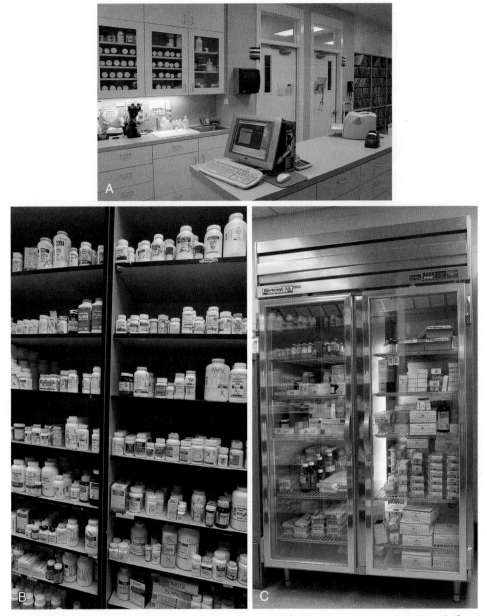

FIGURE 7-11 A, Pharmacy is located near examination rooms and inpatient treatment area. B, Drug shelf storage in pharmacy. C, Glass door refrigerator for storage of vaccines and biologics. (From Bassert JM, McCurnin DM: *McCurnin's clinical textbook for veterinary technicians,* ed 7, St Louis, 2010, Saunders Elsevier.)

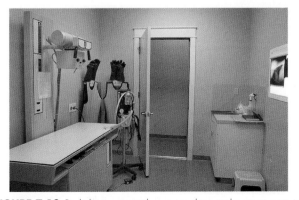

FIGURE 7-12 Radiology room with x-ray machine and protective equipment hanging on the wall. The automatic film processor is not visible through the open door. (From Bassert JM, McCurnin DM: *McCurnin's clinical textbook for veterinary technicians,* ed 7, St Louis, 2010, Saunders Elsevier.)

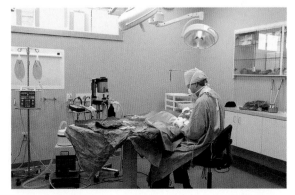

FIGURE 7-13 Surgical room with one door for both entrance and exit, ceiling-mounted lights, and minimal countertops. (From Bassert JM, McCurnin DM: *McCurnin's clinical textbook for veterinary technicians,* ed 7, St Louis, 2010, Saunders Elsevier.)

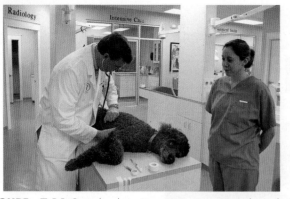

FIGURE 7-14 Centralized treatment area accommodates both outpatient and inpatient treatment. (From Bassert JM, McCurnin DM: *McCurnin's clinical textbook for veterinary technicians*, ed 7, St Louis, 2010, Saunders Elsevier.)

REVIEW QUESTIONS

1. What is the goal of motion economy?
2. What are the principles of time and motion?
3. What is ergonomics?
4. What factors contribute to ergonomics?
5. Why is creating a comfortable reception area so important?
6. What is the correct definition of the term *ergonomics*?
   a. The science that studies the relationship between people and their work environments
   b. The outward appearance of a place of business
   c. Factors contributing to physical injury while working
   d. Acoustical difficulties pertaining to the design of buildings
7. What does the *middle area* in a practice consist of?
   a. Reception area
   b. Doctor's offices
   c. Radiology room
   d. Pharmacy
8. What does the treatment area in a practice consist of?
   a. Laboratory area
   b. Exam rooms
   c. Consultation rooms
   d. Surgery room
9. What can a consultation room be used for?
   a. Euthanasia
   b. Consults over patient care with owners
   c. Discuss laboratory outcomes (radiology, blood work, etc.)
   d. All of the above
10. Where is an ideal place for a client bathroom?
    a. Front office
    b. Middle area
    c. Reception area
    d. The back

Recommended Reading

Bridger RS: *Introduction to ergonomics*, ed 3, Boca Raton, FL, 2008, CRC Press.

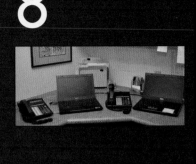

Technology in the Office

OUTLINE

Information Systems, *156*

Hardware, *159*

Software, *159*

Selecting Hardware, *160*

   Location, Location, Location, *160*

   Types of Computers, *160*

   Processor Selection, *160*

   Printer Selection, *160*

   Servers, *160*

Selecting Software, *160*

Cost Analysis, *162*

Software Implementation, *162*

Internet Security, *163*

Backing up the System, *164*

Other Technology, *164*

   Digital Cameras, *164*

   Scanners and Copiers, *165*

KEY TERMS

Adware

Backup Devices

Broadband

Card Reader

CD

CD/DVD

Cookies

Cost Analysis

CPU

Data

Data Conversion

Desktop

Digital Camera

Docking Station

DSL

DVD

External Hard Drive

Firewall

Gigabyte

Graphics Card

Hacker

Handwriting Recognition

Hard Drive

Hardware

Host

Internet

Inventory Management
  Software

IP Address

Keyboard

Label Printer

Laptop

Megabyte

Microphone

Modem

Monitor

Mouse

LEARNING OBJECTIVES

When you have completed this chapter, you should be able to:

1. Differentiate between hardware and software.
2. Determine the appropriate computer hardware to meet the requirements of the practice.
3. Identify veterinary software that will best serve the practice.
4. Create an appropriate hardware and software implementation schedule for the staff.
5. Define methods used to protect the computer system with appropriate security features.
6. Explain the importance of daily backup procedures.
7. Discuss methods that allow office technology to be used to the fullest potential.

CRITICAL COMPETENCIES

1. **Adaptability** - being open to change and flexible work methods; the ability to adapt behavior to changing conditions or new information.
2. **Analytical Skills** - the ability to analyze information and use logic to address problems; the ability to quickly and accurately grasp complex information and concepts and to make correct inferences.
3. **Continuous Learning** - a curiosity for learning; actively seek out new information, technologies, and methods; keep skills updated and apply new knowledge to the job.
4. **Creativity** - the ability to think creatively about situations, to see things in new and different ways; use imagination and creativity to develop innovative solutions to problems.
5. **Critical and Strategic Thinking** - the ability to think critically about situations and to understand the relevance of information for different problems; use critical reasoning to generate and evaluate alternative courses of action or points of view relevant to an issue.
6. **Decision Making** - the ability to make good decisions, solve problems, and decide on important matters; the ability to gather and analyze relevant data and choose decisively between alternatives.
7. **Leadership** - a willingness to lead and take charge; the ability to motivate others and mobilize group effort toward common goals.
8. **Planning and Prioritizing** - the ability to effectively manage time and workload to meet deadlines; the ability to organize work, set priorities, and establish plans for achieving goals.

Network Card
PC
Pop-ups
Printer
Processor Speed
RAM
Scanners
Server
Software
Sound Card
Spam
Spam Filter
Speakers
Spyware
Tablet
Trojan Horse
USB
Video Graphics Card
Virus
Voice Recognition
Wireless LAN Access
  Point
Worm
Zip Drive

9. **Relationship Building** - the ability to develop constructive and cooperative working relationships with others and maintain them over time; must also be able to settle disputes, resolve grievances and conflicts, and negotiate with others.

10. **Resilience** - the ability to cope effectively with pressure and setbacks; the ability to handle crisis situations effectively and remain undeterred by obstacles or failure.

11. **Resourcefulness** - the ability to understand what it takes to complete the job; apply knowledge, skills, and expertise to perform tasks quickly and efficiently.

Over the last decade, the veterinary profession has benefited from the advances made in computer technology, including faster processors, increases in the amount of information that can be stored, and greater networking capacities. The prudent selection of technology equipment is a major component of veterinary practice productivity and efficiency. The ultimate goal is to develop effective, automated information and processing system that can evolve with practice growth and that will be able to use new technology as it is developed.

Computers are used to maintain the functions of the practice on several levels. The electronic office is a workplace where computers and other electronic equipment carry out many of the office's routine tasks. This equipment also provides more options for gathering, processing, displaying, and storing information. Box 8-1 gives some examples of applications of technology that are used daily in veterinary practices.

Veterinary practice managers are responsible for technology systems and policies (establish policies for use of technology in the practice, including computer networks).

The technology revolution that led to the information age has had a profound effect on the business office. The use of electronic office technology in the veterinary practice allows the team to be more efficient and organized. It can help automate routine tasks, improve cash flow, and increase accuracy.

| BOX 8-1 | Applications of Technology in the Veterinary Practice |

- Online continuing education
- Computerized appointment system
- Consultation with specialists and experts
- Credit card processing
- Digital photographs
- Digital radiographs
- Electronic/paperless medical records
- Email reminders
- Online office procedural manuals
- Supply purchases
- Web page design and maintenance

Today, a patient's radiograph can be sent virtually (i.e., by computer) to a specialist as soon as it is taken and before the client leaves the practice. This results in improved patient and client care, increased productivity, and reduced stress on team members.

Information Systems

An information system is a collection of elements that provide accurate, timely, and useful information. To understand the procedure of an information system, one must understand the basic terminology related to the concept. A glossary of terms, definitions, and pictures helps define electronic office equipment and is useful when selecting products (Box 8-2).

BOX 8-2 | Technology Terms

Backup Device: Device that copies information from the CPU and stores it for retrieval in the event of computer malfunction. Backup devices can be either internal or external.

Broadband: High-speed Internet connection that can transmit information 40 times as fast as telephone and modem connection.

Card Reader/Writer: A card reader/writer is useful for transferring data directly to and from a removable flash memory card. Examples of flash cards are those used in a camera or music player.

Central Processing Unit (CPU): The brain of the computer; located in the main unit.

CD: Device for storing data; stores approximately 650 to 700 MB (megabytes) of information.

CD/DVD Drives: Computers are built with a DVD drive that can read CDs or DVDs. CDs or DVDs cannot be recorded or written over; they can only be read by the driver. If one plans to write music, audio files, or documents onto a CD or DVD, then CD/RW or DVD/RW should be considered. RW stands for rewritable. This allows the CD or DVD to be rewritten once the information has been recorded once. A DVD has a capacity of at least 4.7 GB (gigabytes) versus the 650 MB capacity of a CD. Drives can be either internal or external.

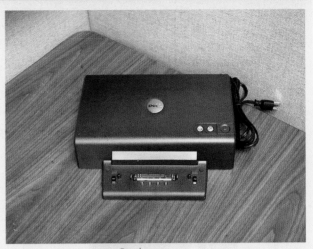

Docking station

External Hard Drive: An external hard drive is a storage drive that allows data to be stored outside the computer. External hard drives are protected in heavy black cases and can create an extra storage space or contain a complete backup of the computer system.

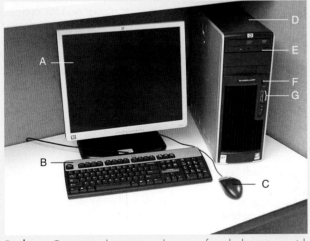

Desktop: Computer that sits on the top of a desk; not considered a portable unit. **A,** Monitor. **B,** Keyboard. **C,** Mouse. **D,** Computer. **E,** CD/DVD drive. **F,** Power. **G,** USB ports.

Digital Camera: A camera that can capture images without the use of film. Images are then transferred to the computer. Photos can then be printed from the computer or stored for future use. Digital cameras come in a range of megapixels. The higher the megapixel count, the better the resolution of the photo. A digital camera can be an effective marketing tool in a veterinary practice.

Digital Subscriber Line (DSL): High-speed Internet connection that uses the same wires as a telephone.

Digital Versatile Disc (DVD): Device for storing data that can hold more information than a CD.

Docking Station: Stationary device that allows a tablet to function as a desktop computer.

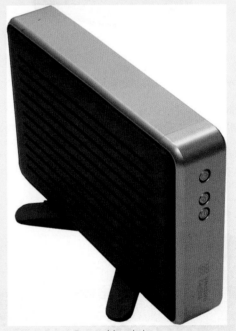

External hard drive

Gigabyte (GB): Measure of computer data storage; approximately 1 billion bytes.

Graphics Card: Card inserted into the CPU that determines the level of detail at which video images will appear on the monitor.

Handwriting Recognition: Technology that allows the computer to convert touch screen writing into printed words.

Hard Drive: A hard drive stores all data and can hold more than 100 GB of information.

Continued

BOX 8-2 | Technology Terms—cont'd

Keyboard: The keyboard is one of the most important devices used to communicate with the computer. It should have at least 101 keys on it and have a USB connection to plug into the computer. Some users prefer wireless keyboards, especially when a smaller desk space is being used. For team members who use the keyboard for a majority of the day, an ergonomic keyboard may be considered.

Label Printer: Printers designed to produce labels for bottles, containers, or envelopes.

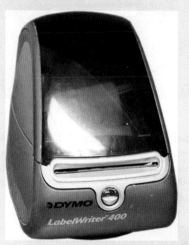

Label printer

Laptop: A portable computer.

Megabyte: Measure of computer data storage; approximately 1 million bytes.

Microphone: Used to record sound.

Modem: A device used to connect to the Internet as well as send and receive faxes via a phone line. The modem converts digital data to analog data to send to the end user; the modem also converts analog information back to digital when it is received.

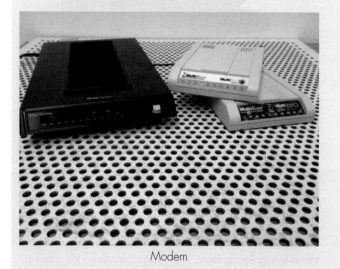

Modem

Monitor: The monitor is used to view documents, read email, and view pictures. A minimum of a 17-inch screen is advised; however, if digital photos will be reviewed, a 19- or 21-inch monitor is recommended. Flat panel screens are excellent space savers and provide a high-quality picture.

Mouse: A mouse allows navigation through applications on the computer. The mouse allows the user to point and click. A mouse can be cordless, which may benefit some users. Others prefer a mouse with an ergonomic design and an optical sensor. An optical sensor allows the mouse to be used without a mouse pad, which may be useful if working in a small desk space.

Network Card: A network card allows connection to a network or DSL for Internet connection. If a server is in use for the practice software system, each computer will need to have a network card to allow the computers to communicate with each other.

Printer: Laser and inkjet printers are available. Laser printers print faster and with higher quality than an inkjet printer, and the ink generally costs less for a laser printer. Photograph printers are more expensive and print with a higher resolution. Printers should have a USB connection.

Processor Speed: The processor speed is the speed at which the brain of the computer can sort information and produce results.

Random Access Memory (RAM): The short-term memory of a computer. RAM plays a vital role in the speed of the computer. 512 MB or more is recommended for optimal use.

Scanner: A scanner can be used to scan documents or photos into the computer. Scanners are generally flatbed scanners; they should have a color depth of at least 48 bits and a resolution of at least 1200 × 2400 dpi. The higher the color depth, the more accurate the color. A higher resolution picks up more subtle gradations of color.

Server: A server serves information to the computers to which it is connected. When users connect to a server, they can access programs, files, and other information.

Sound Card: Sound cards are responsible for playing sounds and recording audio. Most sound cards available today are capable of recording and playing digital audio. If the computer will be used extensively for game playing or as an entertainment system, the sound card can be upgraded.

Speakers: Speakers emanate sound and, as mentioned, if the computer will be used for game playing or used for presentations, the speakers can be upgraded for a higher quality sound.

Tablet: Portable computer that allows touch screen and handwriting recognition.

Video Graphics Card (VGC): A video graphics card enables the computer to display high-quality and clear graphics. If the computer will be used for extensive graphic work, the VGC may be upgraded for enhanced performance.

PC Video Camera: A PC video camera is a small camera that allows the capture of images and display of live video. Cameras sit on a monitor or desk or are embedded into the hardware of the computer monitor.

USB (Universal Serial Bus): The most common type of computer port used to connect keyboards, printers, scanners, Internet, or external drives.

BOX 8-2 | Technology Terms—cont'd

USB Flash (Jump) Drive: A USB drive allows information to be stored on it and used on different computers. The drive fits into the USB port and can hold up to 4 GB of information.

Voice Recognition: Technology that allows a computer to input information from spoken commands.

Wireless LAN Access Point: A wireless LAN access point allows several computers to access a network or Internet connection though a single cable modem or DSL connection. Each device requires a wireless card.

Zip Drive: A zip drive allows the backup of data and important files. An alternative to backing up files on a zip drive is to back up files on a CD-RW or DVD-RW.

Several components make up a computer system. Hardware, software, and data are important and can factor into the decision-making process when choosing to purchase either of the first two. A computerized hospital information system is a significant investment, and the overall plan must integrate hardware, software, training, and ongoing management control. To receive an excellent return on investment, the integration of these elements is crucial.

Hardware

Hardware refers to the actual physical equipment of a computer. The central piece of hardware in the information system is the computer. A computer is a device that electronically accepts data, processes the data arithmetically and logically, produces output from the processing, and stores the results for future use. The word *computer* is often used as a general term for the entire system. In reality, the computer is the actual workhorse of the system.

Computers are generally classified in three categories: mainframes, minicomputers, and microcomputers. The mainframe computer is a large system that handles numerous users, stores large amounts of data, and processes data at very high speeds. This type of computer may be found in a veterinary sales distribution office in which many sales are processed at the same time.

A minicomputer is compact and has a lower processing speed and more limited storage capacity than those of a mainframe. It is, however, more powerful than a microcomputer. This system is generally found in veterinary practices in which computer resources are shared. This system may be implemented in a centralized area, with several computers in outlying areas of the practice linked into it.

A microcomputer, or personal computer, is the smallest of the computer systems and is self-contained with regard to the circuitry and components. These systems are also popular in smaller veterinary practices and can be connected to form a local area network (LAN).

PRACTICE POINT Place all computers on a surge protector and battery backup system, preventing damage and loss of information.

Most computers are made up of a central processing unit (CPU), monitor, keyboard, mouse, graphics and video cards, CD and DVD drives, backup devices, and printers. It is also imperative to consider a power supply that has a surge protector included as well as a backup battery system if the electricity fails for more than a few minutes. The CPU is the central unit of the computer, and the monitor allows visualization of software applications. A mouse allows navigation through software applications, and a keyboard allows the user to type commands for the software. Graphics and video cards are used to produce outstanding quality and detail in the monitor. CD and DVD drives allow programs to be installed or information to be saved. Other backup devices may already be part of the machine or can be connected externally; they can save large amounts of information as needed. Regularly backing up the entire system onto an external device is recommended in case the computer system crashes. A power supply should always have a surge protector; if the electricity surges, it may short out the computer system and cause any stored information to be lost.

Software

Software is the system or program the computer follows. Each software company has different recommendations for hardware guidelines. Microsoft Windows supports most veterinary practice applications. Computers that use this operating system are generally referred to as *PCs*, as opposed to Macs, which are made by Apple Inc., and use a different operating system. Some veterinary practice software applications can also be run on a Mac; the relevant software company should be consulted to ensure compatibility.

Operating outdated software on outdated hardware decreases the efficiency of a practice. Older hardware is slower and less compatible with the technology that is available today. Modern software selection and high-tech hardware will have a positive impact on every aspect of the practice. Compatible hardware and software packages can streamline the business and increase the efficiency of every team member, including the veterinarian. Reports can be developed that have a positive effect on the marketing aspect of the practice, education materials can be developed for individual clients, and reminders can be generated at a faster pace than with previous methods. Software and hardware investments will show a greater return on investment than any other capital expense in the veterinary practice.

Selecting Hardware

It is better to start out small and simple, knowing that computer technology changes constantly. Computers can become outdated in 6 months; therefore it is advisable to buy only for the immediate need. Once the user is comfortable with the computer and wishes to upgrade, a higher quality computer and more complex system can be researched and purchased.

Location, Location, Location

If a practice wishes to buy several computers and place them throughout their operating space, terminal locations must be determined. Common locations include the receptionist station, pharmacy area, doctor's office, practice manager's office, and treatment area. Practices that are preparing to go paperless should also place a computer in each exam room, surgery laboratory, radiology room, and doctor(s) office. Practices should ask team members which locations would best increase efficiency and decrease wasted time. Teams should also determine the number of computers needed to increase efficiency while also maintaining budget requirements.

> **PRACTICE POINT** The placement of computer workstations is critical to increasing staff efficiency.

Types of Computers

Three types of computers may be considered for use in the practice: desktop, laptop, or tablet. Desktop computers are the most durable and least expensive. They are large and bulky and may take up more room than a space has to offer. Laptops are more expensive and fragile, but they are portable, smaller, and great for a practice that needs to be mobile. Tablets, a newer technology, are handheld and offer handwriting recognition as well as touch screen capability. Again, teams should determine the type of computer that will provide the most efficient use of space and time while remaining within budget guidelines.

Processor Selection

Once the type of computer has been chosen, the user must determine which type of processor will be the best option for the practice. Slower processors are cheaper (therefore not recommended); faster and more expensive processors include Pentium 4 and Pentium D. Software companies will verify the type of processor recommended to run their veterinary software. The difference in cost may be minimal, making it worth purchasing a higher quality and faster processor.

Printer Selection

A decision must also be made as to which type of printer will suit the practice best. Laser and inkjet printers are the most efficient in terms of speed and ink usage. The printers responsible for invoices should be durable, quick, and use the smallest possible amount of ink. Color printers are generally more expensive to purchase, and ink refill cartridges can be costly (but clients love to see their pets picture in color, on their invoice). Printers should also be placed in the pharmacy area for increased efficiency. Veterinary software packages will make recommendations of label printers to use with their particular software.

Servers

If a practice chooses to have several computers in the hospital, it is best to have them linked together. Each computer should have its own CPU; however, to allow the computers to work well together, they should be linked to a shared CPU for more efficiency. If only two computers are linked together, then the computer with more memory and a faster processor should be the main server. In practices where five or more computers are linked, it is advised to use a separate server. This will allow information to be processed at a quicker, more efficient rate. A desktop computer is designed to run Microsoft Word and Excel, access email, and support a Web browser. However, to efficiently serve the needs of a busy veterinary practice with practice management software, a server is highly recommended. It is engineered to run many applications at the same time, from all locations connecting to it.

> **PRACTICE POINT** Servers are critical for improving the efficiency of the veterinary practice software.

Computers can be linked together via a wireless Internet or through cabling that may be run through the walls of the building. A computer consultant should be contacted to determine the best method for each practice. Many older buildings have thick walls that can prevent efficient transmission of wireless waves; therefore wired terminals may be necessary. If a practice has an attic crawl space, wires can be dropped in almost any location, allowing the installation of computers anywhere the practice deems helpful.

Selecting Software

Many factors should be considered when researching software applications for veterinary practices. Hardware requirements, software support, education, and customization of software are a few elements that should be taken into account. Support is defined as the technical assistance offered by the company that helps facilitate the proper use of the software. This includes troubleshooting and problem resolution. Two of the most important factors include the hours of availability for tech support and how long it takes for the company to respond to practices in need of help (Box 8-3).

The company must provide training for team members to properly use the software and maximize its efficiency. Training can vary, from "Here's the manual," "go to this Web site," or an on-site trainer. On-site training is going to provide the best "bang for your buck" and should be budgeted (if not included) when selecting software.

Customization is defined as the ability of the software to adapt to the specific needs of the practice. For optimal efficiency, team members should be able to modify features with little or no assistance from the company. If the company needs to modify features, additional costs may be incurred and the team efficiency may be decreased.

BOX 8-3	Suggestions for Successful Software Selection

- Accessible client account data
- Accessible management data
- Clarity of user manuals
- Client education–based documents
- Complete audit trail
- Cost
- Data conversion abilities
- Interaction with other software applications
- Inventory management
- Long-term company
- Medical records
- Payroll
- Recalls/reminders
- Reduction of paperwork
- Reports generated
- Security features
- Technical support
- Training
- User friendly
- Veterinary software

BOX 8-4	Veterinary Software Web Addresses

AVImark	www.avimark.net
Animal Intelligence Software	www.animalintelligence.com
CornerStone-Idexx	http://www.idexx.com//view/xhtml/en_us/smallanimal/practice-management/practice-management-systems/cornerstone.jsf?conversationId=20649&SSOTOKEN=0
ImproMed	www.impromed.com
IntraVet	www.intravet.com
VetOfficeSuite	www.vetofficesuite.com
VetBlue	www.eveterinarysoftware.com
ClienTrax	www.clientraxtechnology.com
VIA Sound-Eklin	www.viainfosys.com
Alisvet Software	www.alisvet.com
eVetPractice	www.evetpractice.com

This is not an exclusive list.

Many practices may need to use multiple types of software packages to meet their needs, as many applications do not cover all aspects needed. Veterinary software is excellent at providing medical records, transactions, and reports relating to production. Accounting and management software may be needed to handle budget planning and payroll administration, whereas picture archival and compression software may be needed for digital radiography and ultrasonography (Box 8-4).

To help determine the type of software that would best suit a practice, a list should be developed of the practice's needs and wants. Team members can brainstorm for ideas to increase the efficiency of the team, and then research can be undertaken on software that meets those needs. What are some areas in which problems always occur? Lost records? Incomplete records? Lost charges? Clients having to wait for invoicing? Inventory management? Forgotten reminders? These are all questions that can be asked of team members.

It is wise to use software companies that have been in business for a number of years because technical support and upgrades in the future are imperative. Many practices have purchased cheap software from fly-by-night companies that are no longer in business. Recommendations can be solicited from other practices, and software applications can be reviewed online and at veterinary conventions. Sales representatives should be willing to give demonstrations of their product in the practice, allowing all team members to ask questions and determine the effectiveness of the software.

Demonstrations can also be loaded onto the computer with a CD or DVD or via the Internet. Those given by a representative in person will be more thorough; however, demonstrations given by a DVD may allow more interaction with the software. If a user can figure out the software without a personal demonstration, then the software is probably very user friendly. This is another benefit that should be seriously considered. Many team members, especially those who are of an older generation, do not have the computer skills that most members of the younger generation possess. A program must be user friendly and easy to navigate to be efficient for all team members.

Sales representatives should be asked for a list of practices that currently use their software. These practices should be called to verify their experience with the company's technical support, the years of service that the company has been in business, and the extent of satisfaction that the practice has with the software.

PRACTICE POINT	Explore all options before deciding which software to purchase.

Based on the information received from several demonstrations, the needs and wants list may need to be changed and updated. Security features should be a top concern as well. Access should be limited to certain areas of the software. Only managers and owners should have access to passwords, pricing, and confidential information and have permission to delete certain items. It is important that these areas are protected so that malicious activity or accidental changes cannot occur.

Medical records entry, storage, and retrieval may vary from one software product to the next, but none will be as flexible as a handwritten medical record. Chapter 14 offers more detail on computerized medical records. Practices wishing to go paperless tend to be more efficient and knowledgeable with computer systems. Paperless records prevent the loss of records and allow all radiographs and lab work results to be downloaded into the patients' files. Radiographs and lab work can be pulled up in any exam room for clients to view. The only paper required is for printing invoices for clients. A major disadvantage is the possibility of a computer malfunction or power outage, either of which could cripple the practice. It is therefore imperative to back up computers on a daily basis, both on site and off site, and have backup generators available, should power be lost.

Inventory management can be accomplished with most veterinary software versions. Chapter 15 offers great detail on inventory management and methods to implement a successful system. Veterinary inventory software will allow the input of invoices when supplies are received and will deplete quantities when clients are charged out. This is an excellent system for products that are sold outright but can create problems for supplies that are used to produce a service. An example might be an injection: a solution is drawn up into a 3-mL syringe, but the doctor prefers a new needle to be placed on the syringe for the administration of the injection. How does one keep track of the extra needle used for the injection? This is why it is imperative that physical inventory be reviewed before placing inventory orders.

Reports can be generated from software management but will usually need to be exported into another type of accounting software for financial management. Veterinary software reports are great for reporting the average doctor and client transactions, determining areas of profit in the practice, or comparing data from year to year. However, to produce profit and loss statements or any other financial reports, information may need to be exported into accounting software, such as QuickBooks or Sage 50.

Cost Analysis

When considering hardware and software requirements, it is important that a budget be determined. Efficient software systems can be costly, and it should be remembered that cheaper software systems might not produce the best results.

PRACTICE POINT   Cheaper software is not better; invest in software that can help your practice grow.

Costs should also be included when preparing the practice for a new computer system or upgrade. The cost of running new cables or electrical lines must be considered as well as the actual computer installation costs. Both hardware and software configuration may need to be completed by a local computer master to ensure they are compatible.

Most software companies offer data conversion as an option to transfer records into the new software. Team members may still need to make small adjustments to client and patient records during the transition.

Other initial costs may include any remodeling that needs to be completed to accommodate the new computers and/or printers and any additional supplies needed to start up the new system.

Recurring costs may include maintenance and support fees for the software system, and the replacement of any hardware components that fail in the future. The average life of a computer system is generally 3 to 5 years, after which time new technology will likely be available to once again increase the efficiency of the practice.

Many companies offer software that "will be able to complete" tasks in the future; however, those features are currently unavailable. Practices should use caution when looking at applications such as these. The company may not be around in the future; furthermore, a practice needs those applications now as well as in the future

Computer hardware should be supported locally; software can be supported over the phone and via an Internet connection. It is impossible to run software on hardware that is broken, and it is essential to have a computer technician available to repair or replace computer hardware when needed. Occasionally, it may be cheaper to replace a computer than to try and repair it. Unfortunately, the downside is having to reload software applications. Software issues can be handled by technical support via the Web. Most computers are or can be connected to the Internet by broadband or DSL. This allows technical support to diagnose and fix software hazards immediately, usually within a few minutes of connection.

Information should be backed up onto a DVD, external hard drive, or off site e-storage at the end of each day. Power surges or computer failure may occur at any time and can be due to multiple problems. It cannot be assumed that because a computer system is new, failures will not occur. It is also recommended to back up information off site on a daily basis in case something should happen to the building, such as theft or fire. This would allow immediate information retrieval and reloading in the event of a catastrophe.

Software Implementation

A change in software can cause great anxiety for a veterinary team. Team members who have been a part of the practice for an extended period will have the most difficulty with the change. Those who do not have extensive experience with computers may also have a hard time with the new process and may need extra assistance regarding training.

The software company should provide in-house training for a predetermined amount of time for all team members. Half-day or full-day training seminars are needed so that the team can learn about the software program. Teams should be able to practice entering client data so that there is little stress on them when the software is up and running. Appointments should be kept to a minimum during this period to allow the staff to adjust. The pace can then be slowly increased back to normal levels.

If many applications are available on the software, practices may wish to add them in phases. Team members can easily become overwhelmed when using new software and make mistakes that would not normally occur. If a practice is changing to a new software program with the ultimate goal of becoming a paperless practice, then the change should take place in either two or three phases. The first phase could be to implement the new hardware in all areas of the practice. Phase two would include the change to the new software program, allowing 6 months to 1 year for the staff to adjust to the new system. The third phase would be to reach the final goal of becoming paperless.

PRACTICE POINT   Develop a phase transition period, when taking the practice paperless.

Practices that have not used computers previously will take more time to implement changes. Team members should first be trained on the use of computers in general and become familiar with the basic Microsoft operations. Courses are available through community colleges to enhance the learning experience. Second, training personnel from the software company should be notified of the slower transition, allowing them to invest more time and proper training techniques to assist in the change. Third, team members should realize the benefit the new computer system will have on the practice and have patience during the transition. Once team members reap the benefits from the increased efficiency, the system will be used with less frustration and anxiety.

Managers should plan to attend continuing education seminars given by the software company to continue learning about the software. Many programs have tools and settings that the practice has never used or even knew existed. Continuing education will allow the continued progressive use of software, integrating new technology every year to help enhance the value to the practice.

Internet Security

Most computer systems will have access to the World Wide Web, especially if the practice maintains a Web site. Doctors may use the Internet to send (and receive) referrals, including radiographs, videos, and blood work results. They may also look up information for complex cases or consult with a specialist.

The Internet can be harmful to computer systems; therefore precautions should be taken to prevent catastrophe. There is no such thing as a completely safe Web site or safe computer system, because hackers have gained access to many of them.

Firewalls, antivirus programs, and different levels of passwords are the major precautions that can be taken to protect a computer system. Emails and attachments from unknown senders should not be opened, and Web sites with uncertainty should not be accessed. Even when all possible protections are used, it is still possible to be victimized by unwanted worms, viruses, and hackers (Boxes 8-5 and 8-6).

Firewalls, which are an excellent source of protection, consist of software (or hardware program) that helps screen out hackers, viruses, and worms that try to wiggle into the computer (system). They check every piece of information that comes in and goes out. Firewalls are often already installed on operating systems; they simply need to be enabled to start their job. It takes a small amount of time for firewalls to become efficient and recognize malicious programs.

Excellent antivirus programs include Norton and McAfee antivirus software. Both programs screen for viruses and include anti-spam programs. Most software programs include a trial period, which must be renewed once it expires. It is important to renew these subscriptions because updates are automatically sent to the computer so that it may recognize newly developed viruses.

Antivirus software should be set up so that it automatically scans all files on a regular basis. This allows continuous scans of files, seeking any viruses that may have downloaded onto the computer system. Neither firewalls nor antiviral software provide 100% protection; therefore it is advised to have both types of security enacted on every computer.

Team members should have limited access to the Internet; it should only be used for veterinary practice business. Facebook, Twitter, and personal email accounts (among others) should be blocked to prevent access and protect the system.

BOX 8-5 | **Internet Security Terms**

Adware: A program or software that installs itself onto the computer without the user's knowledge. Adware plays a role in advertising; it collects information about the user, as well as Web sites visited, and uses this information to display pop-up advertisements that may interest the user.

Cookies: Cookies are messages given to the browser with information that has been collected about the user when visiting Web sites. When the user returns to the Web site, the browser remembers the user and can present the user with a customized Web site.

Firewall: Device that regulates what comes in and out of the computer. The device will reject invalid programs.

Hacker: An individual or group of people that intentionally attempts to break into computer systems and install worms, viruses, or other dangerous software. They may also alter information, cause damage, and erase programs.

Host: A computer that is connected to a network or the Internet. Each host has a unique IP address.

Internet: A network that connects millions of users to various Web sites.

IP Address: A specific number that identifies the user's computer.

Pop-ups: Windows that pop onto the user's screen soliciting unwanted information.

Spam: Emails that are not considered useful and that can be damaging to the user.

Spam Filter: A device that filters spam, preventing it from infiltrating the user's computer.

Spyware: Software that secretly gathers information from the user's computer and transmits it to the source.

Trojan Horse: A destructive program, usually attached to an email that inhibits the computer.

Virus: A program loaded onto a computer and runs against the user's wishes. Viruses are usually able to replicate and send themselves on to other sites. Viruses tend to use up all the memory available on a computer, decreasing the processing speed or stopping the system.

Web Browser: Application used to locate and browse Web sites.

Worm: A program that replicates itself over a computer network and performs malicious actions that can shut the computer system down.

BOX 8-6 | Internet Safety Practices

- Do not open a site if there is any question about its authenticity.
- Do not open email or download attachments from unknown senders.
- Avoid deals that are too good to be true.
- Spybot is software that will search a computer for malicious software and delete it.
- Never use passwords that include personal items such as birthdays, house numbers, or Social Security numbers.
- Change passwords frequently.
- Create passwords that include letters, numbers, and symbols. The greater the combination, the harder it is to hack.

Backing up the System

Backing up the system cannot be emphasized enough. A computer can crash for any reason, including malfunction, electrical surge, theft, natural disaster, or malicious damage. Systems should be backed up each night, after the practice closes, onto a CD, DVD, or external hard drive (software systems will provide a recommendation as to which source to use). This disk should be removed and stored in the safe in case fire, flood, or theft should occur. This disk will allow information to be loaded onto a new system if needed. It is also ideal to back up the system off site. This can be done via the Internet or with a second disk that is taken to a safe storage place off premises.

If a computer crash occurs in the middle of the day, technical support should be called to see if any information lost since the last backup can be retrieved. If information cannot be retrieved, information will need to be re-entered. This is why a daily backup is imperative.

Always check your backups. Is your system actually backing up without error? You don't want to find out this answer when your system has crashed. Also, being prepared and knowing how to restore your system (in case of failure) will make the process seamless in times of high stress.

> **PRACTICE POINT** Always double-check backups; many times, the system has errors, and management does not know about it until they need an emergency backup!

Other Technology

In addition to the computer systems described, other technologies are prevalent in the practice today and include telephone systems, voice mail equipment, fax machines, copy machines, calculators, scanners, digital cameras, and time clocks.

Digital Cameras

Digital cameras and printers are a nice addition to the practice. They can be used to enhance client education, market

the practice, or add information to the medical record. Cameras can be used to take photos before and after dental prophylaxis to show the owners the difference in the teeth once the procedure has been completed. A pet that has a condition that will take time to improve may have a diagnostic photo taken; when it returns for a recheck, the photo can be compared, looking for any signs of improvement. Most veterinary software programs allow the importation of pet photos for the medical record; the photo can be taken each year and imported into the record. One photo can also be given to the owners.

Digital cameras are available in a range of megapixel capabilities; the higher the megapixels, the better the resolution of the photo. Price also increases with the number of megapixels the camera has; therefore choosing the megapixel capability that will suit the practice is important. Some digital cameras are sold with individual printers; others must be purchased separately. Photo printers can be costly, and so can the ink and paper to refill them. Teams should determine to what extent a camera and printer would be used and research the products that are available in the selected price range.

It is important to also check the veterinary practice management software that images will be uploaded to. Some may have maximum megapixels that can be uploaded; also consider the space that each picture will consume on the server.

WHAT WOULD YOU DO/NOT DO?

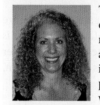

The practice manager receives a call early one morning from the city police department that the alarm had been triggered at the veterinary practice. The manager informs them that nobody should be on premises at this time of night, and she would meet the officers at the practice. Upon arrival, they see that the practice has been vandalized and the computers have been stolen. The phones were smashed, along with the emergency lights. Apparently when the criminals broke into the practice, they thought the emergency lights were the security system and when they could not get the alarm to stop, they broke the lights. Since the alarm continued, they only grabbed the computers and fled the scene. The practice manager panics, thinking they will not be able to operate the business the following day without computers.

What Should the Practice Manager Do?

If backup procedures were followed correctly at the end of the evening shift, the computer system was backed up onto a DVD or an off-site location. A computer can be moved temporarily from an exam room or treatment area to the front office and can provide a temporary practice server for the computer system until another computer can be purchased. The stored DVD can be uploaded into the temporary computer, allowing business to continue as normal; no information was lost in the theft. A plan B should always be available in case emergencies or natural disasters occur. Having a backup plan prevents stress overload in tense situations such as this.

Scanners and Copiers

Scanners and copiers are essential to a veterinary practice on a daily basis. Scanners may be used to scan in previous medical records, authorization forms, or photos. They may also be used to scan laboratory results into a file to email to a specialist. A copier may be used to copy records, client education information, or accounts payable invoices.

The extent that these pieces of equipment will be used will determine the type of product to purchase. If a scanner will be used multiple times a day and needs to capture clearer resolution, then a larger, more expensive scanner should be purchased. If many copies will be produced on a daily basis, then a larger, more efficient copy machine will be required. If smaller machines are purchased to save money, the level of satisfaction will be low. Smaller machines are not equipped to handle large workloads and will stop working sooner. Smaller machines also provide lower quality and take longer to process. This decreases the overall efficiency of the team as well as profits because another machine will need to be purchased sooner.

⚖ VETERINARY PRACTICE and the LAW

As more client and patient information is stored on computers and shared on computer networks that can often be accessed from a veterinarian's home, security and privacy has become a major issue. Social security numbers and driver's licenses numbers should never be stored on a shared network.

Each individual who has access to a computer should have a unique password, which should be changed on a regular basis. The password is a set of alphanumeric characters that allow a user to log on the system or specific parts of the computer system. Individuals should not share passwords with others.

Each individual should have access to only the types of information or applications that fall within their job description. System security should be designed in such a way that each security level permits access to only the applications and databases that are required for the team member to complete job duties.

REVIEW QUESTIONS

1. What is a CPU?
2. What is a server?
3. What is the benefit of having computers connected to each other?
4. What comprises a computer?
5. What considerations should be given when selecting software?
6. What is Spybot?
7. Why back up the system daily?
8. Which is more efficient, a CD or DVD? Why?
9. What benefits would the practice receive from the implementation of a digital camera?
10. What does the acronym *CPU* stand for?
    a. Certified practice units
    b. Central processing unit
    c. Cost prevention unit
    d. Customer protection unit
11. How many bytes are in a megabyte?
    a. 1000
    b. 1,000,000,000
    c. 1,000,000
    d. 100
12. What does the acronym *RAM* stand for?
    a. Radiology access machine
    b. Random access memory
    c. Recognition application modem
    d. Reduced adware memory
13. What is the correct definition of the term *Adware*?
    a. Messages given to the browser with information that has been collected
    b. The software chosen to be installed onto a computer
    c. A program or software that installs itself onto the computer without the user's knowledge
    d. Software that secretly gathers information from the user's computer and transmits it to the source
14. What does a worm do to a computer system?
    a. Filters out harmful or potentially hazardous programs on a computer
    b. Destroys information stored on a computer after being delivered by an email
    c. Protects the computer from harmful viruses.
    d. Replicates itself over a computer network and performs malicious actions

Recommended Reading

Gookin D: *PCs for dummies*, ed 12, Hoboken, NJ, 2013, John Wiley.

Heinke MM: *Practice made perfect: a guide to veterinary practice management*, ed 2, Lakewood, CO, 2012, AAHA Press.

Nash M: Selecting veterinary practice management software, *My EVT*, August 2012.

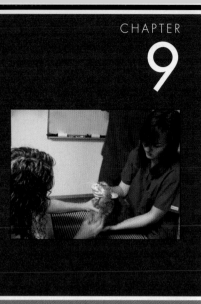

CHAPTER

9

Outside Diagnostic Laboratory Services

KEY TERMS

Aerobic
Anaerobic
Anticoagulants
Clinical and Laboratory
  Standards Institute
  (CLSI)
Cytology
EDTA
Formalin
Histopathology
Plasma
Serum
U.S. Food and Drug
  Administration (FDA)

OUTLINE

Choosing a Diagnostic Laboratory, 167
Sample Submission, 167
Laboratory Forms, 168
Sample Shipment, 173
Sample Pickup, 174
Results, 174
Fees, 175
Client Service, 175

LEARNING OBJECTIVES

When you have completed this chapter, you should be able to:

1. Identify the correct sample needed for specific testing.
2. List methods used to preserve samples correctly.
3. List methods used to label samples correctly.
4. Identify laboratory forms.
5. Define methods used to submit samples safely to the lab.
6. Describe an appropriate fee structure for outside laboratory services.

Outside laboratories are any laboratories to which patient samples are submitted. Some practices may use several outside labs for a variety of tests. It is important that measures are implemented to ensure that the correct forms are sent to each lab and that samples are prepared according to lab standards and sent correctly, either on ice or dry. Samples must also be packaged correctly so that they do not break during shipment. If procedures are not implemented, team efficiency decreases and client frustration increases as results are delayed, or tests are not completed as indicated by the veterinarian.

Many practices continue to use in-house laboratory services for general chemistries and complete blood counts (CBCs). In-house laboratory equipment is essential for receiving immediate results, especially in critical cases. For optimal results, in-house equipment must be consistently checked for quality control while performing maintenance. Many in-house laboratories can increase the bottom line of the practice, and equipment must be chosen with that in mind. For all tests that cannot be completed in-house, an outside service must be chosen.

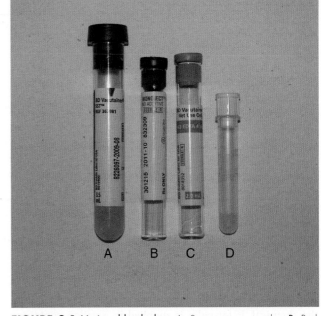

FIGURE 9-1 Various blood tubes. **A,** Serum separator tube. **B,** Red-topped tube. **C,** Lavender-topped tube. **D,** Green-topped tube with serum separator.

Choosing a Diagnostic Laboratory

Choosing a diagnostic laboratory can be a challenge because many factors are involved in the decision. First and foremost, the diagnostic laboratory must offer services and tests that the veterinarian is looking for. Some laboratories specialize in specific tests and have the newest technology available. For example, the Gastrointestinal Laboratory at Texas A&M University specializes in gastroenterology-related tests, and many other diagnostic laboratories will submit samples to this specific lab because of their testing protocol and results.

Standard laboratory services should include analysis for biochemical profiles, CBCs, cultures, cytology, and histopathology. Many laboratories offer services that extend beyond those listed, enabling veterinarians to provide better service to their clients.

Laboratories should abide by guidelines set forth by the Clinical and Laboratory Standards Institute (CLSI) and adhere to the strict guidelines outlined by the U.S. Food and Drug Administration (FDA). All labs being considered should continually monitor and perform quality controls for accuracy and reproducibility by internal and external quality assurance programs.

> **PRACTICE POINT** Laboratories should conform to guidelines set forth by the National Committee for Clinical Laboratory Standards (NCCLS) and the FDA.

Sample Submission

Correct sample submission is absolutely critical for the tests required. Many tests require serum, not plasma, for accurate

testing. Serum is produced when a red-topped tube is centrifuged, separating the red blood cells and coagulation proteins from the liquid portion of the blood. Red-topped tubes should be allowed to clot for 15 to 20 minutes before centrifugation. The sample can then be spun for 10 to 15 minutes at 2500 rpm. The serum can then be removed from the clot and placed in a plain glass red-topped tube for transport. If a serum separator tube (SST) has been used, there is no need to remove the serum. Do not use serum separator tubes for therapeutic monitoring, such as for digoxin, phenobarbital, or theophylline levels.

Tests that require plasma may require the sample to be spun with a specific anticoagulant. EDTA (ethylenediaminetetraacetic acid) is an anticoagulant that is added to a lavender-topped tube, preventing clotting of the blood. Plasma can then be obtained by centrifuging the sample and removing the liquid portion of the sample without any red blood cells. Other common anticoagulants include lithium heparin, sodium heparin, and potassium citrate (Figure 9-1 and Table 9-1).

Tissue samples submitted to the lab for histopathology require fixation. Formalin is a preservative that maintains the tissue characteristics for transport. Larger tissues may be partially cut, allowing the formalin to penetrate thicker tissues. The specimen container should contain 10% formalin at 10 times the volume of the tissue. Never reuse a sample submission jar because it may contain residuals of the previous specimen and is often labeled with the old patient information.

Formalin should be used with caution because it is a known carcinogen. It should not be inhaled, and gloves and

TABLE 9-1	Common Laboratory Tests			
TYPE OF TESTING	SPECIMEN	CONTAINER	ADDITIVES	STORAGE
Chemistries	Serum	RTT	None	Refrigerate
	Serum	SST	None	Refrigerate
Immunology	Serum	RTT, SST	None	Refrigerate
Endocrinology	Serum	RTT	None	Refrigerate
Phenobarbital	Serum	RTT	None	Refrigerate
Digoxin	Serum	RTT	None	Refrigerate
Theophylline	Serum	RTT	None	Refrigerate
Hematology	Whole blood	LTT	Anticoagulant EDTA	Refrigerate
Coagulation	Citrated plasma	BTT	Anticoagulant	Frozen
PT and PTT			Sodium citrate	

BTT, Blue-topped tube; *LTT*, lavender-topped tube; *PT*, prothrombin time; *PTT*, partial thromboplastin time; *RTT*, red-topped tube; *SST*, serum separator tube.

eye protection should be worn when handling the chemical. Most laboratories provide practices with prefilled formalin jars, which decrease the risk to the team members handling the chemical. If formalin is supplied in a gallon container, jars should be filled under a hood or in a well-ventilated area. See Chapter 21 for more information regarding the safe handling of formalin.

Cytology samples submitted to laboratories may need to be stained or unstained, depending on the test and the facility. Laboratory procedure books should be consulted before sample preparation to ensure the correct cytology is submitted. Cytology slides should never be shipped in the same bag as a formalin container because the fumes are known to degrade cytology samples.

> **PRACTICE POINT**   Cytology samples should not be submitted with a formalin sample, because formalin fumes are known to degrade samples.

Samples submitted for cultures must also indicate the source of the sample as well as specify whether an anaerobic or aerobic culture should be performed. Anaerobic is a technical word that literally means *without air,* whereas aerobic refers to *with air.* The veterinarian should indicate which culture is preferred, depending on the location of the sample. Aerobic samples should be kept refrigerated until pickup, and then shipped with a cold pack. Anaerobic cultures should be kept at room temperature and processed within 48 hours of sample collection.

Each sample (blood tubes, biopsy jars, and slide containers) must be clearly marked with the patient's name, date, and type of specimen (urine, serum, plasma, etc.). All lids and/or caps must be secured to prevent the sample from leaking or formalin from spilling. A protective, absorbent material should be wrapped around individual samples to prevent the sample from being broken during shipment. Slides should be packaged in a slide container to prevent the glass from breaking.

WHAT WOULD YOU DO/NOT DO?

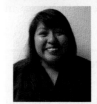 Harry, a 13-year-old Chihuahua is presented for lethargy and weight loss. Dr. Dreamer examines the dog and advises the technician to pull blood for a CBC/chemistry panel to be sent to the lab. Sophia pulls the blood as told and prepares the sample for submission to the lab. All laboratory work is sent by a courier service to a lab outside of the state; therefore it must be packaged well to prevent damage during shipment.

The following morning, the results are received on the fax machine; however it indicates one of the blood tubes broke during shipment, preventing the chemistry samples from being run. Dr. Dreamer is furious at Sophia and insists that she call the owner herself.

What Should Sophia Do?
Sophia knew the importance of protecting samples during shipment; she must call the owner and inform them of the broken sample. She must ensure the owners that Harry has enough blood for a second sample and she will wait for them on her lunch hour, because it is a convenient time for them to bring Harry in to obtain the new blood sample. She should then package the sample correctly, ensuring protection while shipping.

Laboratory Forms

Forms must be filled out correctly for the lab to return correct and sufficient data. Vital information includes species, age, gender, breed, patient name, client name, date, and the submitting doctor's name. The specified test must be marked correctly. If pathology samples are being submitted, the history of the pathology is very important. Pathologists look at the history as well as the patient to help determine a diagnosis. Without this critical information, a misdiagnosis may be made. Various submission forms are shown in Figures 9-2 to 9-4.

ANTECH DIAGNOSTICS

LAB USE ONLY

PLEASE LABEL ALL TUBES WITH PT. NAME & ACCT. NO.

☐ **CRITICAL**   **1W**

REORDER FORM →

CHART NUMBER

DATE	CLIENT	
/ /	PET NAME	

CLASS	CANINE FELINE	EQUINE OTHER	BREED	SEX M CM	AGE
			EXPORT Y N	F SF	

FOR LAB USE ONLY: UNSS   SS   S   R   L   SL   B   P   U   UC   RU   F   FC   CULT   RF   LF   ST   OTHER _____

DOCTOR

CUSTOM PANELS / OTHER REQUESTS
Please write test code and name.

GENERAL PROFILES

SA010	SuperChem	(S)
SA025	Vet-Screen	(S)
SA020	SuperChem, CBC (D2)	(S, L)
SA030	Vet-Screen, CBC (D3)	(S, L)

SA050	Pre-op Profile	
	Pre-op Chem, CBC, PT, PTT	(S, L, B)
SA070	Mini Screen, CBC	(S, L)

SA120	Total Body Function Superchem, CBC, T4	(S, L)
RECHECK	Recheck Profile Superchem, CBC	(S, L)
#		
	PREVIOUS ACC #	

ADD-ONS

ADD04	Coccidioides	(S)
ADD05	Ehrlichia canis	(S)
ADD06	FeLV (ELISA)	(S)
ADD07	FeLV, ELISA & FIV (ELISA)	(S)
ADD15	FIV (ELISA)	(S)
ADD50	Free T4 (ED)	(S)
ADD70	HWAG	(S)
ADD140	Retic Count	(L)
ADD190	T4, Total	(S)
ADD210	Urine Culture & MIC	(U)
ADD220	Urinalysis	(U)

ENDOCRINOLOGY

T435	ACTH, Endogenous	(AP)
ACTH	ACTH Response	(S)
	# of samples _____ Times: Pre _____ Post 1 _____ Post 2 _____	
T445	Cortisol, Resting	(S)
DEX	DEX Suppression	(S)
	# of samples _____ Times: Pre _____ Post 1 _____ Post 2 _____	
T470	Insulin/Glucose	(S)
S16595	PTH/Ionized Calcium	(2FS)
T475	Progesterone	(RS)
T495	T4, Total	(S)
5636	T4, Post Pill	(S)
T460	Free T4 (ED)	(S)
SA360	T3/T4 (Thyroid 1)	(S)
SA370	T4/Free T4 (ED) (Thyroid 2)	(S)
SA380	T4/Free T4 (ED) / TSH	(S)
SA390	TSH/Free T4 (ED)	(S)
T510	cTSH	(S)

SEROLOGY/IMMUNOLOGY

T515	ANA	(S)
S85889	Bartonella henselea (ELISA)	(S)
T530	Brucella	(S)
T535	Coccidioides	(S)
T540	Coombs'	(L)
T555	Distemper, Ab (Canine)	(S)
T570	Ehrlichia canis (Canine)	(S)
T580	FELV (ELISA)	(S)
T585	FELV, IFA	(SL)
T595	FIP (FCV)	(S)
T605	FIP 7b (ELISA)	(S)
T610	FIV (ELISA)	(S)
S16865	FIV Western Blot	(S)
T615	HWAG, canine	(S)
T620	HWAG, feline	(S)
T625	HWAB, feline	(S)
T630	HWAG/AB, feline	(S)
S16510	Leptospirosis	(S)
T670	Lyme IgG	(S)
85030	Toxo IgG/IgM, Canine	(S)
T720	Toxo IgG/IgM, Feline	(S)

CANINE PROFILES

SA090	Senior Comprehensive	Superchem, CBC, T4, FT4 (ED)	(S, L)
SA100	Canine Comp. (D1)	Superchem, CBC, T4, T3, FT4 (RIA)	(S, L)
SA150	Canine Vaccine Titer	Distemper Vaccine Titer, Parvo Vaccine Titer	(S)
SA170	Canine Autoimmune	CBC, Plt Ct, ANA, Coombs, RA	(S, L)
SA330	Canine Tick Serology 1	Ehrl, Lyme, RMSF	(S)

FELINE PROFILES

SA190	Feline Total Health Check	Superchem, CBC, T4, FeLV, FIV, FCV, Toxo IgG, IgM	(S, L)
SA200	Feline Comprehensive Plus (C1)	Superchem, CBC, T4, FT4 (RIA), T3, FeLV, FIV, FCV	(S, L)
SA220	Cat Scan Plus	Superchem, CBC, T4, FeLV, FIV	(S, L)
SA235	Feline Hyperthyroid Profile	Superchem, CBC, T4, FT4 (ED)	(S, L)
SA260	Feline Retroviral	FeLV, FIV	(S)
SA265	Feline Serology 1	FeLV, FIV, FCV	(S)
SA280	Feline Autoimmune Profile	CBC, Platelet Count, ANA, Coombs	(S, L)
S16581	Feline Vaccine Titer	Panleukopenia, Rhino., Calicivirus	(2S)

CHEM / SPECIAL CHEM

T050	Amylase/Lipase	(S)
T105	BUN/Creatinine	(S)
T200	Sodium/Potassium	(S)
T220	Bile Acids, Pre & Post	(2S)
T225	Bile Acid, Resting	(S)
T230	cTLI (canine)	(S)
S16800	fTLI (feline)	(S)
S16345	Fructosamine	(S)
S16195	Cobalamine/Folate	(S)
T240	Protein Electrophoresis	(S)

EARLY DETECTION/WELLNESS PROFILES

1620	Senior Wellness Profile 1	Superchem, CBC, T4, UA	(S, L, U)
85351	Senior Wellness Profile 2	Superchem, CBC, T4, FT4(ED), UA	(S, L, U)
85424	Canine Early Detection Profile	Chem Panel, CBC, HWAG	(S, L)
85425	Feline Early Detection Profile	Chem Panel, CBC, HWAB	(S, L)
85476	Early Detection Profile with O&P	Chem Panel, CBC, Ova & Parasites	(S, L, F)
86284	Early Detection Profile with O&P/Giardia	Chem Panel, CBC, O&P/Giardia	(S, L, F)

HEMATOLOGY / COAG

T330	CBC	(L)
1481	CBC w/Path Review	(L)
T400	Platelet Count	(L)
T415	PT/PTT	(B)
T425	Reticulocyte Count	(L)
S17123	Von Willebrands	(L or B)

THERAPEUTIC DRUG MONITORING

T730	Bromide	(RS)
T735	Digoxin	(RS)
T750	Phenobarbital	(RS)
85711	Diabetes Monitoring Panel	(S,L,U)

85712	Hyperthyroid Monitoring Panel	(S,L)
85714	NSAID Monitoring Panel	(S,L,U)
85851	Phenobarbital Monitoring Panel	(RS,L)

DIAGNOSTIC PROFILES

SA290	Coag Profile 1	(Full B, L)
SA300	Coag Profile 2 (minus CBC)	(Full B, L)
SA310	Renal Profile	(S, L, U)
SA320	Liver Profile	(2S, L)
SA340	Fungal Serology	(S)
T960	PCR Canine Tick Borne Panel	(L)
T965	PCR Feline Tick Borne Panel	(L)

URINE / FECAL

T760	Urinalysis	(U)
T830	Microalbuminuria (MA)	(U)
T775	Urine Prot/Creat	(U)
T770	Urine Cort/Creat	(U)
S16735	Urine Calculi Analysis (Stone)	(U)
T695	Parvo Ag	(F)
T805	O&P	(F)
85862	O&P/Giardia	(F)
T16007	Cl. perfringens Enterotoxin	(F)
T790	Crypto/Giardia (IFA)	(F)
T820	Giardia (ELISA)	(F)

MICROBIOLOGY

M020	Aerobic C & S (Non-urine)	(C)
M030	Anaerobic Culture	(C)
M040	Aerobic C&S, Anaerobe Cult	(2C)
M061	Blood Culture	(2BCB)
M070	Culture ID only	(C)

85072	UA & U. Cult if indicated	(2U)
M160	Fecal Culture	(F)
M080	Fungal Culture	(C)
M090	Gram Stain	(SL or C)
M130	Urine Culture & MIC	(U or C)

SOURCE: _____

SPECIMEN REQUIREMENTS

S	Spun Serum Separator	SL	Slide	G	Green Top
L	Lavender	P	Plasma	AP	Aprotinin Plasma
U	Urine	F	Feces	RS	Red Top Serum
C	Conen Swab	B	Blue Top		

BCB Blood Culture Bottle   FS Frozen Serum

KEEP 2ND COPY FOR YOUR RECORDS.

LABORATORY COPY

Rev. 9/08

A

FIGURE 9-2 A to C, ANTECH lab submission form. (Courtesy ANTECH Diagnostics, Los Angeles, Calif.)

Continued

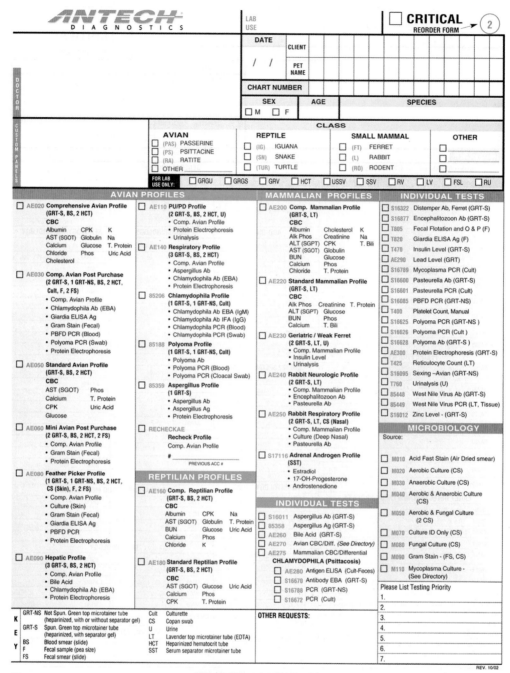

B

FIGURE 9-2, cont'd

ANTECH
D I A G N O S T I C S

| LAB USE ONLY | | | | | | | | | | | REORDER FORM → | 3W |

DATE	CLIENT								
/ /	PET NAME								
DOCTOR									
CHART #									

SPECIES	☐ CANINE ☐ EQUINE	BREED	AGE	SEX
	☐ FELINE ☐ AVIAN			☐ M ☐ CM
	☐ Other _____			☐ F ☐ SF

| CHOOSE A PATHOLOGIST: | If you would like to direct this case to a specific pathologist, please write name in this box. Please note that this is subject to the availability of the pathologist at the time of sample receipt. If the pathologist is unavailable, it will be forwarded to another Antech pathologist. | REQUESTED PATHOLOGIST 1. 2. 3. |

HISTOPATHOLOGY / CYTOLOGY | PATIENT HISTORY

☐ CYTO Cytology (Source: _____)

☐ FLUA Fluid Analysis with Cytology (_____)

☐ CSF CSF with Cytology

☐ BONE Bone Marrow Cytology

☐ BUFFY Buffy Coat Smear

☐ FBX Biopsy, Written
(Includes Microscopic Description, Microscopic Findings, Prognosis & Comment)

☐ MBX Biopsy, Mini
(Includes Microscopic Findings, Prognosis & Comment)

☐ BMCB Bone Marrow Core Biopsy
(Includes Microscopic Description, Microscopic Findings, Prognosis & Comment)

☐ STAT BIOPSY STAT FEE (see Service Directory for details)

☐ DERM Dermatopathology
(Biopsy & Dermatologist Recommendations)

Type of Biopsy: ☐ Excisional ☐ Incisional
☐ Needle ☐ Endoscopic

All tissue(s) submitted? ☐ Yes ☐ No

Number of Containers Submitted: _____

☐ 30 mL ☐ 60 mL ☐ 100 mL ☐ 32 oz.

Number of Specimens Submitted: _____

Source/Site: _____

Previous Biopsy/Cytology Submitted? ☐ Yes ☐ No

Reference Number: _____

LOCATION

DORSAL VIEW

R   L

VENTRAL VIEW

PATIENT HISTORY

PLEASE NOTE:
This section is critical for Biopsy/Cytology interpretation.

_____
_____
_____
_____
_____
_____
_____
_____
_____

FOR LABORATORY USE
(Please do not write in this space)

1. No. of containers received: _____

2. Tissues received: _____

_____
_____
_____
_____
_____
_____
_____
_____

*LABEL EACH CONTAINER SUBMITTED WITH CLINIC NAME, CLIENT AND PATIENT NAME, AND TISSUE SOURCE. (Rev. 7/03)

C

LABORATORY COPY

FIGURE 9-2, cont'd

FOR LAB USE ONLY

COLLECTION DATE

Mark an "X" here for ASAP

IDEXX LABORATORIES
Customer Service
888-433-9987

C601923

Please send duplicate results to:
Account # ____
Practice Name ____
Patient ID# (optional)

OWNER LAST NAME

PATIENT NAME

SEX: Male / Female / Spay/Neut.

SPECIES: Canine / Feline / Avian / Equine / Other

AGE: ____ Years ____ Months

BREED ____

VETERINARIAN(S)

[ ] SOULES
[ ] ____

Check here for BASIC CBC

CANINE / FELINE GENERAL PROFILES
All profiles require serum and lavender top

- 53 Comprehensive Canine (R/S, L) — *Chem 25, Amyl/Lip, CBC, T4, HW*
- 66 Feline Viral Plus (R/S, L) — *Chem 25, CBC, T4, FeL V, FIV, FIP*
- 54 Feline Combo (R/S, L) — *Chem 25, CBC, FeL V, FIV*
- 74 Feline Combo Plus (R/S, L) — *Chem 25, CBC, T4, FeL V, FIV*
- 885 Comprehensive Feline (R/S, L) — *Chem 25, Amyl/Lip, CBC, T4, FeL V, FIV, FIP*
- 75 Total Health Plus (R/S, L) — *Chem 25, Amyl/Lip, CBC, T4*
- 46 HealthChek Plus *Chem 25, CBC, T4* (R/S, L)
- 1 HealthChek *Chem 25, CBC* (R/S, L)
- 1013 Total Health *Chem 25, Amyl/Lip, CBC* (R/S, L)
- 1294 Chem 11, CBC (R/S, L)
- 1272 Chem 21, CBC (R/S, L)
- 1850 Adult Screen *-Chems 25, CBC, UA* (R/S, L, U)
- 865 Senior Screen *-Chems 25, T4, CBC, UA* (R/S, L, U)

SPECIAL TEST REQUESTS
Code # Test Name

FECALS/WELLNESS
- 5010 Fecal Ova and Parasites
- 72440 Lab 4Dx
- 26049999 Canine Easy Annual 1 *(Chem 10, sCBC, Lab 4Dx, Fecal O & P)*
- 26139999 Feline Easy Annual *(Chem 10, sCBC, Feline HW Ab)*
- 2463 O & P, Giardia Antigen by Elisa

CANINE TESTS
- 7246 Lyme Quant C6
- 1849 Spec cPL
- 2337 HealthChek with Spec cPL
- 2625 Canine Diarrhea Panel

FELINE TESTS
- 2626 Feline Diarrhea Panel
- 2512 Feline Upper Respiratory Panel
- 1717 Feline Hemotropic Mycoplasma

HEMATOLOGY
- 300 CBC - Comprehensive (L)
- 319 Buffy Coat Smear (L)
- 309 Platelet Count (L)
- 6 Coag Profile (BTT, L) — *(CBC, PT, PTT, PLT, FIB Quant)*
- 56 Coag Panel #1 *(PT, PTT, PLT)* (BTT, L)
- 311 PT (BTT)
- 312 PTT (BTT)

ENDOCRINOLOGY
- 13 Thyroid Panel #1 *(T3, T4)* (R/S)
- 851 Thyroid Panel #2 *(T4, FT4 ED)* (R/S)
- 804 T4 (R/S)
- 849 FT4 ED (R/S)
- 119 ACTH Stimulation (pre & post) (R/S)
- 274 Dex Suppression (pre & post 8 hr.) (R/S)
- 275 Dex Suppression (pre & post 4 & 8 hr.) (R/S)
- 245 Fructosamine (R/S/L/GN)
- 806 Progesterone (R)

GENERAL CHEMISTRIES
- 257 Bile Acids Panel (Pre & 2 hr Post) (R/S)
- 111 Chem25 (R/S)
- 1113 Chem27 (R/S)
- 1271 Chem21 (R/S)
- 1293 Chem11 (R/S)

LARGE ANIMAL PROFILES
- 11 Large Animal Profile (R/S, L) — *Chems, CBC, FIB*
- 316 Inflammatory Profile (R/S, L) — *CBC, Plasma Protein, FIB*

ADD TO ANY PROFILE *(R/S unless otherwise indicated)*
- 8531 TSH
- 7231 Canine Heartworm Antigen
- 850 Free T4 ED
- 1045 FeLV Ag + FIV Ab
- 2570 Bile Acids (single)
- 997 Urine Pro/Creat Ratio (U)
- 9101 Urinalysis / Cysto / Other (U)
- 22 T4
- 7101 FeCoV (FIP)
- 72461 Lyme Quant C6
- 18491 Spec cPL

IMPORTANT! Please provide history:

HISTOPATHOLOGY
- 601 Biopsy with Microscopic Description
- 608 Biopsy (No Microscopic Description)

# of sites/lesions/organs ____

# of specimens/tissues submitted ____

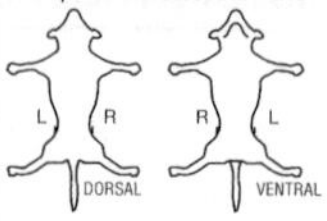

Prev. Date & Accession # ____

CYTOLOGY
Source required: ____
- 605 Cytology with Microscopic Description
- 600 Cytology (No Microscopic Description)
- 607 Bone Marrow with Microscopic Description
- 900 CSF Analysis (Includes Cytology)
- 905 Fluid Analysis, Body (Includes Cytology)
- 906 Fluid Analysis, Joint (Includes Cytology)

THERAPEUTIC DRUG MONITORING
- 1000 Phenobarbitol (red top only)
- 1001 Digoxin (red top only)

URINE / STONE ANALYSIS
- 909 Stone Analysis (Chemical) (STN)
- 90900 Stone Analysis (Crystallographic) (STN)
- 910 Urinalysis / Cysto / Other (U)
- 910 U/A / 943 Culture if indicated (check both boxes) / Cysto / Other
- 4035 Culture ONLY / Cysto / Other
- 994 Urine Protein / Creatinine Ratio (U)
- 946 Urine Cortisol / Creatinine Ratio (U)

MICROBIOLOGY
Source required: ____
- 400 Aerobic Culture & Suscept (C)
- 427 Aerobic Culture ID only (C)
- 401 Anaerobic & Aerobic C & S (ANC, C)
- 4022 Salmonella & Campylobacter Fecal Culture (F)
- 4035 Urine Culture & MIC / Cysto / Other (U)
- 405 Fungal Culture (C/SC)
- 1394 Comprehensive UA & Culture / Cysto / Other (U)

IMMUNOLOGY / SEROLOGY
- 24 FeLV Ag (ELISA) & FIV Ab (ELISA) (R/S)
- 723 Heartworm Ag - Canine (R/S, L)
- 707 Coggins, EIA (AGID) (R/S)
- 7077 Coggins, EIA (ELISA) (R/S)
- 303 Coombs (L)
- 709 FeLV Ag (ELISA) (R/S)
- 717 FeLV Ag (IFA) (L)
- 710 FeCoV (FIP) (R/S)
- 702 Brucella Screen (K9) (R/S)
- 7246 Lyme Quant C6 (K9) (R/S)
- 1849 Spec cPL (K9) (R/S)

AVIAN / EXOTIC
- Panel # ____
- 435 Avian / Reptile Aerobic C&S (C)
- 415 Exotic Respiratory Screen (C&S, Fungal) (C)
- 4023 Avian Fecal Culture (C&S, Gram Stain) (C/F)

WHITE COPY - LABORATORY • YELLOW COPY - HOSPITAL

REV 06-08

FIGURE 9-3 IDEXX lab submission form. (Courtesy IDEXX Laboratories, Inc., Westbrook, Me.)

GASTROINTESTINAL LABORATORY

CLINIC DETAILS

Veterinarian: _____

Clinic/Hospital: _____

Address: _____

City:_____ State:_____ ZIP:_____

Clinic E-mail Address:_____
(E-MAILED RESULTS WILL OFTEN BE AVAILABLE SEVERAL HOURS BEFORE FAXES ARE SENT)

Telephone:_____ Fax: _____

Preferred reporting method: ☐ **E-mail**   ☐ **Fax**   ☐ **Fax & E-mail**

DATE: _____

LABORATORY USE ONLY

Date Received: _____

Accession #: _____

Check #: _____

Charges: _____

Amt. Received: _____

PATIENT DETAILS

Owner's Name: _____

Animal's Name: _____

Species (circle):   Dog   Cat   Other (   )   Breed:

Age:_____ Years   Sex: M   F   MC   FS

Your Internal Identifier: _____

IMPORTANT NOTES

Most assays are species-specific; you **MUST** indicate a species in patient details.

SEPARATE SERUM FROM CLOT BEFORE SHIPPING

Both hemolysis and lipemia may interfere with test performance.

TEST(S) ORDERED - PLEASE CHECK BOXES

Test	Price	
Serum TLI, PLI, Cobalamin, Folate (2.0 mL serum, fasting)	$ 00..............	☐
Serum TLI, Cobalamin, Folate (1.0 mL serum, fasting)	$ 00..............	☐
Serum PLI, Cobalamin, Folate (1.0 mL serum, fasting)	$ 00..............	☐
Serum TLI, PLI (1.0 mL serum, fasting)	$ 00..............	☐
Serum Cobalamin, Folate (1.0 mL serum, fasting)	$ 00..............	☐
Serum TLI (1.0 mL serum, fasting)	$ 00..............	☐
Serum PLI† (0.5 mL serum, fasting)	$ 00..............	☐
Canine C-Reactive Protein (0.5 mL serum, fasting)	$ 00..............	☐
Serum Bile Acids: Pre-feeding (1.0 mL serum, fasting)	$ 00..............	☐
Post-feeding (1.0 mL serum, 2 hours postfeeding)	$ 00..............	☐
Serum Gastrin (0.5 ml serum, fasting)	$ 00..............	☐
Triglycerides (0.5 ml serum, fasting)	$ 00..............	☐
PCR testing: *Tritrichomonas foetus*	$ 00..............	☐
Campylobacter spp. (*C. jejuni, C. coli, C. upsaliensis, C. helveticus*)	$ 00..............	☐
Heterobilharzia americana	$ 00..............	☐
Clostridium perfringens enterotoxin gene	$ 00..............	☐
Fecal α₁-Proteinase Inhibitor (**Canine or Feline**)*	$ 00..............	☐

For ordering supplies please fill out the line below and fax to the laboratory:
5 sets of three preweighed fecal tubes: (   ) boxes at $25.00 each for α₁-PI

Use ONLY FedEx or UPS for all shipping. **Do not use the U.S. Postal Service; this may cause delay in deliveries.**

*Fecal specimens for α₁-Proteinase Inhibitor are **only** accepted in our containers. Samples must be **frozen** in these tubes and **shipped frozen** to the laboratory by overnight carrier. **This test is species specific; indicate species in patient details.**

†Serum PLI (Spec cPL or Spec fPL) will be run only within panels or alone as a follow-up test.

TOTAL CHARGES FOR THIS ANIMAL   **$**

PAYMENT METHOD: ☐ Check Enclosed (make payable to GI Lab - TAMU)   ☐ Please Bill Me

We can not accept packages that are marked "Bill Receiver". Please use our pre-printed shipping labels to save on shipping! Call (979) 862-2861 for more information.   Prices valid as of 01/01/2009

FIGURE 9-4 Texas A&M lab submission form. (Courtesy Jörg M. Steiner, Texas A&M University, College Station, Tex.)

Copies of submission forms should be kept for records. IDEXX and ANTECH provide carbonless submission forms, whereas others may not. Copies should be made so that the team will know which laboratory was selected, where tests were submitted, and on which date. Samples may become lost in the mail, the wrong test may be performed, or results may not have been received. This allows team members to track samples and results, or hold team members accountable if the wrong test code was submitted.

Sample Shipment

Proper sample shipment is absolutely critical when submitting samples. Instructions must be followed for various tests to be completed. Some samples only need to be submitted with an ice pack to keep the sample cool during shipment. Other samples must be sent frozen, and some do not need to be chilled at all. Samples with no specific holding requirements (freezing or room temperature) should remain in the refrigerator for storage until the courier has arrived to pick them up. Keeping the samples chilled preserves cell function. During the winter months, samples must be protected from freezing during shipment. Samples may be submitted with a bag of hot saline solution and can be insulated by wrapping them in layers of newspaper or bubble wrap (Figure 9-5).

Depending on the laboratory and the veterinarian's need for rapid results, some shipments may need to be sent

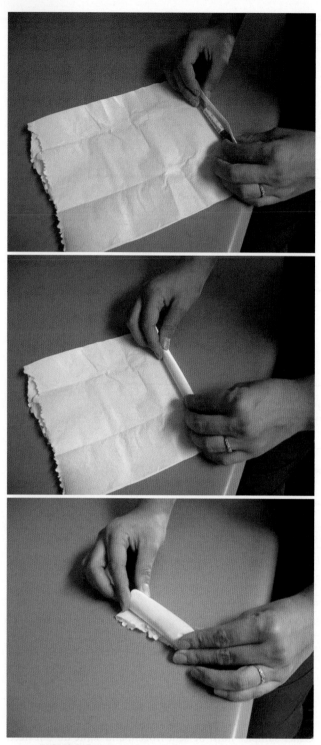

FIGURE 9-5 Protecting samples sent to the laboratory.

overnight to the lab, whereas others may simply be sent by Priority Mail. Team members should verify shipping procedures with the laboratory to ensure the best sample submission and result turnaround time.

> **PRACTICE POINT**   Ensure samples are packed for shipment correctly; reduce the possibility of broken blood tubes or slides.

Sample Pickup

Sample pickup is also an important factor in submitting samples to labs. If most samples are sent to one lab in particular, the lab should provide a courier service for sample pickup. Depending on the location of the laboratory facility, the lab may send its own courier, or another agent, such as FedEx, UPS, or DHL, may ship samples. Timing of sample pickup can also help a practice decide which lab to choose. It is ideal to have samples picked up late in the day, allowing any samples collected during the day to be sent. Ideally, results should be received the following morning. When samples are picked up midday, anything collected after pickup must wait until the following day to be sent to the lab. This causes delayed results, potentially decreasing the quality of patient care. Studies indicate that red blood cell morphology and platelet parameters change with delayed analysis. Laboratories strive to provide the best service available, and courier pickup is one of those services. Ask the laboratory representative for the latest possible pickup; if that time is not ideal, search for other labs and ask what they can offer as far as sample pickup.

Results

Results should be received in a timely fashion. Specialized tests may take longer to run; however, laboratory description books should indicate the time frame required. If results are delayed, a lab representative should call the practice and communicate the delay. Team members should also review forms that have been submitted and watch for results that have not been received. Reviewing these forms can prevent a doctor (and client) from becoming upset; the team member can be proactive and search for results before it becomes a problem.

Results should offer a variety of information. Alongside the patient results, a reference range will be listed. This reference range indicates the normal ranges for that particular piece of equipment. Flags can also indicate patient results outside the normal range, drawing attention to specific abnormalities. If a patient's CBC appears abnormal, a pathology review should automatically be indicated. Having a pathologist review the smear can increase the time until results are received. Some labs require the veterinary practice to request a review when abnormalities are present. This can increase the time for patient diagnosis and treatment; therefore it is beneficial when a laboratory automatically initiates a pathology review. Cytology and histopathology reviews should be received by the practice in a timely manner. All tissue samples should automatically have the margins reviewed, indicating whether tumor cells have spread beyond the margin of the tissues.

Laboratory reports should be detailed and provide current, progressive information for the veterinarian, especially in pathology cases. It saves the veterinary team time when lab reports include specific disease and treatment indicators with regard to sample results (Figures 9-6 to 9-8).

Patient results may be reported by fax, phone, or Internet. Practices with electronic medical records may choose to have results automatically populated into the

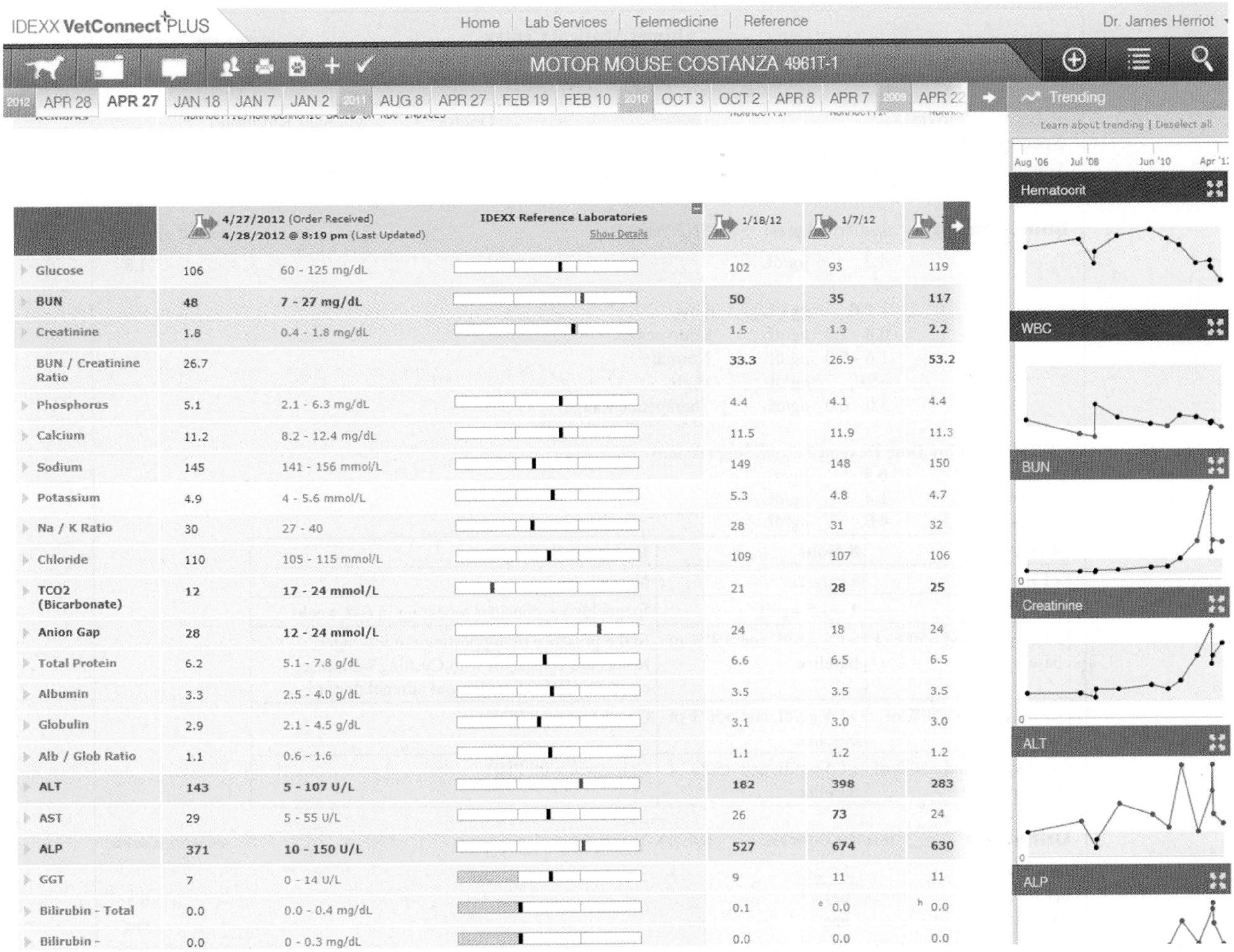

	4/27/2012		1/18/12	1/7/12	
Glucose	106	60 - 125 mg/dL	102	93	119
BUN	**48**	**7 - 27 mg/dL**	**50**	**35**	**117**
Creatinine	1.8	0.4 - 1.8 mg/dL	1.5	1.3	**2.2**
BUN / Creatinine Ratio	26.7		**33.3**	26.9	**53.2**
Phosphorus	5.1	2.1 - 6.3 mg/dL	4.4	4.1	4.4
Calcium	11.2	8.2 - 12.4 mg/dL	11.5	11.9	11.3
Sodium	145	141 - 156 mmol/L	149	148	150
Potassium	4.9	4 - 5.6 mmol/L	5.3	4.8	4.7
Na / K Ratio	30	27 - 40	28	31	32
Chloride	110	105 - 115 mmol/L	109	107	106
TCO2 (Bicarbonate)	12	**17 - 24 mmol/L**	21	**28**	**25**
Anion Gap	28	**12 - 24 mmol/L**	24	18	24
Total Protein	6.2	5.1 - 7.8 g/dL	6.6	6.5	6.5
Albumin	3.3	2.5 - 4.0 g/dL	3.5	3.5	3.5
Globulin	2.9	2.1 - 4.5 g/dL	3.1	3.0	3.0
Alb / Glob Ratio	1.1	0.6 - 1.6	1.1	1.2	1.2
ALT	**143**	**5 - 107 U/L**	**182**	**398**	**283**
AST	29	5 - 55 U/L	26	**73**	24
ALP	**371**	**10 - 150 U/L**	**527**	**674**	**630**
GGT	7	0 - 14 U/L	9	11	11
Bilirubin - Total	0.0	0.0 - 0.4 mg/dL	0.1	e 0.0	h 0.0
Bilirubin -	0.0	0 - 0.3 mg/dL	0.0	0.0	0.0

A

FIGURE 9-6 A and B, IDEXX patient results. (Form courtesy IDEXX Laboratories, Inc., Westbrook, Maine.)

medical record. Alerts are set for the team when results are available. It is imperative that correct patient information be submitted when this option is chosen or results will become lost if they are autopopulated into another patient's record.

Fees

Fees vary from lab to lab. Some labs may compete for the practice's business, thereby allowing special pricing on the most common profiles. Specialized testing can become fairly expensive, especially when one lab forwards the sample to another. Research may be done to find the "best" lab available for running specific tests. A team member can call that lab and receive specific pricing information as well as details on shipping the sample and the turnaround time for results. This can save the practice and client money, along with being able to receive results quicker.

For the practice to recover hidden costs associated with laboratory analysis, the practice must at least double the cost of the testing to the client. Costs that must be considered include:

- The time it takes the team members to draw and prepare the samples.
- The cost of supplies used to obtain the sample if the lab does not provide them. Supplies may include a syringe and needle, formalin if purchased by the gallon, and slides used for cytological analyses.
- Some laboratories may add a fuel surcharge to the monthly statement.
- Shipping fees if samples are submitted to labs other than those used for general analysis. This may include overnight fees to FedEx or UPS.

PRACTICE POINT Appropriate fees must be collected from clients for laboratory services and the cost of supplies, shipping, and interpretation of results.

Client Service

Client service is a very important factor when choosing outside laboratories. Team members often place calls

Animal Medical Center
123 Main St.
Altoona, PA 16602

IDEXX
LABORATORIES

Patient:	Moxie		Doctor:	Michael Raymond
Species:	Canine			
Client:	Charlie Pollock		Client ID:	72145 Page 2 of 2

Immunoassay   11/14/2013 4:15:00 PM   SNAPshot Dx™   9/6/2012 2:18:00 PM

T_4 1.3   μg/dL   1.8

< 0.8	μg/dL	Low
0.8 - 1.5	μg/dL	Equivocal
1.6 - 5.0	μg/dL	Normal
>5.0	μg/dL	High
3.0 - 6.0	μg/dL	Therapeutic Range

CORTISOL (Low-Dose Dexamethasone Suppression)

Baseline	6.5	μg/dL
4 hour	1.4	μg/dL
8 hour	4.0	μg/dL

4-Hour	8-Hour	Interpretation
<1 μg/dL	<1 μg/dL	Normal
1 – 1.5 μg/dL	1 – 1.5 μg/dL	Inconclusive, consider repeating in 6–8 weeks
>1.5 μg/dL and >50% of baseline	>1.5 μg/dL and >50% of baseline	In the presence of supporting clinical signs, results are consistent with Cushing's Disease; consider HDDST to rule out adrenal tumor
<1.5 μg/dL or <50% of baseline	>1.5 μg/dL and >50% of baseline	Consistent with PDH
>1.5 μg/dL and >50% of baseline	>1.5 μg/dL and <50% of baseline	Consistent with PDH

Urinalysis   11/14/2013 4:15:00 PM   IDEXX VetLab® UA™   9/6/2012 2:18:00 PM

Urine SG	1.020		
pH	6.0		6.5
LEU	neg		neg
PRO	1+		neg
GLU	neg		neg
KET	neg		neg
UBG	1+		norm
BIL	neg		neg
BLD	neg		neg

*Confirm all leukocyte results with microscopy

09-68073-00

B

FIGURE 9-6, cont'd

looking for specific results, lab codes, or supplies. It is important that the call is answered in a timely manner, that lab personnel are friendly, and that they provide the answers needed. Veterinarians often need to consult with a pathologist or specialist regarding cases and results of previously submitted lab work. Most labs will provide a consult free of charge if a sample has been submitted on that case. Once a veterinarian has placed a call to the consult line, the lab should return the call to the veterinarian within one business day. Again, laboratories strive to provide the best service available, and consult calls should be returned immediately.

Most laboratories will provide veterinary practices with supplies for submitting samples, free of charge. Supplies may include blood tubes, histopathology jars, sample submission bags, and forms. If any additional materials are needed, a call to customer service should take care of the request (Box 9-1).

ANTECH DIAGNOSTICS 13633 N. Cave Creek Phoenix AZ 85022 Phone: 800-745-4725

Client #
Chart #

Accession No.	Doctor	Owner	Pet Name	Received
PXBC04335299				

Species	Breed	Sex	Pet Age	Reported
Canine	Great Pyrenees	CM	2Y	

Test Requested	Results		Reference Range	Units
SUPERCHEM				
AST (SGOT)	31		15-66	IU/L
ALT (SGPT)	86		12-118	IU/L
Total Bilirubin	0.1		0.1-0.3	mg/dL
Alkaline Phosphatase	19		5-131	IU/L
GGT	1		1-12	IU/L
Total Protein	6.4		5.0-7.4	g/dL
Albumin	3.9		2.7-4.4	g/dL
Globulin	2.5		1.6-3.6	g/dL
A/G Ratio	1.6		0.8-2.0	
Cholesterol	239		92-324	mg/dL
BUN	20		6-25	mg/dL
Creatinine	1.3		0.5-1.6	mg/dL
BUN/Creatinine Ratio	15		4-27	
Phosphorus	4.9		2.5-6.0	mg/dL
Calcium	10.3		8.9-11.4	mg/dL
Glucose	98		70-138	mg/dL
Amylase	540		290-1125	IU/L
Lipase	457		77-695	IU/L
Sodium	153		139-154	mEq/L
Potassium	4.7		3.6-5.5	mEq/L
Na/K Ratio	33		27-38	
Chloride	115		102-120	mEq/L
CPK	84		59-895	IU/L
Triglyceride	66		29-291	mg/dL
Osmolality, Calculated	319 (HIGH)		277-311	mOSm/kg
Magnesium	1.6		1.5-2.5	mEq/L.
COMPLETE BLOOD COUNT				
WBC	5.7		4.0-15.5	$10^3/\mu L$
RBC	6.6		4.8-9.3	$10^6/\mu L$
HGB	16.4		12.1-20.3	g/dL
HCT	47		36-60	%
MCV	70		58-79	fL
MCH	24.7		19-28	pg
MCHC	35		30-38	%
Comment				
RBC MORPHOLOGY	NORMAL			

Differential	Absolute	%		
Neutrophils	3420	60	2060-10600	/μL
Lymphocytes	1653	29	690-4500	/μL
Monocytes	342	6	0-840	/μL
Eosinophils	285	5	0-1200	/μL
Basophils	0	0	0-150	/μL
Platelet Estimate	Adequate			
Platelet Count	290		170-400	$10^3/\mu L$

FIGURE 9-7 ANTECH patient results. (Courtesy ANTECH Diagnostics, Los Angeles, Calif.)

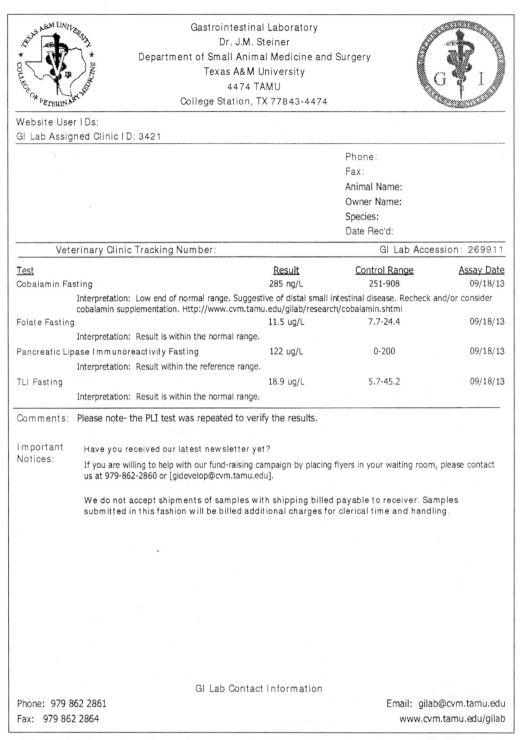

Gastrointestinal Laboratory
Dr. J.M. Steiner
Department of Small Animal Medicine and Surgery
Texas A&M University
4474 TAMU
College Station, TX 77843-4474

Website User I Ds:
GI Lab Assigned Clinic I D: 3421

Phone:
Fax:
Animal Name:
Owner Name:
Species:
Date Rec'd:

Veterinary Clinic Tracking Number: GI Lab Accession: 269911

Test	Result	Control Range	Assay Date
Cobalamin Fasting	285 ng/L	251-908	09/18/13

Interpretation: Low end of normal range. Suggestive of distal small intestinal disease. Recheck and/or consider cobalamin supplementation. Http://www.cvm.tamu.edu/gilab/research/cobalamin.shtml

| Folate Fasting | 11.5 ug/L | 7.7-24.4 | 09/18/13 |

Interpretation: Result is within the normal range.

| Pancreatic Lipase Immunoreactivity Fasting | 122 ug/L | 0-200 | 09/18/13 |

Interpretation: Result within the reference range.

| TLI Fasting | 18.9 ug/L | 5.7-45.2 | 09/18/13 |

Interpretation: Result is within the normal range.

Comments: Please note- the PLI test was repeated to verify the results.

Important
Notices:

Have you received our latest newsletter yet?

If you are willing to help with our fund-raising campaign by placing flyers in your waiting room, please contact us at 979-862-2860 or [gidevelop@cvm.tamu.edu].

We do not accept shipments of samples with shipping billed payable to receiver. Samples submitted in this fashion will be billed additional charges for clerical time and handling.

GI Lab Contact Information

Phone: 979 862 2861
Fax: 979 862 2864

Email: gilab@cvm.tamu.edu
www.cvm.tamu.edu/gilab

FIGURE 9-8 Texas A&M patient results. (Courtesy Jörg M. Steiner, Texas A&M University, College Station Tex.)

BOX 9-1	Outside Laboratories and Their Specialties

Michigan State University (endocrinology)
Diagnostic Center for Population and Animal Health
4125 Beaumont Road
Lansing, MI 48910
www.animalhealth.msu.edu

Kansas State Veterinary Diagnostic Lab (rabies antibody titer)
1200 Denison Avenue
Manhattan, KS 66506
www.vet.k-state.edu/depts/dmp/service/rabies/

Colorado State University Veterinary Diagnostic Laboratories (serology/PCR)
300 West Drake
Fort Collins, CO 80523
http://csu-cvmbs.colostate.edu/vdl/Pages/default.aspx

Cornell University (drug levels, serology, parasitology)
College of Veterinary Medicine
Animal Health Diagnostic Center
Upper Tower Road
Ithaca, NY 14853
https://ahdc.vet.cornell.edu/

Midwest Animal Blood Services (blood typing)
4983 Bird Avenue
Stockbridge, MI 49285

University of California-Davis (serology/polymerase chain reaction)
Endo Lab: Department of Population Health and Reproduction
Tupper Hall, Room 114
School of Veterinary Medicine
Davis, CA 95016

Texas A&M University
Gastrointestinal Laboratory
4474 TAMU
College Station, TX 77843
http://vetmed.tamu.edu/gilab

Vita-Tech Laboratories (parasitology)
2316 Delaware Avenue
Buffalo, NY 14216

⚖ VETERINARY PRACTICE and the LAW

Certain hazardous and perishable items may be mailed through USPS, UPS, FedEx, or other common courier, but are subject to specific packaging and labeling requirements. Diagnostic clinical samples that are liquid or contained in a liquid must be mailed in a sturdy, securely sealed watertight container cushioned in a secondary container. There must be enough cushion to absorb all of the material if the primary container were to break. If hazardous chemicals are used (formalin), the container must be marked with a biohazard symbol.

Numerous instances have occurred when such materials were so inadequately packaged during shipping that they contaminated the transport vehicles and their cargo and created potential public health hazards.

There is no health hazard or sanitation problem associated with laboratory specimens when they are properly packaged to prevent leakage or breaks in the containers. Proper packaging and labeling of such materials will facilitate accurate diagnostics, assure continued service by common carriers, and eliminate any adverse public health or perception problems. Team members are urged to review their methods of preparing diagnostic specimens and ensure that they are in compliance with all applicable guidelines and federal and state laws.

REVIEW QUESTIONS

1. How should lab samples be packaged for shipment?
2. What is serum?
3. What tests use serum?
4. What is plasma?
5. What is an anaerobic bacterium?
6. Why should cytology samples be submitted separately from samples preserved in formalin?
7. Why should samples be submitted on ice?
8. What information needs to be recorded on the laboratory sheet?
9. What factors should be considered when choosing an outside laboratory?
10. What does RTT stand for?
    a. Refrigerate test time
    b. Red-topped tube
    c. Result target time
    d. Report thromboplastin time
11. What does an *LTT* contain
    a. Anticoagulant EDTA
    b. Sodium citrate
    c. Nothing
    d. Serum separator gel

12. What testing lab can a GI panel be sent to?
    a. Colorado State University
    b. Vita-Tech Laboratories
    c. Midwest Animal Blood Services
    d. Texas A&M University
13. How much formalin should be added to tissue before submitting it for testing?
    a. 20 times the volume of the sample
    b. 15 times the volume of the sample
    c. 10 times the volume of the sample
    d. 100 times the volume of the sample
14. What blood tubes are required to submit testing for phenobarbital levels?
    a. LTT
    b. BTT
    c. SST
    d. RTT

Recommended Reading

Cowell R: *Veterinary clinical pathology secrets*, St Louis, MO, 2004, Mosby Elsevier.

Duncan JR, Prasse KW, Mahaffey EA: *Veterinary laboratory medicines*, ed 5, Ames, IA, 2011, Wiley-Blackwell.

Hendrix C, Sirois M: *Laboratory procedures for veterinary technicians*, ed 5, St Louis, MO, 2007, Mosby Elsevier.

Sirois M: *Principles and practices of veterinary technology*, ed 3, St Louis, MO, 2011, Elsevier/Mosby.

Marketing

OUTLINE

SWOT Analysis, *183*
   Strengths, *183*
   Weaknesses, *183*
   Opportunities, *184*
   Threats, *184*
Branding the Practice, *184*
Indirect Marketing, *184*
Direct Marketing, *185*
Internal Marketing, *186*
   Reminders, *186*
   Recalls, *187*
   Target Marketing, *188*
   Other Ideas for Internal Marketing, *189*
External Marketing, *190*
Web Sites, *195*
   Developing a Web Site, *195*
   Search Engine Optimization, *196*
   Promoting the Web Page, *197*
   Pet Portals, *198*
   Blogs, *199*
Mobile Media, *199*

Social Media, *199*
   Developing a Plan, *200*
   Managing Social Media, *200*
   Social Media Policy, *200*
Business Cards, *200*
Magnets, *201*
Practice Brochures, *201*
Client Education Materials, *202*
On-Hold Messaging, *203*
Donations, *205*
Gift Certificates, *205*
Implementing a Marketing and Training Program for Team Members, *205*
   Exam Rooms, *206*
   Human-Animal Bond, *206*
   Body Language, *206*
   Specific Recommendations, *206*
Managing Reviews, *207*
Seize the Opportunity!, *207*
   Creating and Implementing a Marketing Plan, *207*

LEARNING OBJECTIVES

When you have completed this chapter, you should be able to:

1. Define different methods of marketing.
2. Identify effective marketing techniques.
3. Explain and implement ethical marketing.
4. Compare marketing plans.
5. List effective methods for Web site development.
6. Describe a pet portal system.
7. Discuss the benefits of gift certificates.

KEY TERMS

Assertive Marketing
Blogging
Brand
Community Service
Company-Supported Web Site
Cost-Benefit Analysis
Direct Marketing
Domain Name
External Marketing
FTP
Host-the-Site Web Site
Indirect Marketing
Internal Marketing
Mobile Media
On-Hold Messaging
On-Site Hosting Web Site
Open House
Pet Portals
SWOT Analysis
Target Marketing
URL
Web Site

CRITICAL COMPETENCIES

1. **Adaptability** - being open to change and flexible work methods; the ability to adapt behavior to changing conditions or new information.
2. **Compliance** - being reliable, thorough, and conscientious in carrying out work assignments; has an appreciation for the importance of organizational rules and policies.
3. **Creativity** - the ability to think creatively about situations, to see things in new and different ways; use imagination and creativity to develop innovative solutions to problems.
4. **Critical and Strategic Thinking** - the ability to think critically about situations and to understand the relevance of information for different problems; use critical reasoning to generate and evaluate alternative courses of action or points of view relevant to an issue.
5. **Decision Making** - the ability to make good decisions, solve problems, and decide on important matters; the ability to gather and analyze relevant data and choose decisively between alternatives.

6. **Integrity** - honesty, trustworthiness, and adherence to high standards of ethical conduct.
7. **Leadership** - a willingness to lead and take charge; the ability to motivate others and mobilize group effort toward common goals.
8. **Persuasion** - the ability to change the attitudes and opinions of others and to persuade them to accept recommendations and change behavior.
9. **Planning and Prioritizing** - the ability to effectively manage time and workload to meet deadlines; the ability to organize work, set priorities, and establish plans for achieving goals.
10. **Resilience** - the ability to cope effectively with pressure and setbacks; the ability to handle crisis situations effectively and remain undeterred by obstacles or failure.
11. **Resourcefulness** - the ability to understand what it takes to complete the job; apply knowledge, skills, and expertise to perform tasks quickly and efficiently.
12. **Writing and Verbal Skills** - ability to comprehend written material easily and accurately; the ability to express thoughts clearly and succinctly in writing.

In the marketing and client relations domain, the veterinary practice manager plans and coordinates marketing, public relations, and client service programs. In terms of marketing, the manager develops internal and external marketing plans and monitors results of marketing efforts.

Knowledge Requirements

In the marketing and client relations domain, the veterinary practice manager plans and coordinates marketing, public relations, and client service programs. In terms of marketing, the manager develops internal and external marketing plans and monitors results of marketing efforts.

Marketing is an integral part of the success of a practice. Various forms of marketing occur on a daily basis without conscious thought. Client education, clean facilities, and a superb team all contribute to indirect forms of marketing. Direct marketing may include Web pages, social media, blogs, Yellow Page advertisements, newspaper advertisements, and newsletters. Internal marketing is directed toward current clients and includes reminders, postcards, and recalls. External marketing is geared toward potential clients and educates them about the services the practice offers. As one can see, the practice's Web page and social media apply to every facet of marketing—direct, indirect, internal, and external.

Marketing budgets average 2% to 3% of gross revenue, whether for internal, external, direct, or indirect services. This includes community service events, reminder cards, Web page design, phone book advertising, and social media development.

Team members may not be aware of the marketing skills they already possess; these skills can be enhanced on a daily basis, and although the marketing dollars spent only increase slightly, gross revenue can nearly double. Team members directly affect clients through relationship building, client education, superb customer service, and a spotless facility.

Practices must determine what qualities make them unique. Great medical and professional services no longer set one veterinary hospital apart from another. Every practice provides professional service and good medicine. Is the staff unique in a practice that employs several credentialed veterinary technicians or veterinary technician specialists (VTSs)? Do the practice hours differ from those of other veterinary hospitals in the area? What services are offered that are not offered anywhere else? Determining what makes the hospital unique will help make any marketing program a success.

PRACTICE POINT Practices must differentiate themselves from other hospitals in the area.

Each practice may want to consider an analysis of its strengths, weaknesses, opportunities, and threats (SWOT), which can help a practice determine what differentiates it from other veterinary practices within the area (review the SWOT analysis in the next section of this chapter).

Practices may also wish to consider gathering competitive intelligence information from other practices in the area to learn how to differentiate themselves from others. This

differentiation can set the practice apart from other hospitals and ultimately increase sales and profits by attracting new clients as well as retaining old clients.

Practices must strive to create a signature customer service. Poor client service is not an option. Clients understand and know what good customer service is; they expect it (and demand it). They may not know when veterinary medicine is substandard, but they certainly know when customer service is subpar!

Positive word-of-mouth referrals are the most successful form of free marketing. Team members must drive home the value of the service to each and every client, resulting in referrals of friends and family. Client confidence in the medical skills and professional services provided by a team is the primary driver of value, along with friendly staff, compassion, education, and cleanliness. These all lead to superior customer service and client satisfaction.

Product marketing includes both professional services and products that the practice sells. The team must understand and believe in the services and products provided; otherwise, the marketing effort could fail. An example would be acupuncture. Many veterinarians and team members are unaware of the benefits acupuncture may provide to patients. If one veterinarian in the practice promotes and provides acupuncture services but the remaining team members are unaware of the benefits, then the service may fail in the practice. Products are just the same. Team members should receive training on the products that the practice wishes to carry. These include diets, ear cleaning supplies, and shampoos. Manufacturer and distributor representatives love to provide education to practices. Ask the representative to provide a luncheon seminar to help educate the team regarding new products the practice carries.

The location of a hospital is no longer as important as it once was, because Google and GPS help clients locate practices. However, what our "place" looks like is just as important as it has ever been. Parking lots should be easy to pull into, without any barriers or obstructions to avoid. If the parking lot is always overflowing, additional lot space may be acquired, allowing additional parking spaces to be added. The parking area should be clean, free of weeds, dog feces, and trash. The signage should be modern, inviting, and contain the logo and name of the hospital.

Price can be a factor for some clients, and the practice can decide on which services it wishes to provide at competitive prices. Price shoppers generally shop for the best prices on routine surgeries, dental prophylaxis, examinations, preventative medications, and vaccinations. Diagnostic testing and hospital procedures are not shopped services, and relationships should have been developed by the time they are recommended. Clients will accept or decline services at this point, regardless of cost. Practices do not want to be the cheapest service in town, nor should they offer less service in order to compete. If a practice believes in high-quality medicine, then clients should be charged for it. Once clients perceive the value of the excellent service and medicine, they will be clients for life.

Promotion is the mechanism used to recommend products and services within and outside the veterinary practice. This can include direct and indirect marketing or internal and external marketing. All are discussed in the following sections. Many veterinary manufacturers or distributors will support clinic marketing techniques with additional incentives. Some companies may provide free product samples, whereas others will provide incentives to the staff to increase sales.

It should be remembered that the goal of the practice is to offer high-quality medicine (professional, medical, and client oriented) regardless of the specials that may be offered by companies. Marketing techniques and specials should be analyzed to ensure they are in line with the practice's mission, goals, and practice philosophies (see Chapter 3).

Practices should analyze their marketing strategy on a yearly basis. Are current methods working? Have service and sales increased with current marketing techniques? If not, where has the marketing failed? Internally? A decrease in the number of new clients? Practice managers should be able to track before-and-after results and make changes as needed. It is important to track the return on investment (ROI); if one marketing technique did not work, another should be tried.

SWOT Analysis

SWOT is short for strengths, weaknesses, opportunities, and threats. Ideally, any marketing plan must incorporate a SWOT analysis, and it should be part of any strategic business plan on a yearly basis. SWOT analyses are a great team-building event; many times, team members see strengths and opportunities that management overlooks. Take a look at each of the following in more depth.

> **PRACTICE POINT** Complete a SWOT analysis on the practice to help determine where a marketing plan can best be used.

Strengths

Consider the strengths the practice has. Who makes up the team? What do clients like about the practice? What services does the hospital offer that no other hospital offers? Why do clients refer friends and family to the practice? The strengths that are identified will often help overcome the weaknesses that will be found.

Weaknesses

Weaknesses can be hard to determine; it is easier to identify strengths and opportunities. Consider policies and procedures that could use improvement. What do clients complain most about? What do team members complain about? Why do clients leave the hospital? What do the client surveys indicate? When weaknesses are ignored, they become larger problems; when managed, they often become strengths.

Opportunities

Opportunities are fun, because it allows the team to think outside the box. What could be implemented to strengthen the client bond, retention, or compliance? Include thoughts of continuing education, current trends, social media, technology, and equipment. What resources are available in the community that could increase opportunities to the practice? Identifying and acting on opportunities can take the practice to the next level.

Threats

Threats can be both internally and externally related. Threats may be team member loss, client loss, or a new practice opening down the street. Threats can be detrimental to a business when they are not taken into consideration, and a plan implemented to minimize the threat.

Completing a SWOT analysis can help determine where marketing dollars are best spent. As an internal resource, managers may wish to complete a SWOT analysis on team members, identifying areas that need improvement, and capitalizing on strengths that could improve other team members' weaknesses. Internal building must occur before a marketing program can be implemented.

Branding the Practice

Brand can be defined as the name, design, symbol, or features that identify the distinct nature of the practices products or services. It is often one of the most valuable assets to the practice, and it takes time to develop. Proper branding results in increased client compliance, loyalty, and retention.

Brands can also be referred to as the personality that identifies a service. Thoughts, feelings, perceptions, experiences, and attitudes contribute to brand development. If a client knows that ABC Veterinary Hospital consistently delivers quality medicine and superior customer service, they are going to maintain their relationship with the hospital and continue referring friends and family.

A brand that is widely known in the marketplace acquires brand recognition. When brand recognition builds in communities, clients associate logos, colors, and themes with the practice. Therefore, to help develop and improve a brand, practices must be consistent in their delivery of materials (same colors in logo, Web page, and client education materials) and consistent in their delivery of medical and customer service. All clients must have the same standard of care offered, every time they are in the practice (see Chapter 11 for the development of standards of care). If client experience is negative, the brand recognition suffers.

Indirect Marketing

Indirect marketing centers on the clients the practice currently serves. Client education has been discussed in other chapters and is highlighted later in this chapter. Client education serves as the greatest indirect marketing tool that can be used.

> **PRACTICE POINT**   Indirect marketing is more important than direct marketing, and it must be mastered before moving into a direct marketing plan.

Client education materials must be sent home with every client at every visit. This includes puppy and kitten exams, boosters, yearly exams, and senior exams. All clients must be informed about heartworm disease, internal and external parasites (as well as their zoonotic potential), nutrition, and obesity management. If a patient has been diagnosed with a condition or disease, the client must receive printed materials to take home and review. Materials should include information about the disease as well as treatment options that are available. Clients become overloaded with information when they are visiting a practice and will retain only 20% of the information provided. Sending home information reiterates the information and allows improved communication with other household members (spouse, significant other, children), and will increase compliance.

All team members should receive training on services, procedures, and protocols on a continuing basis. When team members can explain procedures with confidence and without hesitation, clients will accept the services that have been recommended.

Facilities must be kept clean and odor free. Clients perceive value and service, along with cleanliness, as top priorities when seeking service for their pets. If a practice has heavy animal or cleaning agent odors, they may never return. Trash containers should be emptied several times a day because they are a significant contributor to odors circulating in the practice. Smaller trash cans should be used, mandating frequent emptying. Pet eliminations must be cleaned immediately, regardless of whether they occur in the reception, treatment, or kennel area. Odors circulate quickly and, unfortunately, efficiently! Walls, baseboards, and door frames must be washed weekly and pictures and fans should be dusted daily. Anatomic models must be free of dust and lint and counters clear of clutter.

Professional, clean, and friendly team members encourage clients to feel comfortable and ask questions. When clients are comfortable, they will not only return to the practice in the future, they will also recommend the practice to their friends, family, and co-workers. Clients must be greeted upon entry and assisted when leaving. Team members wearing name badges inform the client of who they are as well as their positions within the practice. This is comforting to clients who wish to know who they are working with. Team members wearing clean, wrinkle-free uniforms appear professional and approachable, which encourages client interaction.

Team members can also establish courteous and reliable relationships with clients to help promote indirect marketing. Many businesses do not address clients by name. Addressing clients and pets by name is a very effective customer service/marketing tool. When they are addressed directly by name, they feel special. "Good morning, Ms. Thurman. How are

you and Fluffy doing today?" is an excellent greeting for both the client and pet. When the pet's name and history are addressed, the client's confidence in the practice increases, leading to better overall satisfaction with the practice.

All these factors directly contribute to an increase in client communication. Client communication is the key to increasing client compliance and client retention. As stated previously, communication with clients by client education is imperative. Clients must understand procedures and feel comfortable with the recommendations being made. Team members who maintain eye contact and have an open body posture when talking with owners relay a message of confidence. If eye contact is not made and team members have folded arms, the client may not perceive the value of the service being recommended or have confidence in the team. If there is a lack of confidence, client retention and compliance will decrease.

Creating a staff board that lists all team members and placing it in the reception area allows clients to know who is on the team. A staff board may list the employees' first names along with their credentials. Pictures may also be included (Figure 10-1). Doctors are to be listed with DVM (or VMD, depending on the graduating school) and technicians with RVT, CVT, or LVT, along with any other degrees they have received. Often, team members will have completed a bachelor's or associate's program in college. The practice managers may be a CVPM, and assistants may also be certified. All team members, including kennel personnel, should be listed to inform clients who is caring for their pets. Last names should not be listed for security precautions.

Client compliance is discussed in Chapter 11; however, the key point to remember is that client compliance is the driving force behind client retention, client

recommendations, and client satisfaction. Educating the client is imperative, as previously stated. Team members must make recommendations to every client, regardless of their perception of the client's financial situation. Establishing a written protocol of policies and procedures, along with following up on cases, will help increase client compliance. Recommendations and compliance should be tracked, allowing revisions to be made to help increase client compliance. Indirect marketing to current clients takes many shapes and values; every facet must be explored to maximize each practice's potential (Figure 10-2).

Direct Marketing

For many years, the human medical professions have efficiently leveraged direct marketing tools, whereas the veterinary medical community has been slow to adopt these methods. However, as competition for a successful practice has risen, so has the use of direct marketing techniques. In previous years, many communities have only had one or two veterinary practices serving them, and direct marketing was not needed. In today's world, the number of practices has risen, and working to ensure survival of the business is reality. Direct marketing is now needed more than ever to keep a practice viable.

WHAT WOULD YOU DO/NOT DO?

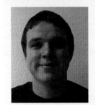

The local association of veterinarians has been approached by the newspaper to provide a weekly veterinary topic that will be printed every Monday in the business section of the newspaper. One specific veterinarian has advised he would be responsible for writing the topics each week. Other veterinarians are concerned that he may use this as an opportunity to promote his veterinary practice instead of the community as a whole.

What Should the Veterinary Association Do?

If more than one veterinarian or practice has concerns with one individual being responsible for the articles, then the concerns must be addressed openly. It is likely that if one practice has concerns, others do as well; but to prevent a confrontation, they will not voice their opinions. Concerned practices may offer a solution: one individual may be responsible to writing the article, whereas others can rotate the responsibility of proofreading the article and add any information that may be needed. This allows several individuals to include their thoughts while educating the community of veterinary medicine topics.

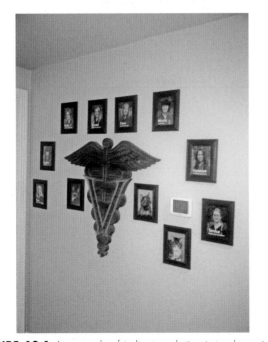

FIGURE 10-1 An example of indirect marketing is to place pictures of team members on the lobby wall for clients to view. (Courtesy of Ben Wilson and Star of Texas Veterinary Clinic.)

Direct marketing is the most popular form of marketing and has been around for years. The Yellow Pages are a classic example of direct marketing; however Web pages and social media have replaced Yellow Page advertising. The practice must make the general public aware of the services that are available as well as the doctors who are on staff. Newspaper

advertising also notifies the public of any specials or notices the veterinary hospital wishes to publish. It is important to keep in mind that the benefit the practice may receive from the advertising must be weighed against the cost of the ad or campaign. It is important to remember that direct marketing is targeted to potential clients the practice wishes to serve and existing clients for whom the practice wishes to expand services.

> **PRACTICE POINT**   Phone book advertising used to be the most popular form of direct advertising, however, it has been replaced with Web pages and social media.

Internal Marketing

Internal marketing has been discussed in previous chapters and includes client education, reminders, recalls, and appointments (among many others). The goal of internal marketing is to retain current clients. Every facet of the client experience must be examined and maximized when building an internal marketing program. The key to successful internal marketing is listening to the client. By listening, team members can determine their wants and needs. Practices can use tools to help implement internal marketing techniques; however, team members must learn to listen and satisfy the needs of each client (Box 10-1).

Reminders

Reminders should appear professional and be free of errors. Reminder cards must have the basic information included on each card: pet's name, the date the reminder is due, and what the pet is due for. The clinic information must include the name, address, phone number, URL of the Web site, and logo of the veterinary clinic. It is also imperative to state that clients should call to make an appointment. Some clients assume that because they received the reminder, they can come any time. They are then upset at the wait time when they arrive as walk-ins. Reminders are discussed in further detail in Chapter 11 (Figure 10-3).

Reminders should be sent no more than 4 weeks in advance of the due date because clients may forget the appointment they have made or simply disregard the reminder because it was sent far in advance. Reminder systems are programmed to delete the reminder if the client has arrived for an appointment before the due date. However, if reminders have been printed too early, the reminder will be sent regardless and the

BOX 10-1	**Examples of Internal Marketing**

- Recalls
- Reminders
- Client education
- Clean, updated, and pleasant-smelling office
- Staff identification
- Staff enthusiasm
- E-newsletter, Web page and social media
- Timely replies to client requests
- Telephone etiquette
- Client acknowledgment
- Professional appearance

Recommendation Compliance Report   **ABC Veterinary Clinic**

Period: 01/01/13-01/01/0/14

Code	Description	# of Recommendations	# of Compliances	%
R0001	Rabies	910	607	66.7
R0002	DHPP	791	298	37.67
R0003	Bordetella	126	61	48.41
R0004	Heartworm Prev	1088	544	50.00
R0005	Dental Prophylaxis	754	398	52.79
R0005	Pre Anesth BW	950	367	38.63
R0006	General Health BW	1589	1061	67.77
R0007	Senior Screening	790	421	53.29
R0008	Therapeutic Food	984	398	40.45

FIGURE 10-2 Sample report tracking client compliance.

client is left feeling confused because he or she just visited the clinic. They may call the reception team and question the accuracy of the staff, because "they were just there."

 Veterinary practice managers develop and manage client reminder systems.

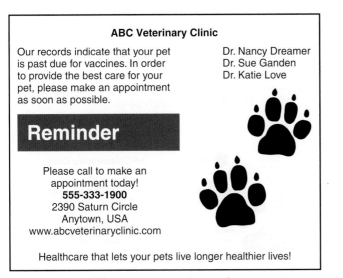

ABC Veterinary Clinic

Our records indicate that your pet is past due for vaccines. In order to provide the best care for your pet, please make an appointment as soon as possible.

Dr. Nancy Dreamer
Dr. Sue Ganden
Dr. Katie Love

Reminder

Please call to make an appointment today!
555-333-1900
2390 Saturn Circle
Anytown, USA
www.abcveterinaryclinic.com

Healthcare that lets your pets live longer healthier lives!

FIGURE 10-3 Sample reminder.

Some reminder systems are also set up to generate second and third reminders for noncompliant clients who have not returned (Figure 10-4). Again, if reminders are printed too early, another reminder will be printed indicating the noncompliance. Clients who do not respond to reminders should be called; this will allow the staff to check on the pet, answer any concerns the owner may have, and schedule an appointment. Often, clients are extremely busy and have not taken the time to schedule an appointment and will appreciate that the practice has called. By making these calls, the practice has added a personalized touch to customer service. Customer service is centered on relationship building, connecting, and engaging with the client.

Email reminders are more popular than ever. Be sure the phone number is embedded in the email reminder, simply allowing the clients to click on the phone number and place a call to make an appointment. The simpler a process is for clients, the higher the compliance rate will be.

Be sure to ask clients if they prefer email or postal card reminders. Again, identifying the needs and wants of individual clients establishes a strong relationship.

Recalls

Recalls should be completed for every patient that has visited the practice in the previous few days, regardless of whether it was for a yearly exam, vaccines, or an ear infection. The team member in charge of recalls can check on a patient after

Print Preview 1/1

Reminder Compliance Report   **IntraVet Animal Hospital**

For period: 8/1/2013 - 9/1/2013

Code	Description	Reminders	Compliance	Percentage
AARCH	AORTIC ARCH PERSISTANT RIGHT	1	0	0
AP005	Comfortis 60-120lbs	1	0	0
TOTALS:		2		0

Find/Next

FIGURE 10-4 Sample reminder compliance report. (Courtesy IntraVet, Dublin, Ohio.)

vaccinations to make sure there was no reaction to the vaccines. If the pet received medications, team members can follow up to ensure the pet is improving and is not having any problems with medications that were dispensed. Many times, antibiotics cause the pet to experience vomiting or diarrhea, and the client then stops giving the medication (however, they never call the practice).

> **PRACTICE POINT**   Recalls on postoperative patients should occur the evening of their surgery, **AND** 3 days later (*not just 3 days later*).

If a pet had surgery, team members should always follow up and review the release instructions, ensuring the client fully understands them (e.g., no exercise for 7 days postoperatively). Postoperative recalls should occur the night the pet has been released from the hospital *and* 3 days later. Clients are most concerned about their pet the night they bring him or her home from the hospital; by day 3, all concerns should be resolved.

Telephone calls allow owners to ask questions that they may not have thought to ask while at the hospital or address new concerns that have arisen. Team members can also verify that the client was satisfied with the visit and schedule a follow-up exam if needed. See Chapter 11 for more information on recalls.

Target Marketing

Target marketing is directed toward current clients with a special breed, species, or age of animal and/or one with a particular disease or condition (obesity, diabetes, and arthritis). Practices can determine the needs, wants, and concerns of a specific group of clients and develop a target strategy based on those results.

If the practice has decided to increase dental awareness for 1 month out of the year, clients with pets older than 5 years may be targeted to receive dental health information. Team members should be able to select a particular species, breed, or age in the veterinary software and create a list with client names, addresses, and pet names. The list can then be exported into a spreadsheet, allowing mailing labels to be generated and affixed to postcards. The dental postcard should educate clients about dental disease and request them to make an appointment for an immediate dental prophylaxis (Figure 10-5).

Another way to benefit from target marketing is to stay attuned to the news media. Team members can listen to breaking news stories regarding veterinary-related issues. For example, tick-borne diseases may be on the increase, with the news media reporting the story. A postcard can be generated listing the risk factors and symptoms of tick-borne diseases and promoting tick-prevention products.

Other ideas of target marketing may include allergy patients and a postcard bringing their attention to the newest dermatologic antihistamine or steroidal drugs available. Practice managers may also consider heartworm disease and a special on a heartworm preventive (Figure 10-6).

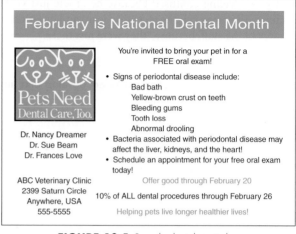

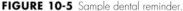

FIGURE 10-5 Sample dental reminder.

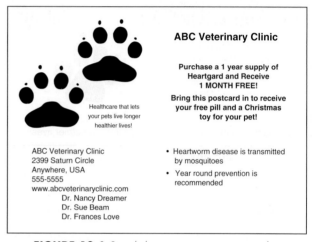

FIGURE 10-6 Sample heartworm preventive reminder.

If postcard or other advertising brochures have been developed, all team members should be made aware of the advertisement. Examples should be given to and reviewed with team members before the mailing. If the information is sent out before a review, a client will inevitably receive it and bring it to the attention of the staff. It is embarrassing and degrading to team members to find out from clients about a special the practice is promoting.

The cost of mailing letters or postcards must be evaluated with a cost-benefit ratio. Producing these items can be expensive, along with the cost of mailing them. It should be determined whether the mailing will produce a greater profit than the cost itself. Email is a much more efficient manner to send materials, resulting in a considerable decrease in costs. Email messages can be bright, colorful, and grab the attention of clients, just as any printed piece of material would. Some clients may prefer to receive email instead of snail mail. Anti-spam laws and legal requirements should be reviewed before sending emails to ensure the practice is within legal boundaries.

Many veterinary manufacturers may sponsor such target programs by providing a postcard and stamp. Team members simply generate an address label, which dramatically

reduces the costs associated with such programs and significantly increases the bottom line. Practices must analyze the information contained in these postcards, ensuring the information contained is in line with the practice's high quality of medicine and marketing techniques. A postcard or newsletter may contain information or phrases that are not supported by the practice, which can be detrimental.

Other Ideas for Internal Marketing

Many practices have been creative in using internal marketing techniques to continue to please their clients. Welcome cards can be sent to new clients, along with a DVD giving the new client a tour of the practice. The DVD can include team members in action, surgery, and client interaction. The DVD does not have to be long; the goal is simply to introduce the client to the practice. DVDs can easily be made with technology available today, and reproduction of the DVD is inexpensive. This idea for internal marketing is very effective at creating a long-lasting relationship and establishing the kind of doctor-practice-client bond for which all practices should strive.

"Thank you for the referral" letters can be sent to current clients who have referred a new client to the practice. Practices may wish to simply send a card, or perhaps include a gift certificate to be used upon the client's next visit at the practice. Any acknowledgement will be greatly appreciated by the client.

Clients always appreciate condolence cards when they have lost a pet. The entire team can sign the card and add a little note expressing their thoughts. Special clients and clients in the top 20% of the accounts should receive flowers, a plant or perhaps a donation to a charity in the pet's name. These clients have obviously spent money helping their pets, and the practice should take the extra step to express their condolence.

Painted paw prints or clay paw imprints are inexpensive and easy to accomplish and are appreciated by owners. Hair from the paw can be clipped and paint applied to the paw. A special piece of paper with the Rainbow Bridge poem printed on it can be applied to the paw, allowing the outline of the paw to be transmitted to the paper. Once dried, it can be mailed to the owner. Clay paw imprints are just as easy to accomplish, but may cost more than paw prints. See Chapter 12 for more ideas on how to remember patients.

A pet that has suffered and survived a traumatic experience or injury might receive a purple heart for its courage (Figure 10-7). Purple hearts make clients feel great and are an excellent conversation piece. Once again, the practice name is brought up in conversation as to why and how the pet received the purple heart. Pet bandannas are relatively cheap to produce, and clients usually put them on pets with excitement (Figure 10-8). Purple hearts or bandannas must have the practice information on it, along with a catchy phrase like, "I survived!" A phrase like this initiates conversations, as friends will ask, "What did Fifi survive?"

A weight management hall of fame can be instituted with before and after photos. A short story can be posted on the

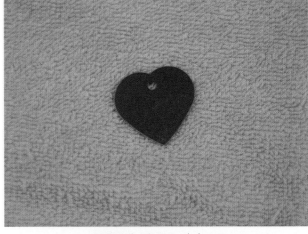

FIGURE 10-7 Purple heart.

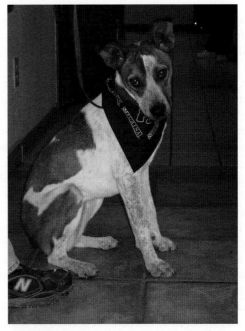

FIGURE 10-8 Pet wearing a practice bandana.

successful endeavor with both the client and the pet posing for the after photo. Halls of fame should be placed in a highly visible area that all clients can see. A weight management hall of fame can engage conversation in the reception area and can motivate other clients to enter their pets in a weight-loss program.

> **PRACTICE POINT** Take before and after pictures of weight loss patients to add to a weight loss hall of fame.

Pediatric toothbrushes can be ordered with the practice name and logo printed on the handle (Figure 10-9). Toothbrushes can be placed in puppy and kitten kits, in dental kits, or simply given to owners when the team is talking about dental disease. Leashes can also be printed with the practice

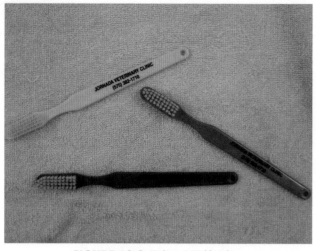

FIGURE 10-9 Pediatric toothbrushes.

name and logo. Luggage tags can be designed with the practice information and placed on animal carriers when cats or small dogs have been dropped off. The client's name can be placed on the back of the tag and tied to the handle of the carrier. The carrier will always have identification on it when the owner returns, and the name of the practice is clearly visible for friends and family to see.

Marketing messages can be printed at the base of receipts to inform clients about important topics. Web site tools, or information regarding puppy classes can be summarized, helping promote the practice's internal marketing tools. The invoice in Figure 10-10 is an opportunity to promote puppy classes that the practice provides.

Social media is another form of internal marketing, and targets many generations of clients. Educating clients via social media foundations is low cost, but requires planning. Review the section, "Social Media," later in the chapter for more details.

"Exam room report cards" can be sent home with clients. Preprinted report cards can easily be marked for normal and abnormal results. Abnormal findings can be summarized. Any procedures or follow-up exams that may be necessary can be prioritized for the client, indicating the most important procedure first. Report cards give clients something to take home. They can review the findings with other family members to better ensure that correct information is communicated. Clients tend to become overwhelmed with information in exam rooms; this will help them remember correct information and increase client compliance (Figure 10-11).

Mailing owners copies of lab work results is also a form of internal marketing. A sheet can be included that summarizes abnormal results and the need to follow up. Electrocardiograms, urinalysis, ultrasounds, and blood work can all be sent to clients. This can also help increase client compliance because the owner may be able to better understand the abnormal results. A preprinted sheet should also be sent, informing the owner which organ each test evaluates. A brief summary may be included regarding what may be causing the abnormality (Figure 10-12).

Clients love to receive copies of radiographs. If a practice has digital radiography, images can be copied onto a DVD for the clients or printed with a high-quality laser printer. Practices that have pet portals may allow clients to review radiographs within their portal, or practices may have their Web page set up to allow clients access to radiographs with a secure password.

Special activities and open houses that celebrate certain events can market the practice to both current and prospective clients. Open houses can be used to promote National Pet Week, National Veterinary Technician Week, the practice anniversary, the welcoming of a new doctor, or the renovation of the practice. Open houses can be simple or elaborate, depending on the budget set aside for the promotion. The American Veterinary Medical Association (AVMA), National Association of Veterinary Technicians in America (NAVTA), and veterinary manufacturers can be contacted for more information, sponsorship, and signage to help promote the celebration. Advertising helps make such events more successful (Figure 10-13).

> **PRACTICE POINT**   Consider hosting an open house during National Veterinary Technician Week, and recognize special team members and patients that have inspired them.

Special events can be hosted during open houses, such as pet walks, pet shows, and talks regarding pet health. Competitions for prizes can be developed with categories such as cutest pet, the pet with the longest nose, or best tricks. Simple, short talks can also be given regarding nutrition, training techniques, and animal husbandry.

Internal marketing techniques can be used in many ways and should be explored to help bring the practice to the next level.

External Marketing

As with direct marketing, the goal of external marketing is to advertise the practice's services to potential clients. Examples include the practice Web site, yellow pages, and newspaper advertising. A large, professional, colorful, and modern sign that is illuminated at night is also a form of external marketing, along with the participation in community service and activities (Box 10-2).

 Veterinary practice managers develop and manage advertising.

The key to external marketing is to determine prospective clients and patients and use the best method to attract them. External marketing does not generally elicit immediate results. Consistent and repetitive messaging must be directed toward potential clients to obtain results; therefore, if the practice wishes to increase business, external and direct marketing approaches are recommended to achieve this goal.

ABC Veterinary Clinic
2399 Saturn Circle
Anytown, USA 89000
555-555-5555

Maria Rogers
6454 Downtown Circle
Anytown, USA 89001   Account # 21312

"Scruffy" Rogers
Age: 9 years
Weight: 45#
Reminders: DHPP due 5/10/15
            Rabies due 5/10/16
            Heartworm Test due 5/10/14

Invoice Number: 10090
Date: 04/28/13
Dr. Nancy Dreamer

Date	Service	Unit	Extended Cost
04/28/13	Exam with Vaccinations	1	$ 0.00
04/28/13	Distemper, Adenovirus,	1	$45.99
04/28/13	Parainfluenza, Parvo	1	
04/28/13	Strongid	1	$ 5.99
04/28/13	HG Puppy Kit	1	$ 0.00
04/28/13	Nail Trim	1	$ 0.00
04/28/13	Biohazard Fee	1	$ 3.00

Subtotal	$54.98
Tax 6.25%	$ 3.44
Invoice Total	$58.42

Puppy Obedience Training Classes Begin May 15, 2013!
Call to reserve your space now!

FIGURE 10-10 Sample invoice with a marketing statement at the bottom.

Client feedback may be used to determine the effectiveness of marketing techniques. "How did you hear about us?" may be listed on a client/patient information sheet or included in a survey offered to clients after their first visit. This and other mechanisms can ultimately be used in a cost-benefit analysis to help determine which marketing techniques may or may not be used in the future.

Client referrals should be the largest method of attracting new clients in an established practice (tracking the previously mentioned information will help determine this). If client referrals are not the largest source, internal marketing techniques need to be revisited, determining opportunities that can be enhanced, used, or created, all of which would drive client referrals. Tracking other sources of new clients is just as important; allowing the manager to analyze where dollars are best spent promoting the hospital.

Marketing must be kept ethical, fair, and professional. The AVMA code of ethics states that advertising by veterinarians is ethical when there are no false, deceptive, or misleading statements or claims. A false, deceptive, or misleading

_____'s Report Card

Owner's Name _____ Date _____

Vaccination Program

- ❏ Up to Date
- ❏ Vac. due: PARVO_____; DHLP-C_____; Bordetella_____; LYME_____;FCVR/C_____; Feleuk_____; FIP_____; Rabies_____
- ❏ Vac. given: PARVO_____; DHLP-C_____; Bordetella_____; LYME_____;FCVR/C_____; Feleuk_____; FIP_____; Rabies_____

1. Coat & Skin
- ❏ Appear Normal
- ❏ Oily
- ❏ Itchy
- ❏ Dull
- ❏ Shedding
- ❏ Parasites
- ❏ Scaly
- ❏ Matted
- ❏ Other _____
- ❏ Dry
- ❏ Tumors
_____

2. Eyes
- ❏ Appear Normal
- ❏ Infection
- ❏ Discharge
- ❏ Cataract: L___ R _____
- ❏ Inflamed
- ❏ Other _____
- ❏ Eyelid Deformities _____

3. Ears
- ❏ Appear Normal
- ❏ Tumor: L___ R___
- ❏ Inflamed
- ❏ Excessive Hair
- ❏ Itchy
- ❏ Other _____
- ❏ Mites
_____

4. Nose & Throat
- ❏ Appear Normal
- ❏ Inflamed Tonsils
- ❏ Nasal Discharge
- ❏ Enlarged Lymph Glands
- ❏ Inflamed Throat
- ❏ Other _____

5. Mouth, Teeth, Gums
- ❏ Appear Normal
- ❏ Inflamed Lips
- ❏ Broken Teeth
- ❏ Loose Teeth
- ❏ Tartar Buildup
- ❏ Pyorreah
- ❏ Tumors
- ❏ Other
- ❏ Ulcers

6. Legs & Paws
- ❏ Appear Normal
- ❏ Joint Problems
- ❏ Lameness
- ❏ Nail Problems
- ❏ Damaged Ligaments
- ❏ Other _____

7. Heart
- ❏ Appears Normal
- ❏ Slow
- ❏ Other _____
- ❏ Murmur
- ❏ Fast
_____

8. Abdomen
- ❏ Appears Normal
- ❏ Abnormal Mass
- ❏ Enlarged Organs
- ❏ Tense/Painful
- ❏ Fluid
- ❏ Other _____

9. Lungs
- ❏ Appear Normal
- ❏ Breathing Difficulty
- ❏ Abnormal Sound
- ❏ Rapid Respiration
- ❏ Coughing
- ❏ Other _____
- ❏ Congestion _____

10. Gastrointestinal System
- ❏ Appears Normal
- ❏ Abnormal Feces
- ❏ Excessive Gas
- ❏ Parasites
- ❏ Vomiting Problem
- ❏ Other _____
- ❏ Anorexia
_____

11. Urogenital System
- ❏ Appears Normal
- ❏ Enlarged Prostate
- ❏ Abnormal Urination
- ❏ Mammary Tumors
- ❏ Genital Discharge
- ❏ Anal Sacs _____
- ❏ Abnormal Testicles

12. Weight _____ lbs
- ❏ Normal Range
- ❏ Thin
- ❏ Heavy
- ❏ Other _____

13. Diet
- ❏ Excellent
- ❏ Vitamins Needed
- ❏ Good
- ❏ Improvement necessary

Dogs
Last Heartworm Test
Date _____
Htwm Prevention
_____
Intestinal Parasites Tested
Date _____
Flea Control
Pet _____
Yard _____
House _____

Cats
Feline Leukemia Test
Date _____ Pos Neg
Feline Aids Test
Date _____ Pos Neg
Intestine Parasites
Checked _____
Outdoors ____ Hrs/day
Flea Control
Cat _____
Home _____
_____
Drug Allergies??
_____
_____
_____

Professional Services
_____
_____
_____
_____
_____
_____
_____
_____
_____
_____
_____

Special Instructions/Recommendations
_____
_____
_____
_____
_____
_____
_____
_____
_____

Examination Needed_____ Days/Months
Next Appointment _____ @____AM/PM

FIGURE 10-11 Sample exam room report card.

Blood Work Summary

Today your pet had blood work completed. Below is a list of the tests that were completed, along with the organ or body part that is being evaluated with that test. You will also find a brief description of what may be causing the abnormality associated with that value. This is not a complete list and is just a summary; please ask our team members if you have any questions.

Pre-Anesthetic Blood Work: An abbreviated profile that is recommended prior to anesthesia.

Test	Organ	Common possible causes of abnormal values
BUN	Kidney	Increased = kidney disease
CREA	Kidney	Increased = kidney disease
ALT	Liver	Increased = liver disease
SGPT	Liver	Increased = liver disease
GLU	Pancreas	Increased = diabetes, stress
Total protein	Various	Decreased = protein loss; increased = dehydration; various causes
WBC	White blood cells	Increased = infection
RBC	Red blood cells	Decreased: various
HCT	RBC volume	Decreased: Iimmune mediated/tick-borne disease
Platelets	Clotting function	Decreased: clotting abnormality

Urinalysis:

Specific gravity	Kidney	Decreased: kidney disease, dehydration
WBC	Bladder	Infection
RBC	Bladder	Inflammation
Glucose	Pancreas	Diabetes
Ketones	Pancreas	Diabetes
Protein	Bladder/kidney	Protein loss
pH	Bladder	Increased or Decreased: urinary stones
Crystals	Bladder	Urinary stones
Casts	Bladder/kidney	
Bacteria	Bladder	Infection
ECG	Heart	Heart disease

FIGURE 10-12 Summary of lab work results and explanation of tests.

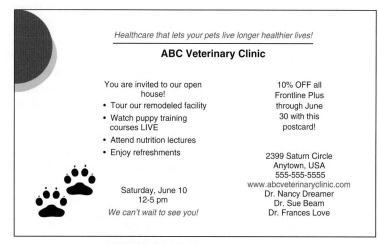

FIGURE 10-13 Open house postcard.

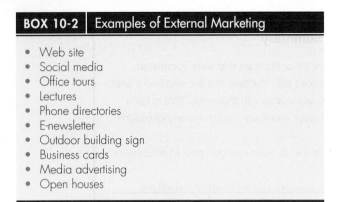

BOX 10-2 | Examples of External Marketing

- Web site
- Social media
- Office tours
- Lectures
- Phone directories
- E-newsletter
- Outdoor building sign
- Business cards
- Media advertising
- Open houses

statement or claim is one that communicates false information or is intended, through a material omission, to leave a false impression. Testimonials or endorsements are advertising, and they should comply with the guidelines for advertising. In addition, testimonials and endorsements of professional products or services by veterinarians are considered unethical unless they comply with the following:

1. The endorser must be a bona fide user of the product or service.
2. There must be adequate substantiation that the results obtained by the endorser are representative of what veterinarians may expect in actual conditions of use.
3. Any financial, business, or other relationship between the endorser and the seller of a product or service must be fully disclosed.
4. When reprints of scientific articles are used with advertising, the reprints must remain unchanged and be presented in their entirety.

The principles that apply to advertising, testimonials, and endorsements also apply to veterinarians and their communication with clients.

Choosing if and how to advertise in the Yellow Pages takes extra thought and consideration. Many factors should be addressed before making a decision regarding this advertisement. What is the return on investment (ROI)? Is the practice really gaining enough clients from the Yellow Pages to continue advertising?

The cost of such ads has become greater than the ROI with the increased use of search engines (Google, Yahoo, etc.) and smartphones. In fact, an overwhelming number of clients no longer use the Yellow Pages, instead using their phones to find veterinary practices (see later section on Web pages).

PRACTICE POINT   Review the return on investment of a Yellow Page ad before signing a 1-year contract.

The overall cost of advertising is relative to the size of the ad chosen. Yellow Pages advertising provides long-term advertising for practices and serves the extended community. Advertisements can range from a single line with the name and phone number of the practice to a large, color, full-page display ad. Practices that are in a small area and have

relatively little competition do not need large ads. Simply stating the facts is all that is needed: hours of operation, doctors on staff, species served, address, phone number, logo, and Web site. If there are several veterinary clinics in the area, then a larger ad may be needed, adding the services that are provided. A large ad can be overwhelming and may cause clients to overlook it. Caution should be used when developing the ad, and all team member opinions should be considered before submitting the ad for publication. In some areas of the United States, several companies produce directories that target the same audience. Practices may have to advertise in each book; therefore a budget should be established for each publication to prevent overspending on advertising. With the increased use of Web pages and social media, a single line entry in each book is sufficient.

Newspaper ads can come in the form of client education. Many newspapers have sections available in which a practice can purchase space and submit an article educating the general public about a particular disease. The ad may state to visit ABC Veterinary Hospital for more information. Other forms of advertising may include a boxed ad introducing a new veterinarian, service, or product. Newspaper ads can have several disadvantages, including the location of the ad in the newspaper. Ads are generally spread throughout the newspaper at the discretion of the graphic development team; this can lead to readers missing the ad due to obscure placement. Some ads can appear dated and reproduce poorly. Unfortunately, the poor quality can reflect on the value of the practice. If an ad is chosen to be run, all team members should be familiar with it.

Community service events create a win-win situation for all those involved. The practice team members may have one or two organizations that they participate in, and in which they can involve the practice as well. The practice owners may have an organization that they wish to donate to within the community. Either way, it is free advertising for the practice and lets the community know that the veterinary team supports community events.

Some ideas of community service may include a "lump and bump" screening at the local farmers' market on Saturday mornings. A veterinarian and technician can educate potential clients about the seriousness of lumps on pets. Many people bring pets to farmers' markets; this is an excellent place to hand out literature and educate. Team members can also participate in dental screenings for pets at local events; many people do not know the significance of dental disease in their pets. Attending career days at local schools is also considered external marketing, in the form of community service. Team members can create "kid packs" that include a surgical cap and mask as well as a business card and literature on heartworm disease or any other potential risks that are high in the area. They can be placed in a bag that has the practice information printed on it.

Veterinary practice managers oversee community outreach.

Speaking at career days can have a lasting impact on children. Showing interesting radiographs and allowing children to auscultate a dog's heart can stimulate interest and help foster their education. Community service at this level is highly recommended and self-gratifying.

Practices may also wish to be more involved in community service events around the holidays, participating in food drives or clothing campaigns for kids, or collecting Christmas presents for a particular family. Instead of buying gifts for each team member, the team can buy a present for a child in a homeless family that the practice adopts through a local homeless shelter. The team can take the presents to the family or shelter; seeing the surprise on a family's faces at this time of year is very rewarding! Shelters generally acknowledge contributors in a local newspaper ad after the holidays.

PRACTICE POINT Participating in community service events shows the community how much you care, and gives back to a community that has helped build the practice.

External marketing can be accomplished in several ways and often at a nominal price. The goal is to increase business by attracting potential clients to the practice. This can be accomplished and be rewarding at the same time.

Web Sites

Technology has accelerated, and many clients use the Internet to search for information. Web sites have become the new phone book ad; clients and potential clients visit Web pages more often than the Yellow Pages. Clients want information on the practice, including professional services that are offered, doctors, hours of operation, and a map to locate the office. Clients also want to be able to refill prescriptions, make appointments, and order products at any time of the day or night. They want reliable information on diseases, vaccination protocols, and procedures recommended by the practice. Web sites allow direct, indirect, internal, and external marketing at all levels.

Veterinary practice managers undertake Web site management.

Web sites can be fun, educational, and a challenge, all in one. They should be visually engaging, attractive, easy to navigate, and interactive. Some practices may elect to hire a design company to develop and maintain a site; others may choose to develop and maintain a Web site themselves. Whichever the practice chooses, it must appear professional, be reliable, and be updated frequently. It should not look like any other veterinary Web site in the vicinity.

PRACTICE POINT Web sites are the new phone book ad! They make the first impression to potential clients and fulfill expectations of existing clients.

| BOX 10-3 | Important Topics for Web Pages |

- Hours of operation
- Doctors
- Staff members
- Achievements/awards
- Procedures
- Professional services offered
- Hot topics: diseases that are prevalent in the area
- Prescription refills
- Appointment requests
- Online pharmacy
- Community service
- Blogs
- Pet of the month
- Client surveys
- Client testimonials
- Virtual tour
- Frequent forms

Developing a Web Site

There are three major options for Web site creation: create and host your own site, use on-site hosting tools, and use company-supported hosting. Hosting the site generally means that it is developed and maintained by the practice, which can be done with the practice server or by renting space on another server. Web site space is very competitive, with many companies offering space, so it is generally cheap to rent space. The pages are created using Web design software and uploaded to the server through file transfer protocol (FTP). Practices have full control over content and can update at will. Many different Web page software applications are available. When looking for software, a top choice is one that is user-friendly, has a tutorial, and has a variety of designs available to build pages. Developing a Web site is time-consuming and takes practice; however, the return on investment is well worth it.

On-site hosting is an option for practices that do not wish to fully design their own Web site. Practices can manipulate predesigned Web formats directly on a preexisting site or upload content that has been previously developed. The advantage is already having predesigned layout; the disadvantage is that other practices will likely have the same or similarly designed Web sites.

A design company typically creates company-supported Web sites, and the practices may have little or no access to the content provided. The company must do updates and changes. Smaller companies that employ webmasters may be able to design practice Web sites and make changes as requested by the practice relatively easily. It is up the practice to submit the information to the webmaster and to ensure that all information that has been included is correct. Any time practice protocols or recommendations change, veterinarians have been added to the staff, or product lines are added the webmaster must be informed with updated content. Box 10-3 lists some important topics that can be included in Web page design. Content is most important

and cannot be delegated to a webmaster without veterinary experience.

Pages should include the same design, colors, and logo on each page. As stated earlier, the logo and phrase should be included on the heading of each page. Pages should be easy to navigate and have a "back" and "home" option on each.

The introduction page is very important. A picture of the front of the building helps introduce the practice to potential clients and refamiliarizes existing clients. A welcome message is an excellent tool that should include the mission of the hospital, core values, and an overview of products and services provided. Videos and music should not be used on the opening Web page, as they can take time to load (depending on the readers connection speed). If a Web page takes too long to load, readers will leave the page and continue searching for information elsewhere.

A variety of pictures (relative to content being covered) should be included in Web design. A site can have too much information listed, and clients will skim over the information and not read it. Pictures should be strategically placed with information bordering them. They should include a variety of species, and be clear and uncluttered. The Web design software or webmaster will recommend what format pictures should be saved in for best uploading.

The Web site address should be the name of the veterinary hospital if at all possible. For example, it would be best if ABC Veterinary Hospital had an Internet address of www.ABCVeterinaryHospital.com. This allows clients to find the address easily and also allows the hospital name to be included in the key words of the address. A URL, or uniform resource locator, is the address of the Web site on the World Wide Web. The address is composed of numbers and periods and is unique to each site. However, the Web site must have a domain name for people to be able to locate it. Many companies sell domain names, all of which are regulated by one nonprofit organization, the Internet Corporation for Assigned Names and Numbers (ICANN). A domain name may need to be purchased to secure the Web site address for the practice. If that particular name is already used by another facility, something creative should be added to the address, such as the city where the practice is located (www.ABCVeterinaryHospitalChicago.com).

Within the design software, the Web page allows key words to be entered that will attract potential clients to the site when they are searching the Internet. Key words to consider include the species of animals the practice treats, professional services that are available, and last names of the doctors on staff. Managers may wish to ask clients for keywords they would use to search the hospital. A compilation of these words should be developed; keywords that are suggested by several clients then become highest priority on the keyword list.

PRACTICE POINT   Keyword lists must be developed and entered to help search engines find the practice Web site.

All Web sites must have an email contact address; email should go to the webmaster or the practice manager in case problems or questions arise. The email address should be checked on a daily basis for any correspondence that may have arrived in the inbox.

Web sites should also include hyperlinks, which are images or highlighted text on a Web page that are linked to other Web pages, either within the same site or another Web site. This allows clients to move to other locations within the Web site more easily, or to move to other Web sites that have been linked with the practice site. In addition, when relevant hyperlinks that site visitors are interested in are embedded in the text content, the site's credibility with search engines is increased.

Practices may wish to provide hyperlinks to businesses that they recommend, such as groomers, pet shops, or boarding kennels. These hyperlinks must be checked regularly to ensure viability of the link. Search engines discredit Web sites that harbor invalid links, thus reducing the Web site's credibility with search engines.

Web sites should follow a three-click rule; information that clients are looking for should be found in just three clicks. Studies suggest that the longer it takes people to find information, the less likely they are to stay on the current Web site. Sites must be informative, fun, and easy to navigate.

To stay in line with the three-click rule, Web pages should be organized well (Figure 10-14). This includes using tabs on the front page, allowing quicker access to information for the reader. Excess text on the front page deters readers.

Search Engine Optimization

Many owners and managers find search engine optimization difficult to understand, therefore they underuse tools available to increase the practice's visibility on the Internet. Search engine optimization (SEO) is defined as the process of affecting the visibility of a Web site or Web page in a search engines' search results. Example of search engines includes Yahoo and Google. When a client searches the Internet, they enter keywords into the search engine, which then scrolls millions of Web pages that match the keywords that have been entered (this is why keyword entry is so critical when developing Web pages). The goal is have the practice's Web page appear in the top three searches that the search engine has found. In order to achieve this goal, Web pages need to strengthen their SEO, which can be accomplished with several methods:

- Keywords: The keywords that have been chosen earlier should be woven into the context of the Web pages. The more often those keywords appear within the Web page, the stronger the SEO.
- Internal hyperlinks: Linking to other pages within the Web site strengthens SEO. For example, a practice may mention digital radiography in the first page, which is then hyperlinked to another page providing the details of digital radiography.
- Inbound hyperlinks: Links from other businesses also drive SEO. For example, consider asking emergency and

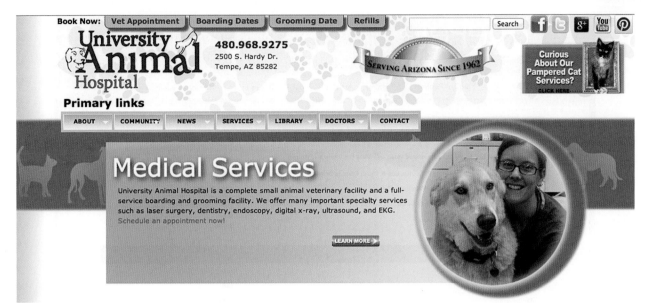

FIGURE 10-14 Example of organization tabs found on Web sites.

referral practices and the Chamber of Commerce to list the practice's Web site on their Web sites.

- External hyperlinks: Linking to other credible Web sites helps strengthen SEO. Consider adding links to the Web sites of such reputable organizations as the AVMA, AAHA, and AAFP (the links are endless). However, one must ensure these links are always viable.
- Update Web page content frequently. Search engines constantly look for new information; therefore the more frequently a Web page is updated, the stronger the SEO.
- Increased Web page traffic: Web pages must have visitors. Without visitors, search engines may find the Web site less credible, hence decreasing SEO.

Promoting the Web Page

Just because a practice has a Web page, one cannot assume clients are going to visit it. Managers must implement methods to drive Web site traffic. Just as indicated earlier, increasing traffic on a Web site leads to a stronger search engine presence. What can be done to drive Web site traffic?

> **PRACTICE POINT** Promote Web page visits to increase SEO credibility.

High-Quality Web Site. Build an excellent Web page that is easy to navigate and full of content. Clients will search the Internet for information; it is up to the practice to provide the correct information for the client and help them find it easily. This comes with great Web design, tabs, and an organizational structure. Start with the top 10 diseases the practice diagnosis, and/or top 10 procedures the practice performs, and develop content about those items. Also consider having a page dedicated to each profit center the hospital has established. The more content that is available for the clients, the more often they will return, therefore driving Web site visits.

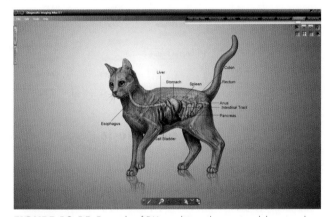

FIGURE 10-15 Example of DIA, a client education tool that can drive Web site visits. (Courtesy Patterson Veterinary Supply, Inc.)

Pet Portals. Pet portals allow clients to access their medical records at any time of the day. They can upload pictures of their pet to their account, request medication refills, make appointments, or print an identification card for their pet. The practice must invest in pet portals; clients love these and are beginning to expect this service from their veterinary hospital. When these portals are linked to the Web site (and clients continue returning to their account), the number of visits increases.

Client Education. Many practices use DIA (Diagnostic Imaging Atlas; available from Patterson Veterinary) (Figure 10-15); when linked to the Web page, DIA helps increase site visits, because clients will repeatedly return to learn more from this revolutionizing method of client education materials.

Client Instructions. Preoperative and postoperative instructions can be placed on the Web page. When appointments for a surgery have been scheduled (although instructions have been provided on the phone) clients can be directed to the Web page for downloadable instructions.

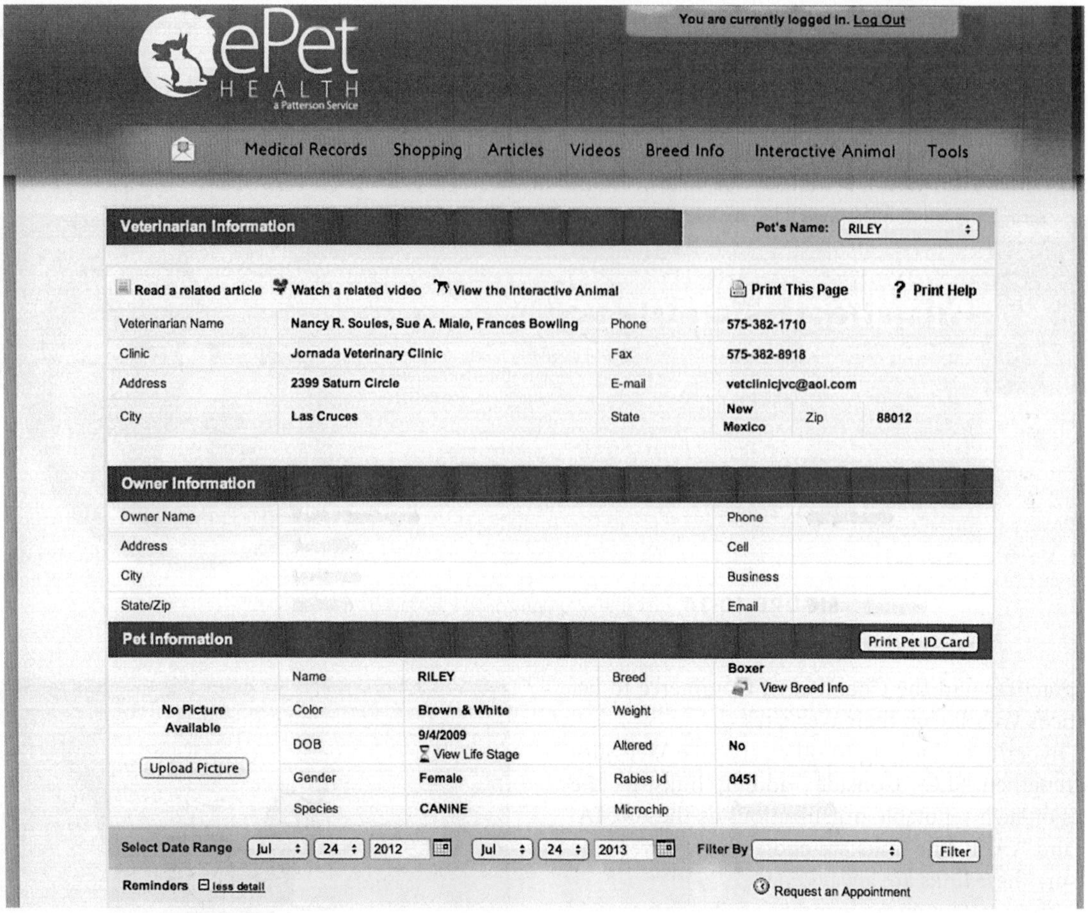

FIGURE 10-16 Example of pet portal. (Courtesy Patterson Veterinary Supply, Inc.)

Downloadable Forms. Consider placing forms clients will need to bring to the practice on the Web page.

Main Page for Practice Computers. All practices are connected to the Internet. Therefore make the practice Web site the home page that opens up (versus Google or Yahoo) when an Internet connection is established. Each time the page is opened, it is classified as a visit, again driving SEO credibility.

Event Calendar. If the practice hosts events such as obesity management courses, puppy socialization dates, or open houses, an event calendar may be considered as a method of informing clients of these upcoming events. Each time an event is entered, an email can be generated and sent to clients informing them of the new event. Each time they click on the event calendar, SEO strengthens.

Clinic Tour. Clients love behind-the-scenes tours. Consider adding a tour of the facility.

Blogs. Blogs are the "new" newsletter that must be linked to the practice's Web page. Keywords in blogs are searchable on search engines, and therefore consistently drive traffic back to the Web page. See the later section on blogs for more information.

Supporting social media links (Facebook, Twitter, Pinterest, etc.), appointment requests, medication refill requests, and the practice's online pharmacy are other options that can drive Web site traffic.

Once the Web site has been developed, the Web address should be published on every business item (along with contact information, logo, and tagline). Business cards, brochures, client education materials, prescription labels, and blogs are a few items managers often forget to list Web addresses on.

Pet Portals

Pet portals are revolutionizing communication in the veterinary industry. As stated previously, clients have learned about these and are demanding them! Pet portals can increase compliance (appointments, services, and products) significantly. Pet portals contain the client's online medical records, use reminders for appointments and surgeries (email, text, and postal), and include an online pharmacy that provides home delivery for clients (Figure 10-16).

> **PRACTICE POINT**   Pet portals are revolutionizing communication in the veterinary industry.

The benefits of an online pharmacy is that the practice does not have to carry *ALL* of the products, therefore allowing the practice to consolidate and decrease ordering, holding, and other inventory-related costs (see Chapter 15 for more details). Clients can shop online at any time (meeting

the clients need for convenience) and feel they can trust the products that are available on the practice's Web site. When products are ordered through the practice's site, they hold the guarantee offered by manufacturers, just as if the products were sold in the hospital.

Blogs

Blogs are an excellent way to communicate with clients (and potential clients). When blogs are attached to Web pages, the content is searchable by search engines. When clients click on a particular blog, it takes them to the practice Web site (once again, driving SEO). A blog is designed to generate new information for the clients, on a frequent basis, and can be in the form of client education, articles, or just simple conversations. The more often a practice posts on its blog, the more frequently the information is updated on the Web site (another method to drive SEO).

Many Web site developers now include an option to produce blogs. If a practice is hosting its own Web site, explore companies such as WordPress (wordpress.org) or LiveJournal (www.livejournal.com) for methods to integrate blogs into the practice Web site. Make sure to place practice name, logo, Web site, and contact information on every blog produced. Also, to help maintain visual consistency with the practice, ensure colors match the Web site design.

Blogs can be public or private (with private blogs, an invitation must be sent); keeping them public for our clients is best. Ideally, content should be kept to a maximum of 400 to 600 words per blog post, ensuring that the audience's attention is maintained. Many clients have multiple tasks they are handling at one time (work, kids, soccer practice, making dinner, doing laundry, etc.) so keeping stories short and sweet is imperative.

Lastly, promote blogs through social media and face-to-face client interactions. Place a few words of the blog on Facebook or Twitter, with a link directly to the blog page. If a client is in the exam room, show them the blogs on the Web page while they are waiting to see the veterinarian.

Mobile Media

Mobile media implies that Web pages are mobile (smartphone) friendly. Many clients (and potential clients) access practice Web pages with mobile devices on a daily basis. However, many Web sites are not accessible with mobile devices, frustrating those that are technologically proficient. Mobile media supports the immediate connection clients want to have with a practice. When electronic reminders are sent, a client opens the reminder and reads it, and wants to book an appointment while the thought is still fresh.

> **PRACTICE POINT**   Ensure the practice Web page is mobile friendly.

As covered previously, ensure the email address and phone number are active, supporting "one click to compliance."

FIGURE 10-17 Example of QR codes.

Some clients love text messaging; others dislike it. The point is that team members need to ask clients how they wish to be communicated with and implement strategies to meet those needs. Text messages can be sent to clients reminding them of upcoming appointments, as well as when their pet has recovered from surgery. One may also send pictures of patients recovering from surgery or while boarding, in hopes that the client will post their pet's picture on their social media page. Team members should indicate in the medical record when text messages were sent and what the message was composed of.

In addition to supporting the compliance feature through emails, mobile media supports geolocation features, such as Foursquare (foursquare.com) and quick response (QR) codes. Foursquare is a game designed for clients to check in while at the practice on their device; checking in alerts their friends and family to their location, and users are usually hoping to unlock a special of some sort. Practices may wish to have a free nail trim for clients when they check in, or other type of service that will drive traffic. Foursquare provides reports that should be analyzed, monitoring ROI for this inexpensive marketing tool.

Facebook users should also be encouraged to check in on their mobile device while at the practice. Facebook only allows clients to "like" the hospital once; however, clients can check in unlimited times and post a comment or recommendation about the hospital.

QR codes allow smartphone users to scan codes with their phone (Figure 10-17). QR codes serve as a quick link feature, and most practices will send QR code users directly to the practice's home page. QR codes can be placed on client education materials, business cards, and medication labels. When clients need a refill of medication, they simply scan the code, taking them directly to the sign-in page of the pet portal.

Social Media

The term *social media* is used to apply to all platforms, which change over time. Facebook, Twitter, Pinterest, Google+, and YouTube are top platforms at press time, but could change within a few years.

Social media has become the new form of communication with clients, and just as with mobile media, supports the one click to compliance theory. Traditionally, practices would have contact with clients once a year, or when the animal became sick. Today, practices have the ability to stay in contact with clients several times a week. Practices can positively influence clients with informative facts, fun trivia, and behind-the-scenes footage of the hospital. If clients like the information they are receiving, they will share it with their friends and family.

 Veterinary practice managers create and manage social media.

In addition to sharing information, clients tend to make recommendations on social media sites. *"Thanks for taking care of Fluffy! Without you, she would have never survived!"* These words are recommendations and serve as referrals for the practice. These referrals are much more powerful than an advertisement could ever be (and they are free!).

Developing a Plan

A social media plan should encompass the overall marketing plan a practice wishes to implement (see "Creating and Implementing a Marketing Plan," at the end of the chapter). If the practice wishes to focus on implementing wellness plans during the first quarter of 2015, the social media platform should support it. Consider methods in which wellness plans will be communicated to clients, such as the Web page, Facebook, Twitter, and YouTube. One may also implement the use of Foursquare (geolocation) to help promote the marketing message.

> **PRACTICE POINT** Clients are more willing to accept recommendations from a social media "friend" than from an advertisement.

Once a plan has been developed, put it in writing, with dates that certain objectives are due (pictures, taglines, and when messages will be released to the clients). Without a written plan, it may not happen!

Managing Social Media

Some practices hire a social media manager, or allow someone without veterinary experience to manage the social media sites. This can be a detriment, because it is no longer "the voice of the practice speaking," and messages that are sent can be confusing, and nonsupportive of practice philosophies. Ideally, a leader on the team should be the social media manager, and should be the only team member allowed to post to the practice's social media sites. Unfortunately, unaccountable team members may abuse the practice's social media pages and post detrimental comments. The practice's social media sites are for business only; personal comments, opinions, and gaming must be saved for personal

pages. Prevent this embarrassing scenario from occurring by appointing one responsible person to be in charge.

Social media does not have to take up a large amount of time, when managed correctly. Once a plan has been developed, key messages, phrases, and pictures can be uploaded to platforms at the beginning of the quarter, with scheduled releases. In general, two to three releases per week is acceptable; anymore than that can overwhelm clients and cause them to disengage.

Store digital photos on the computer, enabling easy access when pictures are needed. Once key messages have been determined, short phrases can be developed with an added picture. Pictures always increase social media traffic; therefore they are a must in every plan.

In addition to time efficiency, social media reports should be monitored. Determine what the clients like and do not like, which topics drove traffic, as well as those that did not drive traffic at all. This will help strengthen the plan for the following quarters. Managers should also determine who follows the practice, and implement strategies that target that particular audience. To do this, visit the reports provided by the social media platform, and break them down to the level of detail needed.

Social Media Policy

A social media policy is a must for both clients and patients. If any pictures are taken of client or team member pets, a social media release must be signed indicating the approval for use of the photo. The term *social media* must be used (rather than specific current platforms, such as Facebook, Twitter, Google+) because the face of social media will change over the years, and the general term, social media, is needed to encompass all platforms.

Team member social media policies are a little more complicated then the client's simple approval for use of pictures. Team members must understand that there are real implications for what they post (pictures and comments), and they must be accountable for their actions. Managers and owners cannot dictate what team members post on their personal social media site, however, professional guidelines can be established, and if violated, implications can occur. Review Chapter 5 for more details on a social media policy.

Managers can, however, mandate that pictures for the hospital's social media platforms be taken on practice approved cameras (never on personal cell phones) and uploaded by approved team members only. This can prevent the wrong person from uploading embarrassing or incorrect information.

Business Cards

Business cards are designed to be an easy reference for clients. They should be professionally printed with minimal information. Cards with too much information appear cluttered and disorganized. The cards should include the basic information: name of the practice, address, phone number,

doctors on staff, Web site address, email, and the practice logo and tagline. If the practice employs more than three doctors, more than one business card may be needed. A professional graphic designer should be consulted to create the best design for the hospital. The back of business cards can be used as appointment cards. The pet's name and appointment date can be listed on the back; this allows clients easy retrieval of both the business information and appointment time.

Team members should also have business cards. This allows each team member to provide clients a contact person should they have questions regarding their pet at any time in the upcoming week. Clients often forget team member's names once they leave the hospital, because they become overloaded with information. Business cards should only have the team member's first name (for security purposes). *Business cards create an identity for team members; an identity results in accountability, which enhances productivity for the team.*

PRACTICE POINT Business cards create an identity for team members; an identity results in accountability, which enhances productivity for the team

Magnets

Business cards can also be placed on magnets. Clients can place the magnets on their refrigerators. Friends and family will see these magnets and may strike up a conversation regarding the practice and the veterinary services offered. This is an excellent way to market the veterinary hospital at minimal cost. Professional printing houses can produce magnets in mass quantities, or packages of magnets can be purchased at local office supply stores, and team members can glue business cards onto the magnets. Team members may try producing their own, asking how clients and team members like them. If it is a good idea for the practice, then a mass production order can be placed.

Practice Brochures

People retain 20% of what they hear and 30% of what they read. Fun and colorful brochures will help clients retain the information the practice wishes to educate current clients about (Box 10-4).

The goal of a practice brochure is to state the mission of the practice, introduce the doctors (and staff if space allows), and list the professional services the practice offers (Figure 10-18). Since many new clients may have visited the practice Web site, they may already be familiar with the services offered by the hospital. However, in order to help them retain information, brochures detailing specific services may need to be developed.

Veterinary practice managers develop and manage practice promotional items (brochures, etc.).

BOX 10-4 | Highlights for Practice Brochures

- State-of-the-art laboratory facility
- Modern surgical facilities
- Radiology services
- Dental services
- Ophthalmology services
- PennHIP certification
- Preventive care
- Intensive care
- Oxygen therapy
- Senior pet health care
- Avian/exotic/reptiles
- Microchip implantation
- Pain management
- Allergy testing
- Artificial insemination
- Early drop-off service
- Variety of specialty foods

Doctors should be listed, including a short biography of each listed next to his or her picture. Clients like to be able to place a name with a face, and knowing something personal about the doctor helps build a trusting relationship from the beginning. Biographies may include where the doctors went to school, how long they have been in practice, and perhaps what their favorite hobbies are. The biography should be short and concise; too much writing can distract the reader, who will skip to the next section of the brochure.

Professional services should be listed with bullet points to emphasize the importance of each service. Current and potential clients often do not know what services veterinary practices provide. This is an excellent area to introduce them to the services that are available to help their pet live a longer life. Services should be limited to one or two words if possible.

The hours of operation are essential, along with the address, phone number, Web address, logo, and tagline. A map can also be placed on the back of the brochure in case a current client passes it on to a friend or co-worker. Do not forget a QR code, linking clients directly to the Web site.

PRACTICE POINT Brochures must appear professionally designed and printed; clients will relate cheap quality brochures with cheap medicine.

Brochures should be a trifold, to the standard brochure size. Pictures should be placed throughout the publication to break up the writing. Again, too much writing can deflect readers' attention and they will not read the brochure. This defeats the purpose of educating clients about the practice.

Brochures should be designed by a professional graphic designer to produce an eye-catching, educational brochure. The purpose of the brochure is to market the practice. Clients

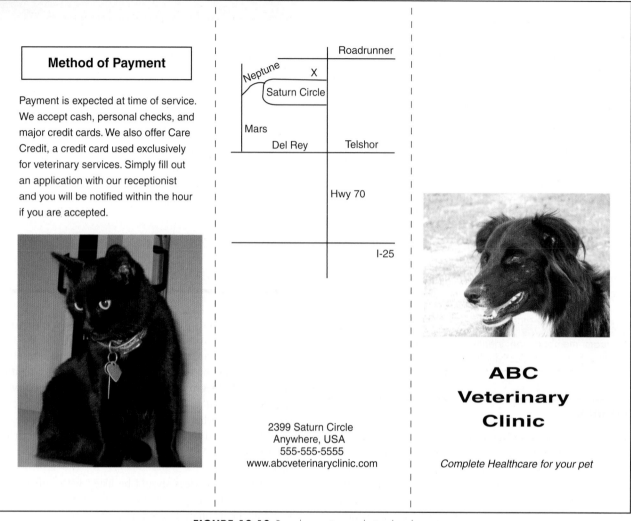

FIGURE 10-18 Sample practice marketing brochure.

will relate a poorly produced brochure to poor professional veterinary service. Strive to have the best brochure possible and spend the extra money (a one-time fee) to have it done correctly.

Professional printing of brochures is also essential. In-clinic laser printers do not print with as high a quality as printing houses do. Brochures should be printed on a thicker stock of paper than copy paper; this will also help draw attention to the brochure. Again, the extra money spent for the professional appearance pays off in the end. Clients relate high-quality brochures and marketing techniques to high-quality medicine. Remember to maintain visual consistency; brochure colors should match the color of the Web site and blogs.

Client Education Materials

As stated earlier, clients retain only 20% of what is told to them but 30% of material they read. It is therefore imperative to send clients home with educational materials. Client education sheets may include preprinted brochures from manufacturers discussing topics such as heartworm disease or preventable diseases. They may also include relevant

information on the health care needs of a client's pet that has just been diagnosed with a particular condition.

Veterinary practice managers manage client education.

Some veterinary practice management software (PMS) versions produce handouts that include the client and pet name, the practice name, the doctor that is seeing the patient, and the date of diagnosis (Figure 10-19). These are informative sheets that explain the disease, symptoms seen with such disease, and the possible treatments. They are professional in appearance, easy to read, and quick to produce. If the practice does not have PMS to produce such handouts, CDs can be purchased, allowing team members to select the disease or condition and print out the information in a Word document format. Visit www.elsevierhealth.com to order a copy of *Small Animal Practice Client Handouts* by Rhea V. Morgan.

When creating these handouts, it is important to keep in mind that they must appear professional, be error free, and

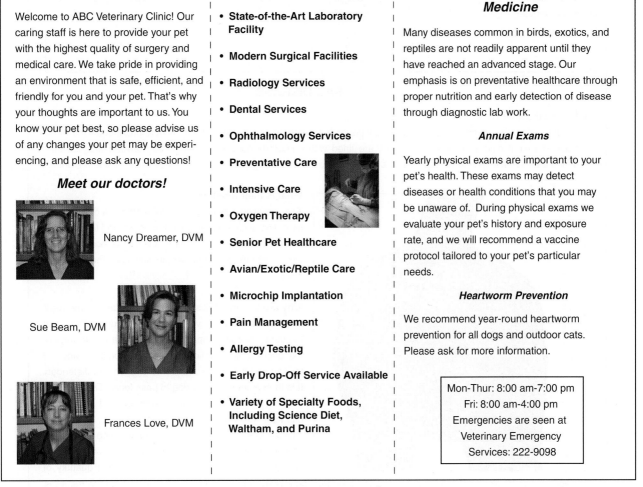

Welcome!

Welcome to ABC Veterinary Clinic! Our caring staff is here to provide your pet with the highest quality of surgery and medical care. We take pride in providing an environment that is safe, efficient, and friendly for you and your pet. That's why your thoughts are important to us. You know your pet best, so please advise us of any changes your pet may be experiencing, and please ask any questions!

Meet our doctors!

Nancy Dreamer, DVM

Sue Beam, DVM

Frances Love, DVM

Services Provided

- **State-of-the-Art Laboratory Facility**
- **Modern Surgical Facilities**
- **Radiology Services**
- **Dental Services**
- **Ophthalmology Services**
- **Preventative Care**
- **Intensive Care**
- **Oxygen Therapy**
- **Senior Pet Healthcare**
- **Avian/Exotic/Reptile Care**
- **Microchip Implantation**
- **Pain Management**
- **Allergy Testing**
- **Early Drop-Off Service Available**
- **Variety of Specialty Foods, Including Science Diet, Waltham, and Purina**

Avian/Exotic Reptile Medicine

Many diseases common in birds, exotics, and reptiles are not readily apparent until they have reached an advanced stage. Our emphasis is on preventative healthcare through proper nutrition and early detection of disease through diagnostic lab work.

Annual Exams

Yearly physical exams are important to your pet's health. These exams may detect diseases or health conditions that you may be unaware of. During physical exams we evaluate your pet's history and exposure rate, and we will recommend a vaccine protocol tailored to your pet's particular needs.

Heartworm Prevention

We recommend year-round heartworm prevention for all dogs and outdoor cats. Please ask for more information.

Mon-Thur: 8:00 am-7:00 pm
Fri: 8:00 am-4:00 pm
Emergencies are seen at
Veterinary Emergency
Services: 222-9098

FIGURE 10-18, cont'd

contain language that clients can understand. They should be short, simple, and easy to read. If clients do not understand the words or if the brochure is too long, clients may toss the information to the side and not read the material once they have arrived home. All client education materials should have the practice name, address, phone number, Web address, and QR code included at the top of the sheet. Some client education sheets may need to be modified when new products or procedures have been developed; it is important to review the materials on a yearly basis looking for needed changes. Practices do not want to make one recommendation when the information they hand out recommends another.

> **PRACTICE POINT** Add QR codes to client education materials, driving them to the practice Web site.

Clients will also share materials with other family members once they have arrived home. Medicine confuses many people, and they may be unable to explain the disease, diagnosis, or medications to others once they have left the practice. If it is in writing, the confusion decreases, communication is clearer,

and fewer mistakes will be made by the client. Clients will also be more likely to follow and accept recommendations because they understand the disease and the treatment options. Practices cannot provide enough education to clients; send every client home with at least one piece of client education material to help improve client knowledge and compliance. Any documents sent home with clients must be recorded in the medical record for future referencing.

On-Hold Messaging

When clients are placed on hold, time seems to pass slowly. The client may only be on hold for 1 minute, but it seems like 5 minutes! It makes sense to be able to use this time to market the services the practice offers. This can be accomplished in several ways. Several companies produce CDs that can be played on a system while clients are on hold. Messages can be developed specifically for the practice and include the practice name as well as the names of the doctors. New messages are produced on a quarterly basis and can change with the seasons. Other CDs may have up to 80 different messages that can be chosen from, and the practice can pick the top

Account number:	Patient:	Age:
Phone number:	Species:	Sex:
	Breed:	Tag:
	Color:	Weight:
	Doctor:	

ANAL SAC DISEASE

What are the anal sacs?

Popularly called anal glands, these are two small pouches located on either side of the anus at approximately the four o'clock and eight o'clock positions. The sacs are lined with numerous specialized sebaceous (sweat) glands that produce a foul-smelling secretion. Each sac is connected to the outside by a small duct that opens just inside the anus.

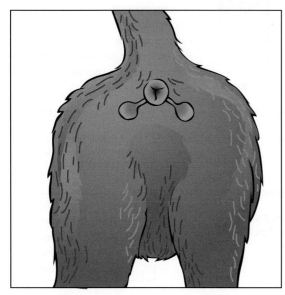

What is their function?

The secretion acts as a territorial marker—a dog's calling card. The sacs are present in both male and female dogs and are normally emptied when the dog defecates. This is why dogs are so interested in smelling one another's feces.

Why are the anal sacs causing a problem in my dog?

Anal sac disease is very common in dogs. The sacs frequently become impacted, usually due to blockage of the ducts. The secretion within the impacted sacs will thicken and the sacs will become swollen and distended. It is then painful for your dog to pass feces. The secreted material within the anal sacs forms an ideal medium for bacterial growth, allowing abscesses to form. Pain increases and sometimes a red, hot swelling will appear on one or both sides of the anus at the site of abscessation. If the abscess bursts, it will release a quantity of greenish yellow or bloody pus. If left untreated, the infection can quickly spread and cause severe damage to the anus and rectum.

How will I know if my dog has anal sac problems?

The first sign is often scooting or dragging the rear along the ground. There may be excessive licking or biting, often at the root of the tail rather than the anal area. Anal sac impaction and infection is very painful. Even normally gentle dogs may snap or growl if you touch the tail or anus when they have anal sac disease. If the anal sac ruptures, you may see blood or pus draining from the rectum.

What should I do?

Problems with the anal gland are common in all dogs, regardless of size or breed. If you are concerned that your pet may have an anal sac problem, call your veterinarian at once. Treatment for impaction involves flushing and removal of the solidified material. Since this condition is painful, many pets will require a sedative or an anesthetic for this treatment.

FIGURE 10-19 Sample client education hand out.

40 to play through the system. Topics may include heartworm disease, special diets, special procedures, dentals, antifreeze toxicity, chocolate toxicity, heatstroke, or plant poisonings. The choice is unlimited and special CDs can be made for each individual practice.

The practice can purchase a one-disk CD player/receiver unit that allows programming. This programming allows the practice to choose the messages to be played and repeats itself when finished playing. The CD plays constantly; therefore, each time a call is placed on hold, the caller will hear a different message. The CD player is plugged into the central phone system, and the volume can be adjusted from the receiver. It is imperative that the message be at the correct volume. If it is too loud, clients will pull the phone away from their ears and not listen to the message; if it is too quiet, they will not be able to hear the message. Team members can call the first

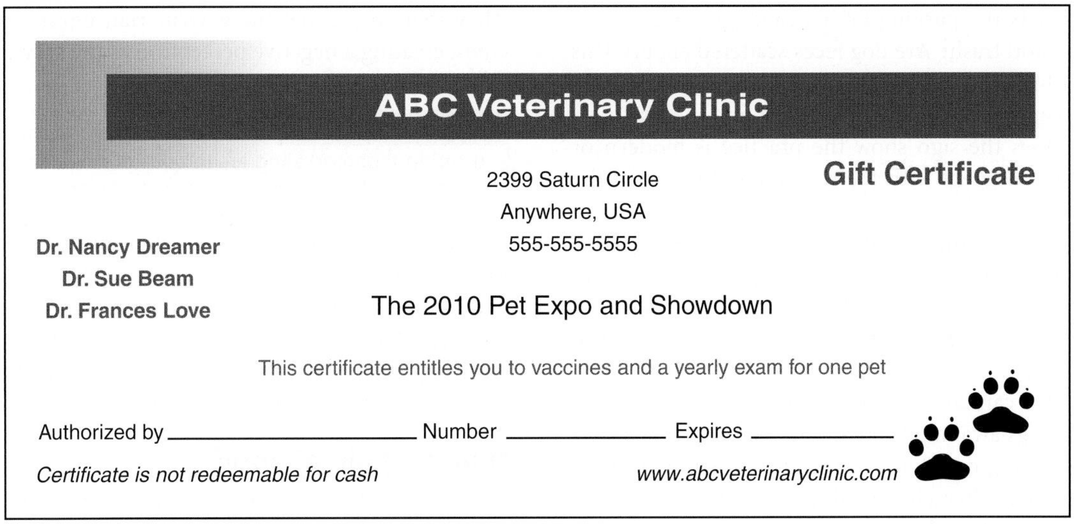

ABC Veterinary Clinic

2399 Saturn Circle
Anywhere, USA
555-555-5555

Gift Certificate

Dr. Nancy Dreamer
Dr. Sue Beam
Dr. Frances Love

The 2010 Pet Expo and Showdown

This certificate entitles you to vaccines and a yearly exam for one pet

Authorized by ____________ Number ____________ Expires ____________

Certificate is not redeemable for cash *www.abcveterinaryclinic.com*

FIGURE 10-20 Sample gift certificate.

phone line of the clinic and place it on hold; while on hold and listening to the message, the volume can be adjusted.

Donations

Many schools, organizations, and individuals will seek donations for events they are sponsoring or attending. Although donations to local events and organizations go to good causes, a predetermined amount should be set aside in the budget each year. It is very easy to go over budget when donating because many students are great at pleading their cases; therefore owners and managers make an emotionally based decision to donate. Spreading the donation budget over a 12-month period will help prevent the practice from donating more than it can afford.

> *PRACTICE POINT* Develop a donation budget, preventing the practice from donating out of emotion and exceeding the limit.

In exchange for donations, it is reasonable to expect some advertising. Some schools may place the contributor's name on a T-shirt or calendar, or recognize larger contributions at sporting events.

When a donation is given to a nonprofit organization, a receipt should be generated for the practice. This receipt should be kept for year-end tax purposes. Donations are an excellent source of external marketing, but a maximum amount should be set each year.

Regardless of where the donation goes, practices must get into the habit of tracking the ROI of such donations. Making good (or bad) decisions can affect the bottom line, either positively or negatively.

Gift Certificates

As with donations, gift certificates can be created to give to nonprofit charities for door prizes, raffles, or drawings. Charities are grateful that the practice would donate gift certificates; in reality, potential clients may or may not use the gift certificates they have won. The practice is the winner in this situation. The name of the practice is announced several times, and they will receive a receipt for the total value of the gift certificates that were given to the organization. The practice may gain a new client, and if a gift certificate is not used, there is no loss (Figure 10-20).

Gift certificates can be used to give away services or products. One example is to print a gift certificate for a yearly exam and vaccines. When a client uses this certificate, he or she is likely to purchase more services or products. He may choose to have a heartworm test and purchase heartworm preventative while at the practice, or may add a collar and a leash while checking out at the counter. Although the exam and vaccines were provided at no cost as a donation, the practice made a profit on the additional services and products the client chose. If the recipient is a new client, then the practice has just gained a new client through the gift certificate.

Implementing a Marketing and Training Program for Team Members

Marketing techniques will not overcome the effects of poor client relations within a practice. If the team is not ready to produce excellent customer service and have high standards, knowledge, and confidence, a marketing plan is wasted time and money. The team has to be ready to deliver in order to produce.

> *PRACTICE POINT* The practice can be marketing intentionally or unintentionally; whichever is chosen, marketing is always happening.

Unintentional marketing is occurring at all times, whether managers realize it or not. Unintentional marketing comes in several forms and can be detrimental when not managed daily.

Parking lot: Is the parking lot appealing, or full of pot-holes, weeds, and trash? Are dog feces scattered about? This is an area of first impression for a client, and it can create a negative perception before they even walk into the practice.

Signage: Does the sign show the practice is modern or ancient? Is it consistent with the mission and vision of the practice?

Smells: What does the practice smell like upon entry? This is another area of potential negative perception. Often, team members are so use to the smell of a veterinary hospital that it is normal to them; however, this smell is not normal to clients.

Audio: What can clients hear when they enter the practice? Crying dogs awaking from anesthesia? Team members yelling at boarding dogs? Team members gossiping? What does it sound like when clients call the hospital? Is the conversation rushed? Does the client hear a monotone or a rude tone of voice? All of these factors MUST be considered on a daily basis.

Relationships: Have lasting relationships been developed with clients? Is time allotted to the team members to establish this relationship? Many times, practices are short staffed, and payroll is the first item that is cut; however, this negatively affects any marketing campaign that is in the stages of implementation.

Listening: Listening to clients is another key component to effective marketing programs. If teams do not listen to clients, they will not understand what their needs are. This ultimately leads to client dissatisfaction and decreased compliance. Client needs and wants may include professional services as well as emotional and consumer needs.

Professional, well-groomed staff: Are uniforms clean, unwrinkled, and stain free? Are team members professional in their word choice, enunciation, and body structure? Clients are less likely to develop a trusting relationship (resulting in decreased compliance) when recommendations are made from a frumpy team.

Compassion and empathy: Does each team member have compassion for pets and their people? Do they show empathy when appropriate?

Exam Rooms

The exam room is the center of marketing efforts. This is where relationships are built, and every step of the client interaction must be evaluated. When veterinary technicians are taking the five vital signs of every patient, the importance of those vitals must be discussed. When the veterinarian enters the room and starts the physical examination, the entire process must be discussed. Many clients perceive that the veterinarian is just petting the patient when in actuality, they are feeling for lumps or bumps (but clients do not know that). Veterinarians must discuss what they are looking for when examining the eyes, ears, mouth, and so on, in order for the client to understand the value of the service. It is the job of the veterinary technician or assistant to hold and distract the pet for vaccinations; they do such a great job that the client does not see that the vaccines have been given

(they then argue that the veterinarian never gave the vaccines, creating a negative perception of the service).

> **PRACTICE POINT**   Evaluate exam room protocols, ensuring that marketing techniques are maximized.

Practices must develop consistent protocols and deliver the same message, which must be repeated several times within the same visit for the client to retain the information. This repeated message starts with the receptionist, continues with the veterinary technician, then the veterinarian, and is followed up one more time at checkout with the receptionist.

Human-Animal Bond

Once communication and client education have been mastered, helping team members to focus on and understand the human-animal bond is a great place to continue developing marketing skills. Many clients do not have a strong support network outside of the veterinary hospital when it comes to their pets. Perhaps the dog is the wife's best friend, and the husband dislikes the dog. The husband will never understand that strong bond that the team members do; when team member's support and reinforce this bond with the wife, client compliance strengthens.

Body Language

Positive body language is just as effective as listening (if not more). Team members should have open arms, wear smiles on their faces, and make eye contact. Folded arms and frowns will prevent clients from asking questions and create a negative atmosphere. Lack of eye contact shows a lack of confidence in the recommendation and can result in client refusal of the service. If possible, maintain physical neutrality; if the client is standing, the team member should also be standing while speaking the client. If a client is sitting, the team member should sit next to the client to prevent speaking (physically) down to him or her.

Specific Recommendations

Assertive marketing can be defined as providing clients with the information they need to accept the practice recommendations (making specific recommendations). Team members should provide the facts about and benefits of the recommended service. Assertive marketing techniques can include showing advantages for the pet and the client, along with explaining the reason for providing the procedure now rather than later, and detailing the consequences of not accepting the recommendation.

Team members should not be shy when making recommendations. Powerful words can be used in conversation. For example, "Fluffy needs blood work," instead of "We recommend Fluffy have blood work ..." will usually convince clients to accept the recommendation. Team members should never be shy or embarrassed about the recommendation they are making; if they are, they need to be educated on the importance of the service they are providing.

Managing Reviews

With the increased role of social media in every day life, online reviews of a practice are available everywhere. Clients may upload reviews while in the exam room, especially when they are upset. It was mentioned previously that recommendations from clients are more powerful than advertising; therefore managing reviews is imperative.

Owners and managers must set up alerts for the practice and each veterinarian via Google, Yahoo, and so on. Alerts will be emailed when any review is posted (usually within 24 hours). It is great to evaluate positive reviews, and negative reviews must be managed as soon as possible. Four steps should be taken to manage negative reviews.

Veterinary practice managers handle client complaints

Step one: When a negative review is found, the initial response is to handle the complaint immediately; however, when an immediate response is formed, it is generally defensive and carries an authoritarian tone. Do not respond immediately. Investigate the complaint; obtain facts from the staff. Take some time and create a planned response that will be perceived in a positive manner.

Step two: Respond to the reviewer with empathy and compassion. Apologize for their experience, and extend the opportunity to discuss the complaint via phone or in person. Do try and reach this client if possible. If one is unable to reach the client, return to the review, and add another response *"We have tried to contact you on multiple occasions with no success; please call us ASAP so that we may resolve this situation."* Clients (and potential clients) will see the practice is attempting to resolve the issue, and will usually discredit the negative review. Do not ever attempt to solve complaints via the review. This will only ignite further negative comments, either from the original complainant or their supporters.

Step three: Promote good reviews. Ask clients to post reviews of the hospital and team members; share stories of success. The more positive reviews that appear, the lower the negative review is posted.

Step four: Be proactive, not reactive (and this should not be considered the last step). Effective managers and leaders that form a positive culture with an excellent team prevent incidents that produce poor reviews. If negative reviews continue to be posted, the manager needs to take a serious look at the culture that is brewing behind closed doors. Remember, positive leadership trickles from the top down. Review Chapter 3 for techniques to create and promote a positive team.

> **PRACTICE POINT** Create a positive culture within the practice to prevent bad reviews from being created.

Seize the Opportunity!

Marketing techniques give the practice the ability to inform the community what the practice is about. Practices should take the opportunity to provide current and potential clients with information regarding veterinary services and recognize the team for their unique abilities. Practices must stand out in the crowd and separate themselves from the rest of the pack. Simply providing veterinary services is no longer good enough. Teams must be creative, informative, and compassionate to help the practice excel at the next level. All these goals can be achieved through some degree of marketing. A professional graphic designer and webmaster can help practices appear more professional, which increases the value to the client. Seize the opportunity while the opportunity exists!

Creating and Implementing a Marketing Plan

A successful marketing plan comes from a variety of analyses, including the mission and vision of the practice, a SWOT analysis, identifying who the target client is, and what their particular needs are. What does the practice wish to accomplish? Is this in line with the practice's mission and values? Will this help reach the practices visionary goals?

Complete a SWOT analysis, and review client surveys and interview team members. Determine the target goal. Goals a practice may consider include increasing client compliance on heartworm preventative, wellness plans, or dental disease prevention. One may wish to increase the number of new clients and new patients, or improve the retention rate of current clients. Once this target has been determined, one must consider what the objectives are and how they will be obtained and measured.

Implement a strategy. What, when, where, why, and how will this plan work? Review the internal team structure. Is the team ready for this marketing plan? Integrate their thoughts and opinions, because these are critical for plan success. Externally, how will this be marketed to clients? Social media, blogs, Web page, postcards, and/or email? Determine the tools or source(s) that are needed for success (use all source's if it will help the marketing plan succeed).

> **PRACTICE POINT** Place a marketing plan in writing, or it may never get accomplished.

Create an action plan that includes a time line and budget and put it in writing. When do objectives need to be met? How much will it cost? What is the ROI for this particular program?

Execute the plan and measure the results. What worked well, and what did not work well? What can be done to improve the next marketing plan? If this plan was a success, what made it a success? Can those strategies be implemented on future plans?

Marketing plans are extremely successful when planned appropriately. One cannot create a strategy and try to implement without the proper planning steps; potholes will be created, adding extra work for the team in the long run.

VETERINARY PRACTICE and the LAW

When marketing products or procedures, it is unethical for veterinarians to promote, sell, prescribe, dispense, or use secret remedies or any other product for which they do not know the ingredient formula. It is also unethical for veterinarians to use or permit the use of their names, signatures, or professional status in connection with the resale of ethical products in a manner that violates those directions or conditions specified by the manufacturer to ensure the safe and efficacious use of the product. Veterinarians cannot prescribe or dispense prescription products in the absence of a valid client-patient relationship.

REVIEW QUESTIONS

1. What is internal marketing? Give an example.
2. What is external marketing? Give an example.
3. What example can be applied to both internal and external marketing?
4. Why is a Web site essential in today's market?
5. What information should be included in client education materials?
6. Why should a practice be branded?
7. What is a pet portal?
8. What is the purpose of reminders and recalls?
9. Why is indirect marketing so important?
10. How would a practice brochure benefit the practice?
11. What does the acronym *SWOT* stand for?
    a. Service with outstanding treatment
    b. Strengths, weaknesses, opportunities, and threats
    c. Service, Web site, office appearance, transactions
    d. None of the above

12. Which of the following is an example of internal marketing?
    a. Lectures
    b. E-Newsletter
    c. Telephone etiquette
    d. Blogs
13. Which of the following can be found on a clinic's Web page?
    a. Virtual tour
    b. Appointment requests
    c. Hours of operation
    d. All of the above
14. How many options are there for Web site creation?
    a. 2
    b. 4
    c. 3
    d. 1
15. What is the correct definition of SEO?
    a. The process of affecting the visibility of a Web site or Web page in a search engines' search results
    b. The key terms that a search engine will use
    c. A search engine's external hyperlinks used to promote a Web site.
    d. None of the above

Recommended Reading

Heinke MM: *Practice made perfect: a guide to veterinary practice management*, ed 2, Lakewood, CO, 2012, AAHA Press.

Roark A: *Marketing your practice, veterinary team brief.* (Web site) www.veterinaryteambrief.com/article/marketing-your-practice-and-yourself. Accessed August 5, 2013.

Tassava B: *Social media for veterinary professionals.* http://www.lulu.com/shop/brenda-tassava-cvpm-cvj/social-media-for-veterinary-professionals/paperback/product-1460, 2011.

## PART II

Communication Management

Clients drive the practice; the team takes the practice to the next level. Without clients, practices cannot make it to the next level. Client communication is essential to the successful practice and must be the number one commitment of all team members. Client communication involves speaking with, educating, listening to, and understanding client wants and needs. If client satisfaction is not met, the client will not return. Not only will they not return, they will tell 10 people why they were not satisfied during their visit.

There are many barriers to client communication and team members must develop methods to overcome these barriers. Some barriers may exist because of ethnicity, gender, or language differences. Others barriers may be factors that are out of the practice's control; the client is having a financially difficult time, is suffering from a medical condition, or is experiencing a divorce or loss of a family member. Whatever the barrier is, methods exist to help the client understand what their pet needs for medical treatment. Treatment plans should always be created for clients, because this is the number one complaint filed with state veterinary boards. Clients often do not know what the charge is going to be, which results in sticker shock, or what the final outcome of the case will be. If clients are fully advised of the services their pet(s) need and they understand the value of the service, receive a plan, and are consistently updated with changes, the satisfaction level of the client will not only be met, but also exceeded.

Verbal image of team members is critical to client communication. If a team member appears to lack confidence in their recommendation, does not have the information to answer client questions, or has decreased levels of eye contact, the recommendations made by the team will likely not be accepted. Team members must be confident in their recommendations, provide information to back up the recommendation, make eye contact, and have excellent body posture. Techniques can be implemented to strengthen each team member's verbal image.

Clients undergoing the grieving process experience a number of emotional conditions, which may be met by the veterinary health care team member. The human-animal bond develops over time and is strong, which explains why clients experience such pain with the loss of a pet. Team members can help clients through this incredibly tough time by providing emotional support.

Client Communication and Customer Service

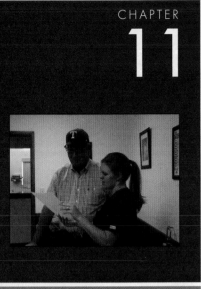

Body Language
Client Communication
Client Compliance
Client Grievances
Client Retention
Client Survey
Estimates
Informational Brochure
Recalls
Reminders
Verbal Image

OUTLINE

Forming a Message, *212*
  Verbal Skills, *212*
  Improving Verbal Image, *212*
  Barriers to Client Communications, *214*
  Putting It All Together, *215*
Writing Skills, *215*
  Email Etiquette, *215*
Client Compliance, *216*
  Reminders and Recall Systems, *216*
  Educational Information, *218*
Treatment Plans (Estimates), *220*
Standards of Care, *222*

Ensuring Client Understanding, *222*
**Understanding Client and Patient
  Needs,** *223*
  What Do Clients Really Want?, *223*
  Client Surveys, *224*
  Handling Client Complaints and
    Grievances, *224*
  Handling Negative Reviews on the
    Internet, *226*
Customer Service, *226*
Client Retention, *226*

LEARNING OBJECTIVES

When you have completed this chapter, you should be able to:

1. Describe the importance of written client materials.
2. Describe the importance of professional verbal skills.
3. List methods used to communicate in a positive, professional manner.
4. Identify methods used to educate clients with a variety of techniques.
5. Describe the importance of providing estimates for clients.
6. Define client needs.
7. Clarify barriers that prevent effective client communication.
8. List methods that can improve verbal image.

CRITICAL COMPETENCIES

1. **Adaptability** - being open to change and flexible work methods; the ability to adapt behavior to changing conditions or new information.
2. **Compliance** - being reliable, thorough, and conscientious in carrying out work assignments; has an appreciation for the importance of organizational rules and policies.
3. **Creativity** - the ability to think creatively about situations, to see things in new and different ways; use imagination and creativity to develop innovative solutions to problems.
4. **Critical and Strategic Thinking** - the ability to think critically about situations and to understand the relevance of information for different problems; use critical reasoning to generate and

evaluate alternative courses of action or points of view relevant to an issue.
5. **Decision Making** - the ability to make good decisions, solve problems, and decide on important matters; the ability to gather and analyze relevant data and choose decisively between alternatives.
6. **Integrity** - honesty, trustworthiness, and adherence to high standards of ethical conduct.
7. **Leadership** - a willingness to lead and take charge; the ability to motivate others and mobilize group effort toward common goals.
8. **Persuasion** - the ability to change the attitudes and opinions of others and to persuade them to accept recommendations and change behavior.

9. **Planning and Prioritizing** - the ability to effectively manage time and work load to meet deadlines; the ability to organize work, set priorities, and establish plans for achieving goals.

10. **Resilience** - the ability to cope effectively with pressure and setbacks; the ability to handle crisis situations effectively and remain undeterred by obstacles or failure.

11. **Resourcefulness** - the ability to understand what it takes to complete the job; apply knowledge, skills, and expertise to perform tasks quickly and efficiently.

12. **Writing and Verbal Skills** - ability to comprehend written material easily and accurately; ability to express thoughts clearly and succinctly in writing.

In the marketing and client relations domain, the veterinary practice manager plans and coordinates marketing, public relations, and client service programs. In terms of client relations, the manager establishes protocols for client communications and monitors client services to facilitate client retention and satisfaction.

Knowledge Requirements

The tasks related to client services and education requires knowledge of the principles and processes for providing customer and personal services, including customer needs assessment and methods for evaluating customer satisfaction.

Communication is one of the most important aspects of working with veterinary clients. It is extremely important that clients fully understand procedures that are being performed on their pets. They must also be educated on the proper care of their animals throughout the various life stages, and all of this must be relayed in a professional manner.

Client communication comes in a variety of forms. It starts in the front office with the reception team. Greeting clients as they enter the practice communicates that the staff acknowledges their presence. Communication should occur in a positive, friendly manner, which enhances the practice image. Communication includes both verbal and written forms in the exam rooms. The veterinarians, technicians, and assistants must educate the client with words that can be understood, but must take care to not offend. Many clients want to learn the information but do not understand medical terminology. The amount of information given to a client can be based on that client's knowledge and skill (Figure 11-1).

Written communication includes all client education materials. Clients should take home information with every visit. After puppy and kitten exams, clients should be sent home with material informing them about internal parasites and vaccination schedules. Clients bringing pets in for follow-up booster examinations may be sent home with information on nutrition as well as on the benefits of spaying and neutering. The last visit may include information on the prevention of obesity and dental disease. Yearly exam patients may need to be educated on weight-loss programs and nutritional and behavioral issues. Senior patients should be educated on the importance of monitoring blood work and frequent, regular exams. Each client should receive a report card explaining the normal and abnormal findings for his or her pet and what follow-up procedures or treatments are recommended (see Figure 10-11).

Surgical patients must receive postoperative discharge instructions. These instructions may vary by procedure, but all clients must be informed as to when to start food, medications, and physical activity.

Boarding clients will appreciate receiving report cards on their pets, which may include information on the pets' appetite, activity level, and attitude (Figure 11-2).

Any patient that is diagnosed with a disease or condition should be given information to take home and review regarding the disease and any treatments available. If the clients have any questions, they can call the practice and verify information before scheduling an appointment for the treatment.

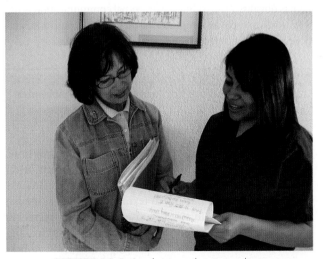

FIGURE 11-1 A technician educating a client.

```
                              Report Card

        For _____        Arrival _____
        Date _____        Departure _____

        How I Ate:                           My Personality:
        _____ I devoured my food!          _____ I was very friendly.
        _____ I ate some of my food.       _____ I was shy.
        _____ I didn't feel like eating much. _____ I was quiet.
                                             _____ I was talkative.

        How I Played:                        Potty Time:
        _____ I was so excited, I played like crazy. _____ I went regularly.
        _____ I was shy.                   _____ I went infrequently.
        _____ It took me awhile to feel comfortable.
        _____ I need to work on my "petiquette."

        My Behavior Was:                     Comments: _____
        _____ Absolutely wonderful!        _____
        _____ Better than most.            _____
        _____ Could have been better.      _____
        _____ Did my best.                 _____
        _____ Forget it. I will be good next time! _____


                        Thank you for boarding with us.
```

FIGURE 11-2 Sample boarding report card.

All of the communication topics covered in this chapter create a path for excellent customer service. Clients have to come to expect value for the services they are paying for, and all these services are enhanced by exceptional communication skills.

Forming a Message

A message has three components when being developed: verbal, paraverbal, and nonverbal. Verbal skills account for 7% of a message, paraverbal skills contribute 38%, and nonverbal skills are the major contributor at 55% of the message. The verbal component is obviously word choice; paraverbal communication is the way words are spoken, emphasizing on tone, pitch and enunciation; and the nonverbal component is body language.

> **PRACTICE POINT**   Messages have three parts: verbal (word choice), paraverbal (enunciation), and nonverbal (body language).

It is important to remember that all messaging has to be professional and be done in a manner that all clients, team members, and colleagues in the industry can understand. As society has started adjusting to texting, using social media, and communicating in short phrases, some team members have implemented that (unnecessary) skill when making entries in medical records and speaking with clients. Abbreviations used in the written messages must be compliant with

veterinary standards (see the abbreviations in the appendices), verbal and paraverbal components must be professional, and the nonverbal aspects must complement these to yield the fully formed message.

Verbal Skills

Team members should be able to communicate well with clients verbally. Specific words may be chosen when talking with clients to project the professional image of the practice. For example, simple words such as "vaccinations" should be used instead of "shots," and "yes, sir" or "yes, ma'am." should be used instead of "yeah."

Many employees do not realize the number of times filler sounds such as "um" are in a sentence until they are counted. A team member may record a conversation and listen to the recording; listening to oneself will help team members realize how much "verbal garbage" fills the conversation. Reducing the number of "ums" in a sentence will increase client trust and compliance.

Team members should be forbidden to say word phrases such as "I don't know." Instead, phrases should be replaced with "That is a great question, let me find out!" "No, we do not accept payments" can be replaced with "we offer payment plans through an outside agency." Enhancing the staff's verbal skills will help take the veterinary practice to the next level.

Improving Verbal Image

Employees should role-play client education topics, because clients will always have questions about their pets' health

care. It is important to remember that clients are asking these questions because they do not know the answers and team members must not judge clients for asking questions.

Team members forget that topics that are very basic to them may be new to an owner. Team members must not get frustrated answering these questions for clients. A client service manual is suggested to help new team members learn the appropriate answers to client questions. This includes correct verbiage, correct pronunciation, and the skill to respond to such questions. Chapter 23 covers the most common diseases and procedures that team members should be familiar with, which will help improve verbal communication.

The success of the veterinary practice depends on client compliance, which in turn depends on client education and acceptance of recommendations. Clients will not accept recommendations from uneducated, unmotivated team members. The client-patient relationship will not be established without confidence, skill, and understanding from team members. By providing continuing education for all employees, team members will be able to discuss procedures, protocols, and diseases much more thoroughly. Team members will learn correct definitions and pronunciations and be able to educate clients with a higher level of confidence. For example, staff members can pick a word of the day and educate others as to the correct definition and pronunciation. Once it has been mastered, team members can use the word in sentences throughout the day. Role-playing and continuing education for team members will help the knowledge, enthusiasm, and proficiency of each individual on the team.

Paraverbal Skills

Lower and deeper voice tones make team members appear more confident and authoritative, whereas high-pitched tones sound insecure and immature. With practice, deeper tones can be established, enhancing each team member's value. Chapter 2 discusses telephone etiquette and effective voice tones as well as how the speed of talking can affect a conversation. Client perception starts when a call is placed to the practice and is definitely affected by the tone of the conversation. Practices have 10 seconds to have a positive impact on a client; when it starts with a phone call, tone of voice may make or break a new client.

Nonverbal Skills

Nonverbal skills are also known as body language. Team members talk with body language a majority of the time and do not even know it! In fact, body language speaks louder than words. Most of this language is subconscious and includes factors such as body posture, hand gestures, facial expressions, and eye contact. These factors can tell someone if the person speaking is stressed, annoyed, or even anxious.

PRACTICE POINT The nonverbal component of a message is the most important and is often deferred to when the listener is confused about the message being sent.

Being able to read a client's body language will help increase client compliance, because team members can alter their verbal conversation. Trust and compliance is also built when clients are able to read team members. Body language is a nonverbal form of communication that plays a key role in client education, trust, and therefore compliance.

Folded Arms

When a person has folded arms, it generally indicates that they are defensive and unwilling to accept recommendations or advice. If a client approaches a team member and the team member has folded arms, the client may feel uncomfortable about asking questions (role-playing will help teach team members to unfold arms while in the practice). A client with folded arms may be unwilling to accept recommendations and may have some underlying issues with the service being provided (Figure 11-3, *A*). A team member can correct this situation easily by handing the client something to hold. A brochure or a model of a joint (e.g., hip, knee, elbow) will force the person to unfold his or her arms; this will gradually open the lines for communication (Figure 11-3, *B*). Once this has occurred, the team member can continue educating the

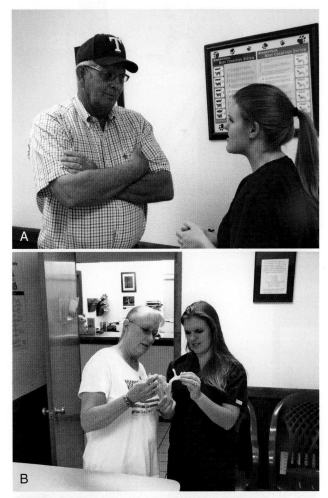

FIGURE 11-3 **A**, A client that has closed arms held close to the body may be defensive and unwilling to accept new information. **B**, Technician educating a client by handing her a model.

client and ask if there is any other information that the client needs. Team members should also make sure at this point that all the client's concerns have been addressed.

Body Posture

A team member's body posture sends a message to the client. If a team member enters an exam room slumped over, with head down and shoulders folded in, the client is going to feel that the team member lacks confidence and skill and does not enjoy his or her job (Figure 11-4). The client may not accept the recommendations that are advised simply because of the team member's poor body posture. Team members who are slumped over are likely to have quiet voices, lack energy, and appear unmotivated. Instead, team members should enter exam rooms with their heads up, a straight body posture, and shoulders back. This attitude will boast confidence, excitement, and skill. Clients will accept the recommendations that are made and develop a firm relationship with the team (Figure 11-5).

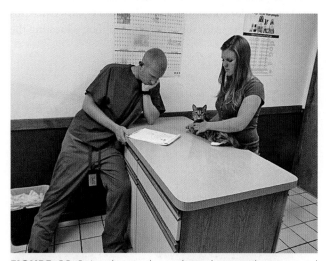

FIGURE 11-4 A technician that is slumped over and not engaged appears unprofessional to clients, resulting in lower compliance rates.

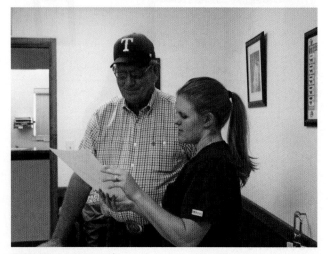

FIGURE 11-5 A professional team member standing up straight with shoulders held back.

Eye Contact and Facial Expressions

Eyes can communicate a large amount of emotion; when clients or team members are annoyed, rolling the eyes may be a subconscious response. Eyes can also show fear, confusion, sadness, stress, and joy.

While educating clients, maintain eye contact with them at all times. Lack of eye contact is perceived as diminished skill, knowledge, and confidence. When team members maintain eye contact, the client will feel more comfortable about accepting recommendations.

Facial expressions include smiling (or lack of) and can reveal the following emotions: happiness, anger, surprise, sadness, disgust, and fear. Other facial expressions include eyebrow movement, which can show the speaker that the listener is understanding the conversation that is taking place. When one is empathetic, the eyebrows are raised and the head tilts; often the listener will nod their head. Tense eyebrows can indicate confusion.

Improving Nonverbal Skills

Characteristics associated with *trust and confidence* include making strong eye contact, maintaining a tall posture and a peppy step (shows enthusiasm and joy), and using hand gestures to help relay information. Characteristics associated with *sincerity* include eye contact, tall posture, and facial expressions (nodding, tilting the head, and raised eyebrows).

> **PRACTICE POINT**   Nonveterinary team members drive 50% of the income in a hospital; effective communication is a large contributor to this number.

Barriers to Client Communications

There are different barriers that must be overcome with clients to increase client communications. Clients may appear nervous, defensive, or embarrassed. They may have language or cultural differences or may be hearing impaired. Team members may prejudge a client and make assumptions before a treatment plan is discussed with the client. This may prevent the best medicine from being offered to the client. Another barrier is listening. Team members must listen to the client (verbal and nonverbal) and be able to understand the client's perspective. Once these barriers have been identified and overcome, the communication can continue and be more effective.

Clients may become defensive or embarrassed when they feel they have not given their pet the best care or cannot afford the best care. Clients may have crossed arms, avoid making eye contact with team members, or only interact with the team when questions are asked. A caring, empathetic team member can easily break this barrier by finding something to compliment the pet on. Suddenly, clients may feel a small sense of pride and may become more open to suggestions and advice.

In various parts of the country, clients will have a different culture or speak a different language than that of team members. It is important to try to understand clients' cultural

differences and elements of their language to provide the best possible medicine to all clients. A specific team member might have a friend or an acquaintance that can educate the staff on a specific culture in the local area, as well as teach a few key terms in that particular language. It may also be of benefit to have a translator available to try to accommodate these clients. Nonverbal behavior varies from culture to culture. Differences are often expressed through gestures, eye contact, interpersonal distance, and touch. A client with folded arms may be insecure of the situation due to cultural differences rather than being upset. Again, this can be overcome by giving the client something to hold while team members are educating them on an important health care topic.

Another barrier to communication can come from team members. It can be extremely difficult to discuss an obese pet with an obese owner. It can also be difficult to discuss dental disease with a client who has bad teeth or no teeth at all. Role-playing different scenarios can overcome situations of this sort. Some clients may have more compassion for their pets than themselves and are willing to place Fluffy on a diet when the health benefits are discussed. By educating the client on the benefits of taking Fluffy outside for daily walks, the client will benefit. Many people show love for their pets by giving treats; however, a team member can show owners other ways to show love for their pets.

Putting It All Together

Listeners can receive confusing verbal, paraverbal, and nonverbal messages from the speaker. When this occurs, the default is to listen to the nonverbal message that is being relayed; hence the importance of knowing what signals team members are sending.

Once a team member has gained experience and knowledge about veterinary medicine, the client notes his or her confidence. Clients begin to feel they can trust the information that has been provided to them, and they develop a relationship with that team member. Clients that build relationships with team members have a higher compliance and retention rate compared to those that only have a relationship with the veterinarian. Nonveterinary team members drive passive income and should be responsible for developing 50% of the gross revenue for the practice. Team member confidence is a great asset to the practice and should be a top training priority for all employees.

> **PRACTICE POINT** Improving communication skills is an excellent continuing education topic that should be brought to the hospital team.

Professional appearance also helps increase client confidence in the veterinary team; clean, unwrinkled uniforms will help project authority and credibility. Team members who are compassionate, concerned, and interested in patients come across as more confident and will stimulate clients to ask more questions.

When delivering bad news to clients, it should be done in a professional, tactful environment. Team members should be empathetic and expect clients to be upset, angry, or emotional. Being prepared for the situation will help the team member diffuse it. Many times, it is the veterinarian that will deliver the news; however, team members should be ready in case they need to take the place of the doctor. Team members should speak slowly and listen to the clients' response. Clients may not fully understand the conversation; therefore it may be necessary to repeat the information. Written information should also be sent home with clients to ensure complete understanding.

Writing Skills

It is extremely important that staff members have excellent writing skills. Chapter 14 reviews the importance of completing medical records in a professional, legible manner. Team members must be able to verbally communicate procedures with clients, along with writing professional, educational, and clear discharge instructions for owners. The goal of written communications is to prevent miscommunications before they occur, prevent the owner from asking the same questions several times, and represent the business in a professional manner.

Team members must be able to write effective letters for different aspects of the practice. Collection letters, vaccine reaction letters, and letters of acclimation are just few letters that a doctor may request. Pets that have had a severe vaccine reaction in the past may have been advised by the veterinarian to withhold vaccinations in the future, and a letter may be required by the city or county as to why the client is not in compliance with the law. Airlines may require a letter of acclimation, indicating that a pet is healthy enough to fly at temperatures below 40° F or higher than 80° F. It is important that the letter only states the facts; do not embellish to make the letter longer.

Letters should include the date, the client's name, the pet's name, and the doctor's name. The pet's species, gender, and whether it has been altered may need to be added depending on what is needed. The problem needs to be addressed, along with the resolution.

All written documents must be proofread for spelling and grammatical errors. A person other than the writer (of the document) should review the document for errors. It is common for the author of a document to miss errors. Once the letter has been proofread, the doctor can then sign the letter.

Email Etiquette

Correspondence by email is becoming a popular choice of communication for clients. Email etiquette is just as important as letter writing and verbal skills. It must always be remembered that email can go anywhere, to anyone. Therefore emails should be kept short and sweet. Clients may take suggestions in email as insults, starting a terrible line of communication. In addition, emotions cannot be read in email; therefore a face-to-face visit is much more beneficial.

If a consultation is needed, the client should be advised to make an appointment with a veterinarian to discuss the case. In general, clients are not charged for the time the team or a veterinarian spends responding to emails.

When responding to an email, it is important to address the client by their name, answer the question(s) asked by the client, and sign the email in a professional manner; this includes the name of the team member who is responding to the email, as well as the practice's contact information, including the Web address and logo.

Client Compliance

There are many categories that contribute to client compliance. Client compliance is defined as the number or percentage of clients who accept recommendations made by the veterinary health care team. Verbal and written skills, reminders and recalls, marketing, education, and understanding client and patient needs are only a few areas that contribute to client compliance.

> **PRACTICE POINT** Client compliance is defined as the percentage of clients who accept recommendations given by the veterinary health care team.

Before client compliance can grow, clients must receive excellent service; they must have a reason to return to the veterinary practice. Trust, satisfaction, and quality of service must be established; the veterinarian-client relationship can span a lifetime and serve a variety of pets. Positive attitudes from team members who believe in the medicine the practice provides will radiate to clients. Excellent medicine and a team-based veterinary practice provide client satisfaction and a high quality of service.

Client compliance can be increased by verbal and written communications. Informing clients about diseases and treatment protocols encourages owners to accept recommendations. This information comes in the form of discussions with the client as well as any client education material available. Following up on the case and regularly sending reminders can also increase compliance.

Managers must track compliance rates in order to continue growing the business. Each profit center that the practice has must be analyzed, ensuring that compliance continues to grow. Areas to focus on include the dental center, surgery, wellness, heartworm and flea/tick preventatives, and preoperative lab work. Compliance can be tracked with a compliance formula (Box 11-1). Information can be obtained from the veterinary practice management software (when codes are used correctly).

Team members should be evaluated for their beliefs, communication techniques (both verbal and nonverbal),

BOX 11-1 | Compliance Formula

\# of patients who received service ÷ # of eligible patients × 100

and knowledge. Team members must believe in the services they are recommending and should be willing to perform the service on their own pets. The practice organization should have an overall evaluation for customer service and follow up with clients (consider having mystery shoppers visit the hospital and provide ratings).

Reminders and Recall Systems

Many software programs can automatically generate reminders and recalls for the veterinary team. Smaller practices may handwrite reminders on a monthly basis. Reminders are simply that; they remind owners that pets are due for a procedure. Practices may elect to send out reminders for a variety of services, including yearly exams and vaccines (based on the current vaccination protocol), heartworm testing, and a fecal analysis (depending on the location of the practice in the United States). Practices may also send out reminders for yearly laboratory work, including testing for hypothyroidism, phenobarbital levels, or bile acids for patients that are on long-term medications that may have potential side effects if not monitored closely. From a marketing perspective, hospitals may send out reminders for senior care exams or dental month (see Chapter 10). Communications can also be sent to remind clients to refill their pets' medications, including heartworm preventive and medications that treat hypothyroidism or hyperthyroidism, seizures, and allergies (Figures 11-6 and 11-7).

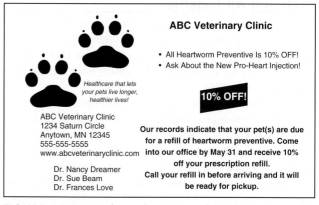

FIGURE 11-6 Reminder cards are a good way to maintain client relationships.

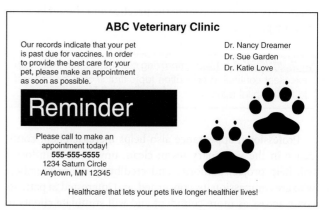

FIGURE 11-7 Reminder cards should grab a client's attention.

Reminders must be clear and concise and indicate what services are needed. They should state if *an appointment needs to be made.* Otherwise, a client may walk into the practice without an appointment, expecting to be seen for the services indicated on the card. Grammar and spelling must be correct, and the message must be inviting.

Reminder cards can be ordered from a variety of software companies or supply houses. Some systems may require a specific type of card to fit system or printer requirements; however, a variety of cards are available to choose from. Dogs, cats, puppies, and horses posing in different outfits and performing different tricks should grab a client's attention. Chapter 10 includes more helpful reminder ideas. Manufacturers also supply reminders for their particular product or service. Merial, Novartis, and Zoetis supply reminders for their vaccines, heartworm preventives, and products.

For practices that use pet portals, reminders can be customized to a particular patient, further enhancing client compliance. Clients feel good about an individualized reminder they receive, which makes them act to provide the best care for their pet. The "act" is the action they take (making an appointment) to enhance the relationship they have with their pet.

> **PRACTICE POINT** Clients are requesting pet portals and an online pharmacy available through the practice Web site.

Reminders can also come in the form of phone calls. Clients should be called the day before their appointments to remind them of surgical procedures or appointments that have been scheduled. Clients can be reminded of the surgical protocol to follow at that time as well. Those whose pets are due for yearly exams, lab work, and vaccinations should also be called as a friendly reminder. If a client needs to reschedule his or her appointment, it can be done at that time, allowing the team to fill the appointment spot with another patient.

In today's high-tech world, veterinary practices can send reminders by email, text message, and cell phone.

This is a relatively inexpensive way to connect with clients and remind them of services that are due for their pets. Computer software systems can be programmed to send either printed cards or email reminders, allowing many reminders to be sent at once. Follow-up reminders can then be generated for those who did not respond to the initial notice.

Reminder systems (whether manual or automatic) must be programmed to remove patients once they have died. It is emotionally distressing for a client to receive a reminder for a pet that has died, especially if the loss occurred at the veterinary hospital. It is not uncommon for a pet to suddenly die at home and for the owner not to inform the hospital of the death until receiving an appointment reminder. Team members should be empathetic, apologize, and guarantee that the owner will not receive another reminder.

Recalls are lists that are generated by veterinary software systems to remind staff to call certain clients to check on patients (Figure 11-8). Recalls can be created for surgical patients, pets that have received vaccines, or any patient that has been in the hospital for a period of time. Software systems allow team members to set a specific number of days for the recall to be generated. Certain charged services can also be linked to a recall generator, thereby creating a recall each time one of those services is entered.

Each day, reception teams can print lists and call clients to see how patients are progressing. This is a great time to ensure that the client was satisfied with the services and answer any remaining questions. If the client has any concerns or the pet has not progressed as expected, an appointment can be made with a specific doctor to recheck the patient. It should always be documented in the medical record when a recall was completed; details of the conversation and how the pet is recovering must be recorded.

Manual recall lists can also be generated by practices that do not use specialized software. A list can be kept in a small notebook with the client information and a brief reminder of the procedure. This is a well-organized way to help follow up with clients. Again, appointments can be made at this time if needed, and these conversations must be documented in the record.

Recall List   ABC Animal Clinic

Printed for dates 3/3/14-3/3/14

Acct no	Client	Patient	Phone	Procedure	Dr
428	Sharon Bean	Miss Kitty	123-458-0901	Fe OVH	ND
17266	Steve Doolittle	Lucky	345-234-1234	K9 OVH	ND
17266	Steve Doolittle	Cookie	345-234-1234	K9 OVH	ND
3427	Desiree Cloud	Scamp	456-123-1234	Dental	SM
6785	Nancy Shade	Wheeler	123-567-8901	K9 OVH	ND

FIGURE 11-8 Recall lists are generated for team members to call and check on patients.

Educational Information

There are many ideas that can increase client compliance, but it must be reiterated that client compliance starts with client education. If a client does not understand a procedure or have a trusting relationship with a veterinary hospital, the recommendations will not be accepted.

 Veterinary practice managers manage client education.

Educational information can come in a variety of forms. Speaking with the client, writing information down, and/or printing out information for the client to take home are the most efficient methods for providing information (Figure 11-9). Providing clients with written materials to take home and read will increase their knowledge and trust of the veterinary practice (Figure 11-10).

Clients will also search the Internet to get more information. Today's Internet is full of information; however, it is

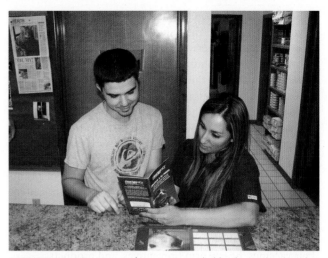

FIGURE 11-10 Written information provided by the veterinary technician will increase client understanding and encourage client compliance.

Dental Report Card

Last name_____ Pet _____ Date _____

Just like human beings, dogs are susceptible to plaque and tartar buildup that can lead to gingivitis and periodontitis, a chronic form of the disease that can be painful.

Stage 1—Gingivitis

Plaque and tartar buildup can lead to an infection causing inflammation of the gums around the dog's teeth. Gum tissue around the teeth can become inflamed and swollen.

Stage 2—Mild Periodontitis

Inflammation progresses to an infection that starts to destroy gum and bone tissue around the teeth. This can lead to discomfort for the dog, and bad breath may be noticeable.

Stage 3—Moderate Periodontitis

The continuing infection destroys more tissue around the teeth, often causing bleeding of gums and loosening of teeth. The discomfort and pain can affect eating habits.

Stage 4—Severe Periodontitis

Extensive infection is tearing down even more of the attachment tissues (gum and bone). Teeth are at risk of being lost.

Periodontal disease, which includes gingivitis and periodontitis, is an inflammation and/or infection of the gums and bone around a dog's teeth. It is caused by bacteria that accumulate in the mouth, forming soft plaque that later hardens into tartar. If untreated, periodontal disease can eventually lead to tooth loss.

Over time, plaque and tartar buildup can lead to inflammation of the gums around the dog's teeth: **gingivitis.**

Periodontitis is a potentially irreversible infection that, if left untreated, can result in the destruction of gum and bone and other tissues around the teeth. In most severe cases, periodontitis can ultimately lead to loss of teeth, fracture of the jawbones, and other serious consequences that can dramatically affect quality of life and overall health. Whenever possible, preventing disease is preferable to treating it!

Dental disease can also lead to cardiac and/or kidney disease. The bacteria that collect in your pet's mouth also circulate throughout the body, contributing to a variety of other diseases.

The good news is that periodontal disease can be prevented with a good dental care program, including:

- Daily home oral care: brushing your pet's teeth can be fun!
- Dental toys: rope toys, rawhides that are dissolvable, and Denta-Bones. Remember, hard toys can fracture teeth. Any chew toy should be slightly pliable.
- NEVER give you pet beef, chicken, or pork bones!
- Veterinary dental cleaning as advised.

FIGURE 11-9 Client education is important to client compliance.

sometimes incorrect. Veterinary team members must understand the client is being proactive on the pet's account in searching for current information; a practice must embrace the idea and filter the information as much as possible. Practice Web sites should contain information for the client to search, both for public access and private access (through their pet portal).

Clients will not remember all the information they were advised of while they were in the clinic. The more printed documentation they receive, the more information they will retain, once they get home and review it. Team members should be available to answer basic client questions; once the client has gained enough experience on the topic, a veterinarian may be needed to answer further questions.

PRACTICE POINT Client educational materials must have a professional appearance. Poorly designed handouts and subpar copies contribute to a negative perception that the client will develop of the practice.

Practices can print customized brochures, handouts, and personalized client instructions to provide the most current and correct information to clients (Figure 11-11). Veterinary software programs have educational materials that print the names of the practice name, client, and patient on a document titled with a specific topic or disease. The benefit to these computer-based documents is the customization that can be done to make them truly client oriented.

Acute Colitis

Acute colitis is a sudden inflammation of the colon. The most common signs are diarrhea and straining to defecate. The stools are often soft and contain blood or mucus. The condition can be caused by infection, eating garbage or foreign materials, intestinal parasites, changes in diet, and even emotional upsets.

Because the exact cause is often difficult to determine, the condition is usually treated symptomatically the first time. If there are recurrences, a more extensive search for the cause is advised.

Important Points in Treatment:

1. Lab tests are often necessary to diagnose the condition and monitor the effectiveness of treatment.

2. Give all medications as directed. Please call the doctor if you cannot give the medication.

3. Diet: _____ Feed a normal diet
   _____ Feed a prescription diet _____
   _____ A special diet: feed mixture of 4 parts boiled white rice to 1 part boiled ground beef, turkey, or chicken. Feed small amounts every 4-6 hours or as follows:_____
   _____
   _____

4. Activity:_____ Allow normal activity
   _____ Restrict activity as follows: _____
   _____
   _____

5. Water: _____ Allow free access to fresh water at all times.
   _____ Restrict water intake as follows: _____
   _____
   _____

Notify the doctor if any of the following occurs:
   - Your pet refuses to eat the recommended food.
   - Your pet's symptoms reoccur after an apparent recovery.
   - Your pet is reluctant to eat and/or loses weight.
   - There is a change in your pet's health.

FIGURE 11-11 Sample client information handout.

Client education manuals are also available for purchase from educational companies. These manuals are either a loosely bound binder or a CD of Word documents; the information needed can be removed and copied (or printed from the CD), then returned to the binder.

Practices can also produce brochures that are unique to the individual practice. Graphic designers can create professional-looking brochures for a nominal fee. Team members with design experience can use Microsoft Publisher to produce professional-looking brochures and print them on a small color printer in the office. Only a small number of brochures should be printed so that changes can be made to the brochure, because procedures may change throughout the course of the year. Chapter 10 includes more information on producing a quality educational brochure.

Practices may also wish to develop a client education center; organizational structures such as those in Figure 11-12 allow easy access to educational materials, promoting the use of such literature.

Messages may need to be repeated several times for clients to retain the information. Clients tend to suffer from sensory overload with all the information they receive in a veterinary practice; therefore it is imperative that information be concise, correct, and simple to read. Studies indicate that 90% of new information learned will be lost within 30 minutes if not reinforced. Repeat, repeat, and repeat. The more clients hear and read a message, the more they will retain the information. The receptionists, veterinary technicians, and veterinarians can drive consistent messages. The more consistent the message, the higher the rate of client compliance.

Manufacturers also provide a variety of professional posters that relate to current medical topics; these come at no charge to practices that use their products (Figure 11-13). These posters should be changed on a regular basis, providing a new look to the clients each time they arrive at the practice.

Treatment Plans (Estimates)

All clients should be provided with an estimate of costs for procedures and services that will be performed on their pets (also referred to as treatment plans). Treatment plans are a major part of client communication and are the most common complaint for state board investigators when clients air grievances against veterinary practices. Clients must be educated regarding the procedures their pets are going to receive. Second, they must fully accept the treatment plan provided. If any charges or procedures change from the original plan, the client should be called and informed.

> **PRACTICE POINT** Treatment plans decrease client sticker shock and improve client communication, both of which increase client compliance.

Treatment plans can be developed and preprinted for simple outpatient procedures such as yearly exams, anal sac expressions, or nail trims, or for inpatient procedures such as routine spays, neuters, and laceration repairs. Patients that are to be admitted to the hospital must have a detailed treatment plan provided, and it must be developed for each individual patient. Further, two separate treatment plans should be provided for patients admitted to the hospital: a diagnostic plan and a patient treatment plan. The diagnostic plan includes all medical services and tests needed to diagnose the problem; the treatment plan should cover all services needed to treat the patient, including medications to go home when the patient is released. Providing two separate plans prevents the team from underestimating, missing charges, or providing an inaccurate estimate when the diagnosis changes as a result of tests.

Knowledgeable, empathetic team members should present treatment plans; veterinarians should be left out of the financial discussion, as their job is to *diagnose, prescribe medications, and perform surgery*, not discuss finances. When presenting treatment plans, the team member must be able to discuss the treatment options with confidence. Using models and brochures to help explain specific procedures will help clients understand what is being recommended for their pet. Body language plays a significant role (along with knowledge and confidence) in client compliance. Along with the positive

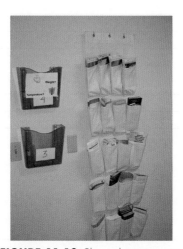

FIGURE 11-12 Client education center.

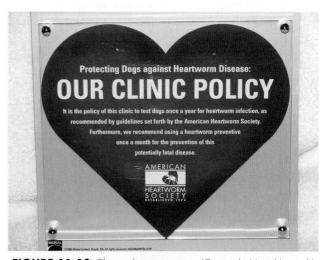

FIGURE 11-13 Client education poster. (Copyright Merial Limited.)

characteristics described previously, team members should stand beside the client to deliver the plan, not across the exam room table (Figure 11-14). The exam table provides a barrier, which indirectly affects client compliance. Other barriers must also be taken into consideration, which were discussed earlier in this chapter.

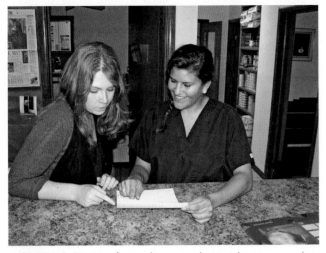

FIGURE 11-14 A professional team member standing next to a client will receive better compliance when presenting a treatment plan.

Estimates should persuade clients to ask questions and encourage discussion regarding the medicine their pets will be receiving. If clients are not asking questions, they may be confused or overwhelmed, and the team member must ask if they understand the procedures being recommended.

Treatment plans can also foster the discussion of deposits and the hospital's payment policy. Some clients will need time to think about the estimate provided and discuss financing options with a spouse. It is advised to present a treatment plan to a client and leave the exam room, giving them time to process the information that have just received. Team members can then go back into the exam room after a few minutes to answer any questions the client may have. For treatment plans presented on the phone, clients may need to call the practice back with approval or decline of diagnostics based on a discussion with a significant other.

Clients should sign estimates, indicating that they agree to the procedures and are financially responsible for the charges (Figure 11-15). They must also be updated both medically and financially, on a (minimum) daily basis. Anytime additional diagnostic tests or treatments are to be added on, the client must be called with an updated estimate of costs.

Managers should monitor delivery of treatment plans and client compliance. Some team members will have

---

ABC Veterinary Clinic
123 Saturn Circle
Anytown, MN 12345
(555) 555-5555

CHARGE ESTIMATION

Account: 19902
Date: 07/31/13
Page: 1

Sharon White	Phone (123) 678-6789		Patient: Marshmallow
Code	Service/Item	Qty	Amount
0216	Office call	1	$35.54
0920	IV catheter	1	$37.90
0924	IV fluids per liter	2-3	$31.28-$46.92
0916	IV care daily	2	$38.48
909	Hospitalization, routine	1-2	$32.48-65.68
4150	Urinary catheter	1	$32.48
0302	Anesthesia	1	$104.36
3815	General health profile	1	$91.24

ESTIMATE TOTAL $403.76-$422.60

THIS IS ONLY AN ESTIMATE AND DOES NOT INCLUDE SALES TAX. The actual diagnostic treatment plan may require more medications and/or procedures. The range of estimate may vary. This estimate is valid for 30 days only.

I have read and understand this estimate. I understand that I must leave a deposit before the procedure, and the balance must be paid when my pet is released from the hospital.

Signature _____ Date _____

FIGURE 11-15 Sample estimate.

exceptionally high rates of success when delivering treatment plans; others may need additional training, either on medical topics or customer service skills. It is also advised to review treatment plans, ensuring they contain client-friendly words. If a client does not understand the line item, they are more likely to decline the service; for example, the word "ovariohysterectomy" should be replaced with "spay" to help gain client acceptance. If the compliance rate is not being managed, it cannot be improved.

When clients decline recommendations that are being made, team members should ask the client why they are declining (this can be an uncomfortable question at first; role-play the scenario to build confidence). Asking clients "why" allows team members to document the reason in the medical record, and allows team members to learn from the experience, helping them improve treatment plan delivery. A study published in the *Journal of the American Veterinary Medical Association* indicated that out of 10 clients, 2 declined the recommendations due to finances; the remainder declined service because they did not feel the recommended treatment was necessary.*

Standards of Care

One of the most important aspects of veterinary medicine is the level of care provided to the patient. Standards of Care must be met, or the veterinarian could be held negligent if a case is not managed properly. Clients expect standards to be met, and patients deserve it. In addition, the veterinary team is guilty of "judging a clients wallet", meaning that the team will offer a sub standard treatment plan because they "feel" the client will not be able to afford the recommended services. This is unfair to the client, and patient.

To prevent this from occurring, Standards of Care (SOC) should be developed for all diseases and procedures recommended by the team. SOCs do not mandate how medicine must be practiced; it instead provides guidelines for all team members to make the same recommendations, to every client, every time.

Some benefits of SOCs include:

- *New doctors will know what is expected in the care of their patients*: Starting out as a new doctor can be nerve racking, and they often feel that they are asking too many questions. SOCs will provide guidance, allowing them to feel more confident, which encourages the client to *feel* better about the person caring for their pet.
- *The addition of new team members*: Since different practices have different protocols and procedures, SOCs will help new team members "get on the same page". The team member will know what to expect, and what to recommend to clients.
- *Protocols in writing help to prevent confusion or misunderstandings, creating team member and client consistency*: When *every* team member knows what the protocol will be, *every* team member can educate *every* client. The client

will hear the same consistent message every time they call or arrive in the practice. Consistent, confident recommendations drive client trust and compliance.

Developing SOCs can seem overwhelming at first. Start simple, and pick the top 10 outpatient procedures (this may include treatment of ear infections, pancreatitis or parasite prevention). Once 10 have been written, create 10 more, until all of the procedures and have been developed. Start the first section with a general description and recommendations that would be made for any patient experiencing this condition (or disease prevention). The second section should include compliance protocols and the third section will include product choices that the practice carries to treat the patient. Since most practices carry two products to treat or prevent diseases, both should be listed.

Because diseases and disease prevention vary (as do recommendations in different parts of the country), the SOCs will also vary in structure. Each SOC should be developed in accordance with the practices values and recommendations made by AAHA and AVMA. Ensure that they are simple to understand (every team member must be able to interpret the recommendations), and are reevaluated on a yearly basis. Protocols, treatments and medications change frequently; therefore updates are required.

Ensuring Client Understanding

Client education is central to client compliance. Clients who do not understand a policy, procedure, or service will not comply with recommendations. Clients cannot ask for services they are unaware of, nor can they ask for services that they do not comprehend. Client education can fail for many reasons, including lack of team member time, concern, or compassion; poorly educated staff; or the unwillingness of clients to comply.

> **PRACTICE POINT** If clients do not understand the need for a service, they will not accept it. Identify areas within the practice that will enhance client education and understanding of services.

Clients, like team members, learn and understand information in a variety of ways. Some may learn better with visual aids, such as pictures, videos, and illustrations. Others may learn better with verbal communication. Team members must be able to determine what the most successful way will be to educate an individual client. Client education should be a positive, enthusiastic experience. Words should be simple and understandable. Many clients are embarrassed to admit that they do not understand medical terms. If they do not understand the terms, they will not comprehend the information provided. A combination of materials should be available to aid in client education. Customized brochures from manufacturers, posters, videos, and CDs that clients can take home will help reiterate information that was presented while the client was in the practice. Skeletal models

* Lue TW, Pantenburg DP, Crawford PM: Impact of the owner-pet and client-veterinarian bond on the care that pets receive. *J Am Vet Med Assoc* 2008 Feb 15;232(4)4:531-40.

and radiographs showing both normal and abnormal findings will help the clients visualize the procedure or abnormality affecting their pets.

WHAT WOULD YOU DO/NOT DO?

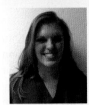 Megan, a veterinary technician is checking in a cat that is 15 years old. Conner has been vomiting for the last couple of days, but still seems to have interest in eating and has normal bowl movements. Megan continues gathering the history on the patient, and begins to take the temperature of Conner. Ms. Coffman abruptly states, "He does not have a fever! He does not need his temperature taken! Why do you guys insist on always taking his temperature? All you do is make him uncomfortable! He already hates coming to this place as it is!" Megan, surprised by the sudden outburst, slowly places the thermometer on the table, collects the medical record and leaves the room, without commenting.

What Should Megan Have Done?

First, Megan may have let Ms. Coffman know that it is hospital policy that the all patients presented to the hospital are required to have a temperature taken, and this must be completed before the veterinarian enters the room. She could explain that body temperature is a vital sign, and that many times, vital signs change with disease. She may also state that it is common for patients to have a fever with an infection; the explanation may have allowed her to continue with the process of taking the temperature.

Alternatively, Megan may ask her supervisor to help her, who can explain the protocol to Ms. Coffman. Megan is already beside herself with the comment and may need someone in a superior position to help explain the procedure in a clearer manner. Having someone else explain the procedure will also prevent Megan from communicating in a defensive manner, which can be perceived as abrasive or rude by the client. Just because the client was abrasive does not give Megan the right to be abrasive in return. Some clients have other issues occurring in their life (recent loss of a loved one, divorce, etc.), which can cause sudden outbursts to unintended targets. This is a client service industry, and every client should be treated with respect, and treated as one would want to be treated.

Understanding Client and Patient Needs

Team members who understand both clients and patients to the fullest extent will have the highest compliance acceptance rates. Many team members can excel at one but not the other, and it takes time, practice, and patience to excel at both. There are different types of clients. Calm, honest, and happy clients may be considered one type. Mean, arrogant, and "know it all" clients can be another. Some can be angry at the world and untrustworthy, and sometimes lack funds. Another type may lack funds but are happy and willing to accept the best recommendations available for their financial situation. Different approaches are needed to best

handle the various types of clients, and patient care must never be forgotten, whichever the client's personality type. Every patient must receive the best possible recommendations, regardless of its owner; determining how to deliver recommendations to each of these types of clients must be mastered.

When communicating with clients, different techniques may be necessary to maximize communications. Some clients may need basic words; others may understand medical terminology. Some clients require choices; others cannot be given options and must be told "what to do." Team members should be able to read clients within 30 seconds and determine the best communication technique for a given situation.

The first type of client (calm, honest, and happy), are the clients every team member dreams of serving. These individuals allow the team to practice the best medicine because they follow recommendations and are polite to work with. They appreciate education and want to learn about their pets' conditions; they will look up information on the Internet and ask questions.

The second type of client (mean, arrogant, and know it all), can be extremely frustrating for team members. These people are perceived as being angry at the world; if team members can remember that, then the comments made by these clients will not be taken personally. Know-it-all clients can be easy to deal with; simply hand them printed client education materials to correct their mistaken information. Once they get home and read the information, they can correct themselves instead of the team trying to make that change.

The angry client who lacks funds can be the most degrading for team members to deal with. These are the clients who may exclaim to team members, "You don't care about my animal! All you care about is the money!" They want to be able to charge the service and then never return to pay. They can belittle the staff quickly; managers should step in and stop this action immediately. Team members do not deserve this treatment, and clients of this mentality should be "fired." Veterinary team members are in their profession because they love animals and *want* to do what is best for patients, regardless of a client's finances.

The final type of clients can be rewarding but sometimes frustrating for some team members. Clients who are lacking in funds cannot follow the best recommendations for their pet. However, these clients love their pets and will do what they can with the limited finances available. These clients are honest about their finances and usually will pay any services that they have charged. Making options available for these clients is rewarding. Finding a solution that works for the client, the pet, and the team can be challenging, but the client will be grateful for the service provided.

What Do Clients Really Want?

Before team members can relate to clients, they must be able to identify what clients really want. Veterinary practices may elect to send out a survey to clients to ask what they want in a veterinary hospital. Typical responses can be classified into

several categories: appreciation, listening, help, honesty, care, and understanding.

PRACTICE POINT Identify client needs through surveys and interviews with the top 10% of clients.

Clients want to be *appreciated* for coming to a specific veterinary practice and not another. Clients want to be appreciated when recommending new clients. Furthermore, clients want to be appreciated for the care they have given their animals. Identify areas where the practice can step up client appreciation, further driving customer service skills.

Clients want team members to *listen*. Clients want to tell stories about their pets (for some, this is their "child") and to be appreciated for telling them. Team members can be poor listeners when they are only thinking of the next question to ask. It is important to listen, remain nonjudgmental, and avoid making assumptions. Listening builds client relationships; long-lasting relationships build compliance and referrals.

Open-ended questions should be asked; who, what, when, where, and why will help the team *listen* to the clients' answers.

Clients want *help* without asking for it. Excellent team members will take the extra step to help clients to the car with their pets or a bag of food. Helping clients establishes an excellent client-practice bond.

Clients want *honesty*. They do not want to be lied to or advised of only one treatment option regarding their pet. They want the clear-cut truth, to receive education about all options available, and be referred to a specialist when needed. If a team member does not know the answer to a question that has been asked, clients want them to honestly find an answer, not just respond, "I don't know."

Clients want to know that the staff *cares* about their pets. They want the receptionist to care when they call, and they want the kennel attendant to care when they pick their pet up. Compassion and empathy are required on the part of the veterinary health care team.

Last but not least, clients want *understanding*. They want the team to understand their particular situation, whether it is financial or personal. The majority of clients are willing to pay for services, regardless of price, if the team satisfies their *wants*. The client has perceived and understood the value of the practice when all of the "wants" have been met.

Focus on identifying client needs and wants when looking to add new clients and increase compliance rates. Offering exceptional customer service will also help meet these goals.

Client Surveys

Surveys can be mailed to clients, given to them as they are checking out with the receptionist, or emailed. Surveys should be kept short and simple, because clients will more likely comply and return the survey. Client surveys are an easy monitoring solution to help understand client satisfaction and level of comfort with the services the practice provides. Surveys should be changed every few months, which

will help managers target specific areas of improvement. Ideas of topics to place on surveys include:

- Value of service: Did the client feel they received the value for what they paid?
- How long was the wait time?
- Was the team knowledgeable and able to answer questions?
- Was the veterinarian courteous and respectful?
- When a practice is focusing on obesity management, an additional question may be: Did you receive information on activities you could do with your pet to prevent or reduce obesity?
- If the practice is focusing on dental disease prevention, an additional question may be: Did you learn about methods you could do at home to help prevent gum disease in your pet's mouth?

Veterinary practice managers obtain and report client feedback on service.

Clients maintain the business; therefore it is imperative to make sure they are satisfied and receive value for the service provided. If clients are unsatisfied, practices want to be notified and given the opportunity to address the problem; unfortunately, many clients will not notify the practice; they just go to another hospital. Practices do not want to lose clients or have negative comments made about them throughout the community. It is very important to strive for a high level of satisfaction from every client (Figure 11-16).

Handling Client Complaints and Grievances

Clients may be frustrated for a variety of reasons that are not related to the medicine itself, but rather, customer service. Others may be frustrated because they do not feel they were provided the best medicine possible. Whatever the client complaint is, it must be handled appropriately, professionally, and quickly.

Veterinary practice managers handle client complaints.

It is imperative that team members not become defensive when discussing complaint issues with clients. When team members get defensive, the intensity and emotion of the conversation rises, and clients become more upset. Team members should immediately take the distraught or angry client to a quiet exam room, away from other clients. Emotions can be more intense when other people are around; therefore taking clients to a quiet room can quickly diffuse the intensity. Team members should listen to what the client has to say. Eye contact should be maintained throughout the conversation. Let the client air the complaint before asking any questions. Once the client has finished, the team member should repeat what was said, ensuring no miscommunication arises. Once the client and team member agree

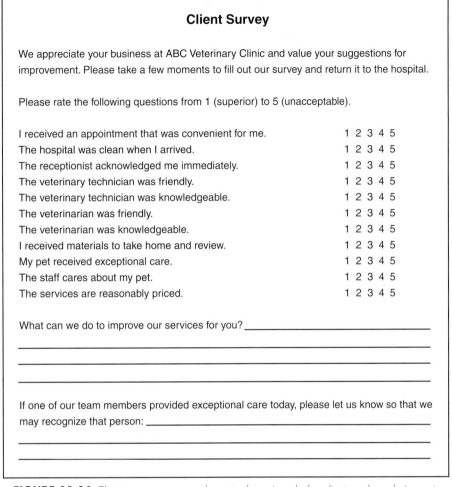

Client Survey

We appreciate your business at ABC Veterinary Clinic and value your suggestions for improvement. Please take a few moments to fill out our survey and return it to the hospital.

Please rate the following questions from 1 (superior) to 5 (unacceptable).

I received an appointment that was convenient for me.	1 2 3 4 5
The hospital was clean when I arrived.	1 2 3 4 5
The receptionist acknowledged me immediately.	1 2 3 4 5
The veterinary technician was friendly.	1 2 3 4 5
The veterinary technician was knowledgeable.	1 2 3 4 5
The veterinarian was friendly.	1 2 3 4 5
The veterinarian was knowledgeable.	1 2 3 4 5
I received materials to take home and review.	1 2 3 4 5
My pet received exceptional care.	1 2 3 4 5
The staff cares about my pet.	1 2 3 4 5
The services are reasonably priced.	1 2 3 4 5

What can we do to improve our services for you? _____
_____
_____
_____

If one of our team members provided exceptional care today, please let us know so that we may recognize that person: _____
_____
_____

FIGURE 11-16 Client surveys are a good way to determine whether client needs are being met.

on the event that has occurred, the team member may offer some solutions to satisfy the client. Once clients are able to voice their concerns, their anger tends to drop a level. Once it is repeated back to them and it appears the team member has understood their side of the story, the anger level drops another level. When solutions are offered, clients feel satisfied that their problem(s) would be handled appropriately.

PRACTICE POINT   Client grievances must be handled immediately and professionally. Those that are not will contribute to a decrease in client retention and compliance and make it difficult to acquire new clients.

Solutions that may be presented to clients may be as simple as adjusting the invoice. Other solutions that may satisfy clients are to let them know a new policy or procedure may be enacted (because of this particular dilemma), that team member education will increase, and/or client education will change to prevent this particular scenario from occurring again. Clients are satisfied when they realize that they can make a difference. Although it may be hard for a team member to say "thank you" after a client discussion of this caliber, it is necessary; *thank you is a powerful phrase to a client.*

At times, the client may not understand a procedure or service that was performed, and regardless of the steps a team member has taken to calm the client, the client will remain irate. It is at this time, the team member must step aside and ask for help from another team member to resolve the situation. Emotions, defenses (nonverbal communication), and communication barriers have prevented client satisfaction from being accomplished. All team members must realize that arguing and confrontation will not resolve a conflict. If a team member has become emotionally involved in an unresolved discussion, another team member must step in and remove the initial member from the confrontation. Emotions will escalate quickly; other clients will hear the argument and staff stress levels will grow. It is important for the entire team to prevent discussions from reaching a higher emotional intensity.

If a client becomes abusive toward a team member despite the team member having taken every step possible to calm the person, the client should be asked to leave the premises. A discussion can continue when the emotions have subsided. If a client will not leave the property when asked, the police

should be called immediately. Staff and client safety should always be a concern. Today's society cannot be trusted to not harm others. A client may be under the influence of an illegal substance or may have some psychological issues that are uncontrolled. Once the client's emotions have subsided, a telephone call can be made by team members to find a solution to the issue at hand.

When clients present problems to team members, it should be taken as a learning experience. Clients perceive actions, conversations, and procedures differently than team members do. If one client perceives an action one way, others may as well. It is important to be proactive and prevent problems from arising, rather than being reactive and solving problems only after clients have become upset.

Handling Negative Reviews on the Internet

With technology today, negative reviews of the hospital can be posted within minutes; hence the importance of addressing negative situations immediately. Every team member should possess the skill and knowledge to satisfy a client if the manager is not present to handle the situation.

However, sometimes as quick as the team is, negative comments will still surface. The recommended response to these online complaints is, *"I am so sorry you have had this experience at our hospital. Please call as soon as possible so that we can resolve this situation."* Do not attempt to defend the hospital or any actions that were taken in the response; doing so will ignite a fury of comments. If the client does not call within a few days, add an additional reply to the complaint indicating you have been waiting for their call, which you have not received, and again, *"please call as soon as possible to resolve the situation."* Please see Chapter 10 for more information regarding the management of online reviews.

If the client returns the call, and the situation was resolved to the practice's (and client's) satisfaction, one may ask the client to post an additional review indicating a solution was reached. Otherwise, practices may solicit other clients to post positive reviews about the practice. As more positive reviews are posted, the negative review will drop lower on the list.

Managers must learn to be proactive rather than reactive, and develop methods to prevent client complaints before difficult situations develop and require resolution. Clients know what good and bad customer service is; the medicine may be spectacular, but if the customer service is poor, negative reviews will be posted. Therefore analyzing all aspects of customer service in the hospital is a must.

Customer Service

There is no question that all of the previously discussed topics contribute to excellent customer service. As stated earlier, clients know what good customer service is, and have grown to expect it when they visit veterinary hospitals.

> **PRACTICE POINT**   Review every facet of the client interaction; identify areas where customer service could be improved, not only to meet the client needs, but to exceed what is expected.

Veterinary practices depend on clients returning to the hospital and referring their friends and family. Without exceptional service, these will not occur.

Team members must strive to make every visit memorable, not just mediocre. If a service is simply mediocre, the hospital down the street may have a better service, and the client will change hospitals. Consider every facet of client interaction and determine what can be done to make that interaction "the best experience." What is it like when phone shoppers call the hospital? Is the receptionist pleasant and informative, or is she too rushed to answer inquiries? What does the hospital look and smell like when clients enter? Are they greeted with compassionate team members? What is the client's experience in the reception area? Can they hear team members gossiping? What is the client's experience in the exam room? How long do they have to wait to be seen? Do team members communicate delays? What is the client's experience at check out? Does every client experience the same medical approach and have the best medicine offered? Review Chapter 2 for more excellent client service tips.

Client Retention

Client development and retention are critical elements that lead to a successful practice. Excellent customer service plays a major role in client satisfaction, resulting in returning clients. The veterinary team plays a significant role in building and maintaining the human-animal bond. Team members educate clients about health care issues from the first visit. Reminders, recalls, and client education can have a positive effect on this bond. It is no secret that retaining clients is much cheaper than obtaining new clients.

Veterinary practice managers monitor client retention.

Some clients will leave a practice for reasons beyond the practice's control. Some clients may move, change jobs, or lose a pet. Some clients may have not established a relationship with the practice and are willing to try another practice because it is closer to their home. In general, a small-animal practice will lose 10% to 15% of clients each year. The goal should be to retain 70% to 75% over a 3-year period.

To retain clients, team members must know the clients' expectations, and practices must meet or exceed those expectations. Positive experiences should be created for each and every client. Once the goals have been met and a positive experience has been created, customers are satisfied, resulting in loyal customers who recommend the practice to family, friends, and co-workers.

VETERINARY PRACTICE and the LAW

When a telephone call concerns an emergency, the team member becomes responsible to provide immediate assistance. The most desirable response for a team member is to place the call with a veterinarian or a team member that can provide assistance. If one is not available, the receptionist may need to provide comfort and ask questions determining the extent of the emergency.

Treatment procedures cannot be given over the phone without the direct consultation with the veterinarian. If a client has a concern, team members must advise owners to immediately bring their pet in for an exam. Any advice given over the phone can be misconstrued, leading to a poor resolution that may place the practice in jeopardy of a malpractice lawsuit.

Each receptionist team should keep an emergency procedural manual in the front office; the manual should list specific questions to ask and specific answers to provide. The name of the client, patient, and a phone number should be written down, allowing record documentation and a follow-up call if the client never arrives at the practice.

REVIEW QUESTIONS

1. Why are verbal and written skills imperative in veterinary medicine?
2. What is client compliance and how can it be achieved?
3. What are the benefits of a reminder system?
4. Create an example that can enhance client education.
5. What would be an appropriate body stance when addressing clients?
6. Why is body posture important?
7. How should an angry client be handled?
8. How can common barriers be overcome?
9. Why are estimates important?
10. How can individual verbal image be improved?
11. The portion of a message that involves facial expressions is:
    a. Verbal
    b. Paraverbal
    c. Nonverbal
    d. Written
12. If a listener receives a confusing message, which portion of the message will they rely on for a better understanding?
    a. Verbal
    b. Paraverbal
    c. Nonverbal
    d. Written
13. The percentage of clients who accept a recommendation is known as:
    a. Compliance
    b. Retention
    c. Turnover
    d. Quantity
14. Client education should be available in which of the following forms?
    a. Web page
    b. Printed materials
    c. Verbal education
    d. Models and videos
    e. All of the above
15. Which team member should present treatment plans to clients?
    a. Veterinarians
    b. Receptionists
    c. Veterinary technicians
    d. b and c

Recommended Reading

Durrance D, Lagoni L: *Connecting with clients: practical communication for 10 common situations,* ed 2, Lakewood, CO, 2010, AAHA Press.
Heinke MM: *Practice made perfect: a guide to veterinary practice management,* ed 2, Lakewood, CO, 2012, AAHA Press.
Klingborg J: *Exam room communication for veterinarians: the science and art of conversing with clients;* Lakewood, CO, 2011, AAHA Press.
Renfrew J: *AAHA's complete guide for the veterinary client service representative;* Lakewood, CO, 2013, AAHA Press.
Smith CA: *Client satisfaction pays: quality service for practice success,* ed 2, Lakewood, 2009, COAAHA Press.

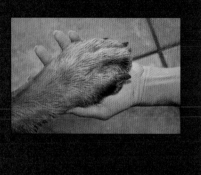

KEY TERMS

Anger
Bargaining
Cremation
Denial
Depression
Euthanasia
Human-Animal Bond

Interacting with a Grieving Client

OUTLINE

Understanding the Human-Animal
   Bond, *229*
Understanding Euthanasia, *230*
The Euthanasia Procedure, *230*

Pet Memorials, *231*
Cremations, *231*
   Owners Picking up Remains, *232*
Understanding and Dealing with Grief, *234*

LEARNING OBJECTIVES

When you have completed this chapter, you should be able to:

1. Define the human-animal bond.
2. Differentiate between quality and quantity of life.
3. Identify the euthanasia process.
4. List types of pet memorials that are available.
5. Define the five stages of grief.
6. Discuss client solutions to help cope with the loss.
7. Explain euthanasia to children.
8. Define pet depression.

CRITICAL COMPETENCIES

1. **Adaptability** - being open to change and flexible work methods; the ability to adapt behavior to changing conditions or new information.
2. **Oral Communication and Comprehension** - the ability to express one's thoughts verbally in a clear and understandable manner, and the ability to actively listen and attend to what others are saying; must have good group presentation skills.
3. **Resourcefulness** - the ability to understand what it takes to complete the job; apply knowledge, skills, and expertise to perform tasks quickly and efficiently.

Understanding the Human-Animal Bond

The human-animal bond is an emotional bond that forms as a benefit to both humans and animals (Figure 12-1). Each party treats the other with mutual respect, trust, devotion, and love. To some clients, pets are their children; to others, pets are their best friends. Whichever connection has been developed, it is generally a long-lasting relationship (Figure 12-2).

This bond is strengthened by the veterinary health care team. Each time the client visits, the bond is strengthened as the owner receives further education on how to help care for his or her pet. Team members who are empathetic and encourage the human-animal bond are cherished and tend to be requested by clients. These team members are usually employed over the long term by a veterinary practice and may have the experience of seeing a pet for its first visit and following its progress until its last visit. These team members will face grieving issues with long-term clients.

Many clients do not have the support of the human-animal bond in their home or work environments. A spouse may feel a pet needs to live outside, whereas the other partner feels the pet should sleep in the bed. In working environments, a client's fellow employees may not understand why the client would need to take the day off work because their pet is having surgery. The veterinary team supports this strong bond; many times, the veterinary hospital is the only place they can receive this support (Figure 12-3).

Sometimes, clients may come to the veterinary practice to euthanize an animal because they are unable to see their current veterinarian. Although these clients have not established a relationship with the staff, team members must remember the clients are grieving. Clients show grief in different ways, and team members may see the worst of the grieving process. Some clients may appear angry with the team when, in reality, this may be the way the client deals with the pain of losing a best friend. If a pet is euthanized or dies in the hospital, clients may appear frustrated and accuse the hospital of not providing the best service possible.

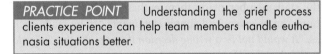

PRACTICE POINT   Understanding the grief process clients experience can help team members handle euthanasia situations better.

An excellent way to handle clients of this type is to listen. Active listeners keep eye contact and nod their heads in understanding. Let the clients talk about their frustrations. Once they can discuss the situation, their anger begins to resolve, especially when they feel team members understand and are empathetic with their frustration. This

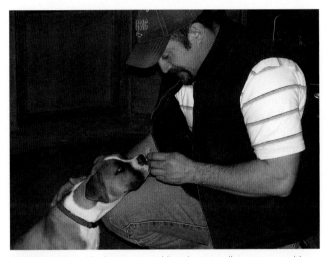

FIGURE 12-1 The human-animal bond is typically a strong and long-lasting one.

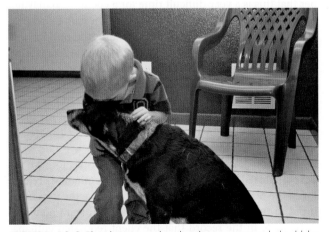

FIGURE 12-2 The decision to bond with a new animal should be left to the client experiencing the loss. Bonding with a new pet should be viewed as a tribute to the love and companionship shared with the previous animal.

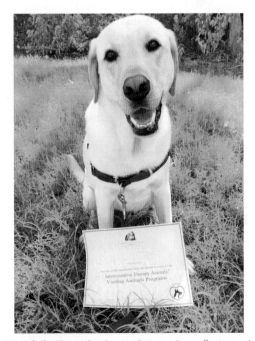

FIGURE 12-3 Clients that lose a therapy dog suffer more than just grief. They also lose the confidence and independence that the pet provided.

is not the time to become defensive for the team; it is the time to listen and respond with simple responses such as, *"I understand your frustration, Mrs. Smith, I will certainly look into this."* or, *"I know you loved Fluffy, Mrs. Smith. She was very special. You provided the best care possible. I will take care of these issues."* The veterinary team provided the best medicine possible, but the state of grief distorts the thought process.

Understanding Euthanasia

Making the decision to euthanize a pet can be extremely difficult for clients. Some clients may not believe in euthanasia, whereas others do not believe in allowing a pet to suffer. The true definition of euthanasia comes from the Greek terms *eu,* meaning good or right, and *thanatos,* meaning death. Therefore euthanasia refers to an easy and painless death.

Clients should be educated regarding the euthanasia process so that they can make well-educated decisions. A team member should never tell a client *"Now is the time to euthanize."* Clients can misconstrue that statement and feel that the staff member made them euthanize their pet. Suggestions can be given, and simple statements can be made such as, *"It would not be a wrong decision if you made the choice to euthanize Fluffy."*

Clients should be able to fully understand and differentiate quality versus quantity of life for their pets. Quality of life being the enjoyable aspect; can the pet can still move around, eat and drink, have normal bowel movements, and urinate appropriately? Quantity of life is the time frame of the animal's life; at times an owner will keep the animal alive for personal reasons or will wait for a specific moment to make the decision. Clients may make decisions based on increasing the length of time the pet can survive rather than the quality of life while the pet survives.

A quality of life scale can be developed and implemented to help clients with this difficult decision (Box 12-1). Dr. Villalobos's quality of life scoring system, HHHHHMM, incorporates measures of hurt, hunger, hygiene, hydration, happiness, mobility, and more good days than bad. It attempts to provide a more objective means to determine quality of life for the client. Owners can be asked to score their pets on a scale of 1 to 10 (1 = poor, 10 = best). When the quality of life score drops below 35, clients can understand the need for euthanasia.

The Euthanasia Procedure

Clients may call and ask questions regarding the euthanasia procedure at the veterinary hospital. They may ask if a house call can be made, if an appointment to bring the pet in is required, or if they can just walk in. Many practices do not perform house calls, and the client can be referred to a veterinarian who does. If a client chooses to come in to the practice, the team member should advise the client of what to expect. Most clients have not experienced a euthanasia procedure and therefore do not know what to expect.

BOX 12-1	Quality of Life Scale
SCORE	**CRITERION**
Hurt: 0-10	Is pain successfully managed?
Hunger: 0-10	Is the dog/cat eating enough? Is a feeding tube required?
Hydration: 0-10	Is the dog/cat dehydrated? Is subcutaneous fluid therapy necessary?
Hygiene: 0-10	The dog/cat should be groomed and cleaned regularly; prevent pressure sores and keep all wounds clean
Happiness: 0-10	Does the dog/cat express interest in its environment? Is it responsive to family, toys, other pets, and so forth?
Mobility: 0-10	Can the dog/cat move without assistance? Are neurologic signs or pain impairing mobility?
More good days than bad: 0-10	When bad days outnumber good days, quality of life may be compromised.
Total	A total of 35 points or more is acceptable for good quality of life

When a healthy human-animal bond is no longer possible, the owner should be aware that the end is near. Euthanasia may be necessary to prevent further pain and suffering

Adapted from Myers F: Palliative care: end of life "pawspice" care. In Villalobos A, Kaplan L, editors: *Canine and feline geriatric oncology: honoring the human-animal bond.* Ames, Iowa, 2007, Wiley-Blackwell.

If team members take the time to educate them before they get to the practice, they are a little more prepared for what is a life-changing experience. Making an appointment may be practice policy; however, some clients may be unable to abide by this policy when it comes to euthanizing their pet. It is an extremely overwhelming decision to make, and having to wait until a scheduled appointment time may be difficult. It is making an appointment for death. Walk-ins should be accommodated when possible.

When a client arrives at the clinic for euthanasia of a pet, every attempt should be made to get him or her into a quiet room as soon as possible. Many practices have separate rooms used only for this purpose. Team members need to remember that this is a very difficult time for a client, who may not understand everything that is explained. The euthanasia process should be explained again, including the options that exist for the body (many hospitals offer private cremations, mass cremations, or burial services at a local pet cemetery). The owner must sign the release form, and all charges should be taken care of at this point. Figure 2-10, *H,* in Chapter 2 is an example of a euthanasia release form. Team members should ensure that the name on the file matches the name on the euthanasia form.

If a pet is hospitalized and its owner wishes to have the pet euthanized but is not present to sign a euthanasia release form, the owner should state the wish to have the pet euthanized to two different team members. Both team members must write in the record that the client requested euthanasia and that this was verified by them. This will protect the practice in the event that a client states that he or she did not authorize the euthanasia.

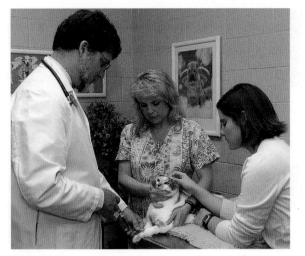

FIGURE 12-4 A client's presence during euthanasia of a companion animal helps say good-bye. Allow the client, with guidance, to make as many decisions as possible about the site, time, and tempo of the euthanasia process; this makes the event more personal and meaningful. (From Bassert JM, McCurnin DM: *McCurnin's clinical textbook for veterinary technicians*, ed 7, St Louis, 2010, Saunders Elsevier.)

> **PRACTICE POINT** Clients that are not present to sign a euthanasia form must tell two team members that they wish to euthanize the pet.

The euthanasia procedure varies from hospital to hospital; however, the same general ideas apply overall. The pet may have a catheter placed intravenously so that the vein is easier to access while in the euthanasia room with the client. Some practices may give a tranquilizer that relaxes the pet. This also allows the owner to stay with the pet and "say good-bye" (Figure 12-4). When the owner is ready, a euthanasia solution is injected into the vein; most solutions are an overdose of a barbiturate. This causes the heart to stop beating and the respirations to cease. When the heart is no longer audible, the patient has died. Clients should be advised that pets may lose control of their bowels and urinate when the muscles relax. They should also understand that pets generally do not close their eyes when they die and that this is normal.

If a patient has died in the hospital and a client would like to visit the pet, every attempt should be made to make the animal as presentable as possible. All catheters and bandaging materials should be removed, and any blood, feces, or urine should be wiped away. The eyes can be glued shut for a more peaceful appearance. The rectal area can be placed in a waterproof sack in case the bowels are released, and the pet should be wrapped in a nice blanket. This will be a lasting memory for the owner; practices do not want to leave negative impressions in the minds of clients.

If owners decide to take the body home, it should be placed in a waterproof bag. Trash bags are not visually appealing, but they may be placed in another bag or box if

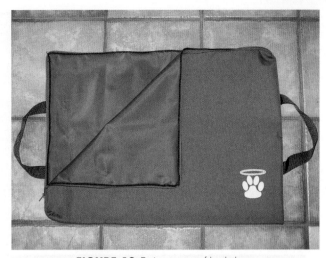

FIGURE 12-5 A waterproof body bag.

needed. "Body bags" are visually appealing and waterproof. Several companies offer a variety of sizes that will usually accommodate even the largest pet (Figure 12-5).

If owners do not take the body, it must be placed in a strong, waterproof bag. Bags must be clearly marked with the patient's name, the client's name, the date, and the name of the practice. The tag must also identify whether the body is to go for mass cremation or private cremation.

Pet Memorials

It is nice to take steps to help clients remember a pet. Many practices will send bereaved clients the poem "Rainbow Bridge." Other practices may make a paw print with paint (Figures 12-6 and 12-7). (To do this, simply clip the hair around the pads and place paint on the pads. Position a nice piece of paper on a clipboard and press the pad firmly against the board. Allow the paint to dry.) Clay paw print kits are available as well.

It is customary to send the client a sympathy card with the team members' signatures within a week of the pet's passing. Some practices may also send flowers to clients; however, this can become expensive. Clients appreciate the extra steps practices take to remember their pets (Figure 12-8).

Cremations

Cremations are available in most places in the United States. Clients can elect to have the pet's remains returned to them (private cremation) (Figure 12-9) or to have the pet be part of a mass cremation (remains are not returned). Mass cremations generally cost less and may be the only option if the client does not want the ashes returned. Many cities and counties have enacted regulations that prevent pets from being buried on private property. City and county regulations should be verified before allowing owners to take the body for private burial. Pet cemeteries are available for

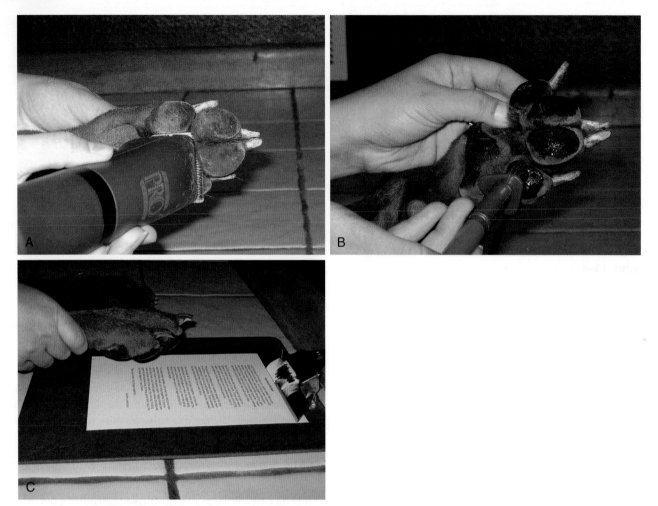

FIGURE 12-6 A, Clipping the paw for the paint. B, Applying paint to the paw. C, Preparing to stamp the paw.

burying pets in many cities. The local Humane Society chapter may have more information regarding the maintenance and upkeep of such places.

Owners Picking up Remains

Owners must return to pick up the ashes of their beloved pet when they have chosen a private cremation. Team members should call the client to state the ashes are ready. A simple and to-the-point statement of, *"Taylor's ashes have been returned and are available for you to pick up when you are ready,"* can be made to the client. It is very hard for clients to return to the practice to pick up remains. Team members must make sure the ashes are easily accessible and that cremation containers and cards are labeled correctly. It is also important for the reception team to be familiar with the names of cremations that are ready for pick up. Often a client will come in to the practice and simply say that he is here *"to pick up Taylor."* The team members automatically assume Taylor is a patient and start looking for an active record. When the client is questioned further (since the file cannot be located), the client must state a request for the ashes. This is a painful statement for the client to make; therefore being prepared and knowing which ashes are ready can eliminate this painful situation.

WHAT WOULD YOU DO/NOT DO?

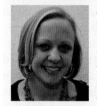

A long-term client, Mrs. Walsh has made the difficult decision to euthanize her dog of 15 years. She and her husband have chosen to have a private cremation, in which they would return to the practice to pick up the remains. The practice receives several private cremation containers at once, along with certificates of official cremation; the names of the pets have been placed on the bottom of the container as well as the card.

A team member calls the Walsh's informing them of Maggie's return; they arrive at the practice and take her home. The following day, Mr. Malcom calls the practice to see if Jeff, his cat that was also cremated, is ready to be picked up. The receptionist comes across a horrible discovery; Jeff had been sent home with the Walsh's, and Maggie was still at the practice.

What Should the Reception Team Do?

The most appropriate, painful task is to call the Walsh's and inform them of the mix up. A team member should deliver the appropriate remains and pick up Jeff, immediately. The team members must sincerely apologize for this awful mistake. The owners will be very upset at first, hopefully becoming grateful for the honesty of the practice.

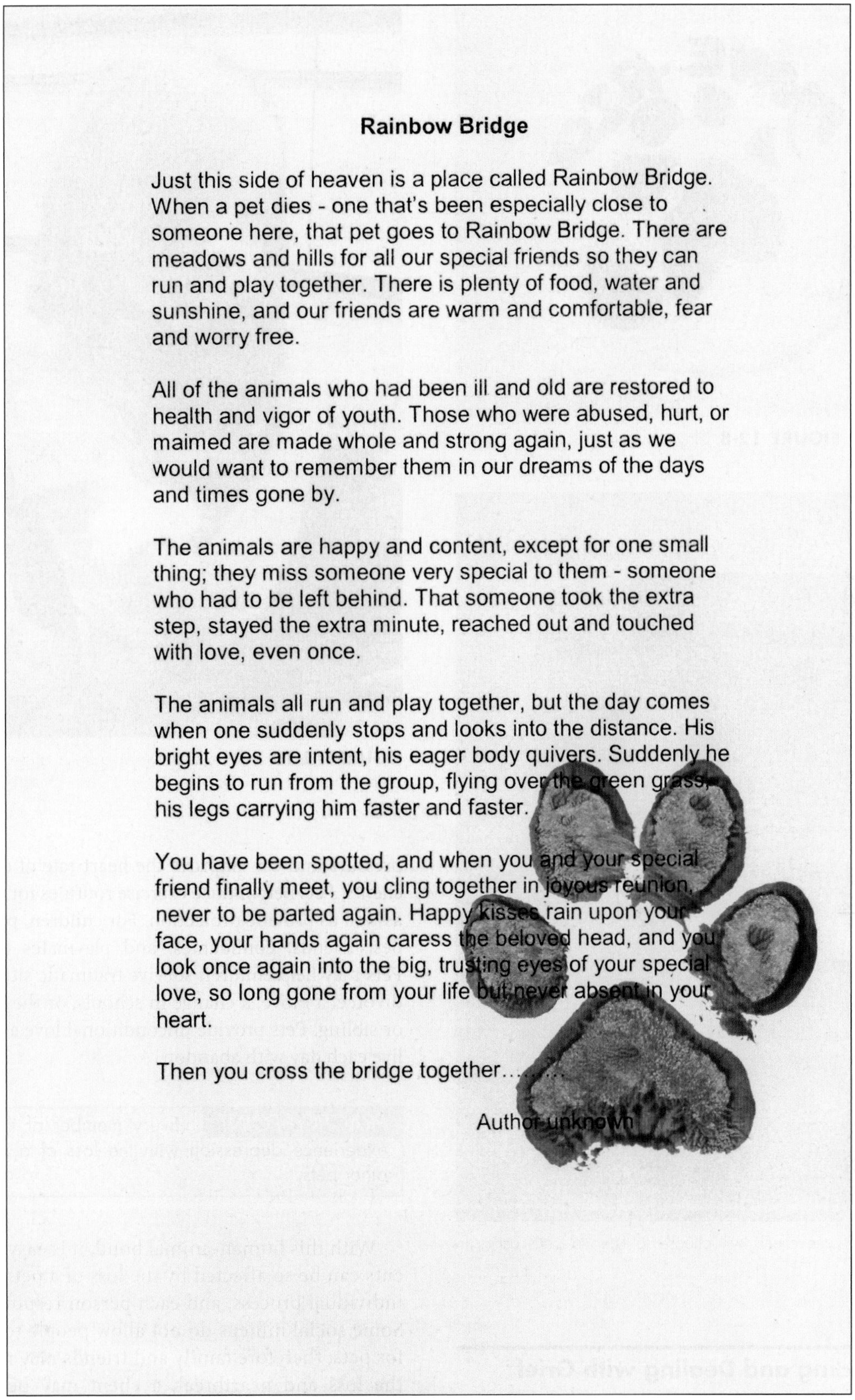

Rainbow Bridge

Just this side of heaven is a place called Rainbow Bridge. When a pet dies - one that's been especially close to someone here, that pet goes to Rainbow Bridge. There are meadows and hills for all our special friends so they can run and play together. There is plenty of food, water and sunshine, and our friends are warm and comfortable, fear and worry free.

All of the animals who had been ill and old are restored to health and vigor of youth. Those who were abused, hurt, or maimed are made whole and strong again, just as we would want to remember them in our dreams of the days and times gone by.

The animals are happy and content, except for one small thing; they miss someone very special to them - someone who had to be left behind. That someone took the extra step, stayed the extra minute, reached out and touched with love, even once.

The animals all run and play together, but the day comes when one suddenly stops and looks into the distance. His bright eyes are intent, his eager body quivers. Suddenly he begins to run from the group, flying over the green grass, his legs carrying him faster and faster.

You have been spotted, and when you and your special friend finally meet, you cling together in joyous reunion, never to be parted again. Happy kisses rain upon your face, your hands again caress the beloved head, and you look once again into the big, trusting eyes of your special love, so long gone from your life but never absent in your heart.

Then you cross the bridge together...

Author unknown

FIGURE 12-7 The Rainbow Bridge poem with a pet's paw print is a nice way to honor a pet.

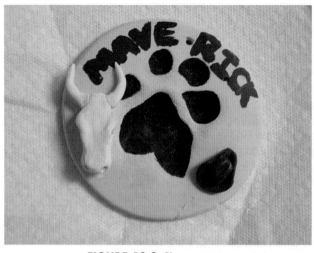

FIGURE 12-8 Clay paw print.

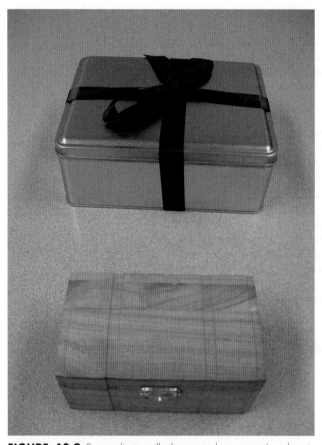

FIGURE 12-9 Some clients will choose to keep a pet's ashes in an urn.

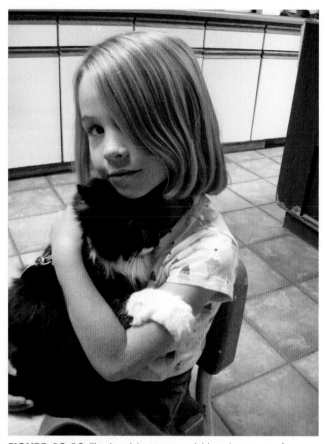

FIGURE 12-10 The bond between a child and a pet is often very strong.

pressure and can improve the heart rate of elderly and sick clients. Pets help induce exercise routines for elderly patients as well as provide protection. For children, pets can be their best friends, confidantes, and playmates (Figure 12-10). Pets may help children survive traumatic situations, such as divorce, a move, a change in schools, or the loss of a parent or sibling. Pets provide unconditional love and support and live each day with abandon.

> **PRACTICE POINT** Every member of the family can experience depression with the loss of a pet, including other pets.

With this human-animal bond, it is easy to see why clients can be so affected by the loss of a pet. Grieving is an individual process, and each person responds differently. Some social milieus do not allow people to openly grieve for pets; therefore family and friends may not understand the loss and heartbreak a client may be experiencing. Other clients may immediately be able to show emotions and grieve openly. It should be shared with clients that grieving is acceptable and that it is a normal process.

There are five stages of grief that should be understood. *Denial, anger, bargaining,* and *depression* are normal steps a grieving person takes before *acceptance* of the loss.

Understanding and Dealing with Grief

The loss of a pet can be as traumatic to some clients as losing a human family member. An animal is often a person's best friend. They are companions and guardians; they are loyal, huggable, and touchable. People can be themselves with their pets; no pretense is needed to gain a pet's trust and love. Pets have many benefits; they decrease stress, tension, and blood

Some clients may be in shock, denial, or disbelief regarding the loss of their pet, especially if it was a sudden death. Traumatic injuries resulting in death, particularly in young animals, may induce client anger. The client may place blame on the staff for not doing a better job or for not having the appropriate equipment to perform lifesaving procedures. The owner may be angry at a family member for leaving a gate open, allowing the pet to escape and be hit by a car. The denial stage generally occurs during the first 24 hours, either after a pet's death or after a terminal illness has been diagnosed. Denial is a coping mechanism to help the mind deal with traumatic news.

Owners may experience guilt that they have failed the pet and express that guilt in anger toward the staff. If a pet has been sick for a longer time, they may be in disbelief that their pet is so sick and may be holding on for some reason. The client may feel guilty for not having done what the doctor had recommended years ago to help the pet live longer. Guilt is the enemy of healing. Clients may try to bargain or reason to keep the pet alive. They may offer vitamins or extra-special food to bargain for extra time. Bargaining is a way to keep hope alive for some clients, allowing time for them to accept the outcome. Many will suffer a stage of depression, then accept the loss and be able to move forward.

Clients must accept that grieving is normal, and that only time can heal the loss. Creation of a personal memorial may help some clients through this difficult time. Some recommendations may be to create a picture collage, plant a tree, or develop a memorial garden.

Special consideration should be given to clients with service dogs. These clients depend on their pets for independence and freedom. The service dog has guided them and provided safety, and suddenly that security is gone. They will have to learn to trust another animal, and only time can build and replace that trust. Another special consideration is for a client who owns a dog involved in law enforcement. This may include a drug-sniffing and/or bomb-sniffing dog or a police dog used for protection. These officers depend on their dogs for their livelihood. The dogs are their daily companions and protectors. Many times, the social circle of law enforcement does not allow grieving and prevents these clients from psychologically accepting the loss. Many officers are unable to continue their duties with replacement dogs and ultimately change positions within the law enforcement department.

Children can have intense emotions and often deal with grief in different ways. Some children may be able to understand the process of euthanasia, whereas it confuses others. Children should be told the truth about euthanasia, and explaining the process will help children comprehend the situation. The child's age should be used to gauge the amount of explanation and detail needed. Words like "put to sleep" should be avoided, as many children associate this phrase with going to sleep at night. It should be explained that euthanasia is not a procedure done to sick and suffering people, that it is only available for animals. It may also help the child to be reassured that the pet will no longer feel pain.

To help clients work through the grief process, team members may recommend that they change their daily routine until the pain from the loss subsides. Clients may go to dinner with friends or go for a walk after work instead of immediately rushing home. Clients should understand that they will never be able to replace a pet, but that a new relationship with another pet is possible, and each relationship is unique. Clients should not be pressured to get another pet. The grieving process can take months, and they should never be surprised with a new pet.

Pets experience depression associated with death as well, regardless of whether they have lost a human or animal companion. Pets may show decreased activity and diminished appetite and may pace. Some may whimper or simply curl up in the corner. Clients can help pets recover from the loss as well. Just as with humans, changing the daily routine can lessen the pain. Owners may take the pet for a walk or go for a ride in the car to the dog park; any new adventure will change the routine. Pets should be shown extra love and attention as well. It must be remembered that both the client and pet are grieving, and any tools that team members can provide will help alleviate the pain associated with the loss of a pet.

VETERINARY PRACTICE and the LAW

The human-animal bond is a mutually beneficial and dynamic relationship between people and animals that is influenced by behaviors that are essential to the health and well-being of both. This includes, but is not limited to, emotional, psychological, and physical interactions of people, animals, and the environment. The veterinarian's role in the human-animal bond is to maximize the potential of this relationship between people and animals.

The AVMA officially recognizes three elements of the human animal bond:

- The existence of the human-animal bond and its importance to client and community health
- The human-animal bond has existed for thousands of years
- The human-animal bond has major significance for veterinary medicine, because, as veterinary medicine serves society, it fulfills both human and animal needs (www.avma.org/KB/Policies/Pages/The-Human-Animal-Bond.aspx).

Veterinary team members must embrace this bond, and understand and support it with superior client service.

REVIEW QUESTIONS

1. What is euthanasia?
2. Why is quality of life important?
3. What are the five stages of grief? Describe each.
4. Why is the human-animal bond so strong?
5. In what ways can a pet be memorialized?

6. How should a pet be presented to an owner after it has been euthanized?
7. What drug is in a euthanasia solution?
8. How does this drug affect the body?
9. How can a team prevent the wrong ashes from being sent home with an owner?
10. Why must a euthanasia release form be signed by the owner?

Recommended Reading

International Association of Animal Hospice and Palliative Care. (Web site). www.iaahpc.org Accessed August 5, 2013.

Lagoni L, Durrance D: *Connecting with grieving clients: supportive communication for fourteen common situations*, ed 2, Lakewood, CO, 2011, AAHA Press.

Shearer TS, editor: *Veterinary clinics of north america, small animal practice, palliative medicine and hospice care* (Vol 41), No 3, St Louis, MO, 2011, Elsevier.

## PART III

Veterinary Practice Systems

Appointments and appointment management are critical factors in practices that use an appointment system; it is essential to maintain a system that keeps appointments on schedule. A client's time is just as valuable as the veterinarian's time; if the practice cannot keep appointments on time, they cannot expect clients to run on time either.

Medical records are not only considered a legal document; they also allow the team to follow cases as they progress. If paper records are used, they must be legible, complete, and initialed by every author that enters information. If they are illegible, steps must be taken to correct the action, because incorrect information and medication may later be derived from the record. Because it is a legal document, a judge should also be able to read and interpret the record. It is imperative that legible medical records follow a SOAP (subjective, objective, assessment, and plan) format, allowing team members and referring veterinarians to follow the case.

Management of the practice inventory is a critical factor. Inventory is the second highest cost in the veterinary practice and the second highest revenue center. Successful management is essential to prevent shrinkage and product expiration. Reorder points and reorder quantities must be developed, leading to effective turnover rates. Effective turnover rates decrease soft costs (also known as holding and ordering costs). Product consolidation is also critical to inventory management; too many products on the shelve increases costs, resulting in greater shrinkage.

Controlled substances are drugs that the U.S. Drug Enforcement Administration (DEA) has classified as having potential for abuse; therefore it is imperative that they are maintained according to law. Every controlled substance that is dispensed must be recorded, and each drug must be balanced yearly or biannually (depending on the state). Losses greater than 3% must be reported to the state board of veterinary medicine and the DEA. Expired medications must be disposed of properly, producing a statement that they were expired and incinerated. Logs associated with these medications must be maintained for several years. Logs can also be maintained for equipment and other products within the practice, including a radiology checkout log (for nondigital practices). This allows radiographs to be tracked in case they were never returned to the practice.

Accounts receivable must be managed just as strictly as inventory, because this is another area associated with loss in veterinary medicine. Accounts receivable should never reach more than a 1.5% of gross revenue. Once these outstanding accounts reach 90 days past due, they can be impossible to collect and must be sent to a collections agency. Those team members responsible for collection of money must be familiar with the Fair Debt Collections Practices Act, which ultimately protects the consumer from harassment. If clients are consistently asking to charge, a third party payment plan may be recommended, such as CareCredit. This credit card is used exclusively for veterinary services and can provide practices an alternative to clients charging at the practice. Pet health insurance should also be recommended, as many procedures and products are covered for pets. Premiums, co-pays and deductibles are required just as in human medicine; however, practices do not file claims.

Preparing and maintaining a budget is essential to practice survival. Practices must plan budgets preventing the overspending of cash, especially during the hospitals slowest months. Preplanning allows for the estimation of production, payroll, and taxes. Budgeting allows the practice to set aside money for team raises, bonuses, and equipment purchases. Excellent planning allows for greater practice reinvestment and a return on investment for the owner.

Zoonotic disease is a real risk in veterinary medicine. Often, veterinary assistants, technicians, and doctors are the first to notice symptoms and come in direct contact with disease. Exceptional personal hygiene must be practiced at all times; team members must be familiar with diseases that are common to the area and practice transmission prevention on all levels. Zoonotic disease prevention should be encompassed in any safety program. Safety programs should cover all aspects of team member safety, including those highlighted by the Occupational Safety and Health Administration (OSHA). In order to satisfy OSHA requirements, practices must maintain a safety program and a hazards safety manual, and they must inform team members of the hazards associated with their job. A safety manager can be appointed, who is responsible for training all team members, documenting the training procedures, and enforcing the use of personal protection equipment. Chemicals should all be listed in a hazards program and include a safety data sheet (SDS) informing team members of the properties of the products and measures to take in case ingestion, contamination, or inappropriate use has occurred.

Safety programs for the staff go beyond OSHA recommendations. Every practice is susceptible to crime and must take all precautions to prevent harm to clients, patients, and team members. Perimeter lighting is very important, deterring

criminal activity that could involve both clients and team members. Staff must be prepared for possible robbery attempts both during and after business hours. Security should also encompass the computer systems. Backup methods must be employed in case a computer is stolen or a hacker interrupts the systems functions. All computer systems should be password protected, adding a second level of security.

Practice and office management go far beyond client and patient care. Behind-the-scenes work must be completed and maintained on a daily basis, allowing the practice to function fully and avert disasters. Preventing problems from arising is much more efficient than resolving problems when they do rise. Veterinary assistants and technicians play an active role in troubleshooting and preventing and solving problems. Skills gained through school, previous employment, and life experiences contribute to the success of the practice as well as each individual on the team.

Appointment Management

OUTLINE

Paper Versus Software Management
  Schedule, *240*
Designing the Appointment Book
  Template, *241*
Factors in Appointment Scheduling, *244*
  Number of Veterinarians, *244*
  Veterinary Technician Appointments, *244*
  Length of Time of Appointments, *244*
  Length of Time for Client Education, *246*
  Surgery, *246*
  Dental Procedures, *246*
  Nonsterile Procedures, *246*
  Holidays, *247*
  Vacation and Continuing Education, *247*
  Type of Appointment, *247*
  Clients, *247*

Scheduling for Productivity, *247*
  Adapting the Schedule for
    Emergencies, *247*
  Habitually Late Clients, *247*
  Management During Busy Times, *248*
  Management of Walk-ins, *248*
  Patient Drop-off, *249*
  No-Show Appointments, *249*
  Clients Who Arrive on the Wrong
    Day, *249*
Appointment Cards, *249*
Entering Appointments, *249*
  Units for Appointment Schedule, *251*
  Reminding Clients of Appointments, *251*
  Training New Employees How to Use the
    Appointment System, *251*
Preparing for the Appointment, *253*

KEY TERMS

Appointment Book
  Template
Appointment Cards
Appointment Scheduler
Appointment Units
Preoperative Instructions

LEARNING OBJECTIVES

When you have completed this chapter, you should be able to:

1. List factors that affect appointment scheduling.
2. Effectively make appointments.
3. Identify appointment cards.
4. Discuss the importance of reminding clients of upcoming appointments.
5. List methods used to increase the production and efficiency of the team by managing appointments.
6. List methods used to manage clients who walk into the practice with minor emergencies

CRITICAL COMPETENCIES

1. **Adaptability** - being open to change and flexible work methods; the ability to adapt behavior to changing conditions or new information.
2. **Analytical Skills** - the ability to analyze information and use logic to address problems; the ability to quickly and accurately grasp complex information and concepts and to make correct inferences.
3. **Compliance** - being reliable, thorough, and conscientious in carrying out work assignments; has an appreciation for the importance of organizational rules and policies.
4. **Creativity** - the ability to think creatively about situations, to see things in new and different ways; use imagination and creativity to develop innovative solutions to problems.
5. **Critical and Strategic Thinking** - the ability to think critically about situations and to understand the relevance of information for different problems; use critical reasoning to generate and evaluate alternative courses of action or points of view relevant to an issue.
6. **Decision Making** - the ability to make good decisions, solve problems, and decide on important matters; the ability to gather and analyze relevant data and choose decisively between alternatives.

7. **Integrity** - honesty, trustworthiness, and adherence to high standards of ethical conduct.
8. **Leadership** - a willingness to lead and take charge; the ability to motivate others and mobilize group effort toward common goals.
9. **Planning and Prioritizing** - the ability to effectively manage time and work load to meet deadlines; the ability to organize work, set priorities, and establish plans for achieving goals.
10. **Resourcefulness** - the ability to understand what it takes to complete the job; apply knowledge, skills, and expertise to perform tasks quickly and efficiently.

Veterinary practices can use an appointment system or accept clients on a walk-in basis; most veterinary practices prefer appointments. A variation of both may work best for some hospitals. Appointments can help control the amount of traffic flow through the veterinary clinic at a given time. All team members should be available on days that the appointments are fully booked, whereas slower times require less staff. It is important to create a schedule that is going to keep the practice running on schedule for appointments; a client's time is just as valuable as the doctor's time, and finding a medium between the two will contribute to a successful practice.

Walk-in practices allow clients to come into the clinic when it is convenient for them; however, this can decrease the efficiency of the team and prevent the regulation of traffic flow. Client wait times will increase, and team burnout will occur quickly. It is important to look at both the advantages and disadvantages of walk-ins versus appointments and decide what is best for the practice, considering both the team and client. The goals of an appointment system should be to maximize productivity, reduce staff tension, and control traffic flow through the veterinary hospital, all while maintaining concern for client and patient needs.

For those practices wishing to convert from a walk-in structure to appointment structure, the transition can be relatively easy. Clients are easy to train and will adapt to the new structure. A client e-newsletter or postcard can be sent to all clients indicating the change. The information contained in this newsletter or brochure can state the advantages to the client of the transition (Figures 13-1 and 13-2). Attractively framed posters in the reception area and exam rooms can also educate clients of the change. Once clients realize that this a better option for them, they will gladly embrace the transition.

Some clinics prefer a slow transition, whereas others prefer to change immediately. An appointment system can start up slowly; they can be made in the mornings and walk-ins can be seen in the afternoons. This can continue for several months until appointments can be integrated into the entire day. Once appointments are scheduled throughout the day, slots can be left available for those walk-ins that have not adjusted to the change. When these clients return, they will know to make an appointment.

Those practices that integrate appointments immediately must schedule and allow for a large number of walk-ins for a

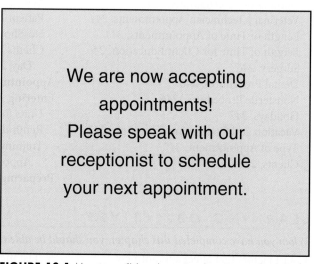

We are now accepting appointments! Please speak with our receptionist to schedule your next appointment.

FIGURE 13-1 Hanging a "Now Accepting Appointments" sign in the practice encourages clients to adapt to the change in the practice.

short period of time. Once the clients have become trained, the amount of time set aside for walk-ins can be reduced. Walk-ins should never be turned away. If it appears that the wait time will be lengthy, team members can offer the client the opportunity to drop off the pet; the owner can then be called when the patient is ready.

PRACTICE POINT Scheduling appointments increases efficiency while also decreasing stress and errors.

During the transition, team members will make mistakes; this can be a positive learning experience for all members. Teamwork, communication, and training among staff and clients will minimize the effect of these mistakes and will prevent errors from occurring in the future.

Paper Versus Software Management Schedule

Some smaller veterinary practices have used a paper appointment schedule book with success and continue to do so. A book may work well with a one-doctor practice, but as the number of veterinarians on staff increases,

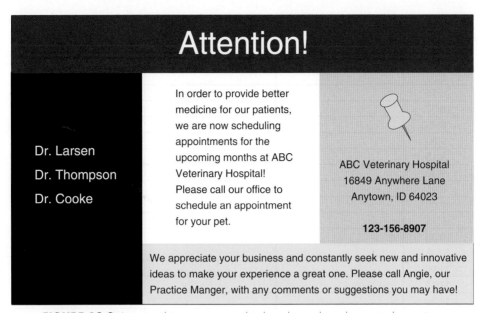

Attention!

Dr. Larsen

Dr. Thompson

Dr. Cooke

In order to provide better medicine for our patients, we are now scheduling appointments for the upcoming months at ABC Veterinary Hospital! Please call our office to schedule an appointment for your pet.

ABC Veterinary Hospital
16849 Anywhere Lane
Anytown, ID 64023

123-156-8907

We appreciate your business and constantly seek new and innovative ideas to make your experience a great one. Please call Angie, our Practice Manger, with any comments or suggestions you may have!

FIGURE 13-2 A postcard is a great way to let clients know about changes in the practice.

appointment books can become difficult to manage and share when multiple clients are waiting to make appointments (Figure 13-3).

If a paper appointment book is preferred, studies indicate that a week-at-a-glance style works best. It will depend on the size of the veterinary practice as to what size book to purchase, the number of columns, and appropriate appointment time slots. For example, a smaller one-doctor practice may use three columns per day. One column can be designated for the doctor's appointments, one column for technician appointments, and another for surgery. A larger number of veterinarians would require more columns.

Software appointment schedulers can be accessed from any computer in the clinic, thereby allowing multiple users to make appointments. This can increase the efficiency of the staff; one team member can make a surgery appointment while another can make an appointment for a yearly exam (Figures 13-4 and 13-5). Access from multiple computers can have one disadvantage. Multiple team members may be viewing one appointment slot available, and when they click on the appointment to secure it, another team member may have already booked it. This is only a minor disadvantage compared with the number of benefits that appointment software can provide.

Software appointment schedulers have far more features than just scheduling appointments. When a team member fills an appointment slot with a current client, the software can show alerts reminding the team of overdue vaccinations, tests, previous no-show appointments, or a poor credit status. When the client account is accessed, all pets owned by that client will be available, and all overdue reminders will show. This allows the reception team to either schedule an appointment for multiple patients owned by the same client or remind the owner of the overdue services (Figure 13-6).

If a client chooses to cancel or move an appointment, software allows the receptionist to cut and paste, keeping all pertinent information together. The receptionist will not have to retype or misinterpret information.

Software allows the veterinary practice to become proactive, instead of reactive, to client needs. Proactive service begins before the client walks in the door. The client is satisfied with the ability to make an appointment, the time available, and the ability to make an appointment with the veterinarian he or she wanted to see. Reactive service is taking care of the client *after* he or she is upset. Perhaps the client had to wait too long, was dissatisfied with the service, or did not get to make an appointment.

Appointment scheduling software can only enhance the experience of a client and make it a more pleasant experience. If the practice is technology proficient and is able to use online Web portals, clients can make their own appointments. New trends show that clients take care of personal business online and prefer to shop, search for information, and make appointments online when possible.

Every veterinary practice software program has an appointment scheduler available, which should be used to its maximum potential. Systems provided by different software companies will have both advantages and disadvantages and vary in their efficiency. Each version of software should be demonstrated before purchase. This will allow the practice to determine which software will integrate best with the practice. User friendliness and compatibility of the programs should top the list of items when looking for software. Refer to Chapter 8 for more information and guidelines on software selection for a veterinary practice.

Designing the Appointment Book Template

The template is the outline of the appointment book and must be established before using a new system. Next, factors that affect appointment scheduling must be considered.

Monday December 29, 2013

	Dr. C	Surgery	Drop Off
8:00			
8:15			
8:30			
8:45			
9:00			
9:15			
9:30			
9:45			
10:00			
10:15			
10:30			
10:45			
11:00			
11:15			
11:30			
11:45			
12:00			
12:15			
12:30			
12:45			
1:00			
1:15			
1:30			
1:45			
2:00			
2:15			
2:30			
2:45			
3:00			
3:15			
3:30			
3:45			
4:00			
4:15			
4:30			
4:45			
5:00			
5:15			
5:30			
5:45			
6:00			
6:15			
6:30			
6:45			
7:00			

FIGURE 13-3 Sample paper schedule.

The hours the clinic is open should be entered into the template first. This includes when the practice opens, closes for lunch, and closes in the evenings as well as any weekend hours. If the practice closes for weekly staff meetings, that should also be entered into the template. Holidays must be added into the system; most systems do not automatically recognize holidays, and practice hours vary by location.

Permanent flextime should also be added so that team members cannot accidentally remove or book an appointment in a slot that has extra time built in. Generally, a practice manager or owner creates the template and is the only one who has access to modify it.

There are many factors that come into play when developing an appointment schedule. There is no written rule

	Dr. A	Dr. B	Dr. C	Dr. D	Surgery	Dental	Techs	Drop Off
Notes				Sx day				
8:00								
8:15								
8:30								
8:45								
9:00								
9:15								
9:30								
9:45								
10:00								
10:15								
10:30								
10:45								
11:00								
11:15								
11:30								
11:45								
12:00								
12:15								
12:30								
12:45								
1:00								
1:15								
1:30								
1:45								
2:00								
2:15								
2:30								
2:45								
3:00								
3:15								
3:30								
3:45								
4:00								
4:30								
4:15								
4:45								
5:00								
5:15								
5:30								
5:45								
6:00								
6:15								
6:30								
6:45								
7:00								

	Dr. A
Notes	
8:00	No Appt
8:15	"Sam" Allen Davis; K-9 Yearly Vaccines
8:30	"Yoshi" Glenda Martin; Fe Boosters
8:45	"Brodie" Kevin Dream; K-9 Yearly Vaccines
9:00	No Appt
9:15	"Wheeler" Keith Davis; K-9 Recheck
9:30	
9:45	"Sophie" Teresa Merril; K-9 Yearly Exam
10:00	No Appt
10:15	
10:30	"Sabrina" Brittany Wise; K-9 Yearly Exam
10:45	
11:00	No Appt
11:15	"Feral" Margie Walters; Fe Recheck
11:30	"Boots" Whitney Sooner; Fe Senior Exam
11:45	"Boots" Whitney Sooner; Fe Senior Exam
12:00	Lunch
12:15	Lunch
12:30	Lunch
12:45	Lunch
1:00	Lunch
1:15	"Pretty" Eva Walters; Avian Wing/Beak Trim/Exam
1:30	"Pretty" Eva Walters; Avian Wing/Beak Trim/Exam
1:45	"Pretty" Eva Walters; Avian Wing/Beak Trim/Exam
2:00	"Macho" Jack Daro; Fe-Yearly Exam
2:15	No Appt
2:30	"KC" Heather Pritchard; K-9 Lame R Fore
2:45	"KC" Heather Pritchard; K-9 Lame R Fore
3:00	"Bird" Albert King; Avian Wing Trim
3:15	No Appt
3:30	"Albert" Mark Valdivia; Fe Senior Exam
3:45	"Albert" Mark Valdivia; Fe Senior Exam
4:00	No Appt
4:15	"Lucy" Chris Reed; Poss. Hip Dysplasia
4:30	"Lucy" Chris Reed; Poss. Hip Dysplasia
4:45	"Sam" Pam Delgado; K-9 Yearly Exam
5:00	"Sam" Pam Delgado; K-9 Yearly Exam
5:15	No Appt
5:30	
5:45	Yearly Exam
6:00	Closed
6:15	Closed
6:30	Closed
6:45	Closed
7:00	Closed

FIGURE 13-4 Sample software schedule. An appointment summary schedule appears on the left, along with a detailed view of Dr. A's appointments (*right*).

stating how many appointments should be made or how long appointments should last. Schedules vary with each practice, and the team determines what is best for both clients and staff. Appointment layout can change as the practice grows and team members identify problems with the current schedule. Once an appointment system has been integrated, it must be aggressively managed. Appointment times, availability, length of time, and available team members should be monitored and revised on a regular basis.

It is absolutely critical to monitor client wait times. If clients are waiting too long to be seen, their patience decreases. This ultimately affects the compliance rate, as unhappy clients will not accept recommended services and procedures. Managers and team members must identify why the wait times are prolonged and implement measures to change the wait time immediately. The most common reasons for extended wait periods include appointment times that are too short, acceptance of walk-ins, emergencies, and critical cases.

PRACTICE POINT Appointment book design may change as the practice progresses, meeting the needs of both the team and clients.

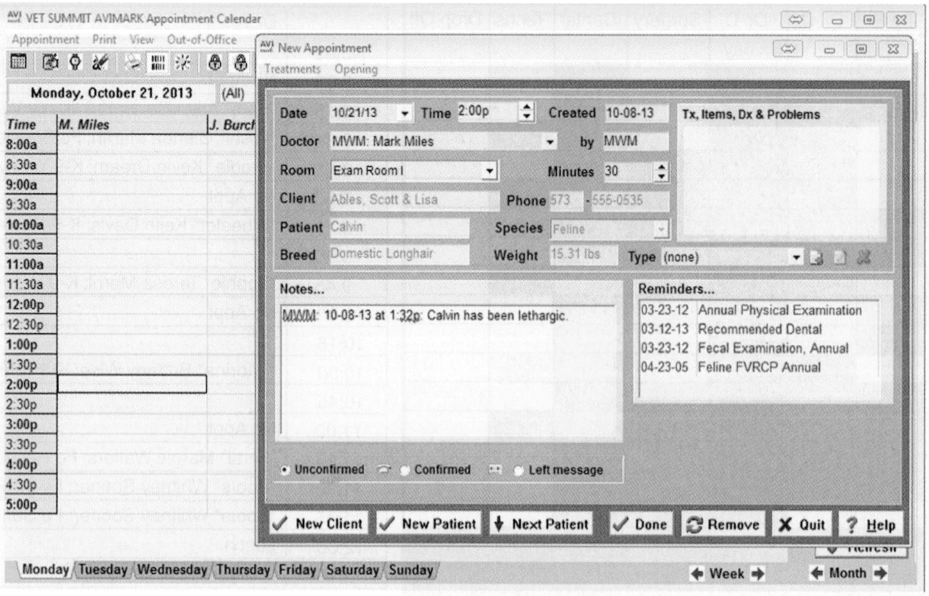

FIGURE 13-5 Sample screen from Avimark's appointment calendar. (Courtesy AVImark, LLC, Piedmont, Mo.)

Patient Medical History		ABC Veterinary Clinic
Teresa Longmower	**Patient:** Jack	**DOB:** 10/01/07
123 Anystreet	**Species:** Canine	**Age:** 6y
Anytown, MI 89892	**Breed:** Boxer	**Sex:** MN
	Color: Brown/White	**Tag:** 123
Acct No: 1234	**Doctor:** Nancy Dreamer	**Weight:** 48.2#
Phone: (555) 555-5555	**As of: 10/10/13**	

Reminders:			
3710	Heartworm Test	Overdue	03/09/13
0690	Canine Yearly Exam	Overdue	03/09/13
0602	DHPP 3 year	Overdue	03/09/13
0601	Rabies 3 year	Overdue	03/09/13

FIGURE 13-6 Sample overdue reminders in a software system.

Factors in Appointment Scheduling

When developing a scheduling system, the following factors should be taken into consideration.

Number of Veterinarians

The number of veterinarians seeing appointments on a daily basis may vary. For example, if three veterinarians are seeing appointments on Monday morning, those times may be staggered so that three appointments do not show up at 9 AM and overwhelm the front reception team. One appointment may be scheduled for 9 AM, the second for 9:05 AM, and the third for 9:10 AM, for Dr. A, Dr. B, and Dr. C, respectively. If appointments are 15 minutes each, Dr. A's next appointment will be scheduled for 9:15 AM, Dr. B's next appointment will be scheduled for 9:20 AM, and Dr. C's next appointment will be scheduled for 9:25 AM (Figure 13-7).

Veterinary Technician Appointments

Some appointments can be scheduled for a technician alone, thereby leaving an appointment slot available for a producing doctor. Nail trims, suture removals, weight-management rechecks, and anal gland expressions (among many other tasks) can be scheduled with a credentialed or skilled veterinary assistant (Figure 13-8). This allows veterinarians to continue to see clients who need to have a diagnosis made. Technicians can always ask a veterinarian for help if they have a question about the case.

Length of Time of Appointments

Team members must decide what length of time an appointment should be to accommodate their clients' needs in the best way possible. Some teams feel that 10-minute slots are too short but have found that they increase the overall practice profit. Thirty to forty percent of small animal practices

Appt Time	Dr. A	Dr. B	Dr. C
8:00	Angela Jones	Block	Eva Marsch "Pat" NT
8:05	"Cassidy" K-9	Sabrina Patterson	Block
8:10	Yearly Exam	"Sheba" Feline	Brittany Wilson
8:15	242-5678	Ear Infection	"Danny" K-9
8:20	Block	876-3334	New Puppy/vaccines
8:25	Nikki Ewing	Block	444-3834
8:30	"Sundance" Hamster	Julie Denamarin	Block
8:35	Vomiting	"Oscar" K-9	Nancy Dallop
8:40	Block	Lame, Left Fore	"Wheeler" K-9
8:45	Sue Biel	889-9098	Growth check 575-9808
9:00	"King" Avian		Block
9:05	Wing/Nail Trim/Exam		Jamie Dunlap
9:10	454-9084	Valarie Goodwill	"Cameron" Feline
9:15		"Sasha" K-9	Senior Wellness Exam/BW
9:30		Consult w/Dr. B	897-3938
9:45	Block	999-8987	
10:00	Denzel Marrow		Block
10:15	"Joy" K-9		Sarah Michael
10:30	Poss. Diabetic	Block	"Enzo" Booster
10:45	242-9098	Linda Block	876-0969
11:00		"Jackie"	Block
11:15		Check Eyes 466-8740	
11:30	Block	Frances Reed	
11:45		"Mike" K9	
12:00		Recheck 575-3493	

FIGURE 13-7 Staggered appointment blocks keep multiple clients from walking in at the same time.

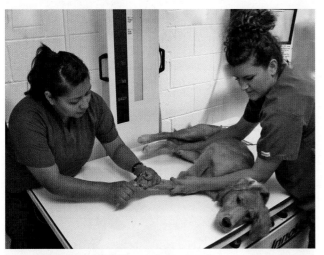

FIGURE 13-8 Two technicians perform a nail trim.

use 15-minute slots. Time and motion studies indicate that it takes approximately 12 minutes to check in a patient, obtain a thorough history, perform a physical exam, prepare the necessary medications and client education materials, and write in the medical record. That leaves only 3 minutes to educate the client about health issues that may be of concern. Some practitioners feel this is an inadequate amount of time to spend with their clients; however, a well-trained staff can educate the client while the veterinarian continues to the next appointment.

Other practices prefer 20-minute appointments. Some practitioners feel that they need to spend the time with the client and educate them personally, not delegate to the staff. By increasing the appointment slot to 20 minutes, the veterinarian has an additional 5 minutes to educate the client. The disadvantage to 20-minute appointments is the reduction in the number of clients seen per day. On the other hand, the average client transaction can rise with the increased amount of time spent with the client. Decreased client volume per day can have a significant impact on the staff and prevent team burnout. The use of 20-minute appointment slots can also improve the practice's on-time performance.

> **PRACTICE POINT** Develop a table of standards lengths of appointments; monitor current lengths of appointments, and make changes as needed to keep the schedule running on time.

A 10-minute flex system is also another option for staff members scheduling appointments. Team members can analyze the client's situation and estimate the length of time an appointment is likely to take. Staff can schedule several

10-minute blocks together to create the perfect appointment time. Each practice must decide what will benefit both the client and the team the best. Team members who schedule appointments must be knowledgeable about diseases, procedures, and clients to schedule effectively. If any question should arise regarding proper time allotment, an informed team member should be consulted; it is better to verify before making the appointment instead of overscheduling the team at a later time.

Length of Time for Client Education

Some practices schedule time for client education alone. Client education does not necessarily need to be given by a veterinarian, but it should be scheduled so that clients do not have to wait. A pet may have just been diagnosed with a serious disease and the client will need to receive lengthy education regarding the patient's disease and health. Scheduling client education can significantly increase client compliance and understanding while establishing a lasting client-practice bond. Client education can be scheduled with a veterinary technician, allowing the veterinarian to continue seeing appointments.

Surgery

The number of surgeries to schedule in a day depends on the team, the length of time it takes the veterinarian to complete a procedure, and the amount of time available to complete the procedures. One veterinarian may be faster at a particular procedure and therefore able to complete more procedures in a day than another. Larger practices may have two surgical tables and are thus able to accommodate a larger number of surgical patients at a time, increasing the efficiency of the team (Figure 13-9).

Dental Procedures

Some teams may have either one or two dental tables and units available, increasing the number of dental procedures a practice can accommodate in one day (Figure 13-10). Practices can have several credentialed technicians performing dental procedures concurrently while nonsterile or sterile procedures are performed on another table.

Nonsterile Procedures

Abscess debridement, anal sac expression, ear flushes, and patients that need to be sedated for radiographs all take time of the treatment team (Figure 13-11). Time should be allotted to complete these procedures; this will help prevent the team from backing up and running late for appointments. Clients do not see the procedures being completed in the treatment area and therefore do not perceive that the hospital is busy. They will not understand why their appointments are late.

An excessive number of nonsterile procedures can increase stress on the team and prevent them from taking their lunches or breaks. Proper scheduling can alleviate this situation, which can ultimately lead to team burnout when it occurs on a daily basis.

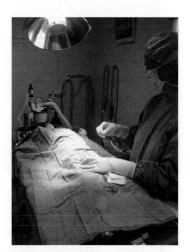

FIGURE 13-9 Surgical procedures may require longer appointment times.

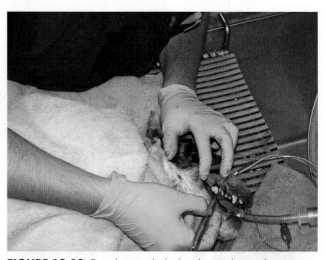

FIGURE 13-10 Completing multiple dental procedures a day increases revenue.

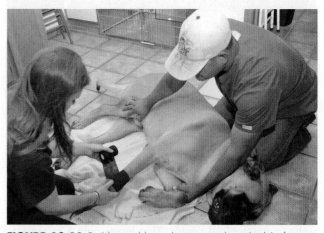

FIGURE 13-11 Building additional time into the schedule for non-sterile procedures keeps the practice from running behind schedule for the day.

Holidays

The owners and manager can decide what holidays to close for and allow the scheduler to accommodate that time off. Team members should remember that business days after a holiday closure are generally very busy and should add flex-time into the appointment scheduler to accommodate minor emergencies and walk-ins that will occur.

Vacation and Continuing Education

Any time doctors or credentialed veterinary technicians take time off, it must be built into the schedule months in advance. It can be difficult and irritating to clients to have to reschedule their appointments. When the practice is short a doctor, the remaining team members must accommodate the veterinary shortage and increased traffic flow. Adjustments must be made to prevent appointments from running behind.

Type of Appointment

Appointment times can vary depending on what they are for. A yearly examination may only take 15 minutes, whereas a limping patient that requires an orthopedic exam can take 30 minutes. Team members should be aware of what types of problems are going to take longer to examine and diagnose and make adjustments when scheduling those appointments. (See Figure 13-14 for examples of appointment units and length of time.) Appointments for new patients may take more time than appointments for existing patients; new clients may take 30 minutes instead of the usual 15 minutes allotted for existing clients.

Clients

Certain clients will always take longer than others simply because of who they are. Team members should be able to identify these clients right away and add extra time for their appointments. These clients may be in the top 10% of the practice's producing clients, or they may like to chat. Whatever the reason, by accommodating these clients, team members can prevent appointments from running behind.

The benefit of appointment software is the ability to create an individual appointment setting for each doctor. If Dr. A prefers 20-minute appointment slots and can complete surgical procedures at a moderately quick pace, then the schedule can accommodate that change. If Dr. B prefers 15-minute appointments but is slower at completing surgical procedures, the software should be able to adjust for that.

> PRACTICE POINT Special clients may need additional time. An alert can be created in the clients accounting, alerting team members to allot additional time.

A clinic will learn what works best for that individual practice and can make changes along the way. Word of mouth spreads quickly as clients say, *"Oh, I have to go to the vet today; you know they will be running late!"* It is better to hear, *"My veterinarian is always on time. It is rare that I have*

to wait more than 5 or 10 minutes for my appointment." However, all practices should be able to accommodate emergencies and walk-ins. Clients may feel their pet is experiencing an emergency regardless of whether it is only an ear infection. It is important to remember client perception; they do not know what is and is not an emergency.

It is also important to realize that clients will often only hear parts of a sentence. For example, a client may call and indicate they need to get their pet in as soon as possible, because the patient is shaking its head. The receptionist politely replies: *"I am sorry Mr. Derk, I do not have any appointments available today; however, I can schedule you for Thursday."* The client has likely only heard *"I am sorry Mr. Derk, we do not have any appointments."* The client will be upset that the practice does not have any appointments and may call another hospital so that his baby can be seen today. A drop-off should immediately be offered as a solution, rather than offering an appointment on another day.

Scheduling for Productivity

Doctors should be able to delegate tasks to a well-trained staff member to continue seeing appointments and increase their productivity. If diagnostic work has been advised, the patient should be turned over to the veterinary technician, who can then complete the tests that the veterinarian has advised. Once results are available, the doctor can be notified and a treatment plan instituted. To keep appointments running as scheduled, the team may ask clients to wait in the reception area (or move to a consultation room) while laboratory work is being performed. This allows the exam room to be freed for the next appointment, preventing a 20- or 30-minute delay.

Adapting the Schedule for Emergencies

Emergencies will always occur. If appointments are scheduled and emergencies arrive, it must be communicated to clients that there has been an emergency. Most clients understand the need to attend to the emergency and do not mind the wait. However, clients should be updated every 5 minutes to let them know they have not been forgotten. The team can offer the waiting client water, coffee, and/or a magazine to try to offset the wait. Remember, 5 minutes seems like 10 minutes to a client!

If an emergency arrives and it is apparent it is going to take more than a few minutes (e.g., the patient needs to go to surgery), reception members can call appointments scheduled for the day and explain that there has been an emergency causing appointments to fall behind. Team members can politely ask to reschedule appointments for a later time in the day or for another day if that does not work with the client's schedule. Yearly exams should always be asked first to reschedule because that appointment has lower priority over a client who has a sick pet.

Habitually Late Clients

There will always be clients who are late. Practices may post a sign indicating that any client who is more than 15

WHAT WOULD YOU DO/NOT DO?

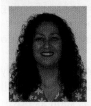

Mrs. Morris calls the practice at 2 PM on a Friday and would like to come in as a walk-in to see if her dog is pregnant. The reception team advises her that all of the appointments have been booked for the day and several emergencies have arrived, placing the team behind schedule. They advise Mrs. Morris to please schedule an appointment for the following week when her wait would not have to be so long. Mrs. Morris schedules her appointment for the following Tuesday, but shows up 15 minutes before closing anyway.

What Does the Reception Team Do?

The reception team must ask Mrs. Morris if something serious has happened that caused her to come in early for her appointment; the client may have a valid concern for her pet's health. If she insists that the pet is feeling fine, "she just can't wait until Tuesday," then the team must inform her of her wait time. Since the practice has had numerous emergencies, the team is still approximately an hour behind schedule and she will be the last client seen. Communication is imperative with the client, making sure she understands the wait for a nonemergency.

Team members should check back in periodically with Mrs. Morris, ensuring her that the veterinarian has not forgotten her. She should be offered coffee, water, or tea (if available). Never make the statement, "the doctor will be right in," when the wait can be extensive; even though the client knows there will be a wait, they have an expectation that the wait is shorter if this statement is declared.

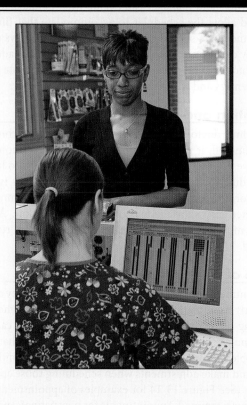

minutes late will be considered a walk-in; they can either be rescheduled or treated as a walk-in and seen as time permits. To enforce this policy, however, practice appointments should run on time or clients will become irate (if clients are expected to respect the doctors time, then practices must learn to respect the clients time).

Once a client has been denied an appointment because of tardiness, it is unlikely he or she will be late for the following appointment. Clients can be politely addressed regarding their constant tardiness. When Mr. Derk, a habitually late client, calls to make an appointment, team members may say *"Mr. Derk, the nature of Fluffy's appointment requires the full time allotted for your appointment. Please remember your appointment is set for Tuesday, June 5, at 3 PM."* This lets the client know that your practice has recognized his tardiness in the past and will be expecting him to arrive on time.

If a client calls ahead and lets the team know he or she will be late, the receptionist should check the schedule to make sure the client can still be accommodated without delaying the rest of the appointments. If it will be a tight squeeze, the appointment can be rescheduled.

Management During Busy Times

Managers can determine the busiest time of a practice. This may be in the morning as patients scheduled for surgery are being checked in along with appointments that are to be seen

by associate doctors. The busy time for another practice may be in the afternoon as clients are picking up patients, walk-ins arrive, and appointments are scheduled. Whichever the case may be, the appointment schedule must be modified to alleviate the busy time. Team member schedules should also be managed to accommodate this schedule fluctuation.

> **PRACTICE POINT**   Managing team member schedules with client appointments can maximize efficiency.

Management of Walk-ins

A veterinary practice is always going to have walk-ins regardless of an appointment policy. The client perception must be recognized as a part of good customer service. Therefore planning for these walk-ins can alleviate the stress associated with them. Time should be allotted in the scheduler for one or two walk-ins per hour, per veterinarian. Clients with appointments should always be assured that they will be seen first, and walk-in clients must be advised that there will be a wait, but the team will do their best to get them in as quickly as possible.

Practices can also hold appointments until the "day of." Appointments that were previously blocked off are made available that day. This allows clients with minor emergencies and walk-ins to be accommodated without having a significant impact on appointments.

Walk-ins set the appointments behind because they are often not routine exams. Practices certainly want to train their clientele that appointments are preferred, but they should never give the impression that their pet is not important enough to be seen. If a client has a concern, the staff must recommend bringing the pet in for an exam. Team members can give the client the option to make an appointment, walk in, or drop the patient off.

Patient Drop-off

Depending on the veterinary team, accepting patients as drop-offs can eliminate the backlog of appointments. Patients that have been dropped off can be fit between appointments, and if blood work or radiographs need to be performed, they can be completed before the owner returns (with owner permission). Technicians must gather a complete history of the patient before the owner leaves and, if possible, provide a preliminary estimate for tests or procedures the doctor might recommend. After the doctor has been able to examine the pet, the owner can be called and decisions can be made regarding the patient's case. Once the case is completed, the owner can be called. This satisfies clients because they do not have to wait for a prolonged period. Certain clients will never leave their "babies" at the clinic, and those clients must always be seen. Some team members may object to drop-offs, but with a well-trained staff this can free up a large amount of time.

No-Show Appointments

All practices have clients who do not show up for appointments. Emergencies may occur, a client may forget, or a pet may disappear for a few hours (cats especially!). Team members should call clients the day before their appointments to remind them of their scheduled appointment times. This can eliminate client forgetfulness; if the client knows that making the appointment will be impossible, the appointment can be rescheduled during the phone call. Clients can also be sent text messages or email reminders, indicating the time and nature of their appointment.

> **PRACTICE POINT** No-show appointments are costly to the practice, and every measure should be taken to minimize them.

If a client does not show up, a team member should call and attempt to reschedule the appointment. It should be noted in the record that the client did not show for the appointment and that a team member attempted to reschedule the appointment. Specific clients may frequently be no-shows. This should be documented in the record. These clients can be nicely advised that they will need to come as walk-ins and will be seen as appointments permit. Veterinary software allows alerts to be entered, informing team members as they access the account to make the appointment.

Clients Who Arrive on the Wrong Day

Every veterinary practice has clients who arrive to the practice on the wrong day but still want to be seen. First, make sure the appointment card was written correctly. A team member may have incorrectly written the date, in which case every effort must be taken to correct the problem. The client should still be seen at the scheduled appointment time, and sincere apologies given to the client regarding the mistake. If a client has made an error, team members may ask the client if he or she wants to keep the original time scheduled (if it has not already passed) or prefers to reschedule the appointment. Otherwise, team members should make every effort to work the client into the schedule. Remember, excellent customer service is the goal, and being able to satisfy a client is very important.

Appointment Cards

Clients should always be given appointment cards when they have made an appointment while they are in the clinic. Appointment cards may have a business card with the veterinary practice name, address, phone number, email and Web address on the front and an open slot for the appointment in the back. The date, day, and time of the appointment should be written in along with the patient's name (Figure 13-12). It is a good idea to include the office policy regarding no-show appointments on the back of the card. This reminds clients that the veterinary practice time is valuable.

If a surgical procedure has been scheduled, instructions for the pet should be given to the owner. These patients are generally held off food and water before surgery, are dropped off at a specific time, and may be picked up at a specific time. Clients should be given this information in writing to take home; this allows them to review the information in a quiet place (Figure 13-13).

> **PRACTICE POINT** Always provide clients with an appointment card.

Entering Appointments

Specific information is needed when making appointments for clients. Obviously, the client's first and last names are essential. The patient's name and the reason for the appointment come next, along with a phone number

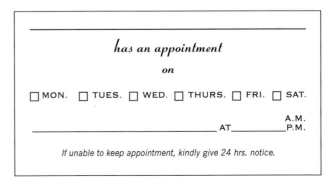

FIGURE 13-12 Appointment cards remind clients of their scheduled appointment times and decrease no-shows.

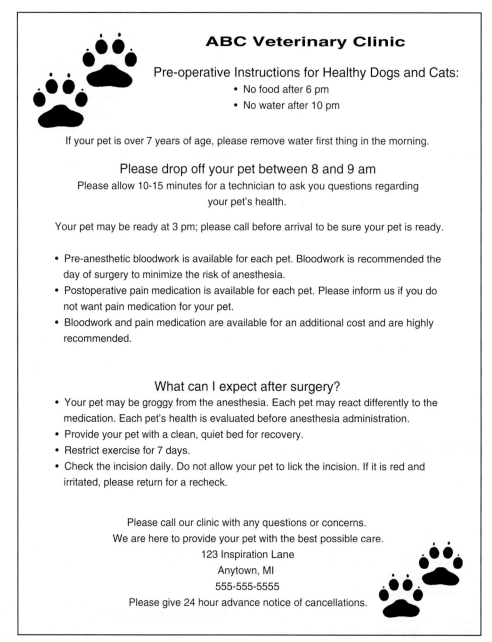

ABC Veterinary Clinic

Pre-operative Instructions for Healthy Dogs and Cats:
- No food after 6 pm
- No water after 10 pm

If your pet is over 7 years of age, please remove water first thing in the morning.

Please drop off your pet between 8 and 9 am
Please allow 10-15 minutes for a technician to ask you questions regarding
your pet's health.

Your pet may be ready at 3 pm; please call before arrival to be sure your pet is ready.

- Pre-anesthetic bloodwork is available for each pet. Bloodwork is recommended the day of surgery to minimize the risk of anesthesia.
- Postoperative pain medication is available for each pet. Please inform us if you do not want pain medication for your pet.
- Bloodwork and pain medication are available for an additional cost and are highly recommended.

What can I expect after surgery?
- Your pet may be groggy from the anesthesia. Each pet may react differently to the medication. Each pet's health is evaluated before anesthesia administration.
- Provide your pet with a clean, quiet bed for recovery.
- Restrict exercise for 7 days.
- Check the incision daily. Do not allow your pet to lick the incision. If it is red and irritated, please return for a recheck.

Please call our clinic with any questions or concerns.
We are here to provide your pet with the best possible care.
123 Inspiration Lane
Anytown, MI
555-555-5555
Please give 24 hour advance notice of cancellations.

FIGURE 13-13 Preoperative instructions should be sent home with clients so they have all the information they need before their pet's procedure.

where the client can be reached. Veterinary appointment software automatically populates all the information except for the reason for the appointment when the client's name is entered. When using a manual appointment book, it may benefit the team to add species, age, and breed of pet. Having all this information allows the veterinary health care team to prepare for the appointment. Team members know which client will be arriving, what procedure to expect, and what equipment or lab work may be required. This increases the overall efficiency of the team, ultimately leading to a satisfied client.

It is important to have a phone number where the client can be reached on the day of the appointment (as well as a cell phone) in case of an emergency or if questions arise.

Veterinarians or team members may get sick or have family emergencies that must be taken care of. Clients will appreciate the phone call notifying them of the delay and may be happy to reschedule their appointment.

Once the appointment information has been completely entered, the team member should read the appointment back to the client, ensuring no miscommunication has occurred. *"Mr. Lockridge, we have Rosie scheduled for her yearly exam on Monday, January 21, at 9 AM with Dr. Dreamer. Is there anything else I can help you with until we see you on the twenty-first?"* is an excellent statement to make because the date has been repeated twice (once while making the appointment; the other while reviewing) for the client.

Training New Employees Appointment Unit List

1 Unit = 15 Minutes

Surgeries

Canine Neuter	2 Units
Canine Spay	3 Units
Feline Neuter	1 Unit
Feline Spay	2 Units
Growth Removal – Ask DVM performing surgery	
Dental	2 Units

Nonsterile Procedures

Radiographs	2 Units
Ear Flush	1 Unit
Anal Sac Flush	1 Unit

Exams

New Client	2 Units
Booster Exam	1 Unit
Yearly Exam	1 Unit
Senior Exam	2 Units
Orthopedic Exam	2 Units
Avian/Exotic Exam	2 Units

FIGURE 13-14 Appointment units make scheduling appointments easier.

Units for Appointment Schedule

Many veterinary software applications name time increments as *units*. When the schedule is set up, the manager assigns a specific time to equal 1 unit. For example, 15 minutes may be classified as 1 unit. If a regular appointment will only take 15 minutes, then one unit is allotted for that patient. Orthopedic procedures can take 30 minutes and possibly more if radiographs are needed. Therefore this particular appointment would be given 2 units (30 minutes total). This can apply to surgical procedures as well. If a canine neuter takes a team 30 minutes from time of injection to time of extubation, then 2 units would be given for that particular operation. Tumor removals that may require extensive time are given more units. The veterinarian performing the surgery can be asked for a time estimate for the surgery. If the doctor requests 1 hour, then 4 units would be allotted for that operation. By giving time a unit, it is easier to schedule appointments, and the efficiency of the staff is increased. Any system implemented by a practice must be easy to understand and user-friendly. Figure 13-14 gives examples of units assigned to specific procedures.

Reminding Clients of Appointments

All clients must be called and reminded of their appointments, regardless of whether it is a surgical or general appointment. Missed appointments represent lost income. Therefore the team should do everything possible to keep missed appointments to a minimum. Many veterinary practices now have the ability to send out reminders and updates by email or text messages. Clients should be asked (during their first visit to the practice) how they wish to be contacted; some clients prefer phone calls, others may prefer a simple text message. This is another example of finding ways to identify and meet the client *needs*.

Clients appreciate the extra effort that team members are willing to put forth regarding their pets. If a procedure or lab work has been scheduled, this is a perfect time to remind clients of their instructions. Clients who don't follow instructions fall in the same category as missed appointments; a canceled surgical procedure is lost revenue.

Training New Employees How to Use the Appointment System

Once team members have experience at scheduling appointments, making appointments becomes an easy, efficient task. However, scheduling appointments can cause anxiety for new employees. A training program should be implemented to ease this stress and decrease the chance of mistakes.

Software systems generally have the usual amount of time allotted for appointments built into the template of the system. However, a list of conditions or diseases and the length of time preferred for related appointments should be made available. A list similar to Figure 13-14 can be created to assist new employees.

A list of clients who need extra time should also be made available to new employees if alerts have not already been added to these client's accounts. This will increase the efficiency of the team and add another element to preventing appointments from running behind.

Selecting, managing, and revising an appointment schedule is an intricate but integral part of the veterinary practice. The schedule must be able to meet the needs of the practice, team members, and clients, while balancing productivity and profitability. Studies indicate that clients regard on-time performance to be a more important factor than the practice fee structure. Compliance rates are also known to drop for

---

ABC Veterinary Clinic – Patient Audit

Client _____ Pet _____ Age _____ Date_____

Puppy/first vaccination series:

DHPP   Yes/No   Booster?   Yes/No

Bordetella   Yes/No   Booster?   Yes/No

Rabies   Yes/No

Leptospirosis or Rattlesnake exposure?   Yes/No

Dewormer?

Puppy Kit?   Yes/No

Fecal   Yes/No   Advised? Yes/No

Heartgard   Sm/Med/Lg; 1 month/6 month/12 month

Home Again Chip   Yes/No

Yearly Exam/Regular Exam

DHPP   Yes/No Due Date _____

Rabies   Yes/No Due Date _____

Bordetella   Yes/No Due Date _____

Rattlesnake   Yes/No Due Date _____

Leptospirosis   Yes/No Due Date _____

Urinalysis   Yes/No   Advised: Yes/No

Heartgard   Sm/Med/Lg; 6 month/12 month

Heartworm/E-Canis/Anaplasmosis/Lyme Test   Yes/No

Home Again Chip   Yes/No

Senior Wellness Canine

DHPP   Yes/No Due Date _____

Rabies   Yes/No Due Date _____

Bordetella   Yes/No Due Date _____

Lepto/Rattlesnake Yes/No Due date _____

Heartworm/E-Canis/Anaplasmosis/Lyme Test   Yes/No

Heartgard   Sm/Med/Lg; 6 month/12 month

General Health Profile/EKG

Urinalysis/Blood Pressure _____

Kitten/first vaccination series:

FeLV/FIV/HWT

FVRCP   Booster?   Yes/No

FeLV   Booster?   Yes/No

Rabies   Yes/No

Dewormer?   Yes/No

Kitten Kit   Yes/No

Fecal   Yes/No   Advise? Yes/No

Heartgard/Revolution

Yearly Exam/Regular Exam

Felv/FIV/HWT

FVRCP   Yes/No Due Date _____

FeLV   Yes/No Due Date _____

Rabies   Yes/No Due Date _____

Urinalysis   Yes/No   Advised: Yes/No

Heartgard/Revolution

Senior Wellness: Feline

Felv/FIV/HWT

FVRCP   Yes/No Due Date _____

FeLV   Yes/No Due Date _____

Rabies   Yes/No Due Date _____

Heartgard/Revolution

General Health Profile/EKG/Blood Pressure _____

Urinalysis/T-4

FIGURE 13-15 Patient audits help team members identify services or products the pet may need while visiting the hospital.

clients that have to wait for a prolonged period of time; irritated clients are not willing to listen or accept recommendations for products or services.

If a patient is going to need further workup, including radiographs or diagnostic tests, it may be advised to leave the patient at the hospital while the workup is being completed. This prevents the client from waiting in the exam room for an extended period of time, thereby making other clients wait in the reception area. If clients do not wish to leave their pet, they may instead choose to make another appointment for their pets when a workup needs to be completed.

It is a common misconception that by meeting the needs of the one client in the exam room and satisfying that client the practice is providing good customer service. Unfortunately, the multiple clients who are waiting are not receiving good customer service; therefore a balance between the two must be developed.

Preparing for the Appointment

Getting the clients into the practice is the first part of the appointment (see Chapter 2, Turning Phone Calls into Appointments); preparing for each appointment is the next step.

> **PRACTICE POINT** Preparing for an appointment can increase efficiency and client compliance and satisfaction.

Each medical record should be reviewed before the patient arrives at the hospital. This allows team members to become familiar with the patient and determine what services and products may be needed for the patient. Many times, practices get busy and overlook standard services that the patient needs. For example, a patient may present for an ear infection. The team focuses on solving the presenting problem but does not notice that the patient is overdue for a heartworm test and is not receiving heartworm preventative. Although administering and requesting heartworm preventative can be seen as an obligation of the owner, it is also an obligation of the staff to follow up with the owner to ensure compliance.

To help team members prepare for appointments, a patient audit may be performed (Figure 13-15). The patient history can be reviewed, looking for any chronic medications that are administered, and determining if any lab work would need to be run to stay in compliance with hospital recommendations. This is also a good time to check for overdue vaccines, previous recommendations for dental prophylaxis, and needed refills for flea, tick, and heartworm preventatives.

Clients would prefer to visit the practice one time for all of their service needs (especially when visiting for anything other than the yearly exam), instead of receiving a reminder 1 month later, indicating what services are due.

⚖ **VETERINARY PRACTICE and the LAW**

Client education time slots should be allotted for clients who have hospitalized pets that will be released. Intense cases require owner communication; they must be informed of the disease or condition, how to treat the disease or condition, as well as the prognosis of the case. If owners are not provided information, the practitioner may be held liable.

If a diabetic patient is released to the owner without client education, the animal could die of hypoglycemia induced by the owner. Owners must be informed of how and when to give insulin injections, the care of insulin, symptoms of hypoglycemia, and the role of the diet with diabetes.

If a time slot is not held for client education, the team member or veterinarian may be rushed and not thoroughly explain the disease or condition. Clients should be provided with written materials that should be verbally reviewed, allowing the client an opportunity to ask questions.

REVIEW QUESTIONS

1. Why should a veterinary practice implement an appointment system if one is not already in place?
2. How can clients be informed of the changes when a practice wants to implement an appointment system? Why create a positive atmosphere when making these changes?
3. What is the benefit of clients dropping off patients?
4. Why should veterinary clinics strive for a proactive environment?
5. Why should an appointment be established for client education?
6. Explain how to handle clients who are always late for their appointments.
7. What factors affect appointment scheduling?
8. Specific clients always take longer for appointments. Why allot those specific clients more time than other clients?
9. Why should walk-in clients be seen?
10. What information is vital when scheduling appointments?
11. The goals of an appointment system include which of the following?
    a. Maximize productivity
    b. Reduce staff tension
    c. Control traffic within the veterinary hospital
    d. All of the above
    e. None of the above
12. The longer a client waits to be seen for his appointment, the more likely:
    a. Compliance with increase
    b. Compliance will decrease
    c. Compliance will not change with appointment wait times
13. To help reduce client overload at the front desk, appointments should be:
    a. Set every 15 minutes
    b. Staggered by at least 5 minutes
    c. None of the above

14. Appointments should be set for:
    a. Client education
    b. Surgery/dental procedures
    c. Technicians
    d. All of the above
    e. None of the above
15. Appointment lengths may vary for all of the following except:
    a. Specific client
    b. Appointment type
    c. Veterinarian
    d. Patient

Recommended Reading

Heinke MM: *Practice made perfect: a guide to veterinary practice management*, ed 2, Lakewood, CO, 2012, AAHA Press.

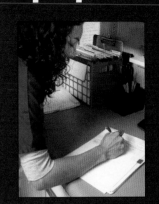

Medical Records Management

OUTLINE

Legibility of Medical Records, *257*
Choosing a File System, *257*
Paper Records, *257*
Computerized Medical Records, *258*
Choosing Medical Record Software, *261*
   Efficiency of Computerized Laboratory
     Requisition Forms, *261*
Medical Records Release, *261*
Establishing a Medical Record, *261*
What is Included in a Medical Record?, *262*
Taking a History, *262*
SOAP and POMR Medical Records, *264*
Herd Health Records, *266*

Purging Medical Records, *266*
Client Discharge Instructions, *267*
Most Common Medical Records
   Violations, *270*
Common Abbreviations, *271*
Radiographs, *271*
Backing Up the Computer System
   Daily, *272*
Management's Role in Medical Records, *272*
   Medical Records Audit, *272*
   Value to the Practice, *272*
   Value of Pet Portals, *272*

KEY TERMS

Client Discharge
  Instructions
Computerized Medical
  Records
Herd Health Records
Legibility
Master Problem List
Paper Medical Records
Primary Complaint
Problem-Oriented
  Medical Record
  (POMR)
Prognosis
Purging Records
SOAP Medical Record
System Backup

LEARNING OBJECTIVES

When you have completed this chapter, you should be able to:

1. Explain methods used to file records.
2. Identify a completed medical record.
3. List the benefits of using labels for medical records.
4. Explain how to purge medical records when needed.
5. Define the advantages and disadvantages of computerized medical records.

6. Develop and provide patient discharge instructions.
7. Identify common abbreviations.
8. Describe methods used to file radiographs.
9. Clarify the importance of backing up computer systems on a daily basis.

CRITICAL COMPETENCIES

1. **Adaptability** - being open to change and flexible work methods; the ability to adapt behavior to changing conditions or new information.
2. **Analytical Skills** - the ability to analyze information and use logic to address problems; the ability to quickly and accurately grasp complex information and concepts and to make correct inferences.
3. **Compliance** - being reliable, thorough, and conscientious in carrying out work assignments; has an appreciation for the importance of organizational rules and policies.
4. **Continuous Learning** - a curiosity for learning; actively seek out new information, technologies, and methods; keep skills updated and applies new knowledge to the job.

5. **Creativity** - the ability to think creatively about situations, to see things in new and different ways; use imagination and creativity to develop innovative solutions to problems.
6. **Critical and Strategic Thinking** - the ability to think critically about situations and to understand the relevance of information for different problems; use critical reasoning to generate and evaluate alternative courses of action or points of view relevant to an issue.
7. **Decision Making** - the ability to make good decisions, solve problems, and decide on important matters; the ability to gather and analyze relevant data and choose decisively between alternatives.

8. **Integrity** - honesty, trustworthiness, and adherence to high standards of ethical conduct.
9. **Leadership** - a willingness to lead and take charge; the ability to motivate others and mobilize group effort toward common goals.
10. **Oral Communication and Comprehension** - the ability to express one's thoughts verbally in a clear and understandable manner, and the ability to actively listen and attend to what others are saying; must have good group presentation skills.
11. **Persuasion** - the ability to change the attitudes and opinions of others and to persuade them to accept recommendations and change behavior.
12. **Planning and Prioritizing** - the ability to effectively manage time and work load to meet deadlines; the ability to organize work, set priorities, and establish plans for achieving goals.
13. **Relationship Building** - the ability to develop constructive and cooperative working relationships with others and maintain them over time; must also be able to settle disputes, resolve grievances and conflicts, and negotiate with others.
14. **Resilience** - the ability to cope effectively with pressure and setbacks; the ability to handle crisis situations effectively and remain undeterred by obstacles or failure.
15. **Resourcefulness** - the ability to understand what it takes to complete the job; apply knowledge, skills, and expertise to perform tasks quickly and efficiently.
16. **Writing and Verbal Skills** - ability to comprehend written material easily and accurately; ability to express thoughts clearly and succinctly in writing.

In the organization of the practice domain, the veterinary practice manager is responsible for general practice management, including maintaining appropriate inventory and medical records systems, establishing protocol for hospital policies and procedures, and coordinating equipment acquisition and maintenance.

Knowledge Requirements

The tasks in this domain require a working knowledge of veterinary medical terminology, the requirements for common veterinary practice procedures (e.g., anesthesia, radiography, IV injections, lab work), and preventative health and risk management protocols. Tasks in this domain also require knowledge of inventory systems and methods, standards for maintaining medical records, and protocols for equipment maintenance and insurance.

Medical records are some of the most important documents in veterinary medicine, and medical record management is one of the most important management tasks. A medical record is a permanent written account of the professional interaction and services rendered in a valid patient-client relationship. Medical records serve many purposes. Obviously, the first purpose is to provide an accurate historical account for the veterinary health care team and owner, enabling any veterinary team member to continue treatment for the patient. It also provides team members a means of communication, alerts them to a patient's special needs, serves as documentation for referrals, serves as evidence in a court of law, and is an asset to the veterinary practice. Records must be complete, legible, and easily accessible at all times. Clinics may choose to have paper records or computerized medical records (often referred to as *paperless medical records*); both have advantages and disadvantages. Inactive records must be kept for a certain length of time, (state law varies regarding

length of time) and can be purged after a set period. Computerized medical records should always be available. It is also important to remember that any written communication with the owner must be in the medical record; the fact that these documents may become evidence in a malpractice suit warrants caution in writing and retaining them (Figure 14-1).

How medical records are maintained depends on each individual clinic. Some medical record systems have evolved with the practice; others may need updating to allow the veterinary practice to become more efficient and provide better patient and client care. The number of veterinarians and team members on staff, along with practice maturity, can affect a medical records system. There can be remarkable differences in medical records between team members, which can decrease the efficiency of the staff. It should be the goal of the team, office, and practice managers to develop a medical records system that allows maximum efficiency as well as excellent client communication and patient care.

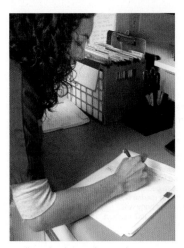

FIGURE 14-1 All medical records must be accurate and complete.

Legibility of Medical Records

Records must be legible and able to be read by anyone. Many team members become proficient at being able to read records written by another team member, but once those records are released to another practice, specialty hospital, or court, the intended audience may not be able to read or interpret them. This can render a record incomplete. If a record was sent to court, a judge may return a decision based on the opinion that a treatment did not occur because he or she could not read the record. A veterinary specialist may not be able to determine if a specific treatment was done because it was not legible. An incomplete, illegible record can be considered an admission of professional incompetence and imply that the service provided was substandard. If records are often illegible, upgrading to paperless records should be considered.

Veterinary practice managers maintain an appropriate medical records system that complies with legal standards.

If legibility is a problem within a veterinary practice, the use of labels or stamps may be suggested for routine procedures. Physical exams, urinalyses, routine dental procedures, and alterations are just a few labels that can be generated in a fill-in-the-blank form to accommodate details. Size of suture material can be easily added on surgical stickers, normal findings can be easily marked on physical exam stickers, and abnormal findings can be clearly defined below the label or stamp (Figure 14-2).

Blank labels can be purchased at a local office supply store relatively inexpensively. Labels can be created within Microsoft Word and can be changed at any time to fit the needs of the practice.

PRACTICE POINT Writing illegible medical records is perceived as an incompetency in veterinary practitioners. Use labels to help increase clarity and interpretation.

BOX 14-1 | Single Line Correction

stopped (N.S.)
Owner ~~started~~ antibiotics 5 days ago.

A medical record is a legal document. Correction fluid cannot be used on any medical record, release, or authorization form at any time. If a mistake needs to be corrected, a one-line strikethrough can be written, with the author's initials indicating the correction (Box 14-1).

Choosing a File System

Practices that use paper records may file records according to different methods. One method is to file alphabetically. All records are filed by the owner's last name, then the first name. Other practices may file by client number. All pets are kept in the same file because many owners have more than one pet. Also included is a client/patient form (see Figure 2-8, *A*; client patient information sheet). Consent forms, patient check-in sheets, treatment plans (estimates), discharge sheets, and any other forms must be kept in this file as well.

Paper Records

Paper records must be full paper records (index card records are no longer considered standard of care). Paper records are written on 8.5 × 11 inch paper and usually fastened into a file folder with a two-hole fastener (Figure 14-3). All lab work results, invoices, consent forms, and miscellaneous documents are kept in this file. Pets can be separated by colored paper. Some clinics may use either blue or pink paper to draw attention to the sex of the patient (preventing team members from offending clients by identifying their pet by the wrong gender). Names can be listed on the colored paper with tabs for quick access. The medical record may also be either blue or pink, indicating the sex of the patient. Some practices maintain one file per pet even when they come from the same household. There is no right or wrong method; however, efficiency and cost must be considered.

File folders can be alphabetized by client name or filed by client number, and colored letters and/or numbered labels can help identify those that are misfiled (Figure 14-4). Color coding the exterior of files can help identify misfiled charts from either the front or the back. Numbers indicating the year on the outside of the file can also help identify the last time a client has been into the practice, making it easier for team members to purge files efficiently.

Alphabetical filing is the most common method used in practice. The last name, then first, along with a client identification number, is generally listed on the exterior of a file; the file is then alphabetized by the client's last name.

Colored warning stickers attached to patient medical records may draw attention to special medical needs (Figure 14-5). Sample stickers may include "Will Bite!" "Anesthetic Alert!" or "Vaccine Reaction." Brightly colored stickers can

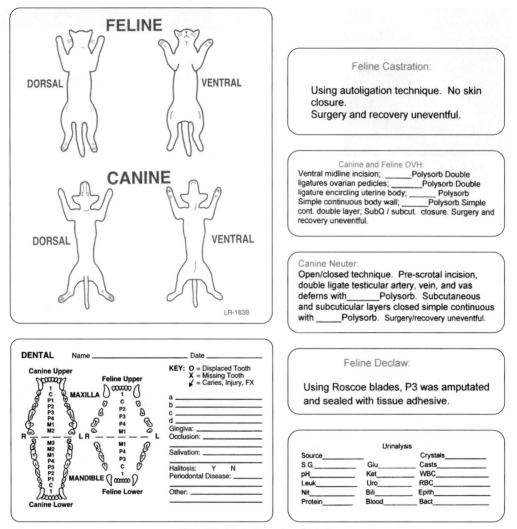

FELINE

DORSAL   VENTRAL

CANINE

DORSAL   VENTRAL

LR-163B

Feline Castration:

Using autoligation technique. No skin closure.
Surgery and recovery uneventful.

Canine and Feline OVH:
Ventral midline incision; _____Polysorb Double
ligatures ovarian pedicles; _____Polysorb Double
ligature encircling uterine body; _____ Polysorb
Simple continuous body wall; _____Polysorb Simple
cont. double layer; SubQ / subcut. closure. Surgery and
recovery uneventful.

Canine Neuter:
Open/closed technique. Pre-scrotal incision,
double ligate testicular artery, vein, and vas
deferns with_____Polysorb. Subcutaneous
and subcuticular layers closed simple continuous
with _____Polysorb. Surgery/recovery uneventful.

Feline Declaw:

Using Roscoe blades, P3 was amputated
and sealed with tissue adhesive.

DENTAL   Name _____ Date _____

Canine Upper
                    Feline Upper
        MAXILLA

R _ _ _ _ _ L R _ _ _ _ _ L

        MANDIBLE
        Feline Lower
Canine Lower

KEY: O = Displaced Tooth
X = Missing Tooth
= Caries, Injury, FX

a _____
b _____
c _____
d _____
Gingiva: _____
Occlusion: _____

Salivation: _____

Halitosis: Y   N
Periodontal Disease: _____

Other: _____

Urinalysis
Source_____   Crystals_____
S.G._____ Glu_____ Casts_____
pH_____ Ket_____ WBC_____
Leuk_____ Uro_____ RBC_____
Nit_____ Bili_____ Epith_____
Protein_____ Blood_____ Bact_____

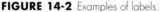

FIGURE 14-2 Examples of labels.

also be used on cage identification cards to alert team members of a patient's special needs. A "Will Bite" sticker is beneficial for alerting team members to animals that require special precautions.

Although patient medical alerts should be obvious, team members can get busy and overlook a handwritten alert. A sticker that is big, bright, and bold will catch the attention of staff members. This is a cheap method for preventing a potential disaster.

Computerized Medical Records

Computerized medical records, also referred to as *paperless records,* are filed in the computer by both client number and last name (Figure 14-6). Any record can be accessed from any computer. Lab work, radiographs, and ultrasound results are stored within the record. All charts, consent forms, and miscellaneous documents must be stored within the record. A practice that is truly paperless does not have any additional client files or folders that store release forms, lab work, or radiographs.

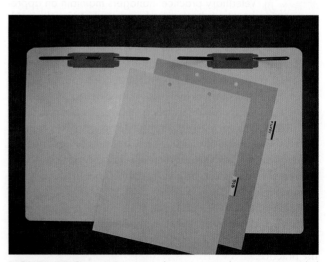

FIGURE 14-3 An 8.5 × 11 inch paper records are recommended over index cards.

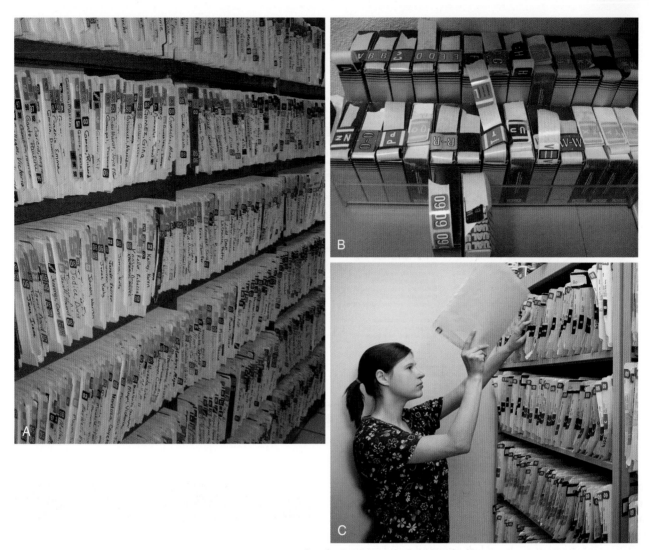

FIGURE 14-4 A – C, Examples of colored letters and numbers for files.

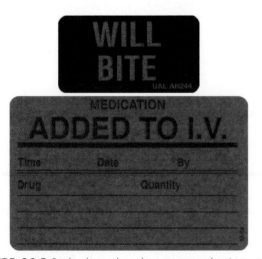

FIGURE 14-5 Bright alert stickers draw team members' attention to special needs patients.

Forms and lab work are scanned into the client's record, or the client must sign the forms electronically, which are then stored in the computer. Radiographs are either in digital form or they are scanned into the record. Most lab work machines will enter results into the client's file once the machine has completed the work. Client identification numbers must be verified before entering lab work to ensure the results will be populated into the correct records. When outside laboratory results are received, they can be electronically filed within the patient's chart. An onscreen notice pops up for the veterinarian or staff when those results have become available.

> **PRACTICE POINT** Computerized medical records are the way of the future and increase the efficiency of every veterinary team.

Computer medical records must be secure, with access limited to authorized individuals only. Computers must be backed up daily and monthly, preferably off-site for the

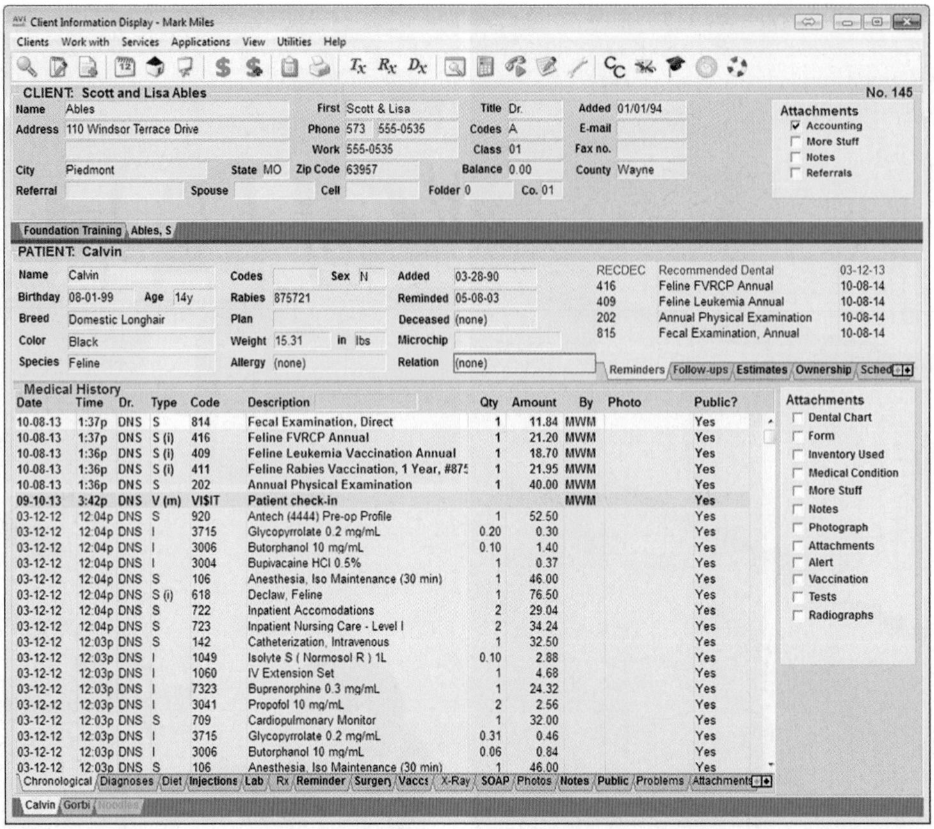

FIGURE 14-6 Sample medical history in a computerized medical record. (Courtesy AVImark, LLC, Piedmont, Mo.)

best security. Software should have an automatic lockout time period, preventing records from being changed after a backup has been completed. Late entries can be added, but a new date will appear with the updates (addendum).

Patient information can be added to computerized records in several ways. Doctors may enter information while they are examining the patient, a veterinary technician or transcriptionist can enter notes written by the doctor to complete the record, or a doctor may use a template that has been generated by the computer to complete the record.

Paper records and paperless records each have their advantages and disadvantages, all of which must be weighed when determining what is best for an individual practice (Box 14-2).

The greatest advantage of paperless records is that they can be accessed from any computer. Most paperless practices have a computer available in every exam room, office, and laboratory area. Records are never lost, misplaced, or misfiled. However, computer systems can fail; therefore records may be inaccessible until the system has been repaired. A "plan B" should be developed in case a system does crash to prevent a major catastrophe from occurring. This may include having a few laptops that serve as backups if a computer becomes unusable. The laptops should have software preloaded, allowing them to be plugged into the server and available for use immediately. If the main server becomes unusable, a second unit should be available, and the storage drive with data from the last daily backup can be loaded. This will keep the practice flowing until the main server has been repaired.

BOX 14-2 | Advantages and Disadvantages of Computerized Medical Records

Advantages
- Easy to capture missing charges
- Easy to access medical records at any computer station
- Can target specific clients quickly and efficiently when promoting specific services
- Takes less time to enter information into the computer than to write it out
- Legible
- Client perceives progressive, higher quality medicine
- Computers take up less space
- Eco-friendly; saves paper

Disadvantages
- Possibility of server crashing
- Records can be lost or altered through computer corruption
- Computer-generated records can lack medical details

One must also consider the possibility of a power outage. Many practices have windows that allow light to enter and emergency lighting within hallways. However, the computer system cannot be forgotten. A backup generator must be considered, preventing this potential catastrophe from occurring. The generator can either be small enough to maintain the computer system, or be large enough to support the major functions of the hospital.

A major disadvantage of computerized medical records is the lack of security to prevent alteration. If a record can be altered, it may be questioned in a court of law. The practice attorney should be consulted regarding the likelihood of problems if a malpractice claim arises. Backing up information onto CDs that can only be written on once may satisfy the court.

Some software companies are excellent at providing medical record lockout periods; these lockout periods prevent medical record alteration after 24 hours (addendums can always be added with the date of the entry). Others do not have a lockout period, allowing records to be altered days or even months later. This disadvantage must be considered when choosing software for the practice.

The advantages and disadvantages of computerized software change annually as new technology is introduced. Computers and software initially can be costly, but their inherent increased efficiency far outweighs the cost. Updates are made available for current software users and should be used to maximum potential.

Choosing Medical Record Software

Veterinary software can have a variety of applications. Some software may be management based, helping maintain inventory and create client invoices, whereas other software may be based on medical record management. Many companies have integrated the two, creating some dynamic choices.

Some practices use a combination of computerized and paper medical records. The computerized medical records can efficiently generate reminders, patient/client alerts, and invoices. Once the patient has been established in the computer system, a paper record is generated for the medical portion of the record. The invoicing system generates a patient history (assuming every procedure was charged for) but lacks the medical details needed to complete a medical record.

PRACTICE POINT Try several different demos of veterinary software before choosing a particular company.

Efficiency of Computerized Laboratory Requisition Forms

Some laboratories work with veterinary practices to generate requisition forms online, creating a unique form and bar code. For example, IDEXX (Westbrook, Me.) LabREXX software (www.idexx.com/labrexx) works with existing veterinary practice software, allowing charges to be captured while ensuring no mistakes are made when submitting the client, patient, and doctor information. To help increase efficiency, a quick guide of the most common tests the practice selects is available, allowing results to be emailed directly to clients and results to be downloaded to patient records. This prevents lost and/or misfiled results. Records are flagged, allowing the team to know that results have arrived in a patient's file.

Chapter 8 gives a brief overview of software that is available in today's market, along with a worksheet to help determine which software will work best for a veterinary practice.

Medical Records Release

Records are confidential and can only be released when the owner has given permission to do so. Clients must sign a records release form that must be kept in the medical record. This includes release to any other veterinary hospital, any boarding or grooming facility, or a new owner of the pet. Any practice can be held liable for the release of records without the owner's consent. It is important to understand the Privacy Act and not release any records without the client's authorization. The Privacy Act of 1974 states in part:

No agency shall disclose any record which is contained in a system of records by any means of communication to any person, or to another agency, except pursuant to a written request by, or with the prior written consent of, the individual to whom the record pertains.

A client is entitled to a copy of his or her record. The original record is the property of the hospital, along with any diagnostic images and laboratory results; however, a client may request copies. Any time a client is referred to a specialist, a copy of the record should be sent (or emailed), along with relevant images that have been taken (if not in digital form, radiographs should be checked out in a log book). If a digital radiograph has been taken, a CD can be generated and sent with the owner, or the image can be emailed to the specialist with a consult form.

All cases must be kept confidential. Cases cannot be discussed by name with clients; the privacy of both the client and the pet must be respected.

PRACTICE POINT All cases must be kept confidential. Cases cannot be discussed by name with clients; the privacy of both the client and the pet must be respected

Establishing a Medical Record

Regardless of the software chosen or whether the records are on paper or computerized, every medical record must follow specific criteria.

- Each patient must have its own medical record. Multiple animals cannot be listed on one sheet of 8.5 × 11 inch paper. It is acceptable for multiple pets to be in one file folder under the name of one owner, but they must be separated with dividers.
- Records must be easy to retrieve. Lost records increase staff and client frustration, time, and labor costs.
- Medical records must be complete and well organized. Each entry should follow a standard SOAP (subjective, objective, assessment, and plan) format that allows the staff to easily follow the progress of the patient.
- Records should be composed as legal documents that can be admissible in court if needed.
- Legibility of records is a must! Illegible records can lead to incorrect dosing of medication and protocols.

What is Included in a Medical Record?

Each medical record must have the same information, regardless of the type of pet, client, or veterinary software used. The organization of the medical record depends on practice preference, but most hospitals use a reverse chronological order system.

The most recent records are placed on top of the file for easy access. Laboratory results, consultation reports, and estimates are placed after the written medical record. The most current laboratory results are placed on top in this section. However a hospital chooses to organize the record, it should be consistent with all medical records throughout the medical record database. The following is required information for each patient record:

- Client/Patient Information Sheet: Some clinics separate these two forms, and others combine them. It is critical that the owner complete the client information in as much detail as possible (see Chapter 2). Client information must be verified at each visit to ensure that the most current information, including the phone number, is kept on file.
- Previous Medical History: If a patient has been seen by another veterinarian and received prior medical treatment, the history should be recorded here.
- Vaccination History: Each patient should have some type of vaccine history unless it is a young puppy or kitten. Dates and types of vaccines administered should be documented. Once the patient has established a history with the practice, vaccine history can be reviewed and updated with each visit. It is important to document where vaccines have been administered on the pet's body for future reference.
- The Primary Complaint: This will accurately summarize the client's complaint and the history of the presenting problem. Team members must listen well to clients and determine the appropriate questions to ask.
- Physical Examination: The results of the pet's physical examination (PE) must be documented for each visit. If the animal is hospitalized, the patient must receive progress exams on a daily basis. These too must be written in the record. Temperature (T), weight (Wt), respiratory rate (RR), heart rate (HR), pain (P), body condition score (BCS), mucous membrane color (mm), capillary refill time (crt), eyes/ears/nose/throat (E/E/N/T), auscultation of the chest (H/L), palpation of the abdomen (Abd), examination of the lymph nodes (LN), musculoskeletal system (MS), and urogenital (Uro) must be documented. Many team members abbreviate terms, descriptions, and abnormalities. Please see the appendixes for common abbreviations used in veterinary medicine. The American Animal Hospital Association (AAHA) also produces an excellent booklet summarizing abbreviations. If a PE is omitted from the medical record, or a particular body system has been omitted, it is assumed that the exam did not occur.
- Diagnosis and/or Possible Diagnosis: Diagnosis is the identification of disease by analysis and examination. The patient may have one or several diseases, and they should all be documented.
- Laboratory Reports: All laboratory results (normal and abnormal), including radiographs, ultrasounds, and

electrocardiograms, must be documented. If a consult was completed with a specialty veterinarian, that also must be documented in the record (date, method of consult, results, and any follow-up communication with the owner). See the following section on the SOAP format for more details of laboratory interpretations.
- Treatment: Any treatment recommendation and/or medications must be written in the medical record. See the following section on the SOAP format for more details on notating medications.
- Prognosis: A prognosis is the prediction of the outcome of the disease. The prognosis must be communicated to the client and documented in the record. The prognosis may help the client decide what medical route to take when treating a pet. The prognosis can change with treatment, laboratory results, and surgery. If it does change, the record must be updated.
- Surgical Report: Any surgical procedure must be described in detail (including anesthesia drugs and duration, type and size of suture material, patient monitoring, and the initials of all technicians and veterinarians working the case) and include complications that might be expected postoperatively.
- Treatment Plans (estimates) and Consent Forms: Each client must give consent to treat a pet. If a treatment protocol has been recommended (it should be documented in the medical record), and clients should also receive an estimate. Both the consent to treat form and the client estimate should be signed and placed in the medical record. If a client declines any of the recommended treatment, that must also be entered into the medical record.

A master problem sheet is an excellent summary sheet to include at the top of all patient files. A master problem list should include the patient name, gender, species, breed, age, diet, allergies (including any to medications, vaccines, or anesthetics), current medications that the pet is receiving, and any vaccinations the pet has received. Although the master problem list is not required to complete the medical record, it helps increase the team's efficiency when refilling medications and determining vaccines for which the patient may be due. Figure 2-11 gives excellent examples of master problem sheets.

Another suggestion for increasing efficiency, although not required, is a laboratory diagnostic flow sheet for patients that return on a regular basis for lab work. The diagnostic flow sheet is a compilation of laboratory data from a patient that shows results in chronological order. These sheets can be of value when monitoring patients with ongoing or chronic diseases, such as diabetes, Cushing disease, renal failure, hyperthyroidism, or hypothyroidism.

> **PRACTICE POINT**   A diagnostic flow sheet helps increase efficiency on patients that have extensive medical workups.

Taking a History

An accurate history is one of the most important aspects of a medical record. All the information the owner has presented

must be summarized in the medical record. This allows the veterinary team to look at the presenting facts and may help the veterinarian diagnose the case more rapidly and more accurately. Many clients will chat with team members and give valuable information that neither the client nor the team member realized was pertinent. For example, a client may indicate that he or she was on vacation in Florida. Fluffy has diarrhea now. Did the pet go on vacation with the owners?

Was the pet exposed to a new environment? Did the pet have a new diet? Did the pet drink any beach water? Did Fluffy eat bird droppings on the beach? Were any special treats given? If the pet did not go on the trip, who stayed home with Fluffy? Did the house sitter stay at the house with Fluffy or did Fluffy go to a boarding kennel? These are all important questions that should be asked during a conversation about a client's recent vacation (Box 14-3).

BOX 14-3 | **List of Questions to Ask During History Taking**

Is the Patient Eating Normally?
- What is the patient fed?
- When was the last meal?
- How much did the patient eat?
- How often does the patient eat?
- Any treats? If yes, what treats? How often?

Drinking
- Is the patient drinking the same amount of water as usual?
- How often?

Vomiting
- How often is the pet vomiting?
- What color is the vomit?
- What does the vomit consist of?
- Has the pet eaten any toys, blankets, or towels?

Bowel Movements
- Is the patient defecating normally?
- What does the stool look like (color and consistency)?
- How often is the patient defecating?
- Any straining to defecate?
- If the patient has abnormal bowel movements, when did the abnormal signs start?

Urination
- How often does the patient urinate?
- Is the patient urinating the same amount as always?
- Is the urine a clear, steady stream?
- Any straining to urinate?
- If the patient is having abnormal urination, when did the abnormal signs start?

Coughing
- Does the patient cough or gag?
- If so, how often?
- When did the coughing start?
- How often does the patient cough?
- How long does the episode last?

Sneezing
- When did the patient begin sneezing?
- Does the patient have any discharge from the eyes and nose with the sneezing?
- If yes, what color is the discharge?

Walking
- Is the patient walking normally?
- If not, when did the abnormal signs begin?
- Is the pet limping or not bearing weight on an extremity?
- If yes, which one?
- Did the owner see any trauma happen to the pet?

Growth(s)
- What is the location of the growth?
- How long has the growth been present?
- Has any previous diagnostic work been completed before?
- Has it increased in size? How much?
- Has the growth changed color? How much?

Miscellaneous
- Swelling: Where is the location of the swelling? When did the client notice the swelling?
- Discharge from the eyes: When did the client notice the discharge? What color is it? Is the pet squinting the eye(s)?

WHAT WOULD YOU DO/NOT DO?

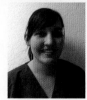

Mrs. Carwell calls the practice because her dog has developed a case of diarrhea. She is advised to bring Domino in, along with a fresh fecal sample to look for intestinal parasites. She advises the veterinarian when she arrives that she just brought home a new puppy from the shelter, which also has diarrhea; however, she attributed the diarrhea to stress and diet change. The veterinarian diagnoses Domino with giardia and dispenses albendazole to treat the parasite. Teresa, the veterinary technician, advises the owner that the puppy probably also has the parasite and needs to be seen in order to receive the correct dose of medication. The owner calls Teresa 4 days later stating that the diarrhea in Domino cleared within 2 days,

so she gave the rest of the medication to the new puppy. Now the puppy is vomiting, and she knows it is from the medication and needs another medicine to treat giardia.

What Does Teresa Do?
The owner must be advised that many parasites and viruses can cause diarrhea, and the puppy must be examined before any medication can be dispensed. Not only can the puppy have vomiting and diarrhea associated with parvovirus, it may also be having an overdosed reaction to the medication, as the albendazole was dosed for a 45-lb dog. Teresa must inform the owner of the possible side effects of the medication and note the discussion in the record. She should also make an appointment as soon as possible for Mrs. Carwell.

SOAP and POMR Medical Records

The problem-oriented medical record (POMR) is the medical record format most commonly used by veterinary health care teams. Each entry follows a distinct format: the defined database, the problem list (also referred to as *master list*), the plan, and the progress section. Within the progress section, a standard SOAP format (*s*ubjective, *o*bjective, *a*ssessment, and *p*lan) is followed. **Subjective** information is the most important element for the reception staff, veterinary technicians, and assistants. Subjective details include the reason for the office visit, the history, and observations made by the client. The opinions and perceptions of the client represent the most subjective information (Figure 14-7).

Objective information is gathered directly from the patient; the physical exam, diagnostic workup, and interpretation are included in this section of the medical record. Objective information is factual information (Figures 14-8 and 14-9).

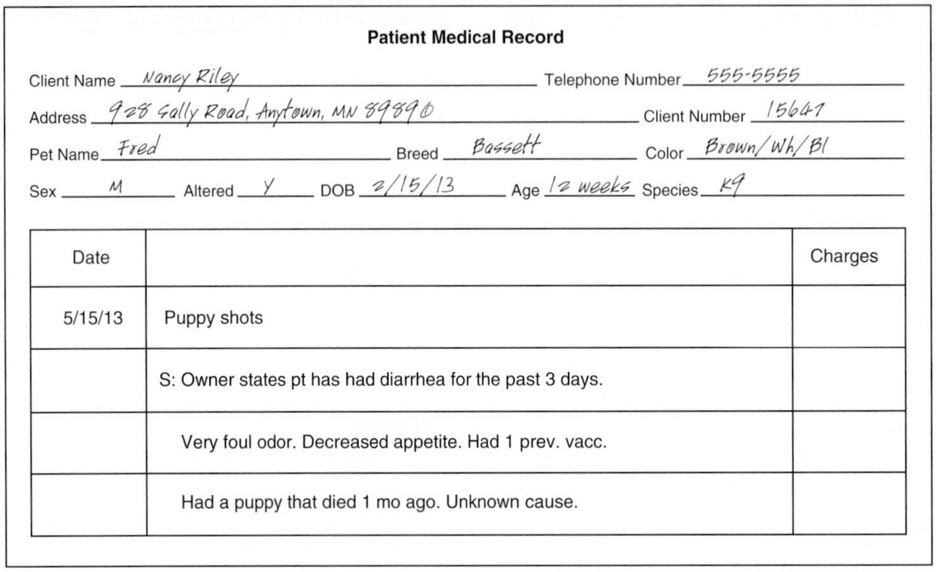

Patient Medical Record

Client Name *Nancy Riley*   Telephone Number *555-5555*

Address *928 Sally Road, Anytown, MN 89890*   Client Number *15641*

Pet Name *Fred*   Breed *Bassett*   Color *Brown/Wh/Bl*

Sex *M*   Altered *Y*   DOB *2/15/13*   Age *12 weeks*   Species *K9*

Date		Charges
5/15/13	Puppy shots	
	S: Owner states pt has had diarrhea for the past 3 days.	
	Very foul odor. Decreased appetite. Had 1 prev. vacc.	
	Had a puppy that died 1 mo ago. Unknown cause.	

FIGURE 14-7 Example of subjective notes in a medical record.

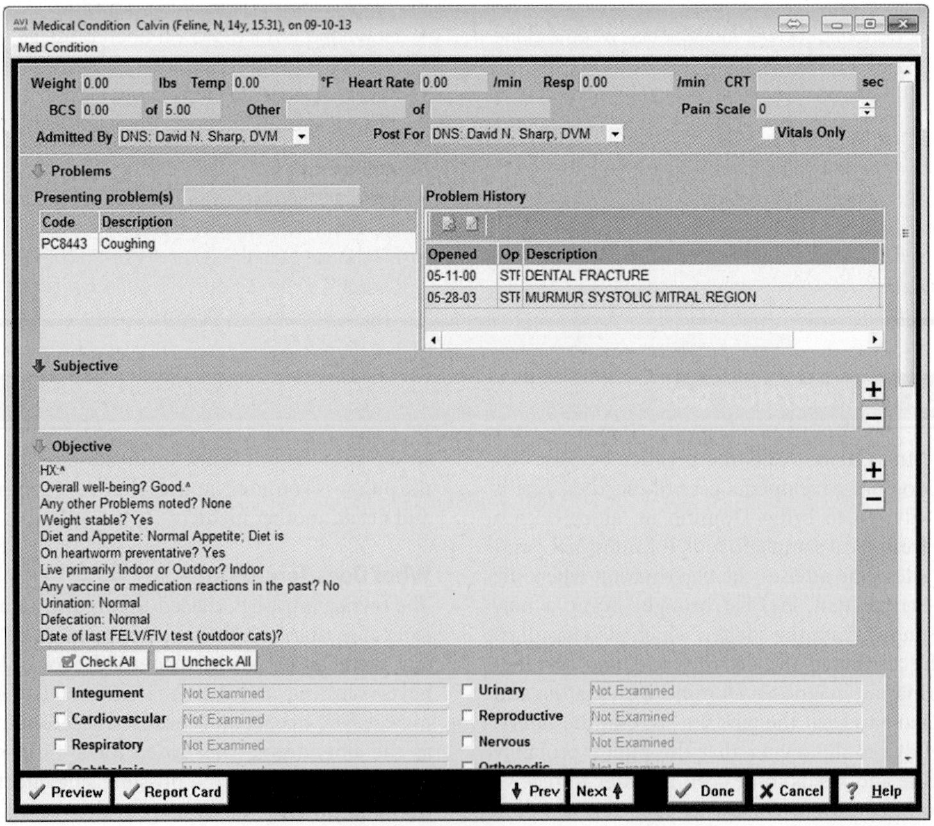

FIGURE 14-8 Example of Avimark's medical record SOAP format. (Courtesy AVImark, LLC, Piedmont, Mo.)

The **assessment** section includes any conclusions reached from the subjective and objective sections, and it includes a definitive diagnosis. If there are multiple or tentative diagnoses, they can all be documented here along with a list of "rule-ins" (R/Is) or "rule-outs" (R/Os). R/Is can be classified as any disease the patient could possibly have as well as diagnostic work that must be done to rule out those particular diseases (Figure 14-10).

A **plan** is developed according to the assessment and includes any treatment, surgery, medication, intended diagnostics, or intended communications with the owner. This can also be a list of options that will be presented to the client (Figure 14-11).

Diligent team members can often catch common errors and omissions in a medical record before the record is filed. Some of the most common incomplete errors include lack of lab work interpretation, progress notes while the patient is hospitalized, preoperative physical exams, anesthetic drugs, and initials of the author(s) writing in the record (Box 14-4).

If previous lab work is being compared with present results, this is also an excellent place to write the comparison. Veterinarians must interpret the results, not just document them! Abnormal lab work values must be written in the medical record. Interpretation is defined as analyzing the results and explaining why those abnormalities may be present. The list of R/Is and R/Os can be completed with the analysis of pending lab work.

Animals should have a daily physical exam while they are hospitalized and receive medications as recommended by the doctor. Results of the physical exam, any medications administered (drug, amount in milligrams, route of administration, who administered, and what time), and any urination, bowel movements, or vomiting must also be documented in the progress notes. Hospitalization sheets can be used to help keep track of patient status while they are hospitalized (Figure 14-12).

Surgical patients must be examined within 12 hours of anesthesia, and the exam must be documented in the medical record. Anesthetic drugs, details of the procedure, the patient's response, and any complications of the procedure must also be documented in the record. The most common error made is not documenting the communication with the owner regarding the prognosis of the patient. The medical record must clearly state if the prognosis is poor, guarded, fair, or excellent.

PRACTICE POINT Preanesthetic exams are a standard of care and should be performed on every patient within 12 hours of the anesthetic procedure.

Medication names, strength, and route given must be accurately written in the medical records. For example, "0.2 mL cefazolin IV" is an incorrect notation. This description does not indicate how many milligrams were given. The entry should read, "0.2 mL cefazolin (100 mg/mL) given IV," or it may read "20 mg cefazolin, given IV."

FIGURE 14-9 Example of objective notes in a medical record.

Patient Medical Record

Client Name _Nancy Riley_   Telephone Number _555-5555_

Address _928 Sally Road, Anytown, MN 89890_   Client Number _15641_

Pet Name _Fred_   Breed _Bassett_   Color _Brown/Wh/Bl_

Sex ___M___   Altered ___Y___   DOB _2/15/13_   Age _12 weeks_ Species _K9_

Date		Charges
5/15/13	Puppy shots	
	S: Owner states pt has had diarrhea for the past 3 days.	
	Very foul odor. Decreased appetite. Had 1 prev. vacc.	
	Had a puppy that died 1 mo ago. Unknown cause.	
	O: PE: General appearance: thin; 5% dehydrated.	
	Lethargic. EENT, LN, MS, NS, all WNL. Abd: tender when palpated.	
	MM = pale and tacky. T - 102.4, Wt - 9.9#	
	HR = 100/min, RR = 20/min, Thermom reveals bloody, loose stool.	
	A: Gastroenteritis	
	R/O Parvo, Giardia, Garbage Gut	

FIGURE 14-10 Example of assessment notes in a medical record.

Many drugs come in different strengths, and it is important to identify and document the correct strength of medication. The same drug can also be administered by different routes (some drugs will have a different dose depending on the route administered); it is therefore important to document by which route the medication was administered (Box 14-5).

If fluids are to be administered to patients, records must clearly indicate the name of the fluids, the amount the pet is receiving, and the route given (IV or SC). If a pet is simply receiving Normosol under the skin, the attending veterinarian or technician can indicate the number of milliliters administered. However, if a patient is receiving a drip intravenously, the rate must be indicated. "Normosol, 66 mL/kg/24 hours = 100 mL/hr IV" would be an accurate entry.

When medications are dispensed, the same principles apply. The name of the drug must be recorded, along with the strength, route of administration, frequency and duration of treatment. If a team member has administered the medication in the exam room, it must be documented in the medical record as well. Team members should always initial labels on prescriptions that they have filled and indicate in the medical record that they filled the request.

Herd Health Records

It is impossible for large-animal veterinarians to have individual records for each food animal they examine. Herd health records refer to the practice of recording information for an entire herd, including medications and vaccinations on one record. Individual records may be kept if surgical procedures or special treatments are completed on one animal.

Purging Medical Records

The length of time a practice must keep an inactive medical record varies from state to state. An inactive medical record is defined as a client who has not been seen by that practice for a year or more. Most states require medical records to be held for at least 3 years; some states may have a requirement to keep them up to 7 years. Because some vaccine protocols have changed to every 3 years, some clients only return when vaccinations are due. Therefore it is more cost-effective for veterinary practices maintaining paper records to keep inactive files in a storage room on premises where records can be easily accessed for a minimum of 3 years.

Many practices have limited space. Purging records on a yearly basis and moving the inactive records to another area

Patient Medical Record

Client Name _Nancy Riley_   Telephone Number _555-5555_

Address _928 Sally Road, Anytown, MN 89890_   Client Number _15641_

Pet Name _Fred_   Breed _Bassett_   Color _Brown/Wh/Bl_

Sex ___M___   Altered ___Y___   DOB _2/15/13_   Age _12 weeks_   Species _K9_

Date		Charges
5/15/13	Puppy shots	
	S: Owner states pt has had diarrhea for the past 3 days.	
	Very foul odor. Decreased appetite. Had 1 prev. vacc.	
	Had a puppy that died 1 mo ago. Unknown cause.	
	O: PE: General appearance: thin; 5% dehydrated.	
	Lethargic. EENT, LN, MS, NS, all WNL. Abd: tender when palpated.	
	MM = pale and tacky. T - 102.4, Wt - 9.9#	
	HR = 100/min, RR = 20/min, Thermom reveals bloody, loose stool.	
	A: Gastroenteritis	
	R/O Parvo, Giardia, Garbage Gut	
	P: Fecal Exam, Parvo Test	ND
5/15/13	O: Parvo Test (+), Fecal (−)	
	P: Discuss Tx plan with owner. 1. Hosp vs home care	
	2. Abx;	
	3. Fluid care: SQ vs IV	
	Owner chooses home care	ND

FIGURE 14-11 Example of plan notes in a medical record.

of the practice frees up space for current records. By reducing the number of records in the active area, the possibility of lost records is decreased. Records can be lost from misfiling, misspelling, and misplacement, which can be irritating to both clients and team members.

Long-term storage can be arranged at an off-site storage facility until state law allows purging. Those records that are purged must be shredded so that confidential information is not available to the public. This includes all lab work results, client informational sheets, and any authorization or release sheets that were signed by the client. The disadvantage of off-site storage is that when a record is needed, it can take 1 to 2 days to retrieve it. This may be too long a wait for the veterinarian who needs the patient's history.

> **PRACTICE POINT** Purged medical records should be shredded to ensure patient and client data never ends up in the wrong hands.

Client Discharge Instructions

Client discharge instructions are very important (Figure 14-13). On average, clients will only remember 30% of the information provided while they were in the practice. Team

members should print out materials for the owner to take home. These instructions and materials must be reviewed verbally with the owner before discharging the patient; it is also a good idea to keep a copy of all materials given to the owner in the record. It may also be of benefit to have the owners sign the bottom of the material to acknowledge receipt of the printed materials. Some clinics will use a carbonless copy set for discharge instructions. This way, the practice is covered when clients state they never received the instructions.

Different types of information may be required for various patient discharges. A patient that is returning home after a normal canine neuter will have different release instructions than a patient that has just had a fractured bone repaired. A patient that has been hospitalized may have a different feeding protocol than that of a surgical patient.

Veterinary practice managers manage client education.

Computer software programs can print detailed release information when the appropriate information has been added to the system. For practices that do not have this ability, sheets can be created with options for team members to highlight for the client. Box 14-6 gives ideas for what to include on discharge sheets for a variety of patient discharges.

Charts, labels, and stamps can help a veterinary team become more efficient at writing in medical records correctly, legibly, and completely. Veterinary team members can place a label or stamp in the record for the veterinarian, who can then chart his or her notes accurately. Some examples of labels and stamps are listed in Figure 14-2;

BOX 14-4 | **Rules for Medical Records**

- Records must be written in blue or black ink only; no other colors, no pencils.
- The author of the entry must date and initial each time an entry is made.
- No correction fluid!
- When correcting an error in a record, make a single line through the mistake and make the correction. The mistake must be initialed.
- Use standard and approved abbreviations only.
- Write in records immediately to prevent the loss of details.
- Records must be legible!
- Each continuation sheet must have all the patient information documented on it, including the owner's name and the pet's gender, breed, and age.

BOX 14-5 | **Routes of Medication Administration**

PO—*Per os*, or by mouth
SC—*Subcutaneously*, or under the skin
IV—*Intravenously*, or into the vein
IM—*Intramuscular*, or into the muscle

Client's last name: _____ Working diagnosis: _____

Pet's name: _____ Primary doctor: _____

Date:	8am	9	10	11	12	1	2	3	4	5	6	7	8
Feed													
Water													
Walk/litter													
Temperature													
Weight													
Appetite?													
Attitude?													
Urine?													
BM or diarrhea													
Vomit?													

FIGURE 14-12 Example of a hospital sheet.

ABC Veterinary Clinic 555-555-5555
Dr. Roe, Dr. Morton, Dr. Larsen
Post-anesthesia Release Sheet

Please provide clean, dry bedding and a quiet place for your pet to recuperate. Please notify the hospital with any concerns.

DIET:

( ) Wait a few hours after arriving home to offer your pet water. Please give only a small amount. If no vomiting occurs, you may offer more water about an hour later. You may feed a small amount (1/4 normal amount) if water stays down.

( ) You may continue to feed your pet normally.

( ) Special diet instructions _____

ACTIVITY:

( ) Restrict exercise for 1 day. NO RUNNING, JUMPING, CLIMBING OR BATHING.

( ) Restrict exercise for 7 days. NO RUNNING, JUMPING, CLIMBING OR BATHING.

( ) Other _____

OTHER:

( ) Please use paper strips or pinto beans in place of litter for 7 days.

( ) Please booster vaccines in 3-4 weeks.

( ) Your pet's metabolism may permanently decrease after surgery. You may need to decrease the amount of food you feed to prevent obesity.

INCISION:

( ) Watch for swelling, redness, or drainage. Prevent scratching, rubbing, and licking of the incision. Please ask for an E-collar if you think your pet will lick the site.

( ) Ice incision for 5 minutes, 3 to 4 times daily for the first 72 hours.

MEDICATION:

( ) Give pain medication _____

( ) Give antibiotics _____

( ) Give other medication _____

_____

( ) Start medication _____

FOLLOW-UP VISITS:

( ) Recheck in _____ days.

( ) There is no need to return for suture removal; the skin was closed with absorbable suture or tissue adhesive.

( ) Not necessary unless you feel there is a problem.

Comments:

Doctor _____ Tech _____ Client _____ Date _____

A

FIGURE 14-13 A and B, Examples of discharge instruction.

Continued

Discharge Instructions

ABC Veterinary Clinic
1001 Any Circle
Boston, MA 88012

Owner _____ Patient _____ Date _____

Diagnosis:_____
_____
_____

Medication: _____
_____
_____
_____

Start Medication: _____
_____

Diet: ( ) Normal ( ) Other_____
_____
_____

Exercise: ( ) No restriction ( ) Other_____
_____
_____

Special Instructions:_____
_____
_____
_____

Recheck _____ Dr. _____

B

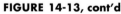

FIGURE 14-13, cont'd

others can be found at various medical and office supply houses. Practices can also design the labels or stamps that will best increase efficiency in their hospital and have them commercially printed or print them with an office laser printer.

Most Common Medical Records Violations

- Euthanasia without consent: This seems like a weird scenario. How can pets be euthanized without consent? Many practices do not have a signed consent form from clients indicating the approval to euthanize their pet. Another increasingly common scenario is the following. A wife usually brings the pet to the hospital for care, and her name is on the medical record. The husband brings the pet in for euthanasia, and provides a reason why the pet is to be euthanized. The practice euthanizes the pet,

and the wife sues the hospital for negligence, because she did not authorize the procedure. The wife wins the case, because her name was on the medical record, not his. The outcome of this lawsuit makes it clear that practices must always have a consent to euthanize form signed by the owner of the pet that is listed on the medical record (see Figure 2-10, *H* and *I*, for examples of euthanasia consent forms).

- The medical record states: "*Routine Castration or Routine Ovariohysterectomy.*" What is routine? What may be routine in one hospital may not be routine in another. Therefore procedures must always be explained in a way that everyone understands and knows what was completed.

- No physical exam: If a PE is not written in the record, it is assumed it was not completed, *at all*. If only the chest was auscultated, then it must be noted.

BOX 14-6 | Discharge Sheet Ideas

Food
- Normal or special diet?
- Restricted-time feedings or feeding intervals, or feed ad lib?
- For what length of time?

Activity
- Restricted or unrestricted?
- For what length of time?
- Physical therapy such as range of motion or pool swimming?

Medications
- What kind? (Antibiotic, anti-inflammatory, etc.)
- Name of the drug and strength
- How much? (How many pills, capsules, or liquid will be given at once?)
- How often will the medication be given?

- What are the side effects?
- When should client start medications?

Miscellaneous Information
- Bandage care
- Vaccine boosters
- Icing the incision area
- Prevent licking (Elizabethan collars if needed)

Rechecks
- When is a recheck needed?
- Do sutures need to be removed? When?
- Any detailed specific patient instructions can be added here.

    All hospital contact information (including an emergency phone number) should be clearly indicated on the discharge sheet, along with the veterinarian and team member who have discharged the patient.

- Client refusals: If a client refuses or declines a service, procedure, or product, it must be indicated in the medical record. If it is not in the medical record, a court of law would assume that the service, procedure, or product was never offered, and the practice does not have proof that it was offered and declined.
- Legibility: Often, illegible records contribute to errors made by the veterinary team.

Many of these violations are easily corrected. Many violations occur because of lack of training, loss of focus, and poor time management. Managers must ensure every team member is trained on the proper procedures of medical record completion, and implement time management strategies to aid in doctor completion.

Common Abbreviations

Abbreviations are used in veterinary practices to help teams become more efficient. It is important to memorize these abbreviations because they are used in everyday practice. Examples of abbreviations are located in the appendixes of this book.

For example, the following instructions have been written for a patient:

IV Normosol fluids maintenance rate; NPO ×12 hrs: sx in am: 12 mg cefazolin IV pre/post sx; increase fluids to sx rate; 3 mg buprenorphine SQ pre/post op.

This can be interpreted as meaning that the patient will be receiving intravenous (IV) fluids with Normosol at the maintenance rate of 66 mL/kg/24 hours. The pet will receive nothing by mouth (NPO) for 12 hours before surgery (sx) and will have a surgical procedure in the morning. The patient will receive 12 milligrams (mg) of cefazolin intravenously (IV) both before and after surgery. The patient will also receive 3 mg of buprenorphine before and after surgery.

Abbreviations greatly increase the efficiency of team members by saving time and space in the medical record.

PRACTICE POINT   AAHA has a small, detailed booklet of all veterinary abbreviations.

Radiographs

Patient radiographs are an integral part of the medical record. Radiographs must be correctly labeled with the veterinary hospital name and address, client's last name, patient's name, date, and a right or left indicator.

If a veterinary practice is paperless, these radiographs can be electronically filed in the patient record. A paper practice will have these radiographs stored in another location on the premises. It is important to be able to locate these radiographs quickly and efficiently when needed; therefore a filing system must be developed. Some practices may use colored letters (as indicated earlier for file folders) to help file radiographs (Figure 14-14). Practices can also purchase a radiograph scanner that scans films into a computer database, allowing clinics to pull

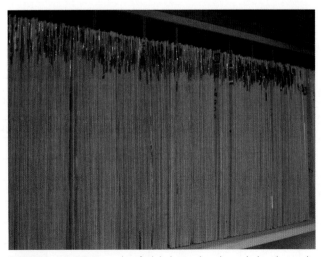

FIGURE 14-14 Example of alphabetized, color-coded radiographs (for nondigital practices).

up the images on a computer monitor. It must be remembered that these are not digital radiographs; it is simply a storage system for films. This allows clinics to use that storage room for other items and prevents the loss or misfiling of films. Images can easily be copied for owners or specialty veterinarians onto a CD; the radiographs will never be lost.

Radiographs are the property of the veterinary practice; therefore practices that do not have a scanner or digital radiographs may provide copies to the client. Copies of radiographs can be made at a local imaging center that has radiographic copying capabilities. If clients are taking radiographs to have them copied or films are being sent to another veterinary clinic, a log should be kept indicating where the radiographs went. This log should include who received the films, the date, and the reason the films have left the practice. Once they have been returned, a single strike line can be made through the entry indicating their return, along with the date and initials of the team member returning the radiographs to radiology. Figure 14-15 is an example of a completed radiograph checkout log. It can be frustrating and time-consuming for veterinary team members when films have become lost or misfiled. Developing an effective file system is as important for radiographs as it is for medical records. Being able to refer to the log is important because owners or other hospitals often have not returned films.

Backing Up the Computer System Daily

The importance of backing up systems on a daily basis cannot be stressed enough. It is best if the system is backed up to both on-site and off-site systems, which increases the safety of the protected information. If a fire or burglary occurs, all records will still be available to reinstall on a new computer. If a computer system fails in the middle of the day, the only information that will need to be reentered is the information from earlier that day. It would be impossible to locate all information that was lost if only a weekly or monthly backup were performed.

 Veterinary practice managers maintain protocols for hospital procedures and risk management plans.

Management's Role in Medical Records

A main priority of a hospital manager has to be medical records. These are the building blocks for a successful practice. If medical records are incomplete, a patient may not receive the treatment it needs, or a client may not receive the communication he or she needs.

Medical Records Audit

The office or practice manager should make it a daily task to pull random records and complete a medical record audit. Practices get busy. The reception team takes the record to invoice the client, and occasionally it does not get returned to the original doctor or team member to be completed. Complete records must include the date of entry, initials of all team members writing in the record, a complete SOAP format, and all authorization forms a client has signed.

> **PRACTICE POINT**   Every practice must implement medical records auditing to catch missed charges.

A medical records template can be developed that allows a manager to capture missing information. Many times, this missing documentation leads to missed charges. Missed charges that occur in a general practice average $64,000 per veterinarian. If a 3-doctor practice produces $1,500,000.00, 10% of gross revenue would be $150,000! This is a huge amount of money that will never be recovered if audits are not completed. See Chapters 3 and 15 for ideas to capture lost charges.

Value to the Practice

Medical records are considered an asset of the practice. When a practice valuation is completed, medical records are evaluated as part of the procedure. Completeness, legibility, and client recommendations/acceptance are reviewed. If any of these items are missing or subpar, the value of the practice is decreased. Incomplete medical records and lack of client recommendations (or proof of) hurt the practice financially.

Value of Pet Portals

Pet portals are an online component of medical records. When practices sign up for this service, clients are allowed

Radiology Checkout Log							
Date	**Owner's Name**	**Patient's Name**	**Check out by?**	**Going to?**	**Initials**	**Return Date**	**Initials**
10/6/13	Pacheco	Cherry	Owner	Crossroads A.H.	LP	12/8/13	MV
10/8/13	Ziehl	Bud	UPS	SW Specialty	CS		
11/1/13	Soules	Blackie	Owner	Arroyo V.C.	SP	12/1/13	DC
12/15/13	Miale	Twinkle	Mail	Tuscon	CS		

FIGURE 14-15 Radiology checkout log.

to view their pets account online. During the setup procedure, practices can indicate what clients can and cannot see in their portal. However, the value in the service is that clients have access to their account. Medical records (especially electronic) play a valuable role in this service, helping clients to remain compliant with team recommendations.

⚖️ VETERINARY PRACTICE and the LAW

Two elements are important for preventing malpractice suits. The first is to implement proper procedures to prevent mistakes. Team members must be trained appropriately to operate equipment and perform tests correctly. Staff must also understand the importance of immediately cleaning spills or urine on the floor to prevent a client or team member from slipping or falling. Safety plans must be instituted for clients, patients, and team members.

A second element for averting malpractice suits is to prevent clients from becoming angry about the care their pet is receiving. Every team member must be respectful and courteous to every client; provide information, both written and verbally, on their pets condition; and communicate effectively on every level. Treatment plans must be given, and clients should receive frequent phone calls with updates on their pet's condition and laboratory interpretation. These actions are essential in preventing lawsuits. All team members must demonstrate respect and concern for all patients and clients at all times.

To prevent malpractice lawsuits, use the following procedures to prevent mistakes:

- Ensure all equipment is in proper working condition.
- Provide a current employee procedure manual that allows team members to review the correct ways to perform procedures.
- Use informed consents; ensure that clients fully understand the risks and benefits of all procedures to be completed on the patient.
- Document conversations, procedures, and recommendation completely and clearly in the record.
- Protect patients from injury.
- Label all specimen samples correctly.
- Post signs indicating a wet floor.
- Never guarantee an outcome.
- Follow up on all patients after surgery or procedures.

REVIEW QUESTIONS

1. Why is legibility so important in medical records?
2. How often are medical records purged?
3. What is the earliest that records can be shredded?
4. Why is history taking critical for a medical record?
5. What is a SOAP progress note? Give an example of each part.
6. What items are mandatory in a medical record? Why?
7. Why are discharge sheets vital?
8. Does a client record belong to the client? Why or why not?
9. Who owns the radiographs of a pet?
10. What is the most common method for filing paper medical records?
11. Legible, complete medical records are an asset to the hospital, and they bring value during a valuation.
    a. True
    b. False
12. Medical records:
    a. Can be released to any person asking for a copy
    b. Must be released to the owner only
    c. Must have an owner's consent to be released to any person asking for a copy
    d. b and c
13. The objective portion of the SOAP format includes:
    a. Chief complaint of the client
    b. Observations of team members upon check-in
    c. Physical exam
    d. Diagnosis
14. Purging medical records:
    a. Increases lost records
    b. Is required by law
    c. Allows inactive records to be shredded
    d. Moves inactive medical records to another storage area
15. Medical record audits should:
    a. Capture missed charges
    b. Identify incomplete medical records
    c. Identify lapses in recommendations
    d. All of the above

Recommended Reading

Heinke MM: *Practice made perfect: a guide to veterinary practice management*, ed 2, Lakewood, 2012, CO AAHA Press.

McCurnin D, Bassert JA: *Clinical textbook for veterinary technicians*, ed 8, St Louis, MO, 2013, Saunders, Inc, Elsevier.

Wilson JF: *Law and ethics of the veterinary profession*, Yardley, PA, 1990, Priority Press.

Inventory Management

OUTLINE

Fundamentals of Inventory, 275
Creating an Inventory Manual, 276
Distributors and Manufacturer Representatives, 276
Designing an Inventory System, 277
Consolidating Inventory, 280
Turnover Rates, 280
Determining Effective Turnover Rates, 280
Reorder Quantities, 281
Determining Effective Reorder Quantities, 281
Reorder Points, 281
Determining Effective Reorder Points, 281
Inventory Storage, 282
Preparing Orders, 282
Developing a Want List, 282
Order Book, 282
Monthly Ordering, 283

Just-in-Time Ordering, 283
Bulk Orders, 284
Receiving Orders, 284
Handling Expired Medications, 284
Returning Products to the Distributor, 285
Effective Pricing Strategies, 285
Break-Even Analysis, 286
Markup, 286
Dispensing Fees, 287
Labeling Fees, 287
Minimum Prescription Fee, 287
Injection Fees, 287
Outsourcing Products, 287
Inventory Protection, 287
Potential Causes of Discrepancies, 287
Safety Data Sheets, 288
Capital Inventory, 288
Decreasing Loss, 288

KEY TERMS

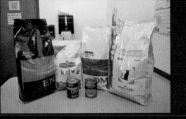

Capital
Central Inventory Location
Distributor Representative
Inventory
Inventory Turns per Year
Just-in-Time Ordering
Manufacturer Representative
Markup
Order Book
Reorder Point
Reorder Quantity
Safety Data Sheet (SDS)
U.S. Food and Drug Administration (FDA)
Want List

LEARNING OBJECTIVES

When you have completed this chapter, you should be able to:

1. Develop an effective inventory system.
2. List methods used to maintain an appropriate amount of inventory on hand.
3. Define and create a central inventory location.
4. Define capital inventory.
5. Identify and use Safety Data Sheets.
6. Calculate an effective price markup for products.
7. Describe methods used to handle expired medications.

CRITICAL COMPETENCIES

1. **Adaptability** - being open to change and flexible work methods; the ability to adapt behavior to changing conditions or new information.
2. **Analytical Skills** - the ability to analyze information and use logic to address problems; the ability to quickly and accurately grasp complex information and concepts and to make correct inferences.
3. **Creativity** - the ability to think creatively about situations, to see things in new and different ways; use imagination and creativity to develop innovative solutions to problems.
4. **Critical and Strategic Thinking** - the ability to think critically about situations and to understand the relevance of information for different problems; use critical reasoning to generate and evaluate alternative courses of action or points of view relevant to an issue.
5. **Decision Making** - the ability to make good decisions, solve problems, and decide on important matters; the ability to gather and analyze relevant data and choose decisively between alternatives.
6. **Integrity** - honesty, trustworthiness, and adherence to high standards of ethical conduct.

7. **Leadership** - a willingness to lead and take charge; the ability to motivate others and mobilize group effort toward common goals.

8. **Oral Communication and Comprehension** - the ability to express one's thoughts verbally in a clear and understandable manner, and the ability to actively listen and attend to what others are saying; must have good group presentation skills.

9. **Persuasion** - the ability to change the attitudes and opinions of others and to persuade them to accept recommendations and change behavior.

10. **Planning and Prioritizing** - the ability to effectively manage time and work load to meet deadlines; the ability to organize work, set priorities, and establish plans for achieving goals.

11. **Relationship Building** - the ability to develop constructive and cooperative working relationships with others and maintain them over time; must also be able to settle disputes, resolve grievances and conflicts, and negotiate with others.

12. **Resourcefulness** - the ability to understand what it takes to complete the job; apply knowledge, skills, and expertise to perform tasks quickly and efficiently.

13. **Writing and Verbal Skills** - ability to comprehend written material easily and accurately; ability to express thoughts clearly and succinctly in writing.

In the organization of the practice domain, the veterinary practice manager is responsible for general practice management, including maintaining appropriate inventory and medical records systems, establishing protocol for hospital policies and procedures, and coordinating equipment acquisition and maintenance.

Knowledge Requirements

The tasks in this domain require a working knowledge of veterinary medical terminology, the requirements for common veterinary practice procedures (e.g., anesthesia, radiography, IV injections, lab work), and preventative health and risk management protocols. Tasks in this domain also require knowledge of inventory systems and methods; standards for maintaining medical records; and protocols for equipment maintenance and insurance.

Effective inventory controls are an important part of the overall profit of a veterinary practice. Creating and maintaining an inventory system takes continuous planning and monitoring. Without proper organization, inventory can easily become a full-time duty. Inventory is the balance between having enough products on the shelves to meet client needs and not running out of product or supplies. Outdated products decrease the practice's profits, as does not having enough product to sell (Box 15-1). Managing inventory requires knowledge of what product is used, how much is used, how often it is sold, as well as how long it takes to reorder and replace the product. A combination of all this information will make it possible to implement an effective inventory management system that takes little time to control (Box 15-2).

It is an advantage to have one team member in charge of inventory. By having one person overseeing the task, mistakes are decreased, duplicate ordering is prevented, and other team members know whom to contact if an item is in short supply. One person can easily organize an inventory system, which will streamline the process. By decreasing the steps and time required to maintain inventory, profits are increased, time is saved, and clients are satisfied.

Fundamentals of Inventory

Although one person should be in charge of inventory, a second team member or manager should be able to fill in as needed. If an emergency happens to the inventory manager, another team member should be able to effectively step up without creating a glitch in the system. Distributor and manufacturer phone numbers, account numbers, and order histories should be readily available.

The front of an order book or an inventory manual is an excellent place to keep a summary of all distributors and manufacturers. Small orders may need to be placed with specialty companies; with easy access to their information, orders can be placed quickly and efficiently.

 Veterinary practice managers maintain appropriate inventory system including controlled substance ordering, tracking, security, and destruction.

BOX 15-1	Losses Associated with Poor Inventory Management

- Too much product sitting on the shelf
- Not enough product on the shelf to sell
- Frequent ordering
- Shrinkage
- Theft
- Backorders
- Expired products
- Wrong products ordered or received
- High costs of overnight shipment for products needed ASAP
- Shipping costs associated with small orders

BOX 15-2	Keys to a Successful Inventory Management System

- Buy in volume from one distributor to reduce shipping costs
- Minimize the number of times ordered per week or month (goal = order top 20% of items monthly)
- Evaluate soon to expire drugs monthly. Can they be returned for credit or replaced?
- Evaluate payment plans. If companies offer a discount when the bill is paid by the tenth of each month, make sure the payment is made!
- Develop turnover rates, reorder points, and reorder quantities
- Limit the duplication of drugs (package size and brand)
- Include soft costs (holding and ordering) when setting product pricing
- Maintain inventory costs between 20% and 26% of gross revenue of the practice

Creating an Inventory Manual

Just as an employee manual is necessary to guide all team members, an inventory manual is also recommended. This manual can provide the guidelines that all team members must follow if and when the inventory manager is absent or replaced. Box 15-3 provides topics that should be covered in this manual. Many team members are unaware of the "science" behind inventory and why it is so critical that this system be created and maintained. An inventory manual will bring this awareness, and keeps all team members on the same page.

> **PRACTICE POINT**   Inventory manuals help the practice manager and inventory manager understand, and outlines the important aspects of proper inventory management.

An organized manager must determine which technique is most effective in maintaining inventory. A variety of techniques are discussed in this chapter; however, the combination of several techniques may work better. Each practice is

BOX 15-3	Inventory Manual Topics

- Define cost of goods
- Calculating inventory needs
- Ordering receiving process
- Invoicing and data entry
- Inventory protection

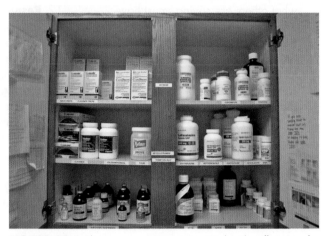

FIGURE 15-1 Pharmacy organization is critical to the efficiency of a team.

different and each manager must be flexible in determining the best technique.

Drugs might be arranged in a pharmacy area in such a way as to help improve the efficiency of a team (Figure 15-1). Drugs may be arranged by category, such as oral solids, oral liquids, injectable, ophthalmic, otic, and/or external topical medications. Other pharmacies may be arranged by type of drug, such as tranquilizers, analgesics, cardiac, diuretics, and so forth.

Distributors and Manufacturer Representatives

Distributor representatives work for a company that carries a full line of manufactured products ranging from pharmaceuticals to equipment and pet foods. *Manufacturer* representatives sell products to distributors or, in some cases, distribute products themselves. Manufacturer and distributor representatives may discuss specials with the inventory manager and educate the veterinary team when new products are launched.

Manufacturer and distributor representatives can provide team members with valuable information regarding products and how they may increase sales for the practice. They can provide a sales history, allowing a prediction for the use of the product for the next year (this is an excellent tool when preparing a budget for the following fiscal year). They can be an excellent source of continuing education for team members and can provide brochures to increase the level of client education.

Caution should be used when companies have sales promotions. Many practices cannot sell the minimum amount of product, and product should not be purchased for the reason of a good friendship. Product should only be ordered when it has been determined that it can sell within a 3-month period.

Working with a limited number of distributors and manufacturers allows larger orders to be placed at one location, usually allowing shipping and handling fees to be waived by the company. These fees are generally imposed on smaller orders and can add up quickly. Most manufactures have set pricing, which means that the distributors will sell the product at the same price, regardless of what distribution center the product is ordered from, or if the practice is a top client. This eliminates the need to "shop around" looking for the best price available (which results in the increased soft costs of inventoried products).

Equipment does not fall under the same guidelines as pharmaceuticals; equipment pricing should always be evaluated. One should consider if the product will need to be installed, what training is provided, and what guarantee comes with the equipment. These factors can increase the price (and can be well worth the expense).

Designing an Inventory System

Veterinary practice management software integrates inventory management into the system and is easily accessible from any computer (Figures 15-2 and 15-3). Veterinary software allows inventory reports to be generated, reorder points and quantities established, and (depending on the software, can place an order for the practice). The accuracy of the reports solely depends on the setup of the system and entry of the invoices. Many issues arise with incorrect data entry.

Correct categories (or departments) and codes must be set up in order for the software to function effectively. For practices just establishing a category system and code entry, this is a simple procedure. For existing inventory systems, a code and category clean up is a must. It is advised that the categories a practice sets up match benchmarking categories, allowing a better evaluation of expenses versus revenue (see Chapter 20). The following categories (at minimum) are recommended:

- Imaging
- Laboratory (in-house)
- Flea/tick/heartworm prevention
- Retail/over-the-counter
- Diets
- Drugs and medical supplies

Drugs and medical supplies can then be further placed into subcategories if the practice desires (injectable, anti-inflammatory, surgical supplies, etc.).

For existing inventory systems, a codes list should be printed and evaluated. Often, drugs are entered into the system multiple times under different names or are classified into the wrong category. At this point, duplicate items can be merged (do not delete, as this will permanently erase the history of the product), or reclassified. Items that are no longer in use can be placed on the inactive list (depending on the software, another term may be used), preventing that code from being used by team members.

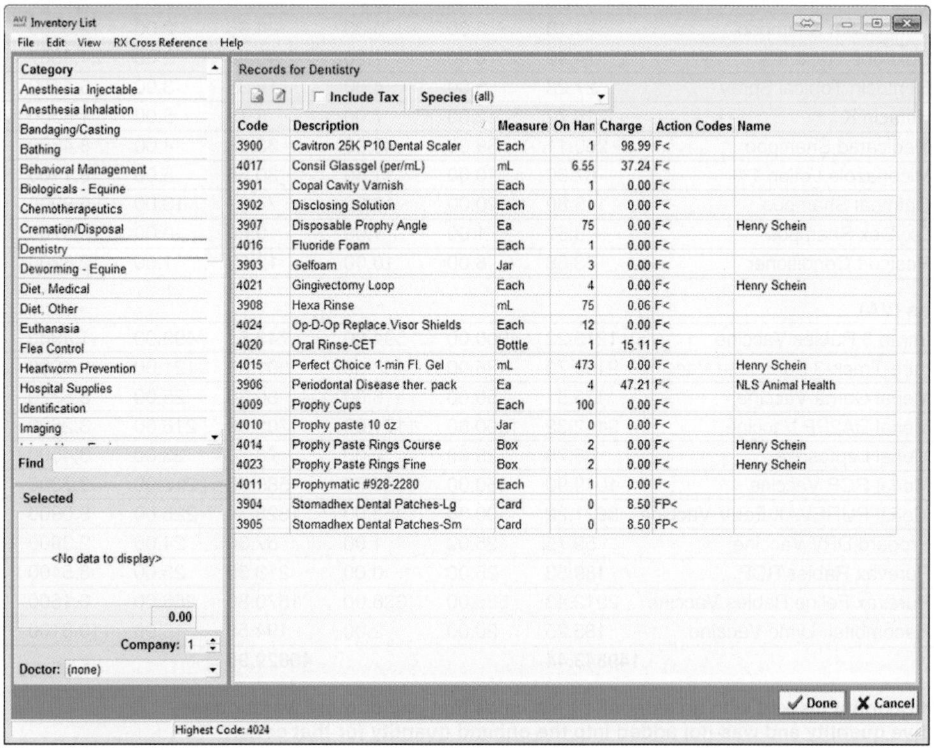

FIGURE 15-2 Example of Avimark's inventory list. (Courtesy AVImark, LLC, Piedmont, Mo.)

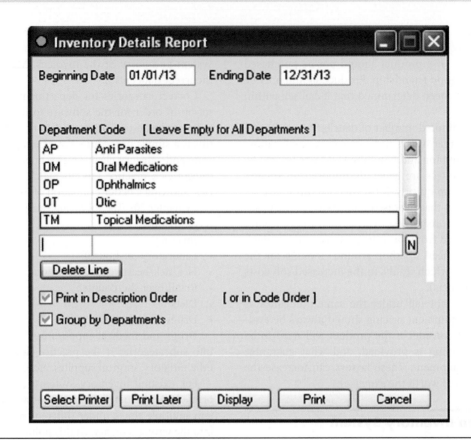

Code	Description	Purchases Amount	Qty	Sales Qty	On hand Amount	Qty	Cost	Percent Markup	Price
Topical medications (TM)									
TM050	Allermyl Shampoo	131.16	12.00	8.00	78.05	7.00	11.1500	10	12.26
TM055	Allermyl Spray	84.56	8.00	3.00	21.58	2.00	10.7900	10	11.87
TM073	Animax Cream 15 ml	177.24	30.00	29.00	99.00	20.00	4.9500	33	6.60
TM075	Animax Ointment 15 ml	156.75	31.00	26.00	80.75	19.00	4.2500	88	8.00
TM125	Corti Sooth Shampoo	24.18	2.00	0.00	24.66	2.00	12.3300	8	13.30
TM220	Doxirobe Gel 8.5%	74.90	3.00	1.00	49.93	2.00	24.9667	0	0.00
TM350	Gentocin Topical Spray	27.25	5.00	4.00	16.35	3.00	5.4500	50	8.18
TM450	Hetacin K	18.72	12.00	7.00	8.15	5.00	1.6300	50	2.45
TM600	Medicated Shampoo	260.11	39.00	43.00	33.68	4.00	8.4200	10	9.26
TM610	Miconazole Lotion 1%	67.30	10.00	11.00	30.55	5.00	6.1100	65	10.10
TM675	Oatmeal Shampoo	115.80	20.00	16.00	77.87	13.00	5.9900	0	5.99
TM690	OxyDex Shampoo	5.57	1.00	1.00	0.00	0.00	5.5700	10	6.13
TM700	Resicort Conditioner	73.68	6.00	10.00	12.52	1.00	12.5200	17	14.61
Vaccinations (VA)									
VA106	Imrab 3 Rabies Vaccine	1216.22	900.00	594.00	743.51	499.00	1.4900	1108	18.00
VA116	Intra-Track-3 Bordetella Vaccine	9193.70	425.00	458.00	301.29	121.00	2.4900	623	18.00
VA118	Merial Corna Vaccine	175.51	50.00	6.00	89.30	25.00	3.5720	404	18.00
VA119	Merial DA2PP Vaccine	3442.32	1200.00	1171.00	702.00	216.00	3.2500	854	31.00
VA138	Merial Leptospira	75.76	25.00	0.00	78.20	23.00	3.4000	429	18.00
VA152	Merial RCP Vaccine	1019.90	450.00	381.00	589.68	216.00	2.7300	559	18.00
VA158	Merial PUREVAX FeLV Vaccine	3621.22	500.00	353.00	1828.34	226.00	8.0900	160	21.00
VA114	Progard DPV Vaccine	59.75	25.00	1.00	57.36	24.00	2.3900	1197	31.00
VA112	Purevax Rabies/RCP	189.53	25.00	0.00	213.50	25.00	8.5400	298	34.00
VA111	Purevax Feline Rabies Vaccine	2912.43	525.00	328.00	1570.80	255.00	6.1600	192	18.00
VA141	Recombitek Lyme Vaccine	185.25	20.00	2.00	194.58	18.00	10.8100	113	23.00
		149843.44			**48829.95**				

An on hand quantity marked with an asterisk (*) indicates that one or more warehouses has a negative quantity and was not added into the onhand quantity for that code.

A

FIGURE 15-3 A and B, Example of IntraVet's inventory details report. (Courtesy IntraVet, Dublin, Ohio.)

Inventory On-Hand Report

Department Code   [Leave Empty for All]

☐ Print in Description Order   [or in Code Order]

☑ Group by Departments

[Select Printer] [Print Later] [Display] [Print] [Cancel]

Inventory On-hand Report   **INTRAVET VETERINARY CARE**

Ophthalmics (OP)

Code	Description	Dept	Tax	Quantity on hand	Reorder level	Reorder quantity	Cost	Percent mark-up	Price
OP100	Atropine Sulfate 1% Ophth Sol.	OP	N	5.00	2.00	4.00	1.05	319	4.40
OP101	Atropine Sulfate 1% Ophth Oint.	OP	N	28.00	2.00	3.00	0.95	387	4.63
OP200	Dexamethasone Drops	OP	N	24.00	2.00	4.00	3.13	468	17.81
OP405	Gentocin Ophth Solution	OP	N	29.00	12.00	24.00	31.00	0	6.40
OP500	BNP Ophth Oint 1/8 oz	OP	N	19.00	2.00	4.00	19.00	0	5.74
OP510	BNP-H Ophth Oint 1/8 oz	OP	N	27.00	2.00	4.00	17.64	0	7.01
OP550	NPS w/Dex Ophth Sol	OP	N	40.00	12.00	24.00	1.73	137	4.09
OP552	*Neo Poly Dex Ophth Ointment	OP	N	24.00	0.00	0.00	1.60	240	5.42
OP600	Optimmune Ophth Oint	OP	N	14.00	3.00	6.00	8.78	184	24.90
OP800	Terak Ophth Oint	OP	N	12.00	0.00	0.00	2.50	190	7.24
OP850	Terramycin Ophth Oint 3.5 gm	OP	N	3.00	3.00	2.00	7.84	62	12.71

Otic (OT)

Code	Description	Dept	Tax	Quantity on hand	Reorder level	Reorder quantity	Cost	Percent mark-up	Price
OT050	Acarexx Otic Solution	OT	N	24.00	2.00	6.00	7.64	102	15.43
OT150	Baytril Otic	OT	N	20.00	2.00	6.00	9.16	100	18.31
OT160	Baytril/Conofite/Dex SP	OT	N	53.00	0.00	0.00	8.40	138	20.00
OT670	Otomax 15 gr	OT	N	32.00	12.00	12.00	8.92	18	10.50
OT830	Synotic	OT	N	8.00	1.00	3.00	8.40	100	16.80
OT832	Synotic w/Banamine	OT	N	8.00	0.00	0.00	19.30	0	4.19
OT834	Synotic w/Gentocin	OT	N	12.00	0.00	0.00	22.30	0	6.19
OT850	Tresaderm	OT	N	62.00	12.00	36.00	8.38	67	13.97
OT855	Trizedta Flush	OT	N	16.00	1.00	2.00	0.61	128	1.39
OT910	Vet Sol Ear Cleaner	OT	N	44.00	12.00	24.00	6.00	50	9.01

Vaccinations (VA)

Code	Description	Dept	Tax	Quantity on hand	Reorder level	Reorder quantity	Cost	Percent mark-up	Price
VA106	Imrab 3 Rabies Vaccine	VA	N	261.00	50.00	200.00	1.56	1054	18.00
VA111	Purevax Feline Rabies Vaccine	VA	N	230.00	50.00	100.00	6.16	192	18.00
VA112	Purevax Rabies/RCP	VA	N	97.00	12.00	25.00	8.72	290	34.00

B

FIGURE 15-3, cont'd

| BOX 15-4 | Disadvantages of a Large Inventory |

- Shrinkage (items missing with no explanation)
- Bottles breaking
- Items expiring
- Doctors wanting to change to another product and being unable to do so because of large quantity of previous product

Consolidating Inventory

Managers will often realize that many products of the same category exist. For example, a plethora of flea and tick preventatives are available, and many practices elect to carry multiple products to satisfy doctor recommendations and client needs. However, carrying multiple products has a negative effect on the inventory system and cash flow of the hospital (Box 15-4). Ideally, practices should carry a maximum of two options of a product. When multiple products are carried, the following effects are seen:

- Increased dollars are spent on products
- Products sit on the shelf and have a decreased turnover rate
- Products expire and the practice loses money
- Team members need additional training to remember the functions of each product
- Client communication and recommendations suffer because specific recommendations are not being made, ultimately decreasing client compliance

> **PRACTICE POINT** Consolidating inventory items can improve practice cash flow.

It can be difficult for veterinary team members to understand why the consolidation of products is critical; it can be even more difficult to determine which products to continue carrying.

How to consolidate (Box 15-5):

- Produce a report of a particular category (e.g., heartworm preventative).
- Determine how many units were purchased and sold of each product.
- Determine how much product expired of each.
- Identify the top two items that were purchased and sold (without expiring) and produce a report showing the profit of each.
- Produce a second report, showing the losses associated with the remaining items.
- Have a team discussion, determining what products the practice will carry.

Number evaluation is important when determining what products to carry or discontinue. The reality is that if the product is not selling, it cannot be carried by the hospital. Veterinarians will have to decide what products they wish to carry in the hospital (low producing products can be scripted out of the hospitals online pharmacy). If a team

| BOX 15-5 | Example of Consolidating Inventory |

PRODUCT	# PURCHASED	# SOLD	ON SHELF	EXPIRED	DISCREPANCY
Trifexis	100	70	20	10	0
Interceptor	50	30	10	10	0
Revolution	150	100	20	Unknown	30
HG Plus	780	750	20	Unknown	10

A table like this can be created when comparing products and determining which products should be kept in the hospital. Additional columns can be added charting the revenue gained/lost and the potential revenue that could be captured as a result of consolidating.

member insists that the hospital carry a specific product, a large enough markup has to be placed on the product to ensure that purchasing the item does not cause the practice to lose money.

Once codes and categories have been corrected and products have been consolidated, a physical count of the inventory must be completed and entered into the computer. From this point forward, all invoices must be entered into the software system when an order is received.

Turnover Rates

Inventory turns per year is a goal every inventory manager should set. *Turns per year* is defined as the number of times a specific product turns over in a practice. This helps determine correct reorder quantities and points. Managers should set a rate for each product, based on the volume purchased and sold. Some products will have a turnover rate of 12, where as others will have a turnover of 6.

> **PRACTICE POINT** Proper inventory turnover rates are essential when trying to maximize inventory profits.

The goal of developing effective turnover rates is to increase the profits of the practice and decrease expired product, shrinkage, and soft costs (holding and ordering costs).

Roughly 80% of the income (from inventory sales) is produced from 20% of the inventoried products (also known as the Pareto principle). Therefore if an inventory manager can spend a consolidated amount of time on managing 20% of the inventory, higher profits will be generated because holding and ordering costs are decreased. The top 20% of items are those that produce a high level of sales, or items the practice cannot function without. Examples of top items include vaccinations, flea/tick/heartworm preventative, parvovirus stool tests, and so on.

Determining Effective Turnover Rates

To determine the inventory turns per year for a specific product, the beginning inventory is added to the ending inventory and divided by two. This gives the average inventory

---

BOX 15-6	Example of Inventory Turns per Year

- *(Beginning inventory + Ending inventory) ÷ 2 = Average inventory*
- *Total units of product purchased during measured period ÷ Average inventory = Number of turns per year*

Example:
- Inventory for eye drops at the beginning of the year was 4.
- Ending inventory was 4.
- Total purchased for the year was 36.

$4 + 4 = 8$

$8 ÷ 2 = 4$ (average inventory)

$36 ÷ 4 = 9$

The product turned 9 times. This is an excellent value!

(More examples available in Chapter 24)

BOX 15-7	Example of Reorder Quantity

- *Average daily use × Turnover goal (in days) = Reorder quantity*

Example:
- Heartgard Plus Small has an average daily use of 3.5 (3.5 boxes sell on a daily basis)
- The turnover goal for this product is 12 (30 days)

$$3.5 × 30 = 105$$

When this product is ordered, 105 boxes should be purchased at once (which is estimated to sell within 30 days). Since Heartgard Plus Small is supplied in 10 boxes per carton, then 11 cartons would be ordered.

---

per year. The total amount of product purchased during that period divided by the average yields the number of turns per year for that product (Box 15-6).

To determine what an effective rate is for each product, print a sales history sheet of all inventoried items, and determine which products are in the top 20%. These items should turn 12 times per year. This means that a particular product should be ordered once a month, and when ordered, the quantity ordered should support the sales of such product for a 1-month period. Therefore this product will be ordered 12 times during the year, equaling a turnover rate of 12.

When ordering monthly, the costs associated with inventory management drop dramatically (also known as soft costs, which will be covered later in this chapter). Products in the previous report that produce the *next 20%* may have a turnover rate of 10. Any product with a turnover rate less than 6 must be outsourced (covered later in this chapter).

Reorder Quantities

It is imperative that correct reorder quantities be determined for each product. If an excess amount of product is ordered, it will sit on the shelf, increase holding costs, and have the potential for expiration and theft. If too little product is ordered, ordering costs increase, a product shortage occurs, and clients and team members are upset. As indicated earlier, correct reorder quantities contribute to a healthy turnover rate.

> **PRACTICE POINT** Developing and using effective reorder quantities decreases stockouts.

Determining Effective Reorder Quantities

Three factors are presented when determining reorder quantities; average daily use, turnover goals, and product expiration (Box 15-7).

When the *average daily use of product is calculated,* one can better determine how many units will sell per day. Average daily use is determined by taking the number of units

sold in the year and dividing by the number of days the practice is open in a year.

Example: A practice is open 365 days per year and sells 550 bottles of Rimadyl, 25 mg, 180 count.

- $550 ÷ 365 = 1.5$
- Rimadyl, 25 mg, 180 count, sells on an average of 1.5 bottles per day

Turnover is important in this equation, because it must be known how long the quantity ordered should support sales (without running out or having excess product).

Product expiration is the last factor to consider. If product is short-dated and will not sell by the end of the turnover goal, fewer quantities must be considered.

Reorder Points

Reorder points is defined as the point at which a product needs to be ordered, and takes into consideration lead time and average daily use (Box 15-8). A reorder point is NOT when the product has run out!

> **PRACTICE POINT** A reorder point is NOT when a product has run out!

Determining Effective Reorder Points

Lead time is defined as the amount of time between when a product is needed and when it gets onto the practice shelf. For example, consider a practice that orders every Monday and the order is received on Tuesday. If a product is noticed to be low on Wednesday, and the next order will be placed the following Monday (to be received Tuesday), then the lead time is said to be 7 days. If a product is noticed to be low on Friday, and the order will be placed on Monday, the lead time will be 4 days.

Lead time multiplied by the average daily use determines the reorder point of a product.

The seasonality of certain products throughout the United States may affect the reorder points and reorder quantities. Creating a list of seasonal products will help the inventory manager overcome this obstacle.

BOX 15-8 | Example of Reorder Point

- Lead time × Average daily use = Reorder point
  Example:
- Heartgard Plus Small has an average daily use of 3.5 (3.5 boxes sell on a daily basis)
- The lead time for this product is 4 days

$$4 \times 3.5 = 14$$

This product must be reordered when 14 units remain on the shelf.

Inventory Storage

Practices that can have storage space available to order bulk supplies and support a 12× turnover rate generally have a higher profit margin than those that do not.

Central inventory locations store additional supplies, and are generally locked, allowing limited access. Pharmacy shelves are stocked on an as-needed basis from the central inventory "closet" or "cage." Items can be checked in when they are received and checked out when a bottle is needed in the pharmacy. New items should be placed behind old items, allowing the older items to be sold first.

Practices may have one cabinet that can be used for excess product. When a bottle is emptied, the new bottle can be pulled and placed in the correct location. This can help prevent overcrowding of products in one area. Overcrowding loses items in the clutter; they may be displaced or overlooked.

Preparing Orders

Once software has been set up correctly (codes, categories, physical inventory entered, reorder points, and reorder quantities determined), managers may learn to depend on inventory reports to help them place an order. It is advised to always double-check physical levels, ensuring the reports are accurate (human error does occur!).

> **PRACTICE POINT** Preparing orders is a soft cost that must be calculated into the selling price of the item.

For practices that do not have an accurate inventory system, another method must be used to help the inventory manager to place accurate orders (it takes a team to make a system succeed).

Medical supplies can be difficult to manage with inventory software. Many services use supplies but do not account for a specific number of gauze, latex gloves, syringes, and so on. Some services (such as vaccinations) can be linked to syringes, but the quantity on hand can be less when team members use syringes to draw blood. Physical spot-checking of these items is mandatory to ensure the practice does not run out.

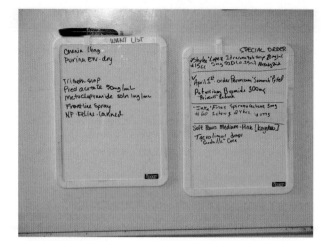

FIGURE 15-4 A want list and special order list are placed on two separate dry erase boards.

Developing a Want List

A want list may be developed for team members who recognize that a specific product is running low. A dry erase board works well for a want list because products can be erased as soon as they arrive. A special order board may be established for those medications that need to be custom-ordered for clients; this may include compounded and/or flavored medication (Figure 15-4). This special order board can provide a quick reference for team members preparing the medication once it has arrived at the practice because it will have the client and pet name listed.

A spreadsheet of items may be developed for the inventory manager to follow as an order is being made. Many times, items are removed from the shelves and team members forget to write the product on the board or place the red tag in the designated place. This spreadsheet allows a third check of the inventoried items. It may not be noticed that a product is missing until a doctor needs it. If a spreadsheet is used, the need can be detected and the product ordered. A spreadsheet may simply contain the name and size of the product. It is useful to have it as a simple reminder of all products that should be on the shelf at all times.

Figure 15-5 is an example of a spreadsheet of inventoried products for a veterinary practice. This specific practice has a pharmacy that is first organized by location (refrigerator, controlled substance, shelf); then the product is alphabetized. The quantity in which the product is supplied is listed in column B, distributor or manufacturer in column C, the quantity to reorder in column D, and the shelf life of that particular product in column E.

> **PRACTICE POINT** Use all team members to help make a reorder system efficient.

Order Book

All orders should be kept together, listed chronologically in a book. This allows the inventory manager to see what products were ordered, how many, from which distributor or

Product	Quantity	Distributor	Reorder #	Shelf Life	Notes
FELV/FIV	30/bx	Patterson	1	30d	
General Health Profile	2/bx	Patterson	6	1d	
Heartworm 3DX	30/bx	Patterson	2	15d	
Parvo	5/box	Patterson	2	10d	
Plasma	1	ABB	1	30d	
Pre-op Profile	4/bx	Patterson	6	1d	
Apomorphine	1	VPA	5	3 mo	
Buprinex	1ml x 10vials	DVM	2	7d	
Butorphenol Inj	50mg	DVM	1	6 mo	
Butorphenol Tabs	100	DVM	1	6 mo	
Diazepam	10ml; 5 vials	DVM	1	6 mo	
Ketamine	10ml; 5 vials	DVM	1	2 mo	
Hycodan	100 tabs	DVM	1	6 mo	
Telazol	5ml	DVM	5	7 d	
Activated Charcoal	1	Patterson	5	30d	
Albon	100	Zoetis	1	30d	
Amoxi Clavulanate	210	Zoetis	1	30d	
Amoxicillin	100	Patterson	1	30d	
Antirobe	100 and drops	Zoetis	1	30d	
Artificial Tears	1	Patterson	5	7 d	
Atropine Ophth	1	Patterson	2	10 d	
Barium Sulfate	1	DVM	1	30 d	
Baytril oral	100	Bayer	1	60 d	
Benedryl Capsules	500, 1000	DVM	1	3 mo	
Benedryl Susp	473ml	DVM	1	6 mo	
Carafate	473ml	DVM	1	6 mo	
Cefa Drops	15ml	DVM	6	10 d	
Cephalexin Caps	100, 500	Patterson	1	7 d	
Chlorpheniramine	1000	DVM	1	30 d	
Deramax	90	Novartis	1	60d	
Doxycycline	100, 500	Patterson	1	7 d	
Droncit	50	Patterson	1	4 mo	
Fenbendazole	Liquid or powder	DVM	1	5 mo	
Genesis	1	Patterson	6	30 d	

FIGURE 15-5 Example of spreadsheet for inventoried products.

manufacturer, the date the order was placed, and the name of the representative who took the order. This is also a great history resource. As a key to decreasing order confusion, the same representative should be called each time. Inside sales representatives become familiar with products the practice prefers and make every effort to ensure the order is 100% satisfactory. If an item is on back order, the representative should notify the manager at that time, and a decision can be made to order an alternative product or to search for the product through another company. The back order should be noted in the book at this time and a notice posted for all team members.

Monthly Ordering

To decrease holding and ordering costs, the top 20% to 40% of products should be ordered on a monthly basis. Team members often spend a large amount of time placing orders on a weekly basis, so by decreasing this to monthly, less time is wasted.

Ordering on a monthly basis can also increase the cash flow of the practice. If a majority of inventory is ordered at the beginning of a distributor's or manufacturer's billing cycle, the practice has an entire month to sell the product before a monthly invoice is produced. Spot ordering can occur throughout the month, but most of the time spent on ordering should occur only once a month.

Just-in-Time Ordering

Just-in-time ordering is defined as ordering a product when it is needed but before it runs out. Just-in-time ordering is needed for products that do not have a high turnover rate in the hospital, but still must be maintained on the shelves.

BOX 15-9 | Example of Bulk Order

Average daily use × # of working days in billing period × % of growth = Bulk order

Example:
- Heartgard Plus Large has an average daily use of 12 (12 boxes sell on a daily basis)
- There are 64 working days in the billing period
- The practice has been experiencing a steady 4% increase in business for the year

$$12 \times 64 = 768$$

$$768 \times 4\% = 31$$

$$768 + 31 = 799$$

In order for this bulk order to be most beneficial, 799 boxes could be ordered. (Because Heartgard is sold in cartons of 10, 80 cartons would be ordered.)

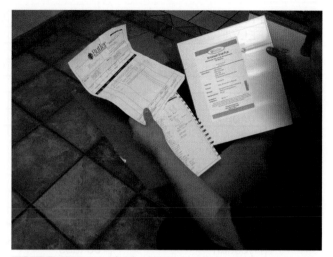

FIGURE 15-6 An order should be compared to the invoice and want list, ensuring that the correct product and quantity were received.

Unfortunately this method does not account for manufacturer or distributor lead times or back orders. If a product is on back order, the inventory manager must find the product from another distributor or find a product that is equivalent. If a match is not available, other team members and veterinarians must be made aware of the back order.

PRACTICE POINT   Just-in-time ordering increases soft costs associated with inventory. The more time that is spent on ordering products, the higher the cost is for the clinic.

Bulk Orders

Some manufactures offer discounts when purchasing large quantities of items. Bulk orders can be a good decision when purchased with the following in mind:
- Quantity is based off of historical sales, within the period being measured
- The quantity ordered must sell before the delayed billing is due
- Product cannot have a short shelf life
- Consider year-end tax implications (cash versus accrual reporting)

To determine an effective quantity for a bulk order, a manager would consider the average daily use of the product, the number of working days in the billing period, and the percent of growth (or loss) the practice may be experiencing (Box 15-9).

Receiving Orders

When a shipment is received, the inventory manager should inspect the order before it is put away. Items should be inspected for damage and compared to the invoice and order book (Figure 15-6). Quantity (e.g., number of bottles), strength of product (e.g., in milligrams or grams), and size

of product (e.g., number of tablets, capsules, or milliliters) should be double-checked. Once it has been determined that the products match the invoice and book, products can be placed in the appropriate location.

These invoices also need to be matched to the monthly statement to ensure that no additional charges were added to the account. A manager may create an open order file. Once packing slips have been checked against the product received, the slip can be placed in an open file; this indicates that the packing slip needs to be matched to the invoices received at the end of each month. Once the match has been completed, the packing slip can be placed in a closed file.

Handling Expired Medications

The U.S. Food and Drug Administration (FDA) requires that all drugs it has tested and approved have an expiration date (Figure 15-7). Drug manufacturers determine this date by performing efficacy tests on the product. Once the efficacy of a drug has dropped below a certain percentage, it is no longer effective. Products must be removed from the shelves once they have expired, and they cannot be sold. Not only is it unethical to dispense expired drugs, it is illegal.

Many practices do not want to lose money associated with expired products; therefore an effective inventory management system must be implemented to prevent medications from expiring. Inventory managers may keep a running list of products and expiration dates that can be completed each time an order is received. If a product bottle is opened that is getting close to expiring, a note should be made for the doctors, allowing them to increase the dispensing of the product. If the bottle is not opened, the distributor or manufacturer may exchange the product at no charge. Return policies should be verified and kept on file for referencing.

When medications have expired, they should **not be** discarded in the trash or flushed down a drain. Pills can be added to a small amount of water and mixed until dissolved. A small amount of cat litter can then be added, and the

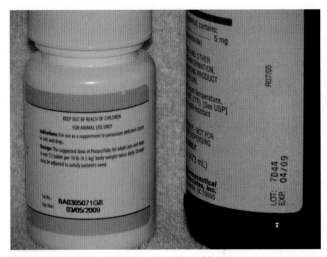

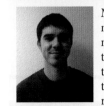

FIGURE 15-7 Expired drugs cannot be sold. Inventory managers must track expiration dates of products and dispose of expired drugs appropriately.

mixture can then be thrown away. Solutions and injectable medications can also be added to cat litter and then thrown away. The U.S. Environmental Protection Agency advises against pouring medications into the toilet to discard them.

Expired controlled substances must be submitted to a facility certified to dispose of controlled substances. A receipt for the controlled substances submitted will then be returned to the clinic and should be kept with the current controlled substance log indicating they were disposed of. State veterinary boards and local or regional offices of the U.S. Drug Enforcement Administration (DEA) offices should have a current list of manufacturers certified to accept controlled substances. Disposing of controlled substances is described in greater detail in Chapter 16.

Returning Products to the Distributor

Products may need to be returned to the distributor for a variety of reasons, including damage, the wrong product being sent, or the wrong product being ordered. Most distributors are happy to return the products, although some may institute a restocking or shipping fee. A call should be placed to the sales representative who handled the order to notify that person of the problem. The representative may ask whether a replacement product or credit is requested. A call tag will be sent for the return of the item. A call tag is an address label produced by the company to be placed on the outside of the shipment box. This label has a special reference number on it so that the returned product can be credited to the appropriate account. Once the tag has been received, it is important to document on the original invoice when the product was returned. A credit should be given to the practice upon receipt of the product, and a credit invoice will be generated. The credit may take a few weeks to be received. Distributors and manufacturers may also take unopened bottles of recently expired product. However, instead of a credit, the product will be replaced. Each company has different policies regarding the expired product, and options should be researched before ordering new product.

PRACTICE POINT Be familiar with manufacturer return policies to maximize the return of expired items.

WHAT WOULD YOU DO/NOT DO?

Ms. Eoff's cat Harvey was recently diagnosed with hyperthyroidism. The veterinarian prescribed 1 month of methimazole tablets, a medication used to treat hyperthyroidism in cats. The owner was advised to return in 3 to 4 weeks to recheck the thyroid values. Ms. Eoff called 2 weeks after therapy started and stated she just couldn't get Harvey to take the pills and wanted another option for treatment. Dr. Dreamer advised her that radioactive iodine was an option at the specialty center; however, the owner declined. Dr. Dreamer offered to special order a transdermal medication that could be applied to the tip of the ear. Ms. Eoff was greatly appreciative of the solution and authorized the ordering of the medication.

Upon arrival of the special order, Alex, a veterinary technician, calls to inform Ms. Eoff that the medication as arrived. He advises Ms. Eoff that he would like to schedule an appointment with Harvey, allowing him to review the medication and show her how to apply the medication. She informs Alex at that time that she has learned how to give Harvey the tablets and will no longer need the specially ordered medication. Alex knows that the inventory manager ordered this medication specifically for the dose that Harvey requires, and that the medication cannot be returned to the company that produces methimazole gel.

What Should Alex Do?
Alex must inform Ms. Eoff that this medication was specially ordered for Harvey, which she approved when she last spoke with Dr. Dreamer. Alex can advise Ms. Eoff that she should try the medication, it may ultimately be easier for her to administer once she tries it; if it does not work she can return to the use of tablets at the end of the month. Ms. Eoff must understand that the medication cannot be returned; and the product cannot be sold to another client because this particular dose was for Harvey.

Effective Pricing Strategies

Before pricing strategies can be determined, team members must understand the replacement costs, soft costs, hard costs, and profits associated with inventory.

Replacement cost is the price a practice would pay to replace an item. The original costs associated with that product may not be the updated price and could have been received with free goods or a bulk purchase.

Soft costs include holding and ordering costs, and are often referred to as hidden inventory costs. **Ordering costs** are human resource related and basically account for all time spent preparing and maintaining an order (Box 15-10). Ordering costs account for approximately 15% to 20% of the

BOX 15-10	Hidden Ordering Costs Associated with Inventory

- Determining reorder quantity and reorder points
- Price shopping
- Visiting with sales representatives
- Requesting an order
- Researching items to replace back orders
- Receiving and unpacking products and supplies
- Entering invoices into veterinary software
- Reconciling statements

BOX 15-11	Hidden Holding Costs Associated with Inventory

- Property tax paid on inventory value
- Insurance
- Utilities to maintain safety of product
- Shrinkage
- Pharmacy licensing/DEA fees
- OSHA training and maintenance

BOX 15-12	Example of Soft Cost Calculation

- Soloxine 0.6 mg 250 count; unit cost $28.35
  - $28.35 × 23% = $6.52 (23% when inventory management is at its peak)
  - $28.35 × 35% = $9.92 (35% when inventory management is at its worse)
- When inventory is being managed well and soft costs are kept to a minimum, $6.52 would be added to the original cost of $28.35
  - $28.35 + $6.52 = $34.87 – the true cost of this product
- When inventory is not being managed and soft costs are high, $9.92 would be added to the original cost of $28.35
  - $28.35 + $9.92 = $38.27 – the true cost of this product

BOX 15-13	Example of Break-Even Analysis

- Unit cost + Hard cost + Soft cost + (Profit × sales price) = Sales price
- Otomax: Unit cost: $12.28
- Hard costs: 15% (predetermined by practice)
- Soft costs: 23% (predetermined by practice)
- Desired profit: 20%

$$\$12.28 \times 0.15 = \$1.84$$
$$\$12.28 \times 0.23 = \$2.82$$
$$\$12.28 + \$1.84 + \$2.82 + (20\% \times \text{Sales Price}) = \$16.94$$
$$\$16.94 + (0.20 \times \text{Sales Price}) = \text{Sales Price}$$
$$\$16.94 = \text{Sales Price} - (0.20 \times \text{Sales Price})$$
$$\$16.94 = (0.80 \times \text{Sales Price})$$
$$\$16.94 \div 0.80 = \text{Sales Price}$$
$$\$21.18 = \text{Sales Price}$$

The absolute minimum price this product could be sold for is $21.18.

BOX 15-14	Average Product Markup

Medicine	150%
Heartworm/flea/tick	90%
Drugs administered	150%
Oncology drugs	150%
Drugs for chronic conditions	100%

Markup as determined by Benchmarks: 2013.

> **PRACTICE POINT** Every product's selling price must include ordering costs, holding costs, a profit, and hard costs (if veterinarians are paid on production).

Break-Even Analysis

Long-term medications and heartworm, flea, and tick preventatives are sold through a variety of markets that some veterinarians wish to be competitive with. In order to determine the lowest cost a medication can be sold for, one would consider a break even analysis.

Break even analysis (Box 15-13):
- Unit Cost + Hard Cost + Soft Cost + (Profit × sales price) = Sales Price

Markup

Markup is a percentage added to the cost of the unit when determining the selling price. Markup percentages can be based on the number of inventory turns or a product category (Box 15-14). Products with a higher turnover rate (10× to 12×) have less of a markup (140% to 175%); those with lower turnover rates (4× to 6×) have higher markups (200% to 275%) to account for the potential expiration of product. Categories that are competitive will have a lower markup than those that are used to treat chronic conditions, cancer, and so on (Box 15-15).

unit cost. **Holding costs** are facility related (Box 15-11) and account for approximately 8% to 15% of the unit cost. Together, ordering and holding costs account for 23% to 35% of the cost of the product (Box 15-12).

Soft costs can be decreased by maintaining effective turnover rates, reorder points, and reorder quantities. These will also indirectly decrease shrinkage and wastage.

Hard costs are the costs associated with paying veterinarians when they are compensated by the production method. Traditionally, veterinarians are paid 10% to 25% of an item (the amount is at the discretion of the practice).

Profits must be made on inventory items; however, the profit may vary, depending on the product or product category. Profit also depends on whether the item is a shopped or competitive item. Profit goals are at least 15% to 20% of the unit costs.

BOX 15-15 | Example of Markup

- Unit cost × 150%
  Otomax: Unit cost: $12.28

$$\$12.28 \times 150\% = \$12.28 \times 1.5 = \$18.42$$
$$\$12.28 + \$18.42 = \$30.70$$

BOX 15-16 | Average Markup of Injectable Drugs

- Chemotherapy   150%
- Compounded   133%
- Long term   100%
- Others   150%

BOX 15-17 | Example of Injection Fee

- Unit cost of Rimadyl injectable: $2.68/mL
- Product markup: 150%
- Injection fee: $15.42

$$\$2.68 \times 150\% = \$4.02$$
$$\$2.68 + \$4.02 + \$15.42 = \$22.12$$

Dispensing Fees

Dispensing fees are added after the markup has been determined. Dispensing fees cover the veterinary technician's time to count the medication, the vial to package the medication, prescription label, and label printer wear and tear. Average dispensing fees are $6.00 to $11.00 (Wutchiett Tumbin and Associates, 2013).

Labeling Fees

Labeling fees are applied to products that are sold in the original container, and a team member does not have to count the medication. This fee covers the veterinary technicians' time to prepare the product, prescription label, and label printer wear and tear. The average labeling fee is 25% to 30% of the dispensing fee.

Minimum Prescription Fee

Many practices have a minimum prescription fee that averages $11.00 to $13.00.

Injection Fees

Injections are priced differently than capsules or tablets. Injections are priced both as an inventory item and as a service item, because a skilled professional must give the injection. Injection fees will have a similar product markup structure that the practice has created for tablets or capsules, with a service fee for the injection (Box 15-16). Injection fees range from $12.00 to $28.00 (Box 15-17).

PRACTICE POINT Injections are priced with both an inventory cost and a service or procedure cost. The product is being used (inventory) and administered by a professional (service/procedure).

Dispensing, labeling, injection, and minimum prescription fees must be blind to the client. They do not understand all of the overhead costs associated with the veterinary practice and would question the hospitals product markup techniques.

More examples of inventory turnover and markup calculations, dispensing fees, and soft costs are in covered in Chapter 24.

Outsourcing Products

As it is stated earlier, products with a low turnover should be outsourced. These are products that the practice rarely sells, and they usually expire before the entire amount can be sold. Outsourcing simply refers to allowing clients to order the medication through the practice's online pharmacy.

The practices online pharmacy is hosted by a known veterinary distributor and ties directly into the practice Web site. Practices regulate what products they will carry as well as their pricing. Manufacturer guarantees on product and efficacy continue through this pharmacy, just as it would if they purchased the product from the hospital. The practice will receive an alert asking for prescription approval, and money is deposited into the practice checking account on a monthly basis. Most companies that host pet portals also host an online pharmacy for the practice.

Outsourcing products is an excellent way to help consolidate inventoried items, reducing the financial burden on the practice.

Inventory Protection

Considering that inventory is the second largest expense of the practice, measures to protect it must be implemented. The top 40% of items that have been previously identified as Pareto's items must be constantly monitored. These are the largest producing products of the hospital, and should have a random, monthly count. These physical counts must be compared to computer reports. If there are discrepancies (and there will be), they must be investigated. The remaining 60% of items must also have random spot-checks, perhaps semiannually. When any item has a continued discrepancy it must have random spot-checks more frequently.

Potential Causes of Discrepancies

Shrinkage – Shrinkage is defined as the loss of product inventory. Shrinkage can be due to product expiration, theft, missed charges, or giving away products without

recording the transaction. Managers must implement measures to decrease shrinkage of inventoried items, because this is one of the largest expenses that a veterinary hospital has.

Missed Charges – Managers must implement measures to prevent team members from missing charges. Missed charges account for (a minimum of) 10% of gross revenue (see Chapter 20 for more information). By managing inventory and investigating discrepancies, managers should be able to determine why team members are missing charges. Reasons may include lack of focus, lack of training, or multitasking (creating a lack of focus).

> **PRACTICE POINT**   Missed charges account for at least 10% of gross revenue!

Incorrectly Invoiced Products – Team members may either enter the wrong product into the computer system, or pull the wrong product to send home with the client.

Medical Supplies – As mentioned previously, some medical supplies will create discrepancies; however supplies used to run in-house lab work should be accountable.

Free Doses – Some promotions include free goods, which are great for the hospital to receive. However, unless they are entered into the software correctly, they can cause discrepancies between the physical and report counts.

In-House Use – Many items are used in-house to treat patients; food is the first item to fall on this list. When items are used in this manner, they should be placed into a log or in-house use account to help clear discrepancies. Errors that occur with laboratory tests could also fall into this account, again, helping to clear discrepancies.

Safety Data Sheets

Safety data sheets (SDSs) (originally MSDS; see Chapter 21 for explanation) are required for all chemical products that are sold or used within a veterinary practice. The Occupational Safety and Health Administration (OSHA) set forth standards for current practice relations. The Occupational Safety and Health Act of 1970 was enacted to ensure safe work environments for all employees. The law is based on the simple concept that all employees have the right to know about any potential hazard to which they may be exposed. Each SDS lists the potential hazards related to that substance and what protective measures can be taken if any hazard occurs.

It is the ultimate responsibility of the veterinary practice to ensure that SDSs are retrieved every time a new product has been brought into the hospital. SDSs are available from either the manufacturer or the distributor, free of charge.

It is important when considering soft costs of inventoried items that the costs associated with creating and maintaining an SDS system be included.

Capital Inventory

Capital inventory includes any equipment purchased throughout the life of the practice. Equipment includes items used to provide veterinary services, along with office printers, credit card machines, and copy machines. A running capital inventory list should be kept in a safe place and added to each time a piece of equipment is received. A spreadsheet can be created that includes the equipment name, manufacturer, model number, serial number, purchase date, where it was purchased from, and the purchase amount. If the building is vandalized or the equipment stolen, this information will be invaluable for the police report and insurance claims. Equipment purchase information is also important for tax purposes. This list is also handy when needing to look up dates for warranty expiration. Figure 15-8 is an example of an inventory list that has equipment purchased before the inventory manager's hire date. The cost and manufacturer of several pieces of equipment are unknown, but the fact that they are listed completes the inventory sheet.

Decreasing Loss

Inventory is the second largest expense to a practice, next to payroll. A large amount of money is invested in this asset, and all areas must be managed well, making changes when necessary to decrease loss. Chapter 3 discusses at length the various means of decreasing loss. Four ways that teams can contribute to decreasing the loss of inventoried items is to use a travel sheet, appropriately set fees, have a structured inventory system, and ensure team member accountability.

Travel sheets must be used by each team member and double-checked by others that all charges have been circled. A good policy to instill into team members is that the one who performs the procedure should circle the code. For example, when the veterinarian does the exam, the veterinarian should circle the exam code. If a technician performs a heartworm test, the technician should circle the heartworm test code. If an assistant gets medication ready, the assistant should circle the medication on the travel sheet. Once the receptionist team receives the record and travel sheet, they compare the travel sheet to the record, looking for any missed charges.

As previously mentioned, fees for both products and services must be appropriately set to cover all of the overhead costs associated with a veterinary practice. Last but not least, effective inventory systems have the greatest impact on decreasing loss of products. Several methods have been discussed in this chapter, which must be used to create and maintain a profitable practice (Box 15-18).

The ultimate goal should be to keep inventory costs between 20% and 26% of the overall income for the practice. If a practice generates $1 million, 20% is $200,000. Costs of products should not exceed $260,000 for the year. This contributes to successfully implementing and maintaining a budget (see Chapter 20 for more information).

Product	Name	Manufacturer	Purchase Date/Price	Model Number	Serial Number
Anal Gland Excision Kit		Jorgenson		J-101	
Anesthesia Machine #1	Anesthesia Machine #1	Matrix		VMS	6380
Anesthesia Vaporizer #1	Anesthesia Vaporizer #1	Cyprane LTD			300437
Anesthesia Machine #2	Anesthesia Machine #2	Matrix	12/24/2010		SN14989
Anesthesia Vaporizer #2	Anesthesia Vaporizer #2	Vet Tech 4	12/24/10, $400 for both	100F	SN BASPOX7
Aspirator	Schuco Vac	Schuco		130	49500008498
Autoclave	Tuttanauer Autoclave	Tuttanauer	04/02/09, $2600	2340M	2110582
Bird Scale		Pelouze		PE5	
Camera	Digital Camera	HP	Aug 2010, $177.52	Photosmart 320	CN318111DG
Cast Cutter		Stryker		9002-210	8H8
Cautery Unit	AA Cautery	Jorgenson		J313	
Centrifuge	MS Centrifuge MicroHCT	Damon/IEC Division		MB	2513
Centrifuge	Sta-o-Spin	Stat-o-Spin	3/14/13, $1026.83 Butler	V0901.22	607V90111962
Centrifuge (lab)	Cinaseal	Vulcon Tech		C56C	6840
Clippers	Speed Feed	DVM	12/15/11, $91		
Clippers Cordless	Oaster	Butler		78400-01A	
Clippers Cordless	Oaster	Butler		78400-01A	
Clippers Cordless	Oaster	Butler		78400-01A	
Credit Card Terminal					
Credit Card Terminal	Care Credit				SN 207-397-407
Copier	Cannon			PC 940	NVX37080
Dental Machine	Ultrasonic Scaler/Motor Pack	Delmarva			C028-647
Doppler, BP	Mini Dop ES 100VX	Hadeco	11/2008, $800		SN-00090054
Doppler Probe		Jorgenson			
Doppler Ultrasound	Grafco Mini Doppler			4070	
Dremel Unit		Craftsman		5 Speed	
ECG PAM	VM8000PAM Cardiac Monitor	Technology Transfer	12/10/08, $2775	VM8000	SN V04408
ECG Printer PAM		Technology Transfer	12/10/2008	930	1029
ECG Biolog		QRS Diagnostic	9/2013 DVM Solutions $2735		2004-054237
ECG Printer Biolog			Came with Biolog	Brother HL-207	U61230M5J5
Glucometer	One Touch Ultra	Walgreens			RHW4E23Ft
Home Again Scanner		Schering Plough			SN 070535
Hair Dryer					
ECG Surgery	KENZ ECG 103	KENZ	GW Gift		9509-2815
IDEXX Electrolytes	VET LYTE	IDEXX	Aug. 2008		U15.9976
IDEXX Lasercyte	Lasercyte	IDEXX	Jun. 2013	93-30002-01	DXBP005586
IDEXX Vet Test	Vet Test 8000	IDEXX	08/01/08, $2700		OA26949
IDEXX Server				PCNE	H1BFQ91
IDEXX Printer				HP Deskjet 5650	MY45F4NOHI

FIGURE 15-8 Sample capital inventory spreadsheet.

⚖ VETERINARY PRACTICE and the LAW

Many people do not think about medications having an expiration date; but the fact is, medications expire much in the same way that food expires. There are people who wouldn't consider drinking milk just one day after the expiration date, but the same people are often unaware that their medicine cabinets contain expired products. All medications, prescription and over-the-counter drugs, have expiration dates and should be discarded when expired.

Expired medications are not always dangerous, but they can become weak and possibly ineffective after the "use-by" date. In addition, if a medication is an antibiotic that has decreased efficacy, the bacteria that are the target of the antibiotic may develop resistance. This can lead to an unresolved case and an unhappy owner. These owners will either seek a second opinion (therefore losing a client) or make a complaint to the board of veterinary medicine. If the investigator for the board determines expired medication was dispensed, the veterinarian could be in hot water.

BOX 15-18 | What NOT to Do with Inventory

- Order large quantities of products that will expire before they are sold
- Order multiple products that provide the same service
- Order more than once per week
- Order on an as-needed basis (for top producing items)
- Run out of inventory
- Store large amounts of products in full view of customers and staff

REVIEW QUESTIONS

1. Why should distributor and manufacturer representatives be seen by the inventory manager?
2. What is the goal of an inventory system?
3. Why should a "want list" be developed?
4. What is an order book?
5. What is an SDS?
6. What is capital inventory?
7. What does an inventory manager do with expired medications?

8. What minimum percentage should products be marked up to break even?
9. What are some losses associated with poor inventory control?
10. How many times should inventory be turned over per year?
11. Improving profits in the primacy revenue center can be accomplished by:
    a. Determining and using effective turnover rates
    b. Determining and using effective reorder points
    c. Determining and using effective reorder quantities
    d. All of the above
    e. None of the above
12. Price shopping for inventory items is a cost-effective method to reduce Cost of Goods.
    a. True
    b. False
13. To help reduce soft costs, orders of top producing items should be placed:
    a. Weekly
    b. Semimonthly
    c. Monthly
    d. As needed
14. Consolidating inventory reduces profits.
    a. True
    b. False
15. In order to determine the least cost that can be charged to a client, a practice must determine the:
    a. Turnover rate
    b. Break-even cost
    c. Markup
    d. Soft cost

Recommended Reading

Heinke MM: *Practice made perfect: a guide to veterinary practice management*, ed 2, Lakewood, CO, 2012, AAHA Press.

Wutchiett Tumbin and Associates: *Benchmarks 2013: a study of well managed practices.* http://www.industrymatter.com/benchmarks2013.aspx, 2013. Veterinary Economics.

Controlled Substances

OUTLINE

Schedules of Drugs, *292*
Registration, *293*
Security and Protection, *295*
Record Keeping, *295*

Management of Controlled Substances, *295*
Loss Reporting, *298*
Substance Disposal, *298*

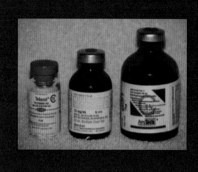

LEARNING OBJECTIVES

When you have completed this chapter, you should be able to:

1. Define controlled substances.
2. Identify drugs available for use in the veterinary practice.
3. Explain the importance of logging all drugs used.
4. Discuss the importance of managing controlled substances.
5. Discuss methods used to inventory controlled substances.
6. Describe methods used to order controlled substances for a veterinary practice.
7. Identify appropriate documents to order Schedule II drugs.
8. List the process used to report the loss of controlled substances.

KEY TERMS

Controlled Substance
Controlled Substances Act
U.S. Drug Enforcement Administration (DEA)

CRITICAL COMPETENCIES

1. **Adaptability** - being open to change and flexible work methods; the ability to adapt behavior to changing conditions or new information.
2. **Analytical Skills** - the ability to analyze information and use logic to address problems; the ability to quickly and accurately grasp complex information and concepts and to make correct inferences.
3. **Creativity** - the ability to think creatively about situations, to see things in new and different ways; use imagination and creativity to develop innovative solutions to problems.
4. **Critical and Strategic Thinking** - the ability to think critically about situations and to understand the relevance of information for different problems; use critical reasoning to generate and evaluate alternative courses of action or points of view relevant to an issue.
5. **Decision Making** - the ability to make good decisions, solve problems, and decide on important matters; the ability to gather and analyze relevant data and choose decisively between alternatives.

6. **Integrity** - honesty, trustworthiness, and adherence to high standards of ethical conduct.
7. **Leadership** - a willingness to lead and take charge; the ability to motivate others and mobilize group effort toward common goals.
8. **Oral Communication and Comprehension** - the ability to express one's thoughts verbally in a clear and understandable manner, and the ability to actively listen and attend to what others are saying; must have good group presentation skills.
9. **Persuasion** - the ability to change the attitudes and opinions of others and to persuade them to accept recommendations and change behavior.
10. **Planning and Prioritizing** - the ability to effectively manage time and workload to meet deadlines; the ability to organize work, set priorities, and establish plans for achieving goals.
11. **Relationship Building** - the ability to develop constructive and cooperative working relationships with others and maintain them over time; must also be able to settle disputes, resolve

grievances and conflicts, and negotiate with others.

12. **Resourcefulness** - the ability to understand what it takes to complete the job; apply knowledge, skills, and expertise to perform tasks quickly and efficiently.

13. **Writing and Verbal Skills** - ability to comprehend written material easily and accurately; ability to express thoughts clearly and succinctly in writing.

In the organization of the practice domain, the veterinary practice manager is responsible for general practice management, including maintaining appropriate inventory and medical records systems, establishing protocol for hospital policies and procedures, and coordinating equipment acquisition and maintenance.

Knowledge Requirements

The tasks in this domain require a working knowledge of veterinary medical terminology, the requirements for common veterinary practice procedures (e.g., anesthesia, radiography, IV injections, lab work), and preventative health and risk management protocols. Tasks in this domain also require knowledge of inventory systems and methods, standards for maintaining medical records, and protocols for equipment maintenance and insurance.

Controlled substances are drugs that have a high abuse potential and that must be regulated to help prevent those abuses (Figure 16-1). The Controlled Substances Act of 1970 was passed to reduce drug abuse by restricting certain substances with a high abuse potential. The act was established by and is controlled by the U.S. Drug Enforcement Administration (DEA) and provides approved means for proper manufacturing, distribution, dispensing, and use through licensed handlers.

Schedules of Drugs

A controlled substance (CS) will have a "C" written on the bottle, with a notation next to it indicating what schedule that particular drug is. Drugs are classified into five schedules according to their abuse potential. Controlled substances include opiates (narcotics), barbiturates, hallucinogens (e.g., ketamine), amphetamines, and other addictive and habituating drugs. Class I drugs have the highest abuse potential; therefore medical use of these substances is not allowed in the United States. Drugs such as LSD and heroin are examples of controlled substances in Class I and are illegal. Class II drugs produce severe psychological and physical dependencies and include drugs such as morphine, oxymorphone, and pentobarbital. Table 16-1 lists drugs and their schedules.

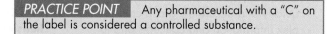

PRACTICE POINT Any pharmaceutical with a "C" on the label is considered a controlled substance.

States can also place drugs on the controlled substance list. For example, tramadol, propofol, and phenylpropanolamine are drugs that are classified as controlled in some states and not others.

If veterinarians write controlled substance prescriptions for clients, a pharmacy can only fill a 30-day supply for classes III, IV, or V. Those prescriptions can have five refills available for 6 months, at which time a new prescription must be submitted to the pharmacy. Class II drugs can only be filled for 30 days and must have a new prescription submitted every 30 days; no refills are allowed on the original script (Table 16-2).

DEA Form 222 must be filled out and sent to distributors or manufacturers that wish to purchase Schedule II drugs. Morphine, oxymorphone, and Sleepaway are examples of drugs that require DEA Form 222 (Figure 16-2 and Box 16-1). These forms must be filled out without error. Any

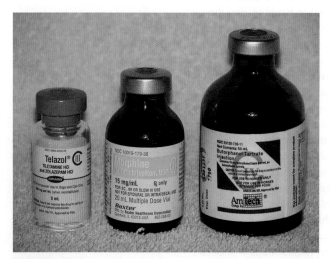

FIGURE 16-1 Controlled substances are labeled with a "C" and a roman numeral.

errors will void the form, and the distributor or manufacturer will be unable to fulfill the order. The name of the company, address, drug name, strength, and quantity must all be correct. The signature and license must match those on file or the order will be denied. Just as the DEA and state board of pharmacy are strict with veterinarians, they are just as strict (if not more) with distributors and manufacturers. The DEA supplies veterinarians with Form 222 to order Class II drugs.

Five areas must be focused on when managing controlled substances: registration, security and protection, record keeping, reporting of losses, and substance disposal.

Veterinary practice managers maintain appropriate inventory system including controlled substance ordering, tracking, security, and destruction.

Registration

All veterinarians are required to have a DEA license to purchase or write a prescription for a controlled substance.

Associate veterinarians are allowed to dispense a product from the hospital inventory without a CS license, if the state allows it. However, some states have a secondary controlled substance license that requires the initial DEA license in order to obtain it (the state license). The owner of the practice can order the controlled substances to be kept in the hospital and is responsible for protecting and accounting for all drugs dispensed. If any discrepancy occurs, the owner is held accountable and can have his or her DEA license revoked by the DEA (and state, if required). It is therefore absolutely critical that all drugs balance on a frequent basis. More details are provided in the record keeping section of this chapter.

Veterinarians are required to submit Form 224 to the DEA for the application of a CS license. Form 223 is then issued to the veterinarian and must be posted within the facility, easily accessible and available for inspection at any time. Form 224a must be submitted every 3 years, for renewal of the CS license.

Some states also have a prescription monitoring plan, in which drugs dispensed must be immediately reported to the state pharmacy board. Each state varies in their requirements and procedures; visit the appropriate state board of pharmacy for more details.

TABLE 16-1	Controlled Substance Schedule			
SCHEDULE	ABUSE POTENTIAL	DISPENSING LIMITS	RESTRICTIONS	EXAMPLES
I	Highest	Research only	DEA Form 222 required	LSD, heroin
II	High	Written prescription, no refills	DEA Form 222 required	Oxymorphone, morphine, pentobarbital, fentanyl
III	Less than II	Written prescription; can refill five times	DEA number	Hycodan, codeine, buprenorphine, hydrocodone, ketamine, Telazol, anabolic steroids
IV	Low	Written prescription; can refill five times	DEA number	Diazepam, phenobarbital, alprazolam, butorphanol, midazolam
V	Low	No DEA limits	DEA number	Lomotil, Robitussin AC

TABLE 16-2	Summary of Controlled Substances Act Requirements		
	SCHEDULE II	SCHEDULE III & IV	SCHEDULE V
Registration	Required	Required	Required
Receiving records	Order forms (DEA Form 222)	Invoices, readily retrievable	Invoices, readily retrievable
Prescriptions	Written prescriptions (see exceptions*)	Written, oral, or fax	Written, oral, fax, or over the counter†
Refills	No	No more than 5 within 6 months	As authorized when prescription is issued
Distribution between registrants	Order forms (DEA Form 222)	Invoices	Invoices
Security	Locked cabinet or other secure storage	Locked cabinet or other secure storage	Locked cabinet or other secure storage
Theft or significant loss	Report and complete DEA Form 106	Report and complete DEA Form 106	Report and complete DEA Form 106

Note: *All records* must be maintained for 2 years, unless the state requires a longer period.
*Emergency prescriptions require a signed follow-up prescription.
Exceptions: A facsimile prescription serves as the original prescription when issued to residents of long-term care facilities, hospice patients, or compounded IV narcotic medications.
†Where authorized by state controlled substances authority.

See Reverse of PURCHASER'S Copy for Instructions	No order form may be issued for Schedule I and II substances unless a completed application form has been received, (21 CFR 1305.04).	OMB APPROVAL No. 1117-0010

TO: *(Name of Supplier)* | STREET ADDRESS

CITY and STATE | DATE | TO BE FILLED IN BY SUPPLIER — SUPPLIERS DEA REGISTRATION No.

	TO BE FILLED IN BY PURCHASER					
LINE No.	No. of Packages	Size of Package	Name of Item	National Drug Code	Packages Shipped	Date Shipped
1						
2						
3						
4						
5						
6						
7						
8						
9						
10						

◀ LAST LINE COMPLETED *(MUST BE 10 OR LESS)* | SIGNATURE OF PURCHASER OR ATTORNEY OR AGENT

Date Issued | DEA Registration No. | Name and Address of Registrant

Schedules

Registered as a PRACTITIONER | No. of this Order Form

DEA Form -222 (Oct. 1992)

U.S. OFFICIAL ORDER FORMS - SCHEDULES I & II
DRUG ENFORCEMENT ADMINISTRATION
SUPPLIER'S Copy 1

104586067

FIGURE 16-2 DEA Form 222. (Courtesy U.S. Department of Justice, Drug Enforcement Administration, Washington, D.C.)

BOX 16-1 Common Questions and Answers Regarding DEA Form 222

Question: How do I obtain additional official copies of DEA Form 222?

Answer: Official order forms may be ordered by calling the DEA Headquarters Registration Unit toll free at 800-882-9539 or the nearest DEA Registration Field Office. The forms will be mailed within 10 working days. Official order forms may also be obtained by submitting a completed requisition form, DEA Form 222a, to DEA, Registration Unit, PO Box 28083, Washington, DC 20038-8083. There is no charge for official order forms.

Question: Can a distributor accept a DEA Form 222 that contains minor misspellings in the registrant's name, address, or drug name?

Answer: Yes, the DEA Form 222 is acceptable if the registrant's name or address contains minor misspellings. The registrant should request corrected official order forms and, if necessary, a corrected registration certificate from DEA. If the drug name has been misspelled and there is no question as to what product has been ordered, then the DEA Form 222 is acceptable.

Question: Can a distributor fill in sections omitted by a registrant on a DEA Form 222?

Answer: *Date of the form:* The distributor may place the date on the form. When possible, the date ascertained from the delivery document should be used as the issue date. The form is acceptable unless the ascertained date of issue is greater than 60 days from the date of receipt.

Size of the package: The size of the package must be completed by the purchaser unless the product is only manufactured in one size. If more than one package size is manufactured and no package size is indicated, then the package size may not be added by the supplier. The line item with the missing package size must be voided by the supplier and the purchaser notified.

Strength of the drug: If the product is only manufactured in one strength, then it is not necessary to indicate the strength in the section "Name of Drug." If the product is available in more than one strength, then the strength may not be added by the distributor. The line should be voided on the DEA Form 222 by the supplier and the purchaser notified.

Last line completed: A distributor may not fill in the "Last Line Completed" area of the DEA Form 222. This section must be completed by the purchaser. If the purchaser enters an incorrect number, such as the total number of packages ordered instead of the last line completed, then the DEA Form 222 is not valid.

Question: Can a distributor accept a DEA Form 222 if the size and strength of a product have been placed incorrectly on the form?

Answer: Yes, the DEA Form 222 is acceptable as long as there is no question as to what product has been ordered.

Security and Protection

The DEA is stringent on the regulations that practices must follow in order to keep drugs safe and secure.

Veterinary practice managers understand and ensure compliance with the DEA and state and local agencies.

The first part of this requirement relates to personnel that have access to the drugs. Employees should undergo background checks and drug testing before employment. Practices may also wish to implement a drug-free workplace, in which random drug testing is completed on all employees. This helps the practice take reasonable guard from hiring and employing risky people.

> **PRACTICE POINT** Employers are required to take reasonable guard when hiring new team members.

Those team members that have access to the controlled substances (should be limited to a few) must be held accountable. Signature cards should be kept on file for those removing and logging drugs (allowing a comparison of signatures if ever needed).

All controlled substances that are kept on the facility property must be kept in a securely locked, substantially constructed cabinet or safe. The cabinet or safe must be secured to the wall or floor, therefore bolted to the wall or floor. If a safe weighs more than 750 lb, it can be excluded from being bolted to the floor.

Drugs in active use can be placed in a less substantially locked cabinet (hospital cabinetry) during open hours. However, these drugs must be placed back into the substantially locked cabinet at night.

Controlled substances for house call and large animal practices are not considered to be substantially secure when in a vehicle. Therefore CSs cannot be stored in vehicles used for these calls (at the time of publication, this action is being challenged, and may change in the upcoming months).

Within the safe, Schedule II drugs must be kept separate from drugs classified as Schedule III, IV, or V. This separation can be a shelf or placement in a box.

Record Keeping

The DEA can inspect records, invoices, inventory, and facilities that house controlled substances at any time. State agencies, such as the board of veterinary medicine or the board of pharmacy, may also inspect at any time and may have stricter rules and regulations than the DEA. The agency that has more stringent regulations takes precedence. Records and invoices must be kept for a minimum of 2 years (after date of use) for any agency to inspect.

Logs for CSs must be kept in a separate location than the drugs themselves (i.e., logs should not be placed in the safe with the drugs). In addition, Schedule II drug logs and invoices must be kept separate from logs and invoices for Schedule III, IV, or V drugs.

Practices that are accredited by the American Animal Hospital Association must use bound logs; however, the DEA will accept logs kept in binders.

Drug logs must include the following information:
- Client name
- Client address
- Patient name
- Reason of use
- Amount of drug administered
- Balance of drug after use
- Initials

Inventory logs must include:
- Product name, strength, and count in a full bottle
- Date of purchase
- Name and address of vendor
- Date and time of inventory
- Log quantity
- Physical quantity
- Any discrepancy found
- Initials

Management of Controlled Substances

An initial inventory must be taken when the business opens, and then taken biennially thereafter (be sure to verify state requirements, which may supersede biennial inventory). However, when considering the potential losses that can (and do) occur in this area of the practice, biennial inventory is not sufficient. Practices should be able to balance their drugs and account for every pill and milliliter (mL) of controlled substances at anytime. Therefore weekly inventory may be required. If managers feel their CS logs are accurate, this inventory may only need to be performed monthly. A closing inventory must also be taken if and when the business closes permanently.

> **PRACTICE POINT** It is advised that practices complete a controlled substance inventory on a monthly basis (minimally).

Anytime a physical inventory is taken, the following information should be documented:
- Drug (name of product, strength, and number of milliliters or tablets that come in a full bottle)
- Physical count of drug
- Name of person completing the inventory
- Time of day the inventory was completed

The time is important; if the DEA completes an audit of the facility drugs, they need to know whether drugs that were used the day of the inventory should be included in the audit.

Drugs must be balanced on a perpetual inventory balance system; this provides a running balance that can be compared with the physical inventory at any time.

A folder should be kept separate from the controlled substance log book to house all invoices that list controlled drugs that have been received by the clinic. Drug listings should

Date	Time	To/From	Bottle #	Initial Amount	Amount Change	Balance	Initials
4-Aug	2:00 pm	DVM Res	100-112	0 Bottles	12 Bottles	12 Bottles	CS
5-Aug	8:00 am	SX Plain	100	12	1	11	NS
8-Aug	10:40 am	SX Plain	101	11	1	10	CS
10-Aug	2:00 pm	SX Plain	102	10	1	9	CS
				9			

Year 2013　　　　　　　　　　　Name of Drug: Telazol 100 mg/mL, 5 mL

FIGURE 16-3 Sample stock supply sheet.

be highlighted on the invoice, along with the assigned bottle numbers. A stock supply sheet, or closed bottle sheet, can help keep track of bottle numbers.

Figure 16-3 shows that 12 bottles of Telazol were received on August 4, 2013. Initially, there were no bottles available for use. Once the 12 bottles were added, the initial amount became 12 bottles. The bottles were assigned the numbers 100 through 112; these were the next numbers in sequence (99 bottles had been previously used). The stock supply list states that bottles were checked out to the surgical plain on August 5th, 8th, and 10th by two team members. Each time bottles are checked out, they must be recorded on this list and initialed by the team member removing the bottle. A form of this nature holds team members accountable and simplifies drug tracking.

Figure 16-4 is an example of a running drug log. Notice the bottle number, date, time, client name, patient name, initial amount, amount used, and balance are all required entries. Each bottle should be fully accounted for before opening another bottle.

Ketamine is the drug being logged in Figure 16-4. The initial amount and bottle number are on line 1, along with the owner's information and the amount of drug used. Each milliliter is accounted for before opening the next bottle. Bottles 1 and 3 balance well. Obviously, bottle 2 is missing 0.7 mL, which is almost 10% of a bottle. This amount of drug must be searched for; surgical records should be examined and team members questioned regarding who may have pulled the drug without writing the information down. If the missing drug cannot be found, management must consider inside theft. This information must be logged and highlighted so that it may be reported as a discrepancy on the annual controlled substance physical inventory list.

Each drug must have an individual log for the year. Each log must be balanced to ensure all drugs that were purchased

are accounted for. An annual controlled substance physical inventory should be performed, allowing inspectors to quickly review use within the practice. Ideally, practices should inventory controlled substances on a monthly basis. Human error occurs, and team members will forget to write down substances used to treat patients in emergency situations or drugs dispensed to clients for their pets. If practices perform monthly inventories and balances of their drugs, discrepancies can be located more easily in a month as opposed to a year (or two, as required).

To complete an annual controlled substance physical inventory, each drug log must be finished, and a physical count of the drug must be completed. The discrepancy is the physical count minus the running balance. The percentage of annual use should be calculated by dividing the discrepancy by the total number of milliliters or tablets (whichever form the drug comes in) and multiplied by 100 to obtain a percentage. If the discrepancy is greater than 3% for the year, the loss must be reported. Figure 16-5 uses Figure 16-4 to calculate the annual use of ketamine. The running balance (the total in milliliters that the practice has received for the year) minus the physical count (inventory performed) gives a discrepancy of −0.7 mL. Therefore 0.7 mL divided by 30 mL (the total use for the year) equals 0.02. To obtain the percentage, 0.02 is multiplied by 100. This gives an annual percentage use of 2.3%. If this number equaled 3% or higher, it would have to be reported to the DEA, the police department, and the state board of pharmacy.

It is expected that there will be a small amount of hub loss associated with each draw. It is advisable to ask the state veterinary inspector or the local DEA office for the best way to account for hub loss. Some departments may allow a small percentage of the total use to be written off as hub loss. If a bottle is broken, two people must initial the log indicating the broken bottle.

Bottle #	Date	Time	Owner's Name	Animal's Name	Initial Amount	Amount Used	Balance	Initials
1	4-Aug	8:00 am	Slatery	Waldo	10 mL	3	7	CS
	4-Aug	8:00 am	Garcia	Baby	7	0.5	6.5	NS
	4-Aug	8:15 am	Jones	Prancer	6.5	1	5.5	CS
	4-Aug	8:15 am	Loving	Tootsie	5.5	0.8	4.7	CS
	5-Aug	8:15 am	Pinto	Wonder	4.7	0.4	4.3	NS
	5-Aug	9:15 am	Adams	Wendy	4.3	2	2.3	NS
	5-Aug	9:30 am	Howard	Bobo	2.3	0.3	2	NS
	6-Aug	8:15 am	Bush	Tristen	2	2	0	CS
2	7-Aug	8:00 am	Evans	Ashley	10	0.6	9.4	NS
	7-Aug	8:00 am	Langford	Bobby	9.4	0.7	8.7	CS
	7-Aug	8:15 am	Smith	Casper	8.7	6	2.7	CS
	8-Aug	8:15 am	Howard	Wimpy	2.7	2	0.7	NS
			MIA	MIA		0.7	0	CS
3	8-Aug	9:30 am	Brown	Blackie	10	1	9	NS
	9-Aug	8:15 am	Hyatt	Lawrence	9	2	7	CS
	9-Aug	8:30 am	Ralph	Ariel	7	2.5	4.5	CS
	9-Aug	9:00 am	Jameson	Taylor	4.5	0.5	4	HP
	9-Aug	10:15 am	Lee	Wheeler	4	1	3	HP
	9-Aug	10:30 am	West	Katie	3	3	0	SM

Year 2013   Ketamine 100 mg/mL, 10 mL

FIGURE 16-4 Sample running drug log.

WHAT WOULD YOU DO/NOT DO?

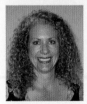

Amber is in charge of controlled substances at the practice but does not have time on a monthly basis to balance controlled drugs. Therefore once a year she sits down and tries to balance the drugs. However, large discrepancies usually exist. Instead of researching records and looking for lost drugs, she creates pets in employee files and falsifies medical records. She creates procedures that were never completed and logs controlled substances that were never given. She completes enough records to meet the maximum 3% loss for the year.

The new practice manager reviews employee medical records and notes that medical records are not complete in several cases and reviews the procedures with the veterinarian who oversaw the case. Several veterinarians did not recall completing procedures on those pets, and the veterinarians then question the team members. They inform the new practice manager that this is how Amber often balances lost drugs and compensates for those that were not recorded.

What Does the New Practice Manager Do?

First, Amber must be called into the practice and informed that falsifying medical records is a crime and unethical. Controlled substances are controlled for a reason, and they must be accounted for. The practice manager must implement new CS inventory procedures, which will ensure drugs are logged and accounted for on a daily basis. An immediate CS inventory must be completed and compared to the physical logs, and discrepancies must be investigated. Whichever drugs cannot be located must be reported (if the discrepancy is greater than 3%). If the DEA investigates, they will likely see that new protocols have been put in place and accountability will be scrutinized; they will also likely follow up, ensuring the new protocols are still in place.

Year 2013

Drug and Strength	Physical Count	Running Balance	Discrepancy ±	Percentage of Annual Use
Diazepam 5 mg Tabs	152 Tabs	155 Tabs	−3	$3/225 = 0.013 \times 100 = 1\%$
Torbutrol 1 mg Tabs	112 Tabs	112 Tabs	0	0
Ketamine Inj 100 mg/mL	29.3 mL	30 mL	−0.7 mL	$0.7/30 = 0.02 \times 100 = 2.3\%$
Sleepaway 100 mg/mL	157 mL	150 mL	+7 mL	N/A

FIGURE 16-5 Annual controlled substance physical inventory summary.

Loss Reporting

Theft or drug loss must be reported to the police and DEA immediately. Ongoing losses can result in loss of license and strict fines. DEA Form 106 should be filled out and forwarded to the local DEA office; another copy may have to be forwarded to the state board of pharmacy. One copy should be maintained for the controlled substance file (Figure 16-6). Verbal reports should be made as soon as possible, followed up with a written notification within 15 days.

PRACTICE POINT   If a practice has not implemented measures to protect CSs, veterinarians can lose their DEA license.

Substance Disposal

Controlled substances cannot be disposed of, as one would for regular pharmaceuticals. They must be sent through "reverse distribution," in which companies are certified to handle and dispose of controlled substances. Schedule II drugs require the use of DEA Form 222, whereas drugs classified as Schedule III, IV, or V simply require an invoice. It is advised to contact the local DEA office to determine who authorized reverse distributors are. The company can be contacted, who will then issue an invoice and call tag for the expired drugs. UPS, FedEx or an authorized transporter will pick up the drugs, deliver them to the reverse distributor where they will be incinerated. The reverse distributor will then issue a receipt and proof of destruction; this receipt should be kept for 2 years and stored with logs and invoices in which they correlate.

U.S. Department of Justice
Drug Enforcement Administration

REPORT OF THEFT OR LOSS OF CONTROLLED SUBSTANCES

Federal Regulations require registrants to submit a detailed report of any theft or loss of Controlled Substances to the Drug Enforcement Administration. Complete the front and back of this form in triplicate. Forward the original and duplicate copies to the nearest DEA Office. Retain the triplicate copy for your records. Some states may also require a copy of this report.	OMB APPROVAL No. 1117-0001

1. Name and Address of Registrant (Include ZIP Code) ZIP CODE

2. Phone No. (Include Area Code)

3. DEA Registration Number
2 ltr. prefix   7 digit suffix

4. Date of Theft or Loss

5. Principal Business of Registrant (Check one)
1 ☐ Pharmacy   5 ☐ Distributor
2 ☐ Practitioner   6 ☐ Methadone Program
3 ☐ Manufacturer   7 ☐ Other (Specify)
4 ☐ Hospital/Clinic

6. County in which Registrant is located

7. Was Theft reported to Police?
☐ Yes   ☐ No

8. Name and Telephone Number of Police Department (Include Area Code)

9. Number of Thefts or Losses Registrant has experienced in the past 24 months

10. Type of Theft or Loss (Check one and complete items below as appropriate)
1 ☐ Night break-in   3 ☐ Employee pilferage   5 ☐ Other (Explain)
2 ☐ Armed robbery   4 ☐ Customer theft   6 ☐ Lost in transit (Complete Item 14)

11. If Armed Robbery, was anyone:
Killed? ☐ No ☐ Yes (How many) _____
Injured? ☐ No ☐ Yes (How many) _____

12. Purchase value to registrant of Controlled Substances taken?
$

13. Were any pharmaceuticals or merchandise taken?
☐ No ☐ Yes (Est. Value)
$

14. IF LOST IN TRANSIT, COMPLETE THE FOLLOWING:

A. Name of Common Carrier

B. Name of Consignee

C. Consignee's DEA Registration Number

D. Was the carton received by the customer?
☐ Yes   ☐ No

E. If received, did it appear to be tampered with?
☐ Yes   ☐ No

F. Have you experienced losses in transit from this same carrier in the past?
☐ No   ☐ Yes (How many) _____

15. What identifying marks, symbols, or price codes were on the labels of these containers that would assist in identifying the products?

16. If Official Controlled Substance Order Forms (DEA-222) were stolen, give numbers.

17. What security measures have been taken to prevent future thefts or losses?

PRIVACY ACT INFORMATION

AUTHORITY: Section 301 of the Controlled Substances Act of 1970 (PL 91-513).
PURPOSE: Report theft or loss of Controlled Substances.
ROUTINE USES: The Controlled Substances Act authorizes the production of special reports required for statistical and analytical purposes. Disclosures of information from this system are made to the following categories of users for the purposes stated:
  A. Other Federal law enforcement and regulatory agencies for law enforcement and regulatory purposes.
  B. State and local law enforcement and regulatory agencies for law enforcement and regulatory purposes.
EFFECT: Failure to report theft or loss of controlled substances may result in penalties under Section 402 and 403 of the Controlled Substances Act.

In accordance with the Paperwork Reduction Act of 1995, no person is required to respond to a collection of information unless it displays a ly valid OMB control number. The valid OMB control number for this collection of information is 1117-0001. Public reporting burden for this collection of information is estimated to average 30 minutes per response, including the time for reviewing instructions, searching existing data sources, gathering and maintaining the data needed, and completing and reviewing the collection of information.

FORM DEA-106 (11-00) *Previous editions obsolete*
Electronic Form Version Designed in JetForm 5.2 Version

CONTINUE ON REVERSE

FIGURE 16-6 DEA Form 106. (Courtesy U.S. Department of Justice, Drug Enforcement Administration, Washington, D.C.)

VETERINARY PRACTICE and the LAW

Controlled drugs have specific laws that regulate their ordering, storage, and dispensing. Failure to adhere to these regulations may cause a veterinarian to lose his or her license. Veterinary team members must be aware of the drug-seeking behavior of clients and the physical symptoms of addiction. Many clients will create a story to get a prescription for their pet, and then take the medication themselves. They will frequently call for refills, often with excuses of spilling the medication, losing the pill vial, or leaving it out of town at a relative's home.

Team members should also be aware of co-workers behavior and report any abnormal behavior to the owner or practice manager. Many co-workers will divert medication for their own use; a tablet here and a tablet there add up, and substance abusers consistently need more chemical to achieve the desired high. Team members under the influence affect the practice in many negative aspects, and they should be terminated immediately for the safety of the patients and clients.

REVIEW QUESTIONS

1. What are controlled substances?
2. What is the abuse potential of ketamine?
3. Why are controlled substance log sheets required?
4. What is the purpose of a year-end physical inventory?
5. What is DEA Form 106 used for?

6. The class with the highest abuse potential is:
   a. II
   b. IV
   c. V
7. DEA Form 222 is used to:
   a. Register a doctor for a DEA license
   b. Report lost CSs
   c. Order Schedule II CSs
   d. Order Schedule IV CSs
8. Logs can be stored with CS.
   a. True
   b. False
9. A loss of _____ or more must be reported to the DEA
   a. 1%
   b. 2%
   c. 3%
   d. 4%
10. A reverse distributor:
    a. Sells CSs to veterinary hospitals
    b. Incinerates expired CSs
    c. Both of the above
    d. Neither of the above

Recommended Reading

United States Department of Justice, Drug Enforcement Administration: *Physicians manual: an information outline of the controlled substance act of 1970*, rev ed, Washington, DC, 2006, GPO. www.deadiversion.usdoj.gov/.

Logs

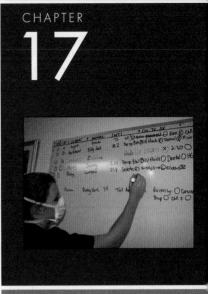

OUTLINE

Controlled Substances Log, *302*
Radiology Log, *302*
Surgical Log, *304*

Laboratory Log, *304*
Miscellaneous Logs, *304*

LEARNING OBJECTIVES

When you have finished this chapter, you should be able to:

1. Define the importance of logs in the veterinary practice.
2. Develop a practical log for each area of the practice.

KEY TERMS

Controlled Substance Log
Laboratory Log
Radiology Log
Surgical Log

Veterinary practices use many log books to help keep items organized, and to some extent these are required by law. Log books should be easy to use and maintain; the more difficult they are to use, the less likely it is that team members will use them. Log books can be created by team members to include information the team may need as well as that information required by law. State laws should be reviewed to determine what logs are required in each state as well as the length of time logs are required to be kept on premises. Logs can be kept in binders in each area identified as having a log book.

Controlled Substances Log

Controlled substances are reviewed in Chapter 16, with an example of a running drug log in Figure 16-4. The U.S. Drug Enforcement Administration and the state board of pharmacy (may) require this log. The state board of veterinary medicine in some states may also require it. These logs must be kept for 2 years beyond the last recorded date

and should be easily retrievable for inspection. Individual controlled drugs must include the date, owner's name and address, pet's name, the amount used, and the initials of the person responsible for the drug. All drugs must be accounted for, and a running drug log must be kept to indicate the balance of each drug at any time.

> **PRACTICE POINT**   Controlled substance logs are required by law.

Radiology Log

Some states may require a radiology log. Hospitals that utilize analog machines should maintain a radiology log, regardless of any requirement. Logs are excellent references when taking radiographs or looking up the history of a radiograph. Technicians taking the radiographs can record the information needed as they prepare for the x-ray (Figure 17-1). Radiology logs should include the

Date	Owner's Name	Patient's Name	Study	Position	kVp	mA	Initials
5/4/13	Patterson	Riley	Abdomen	Lat/VD	78/85	300	HP
5/4/13	Burns	Ariel	Chest	Lat x 2, VD	65/69	300	DB
5/5/13	Montoya	Blue	Right foreleg	Lat, ap	69	300	DB
5/5/13	Valdivia	Twinkle	Cat-o-gram	Lat, dv	72	300	HP

FIGURE 17-1 Sample radiology log.

owner's name, pet's name, the body part being radiographed, position, kilovolts, milliamperes, and the initials of the technician. If a radiograph needs to be repeated several days later, team members can review the log and use the same setting (if comparison radiographs are being taken, it is extremely important to have the same settings).

> *PRACTICE POINT*   Radiology logs are not required by law, but can increase the efficiency of a nondigital hospital.

If radiographs are checked out to owners or are sent out for referral, a log needs to be in place to document the removal of the radiographs from the premises (Figure 17-2). Radiographs are the property of the practice and should remain on the premises at all times. It is acceptable to lend them out for referrals or second opinions, but it should be documented that the radiographs were removed. This also helps when team members are looking for radiographs and cannot find them. Instead of assuming they are misfiled, the log can be consulted to see that they were removed. Checkout logs should include the date, owner's name, pet's name, who took the radiographs (whether the owners checked out the radiographs or they were sent by mail), where they went, and the team member's initials. The last column should be left blank to indicate their date of return, with another area for team member initials indicating that they were returned to the files.

Practices that are digitized do not have to use radiograph logs. Digital radiographs are automatically loaded into a patient's file with all the setting information attached to them. If radiographs need to be sent out for a second opinion, they can be copied to a CD. The film is never lost or misfiled. The log can be printed when needed, if required by the state.

Date	Owner's Name	Patient's Name	Check out by?	Going to?	Initials	Return Date	Initials
10/6/13	Pacheco	Cherry	Owner	Crossroads A.H.	LP	12/8/09	MV
10/8/13	Ziehl	Bud	UPS	SW Specialty	CS		
11/1/13	Soules	Blackie	Owner	Arroyo V.C.	SP	12/1/09	DC
12/15/13	Miale	Twinkle	Mail	Tuscon	CS		

FIGURE 17-2 Sample radiology checkout log.

WHAT WOULD YOU DO/NOT DO?

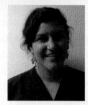

Sarah, a practice manager, balances the controlled drugs on a monthly basis. She finds that drugs are often not recorded when they are taken from the lockbox, and she has recently become very frustrated at the team for not being responsible about writing down the drug information. She has talked to each team member individually but the situation has not improved. Sarah tried to implement a protocol in which only she could remove drugs from the box. However, the system was ineffective when Sarah was not at the practice.

What Should Sarah Do?

Two team members must have access to the lockbox; these two team members must be accountable, and one must be on premises during all open hours. It is then their responsibility to write down drugs as they are taken from the box; however, occasionally the individual is multitasking and may forget to write down the controlled substances. Sarah could place one log sheet on the outside of the lockbox; all drugs could be written on one sheet at the time of removal instead of having to locate the controlled substances binder and recording the drug on the appropriate sheet. Sarah can then record the drugs on the appropriate log sheet on a monthly basis. This prevents the individual from walking away from the box before the drugs are recorded, and the log sheet serves as a simple reminder to log the substances.

Surgical Log

Some states may require a surgery log listing all patients that have received anesthesia within the practice. The surgery log can also be a great reference when looking for a lost controlled substance, when estimating the time an anesthetic machine has been in use, or for reviewing surgical cases (Figure 17-3). Surgical logs should contain the date, time, owner's name, patient's name, the surgical procedure, drugs used, and the initials of the team member overseeing the surgical case. Surgical logs are often referred to as *anesthesia logs* because this is where all anesthetics are recorded.

> **PRACTICE POINT**   Refer to state practice laws regarding the requirements of a surgical log.

Laboratory Log

Some practices may find it helpful to record laboratory tests and results on a sheet for referencing if needed. In-house testing such as fecal examinations, urinalyses, heartworm tests, parvovirus tests, and feline leukemia/FIV tests can be recorded. Occasionally, authors of the medical record will forget to record test results in the record. A log allows the team to locate the sample result without having to run another sample (Figure 17-4). Samples sent to outside laboratories can also be recorded and easily referenced if needed. An outside laboratory log can be used to compare with monthly statements to ensure the practice was billed correctly. If any questions arise, the record can be pulled to verify the charges.

Miscellaneous Logs

Other logs that may be useful in practice but are not required by state or federal agencies include maintenance logs. Radiograph developers, anesthetic machines, autoclaves, and laboratory machines must be cleaned on a regular basis, and a maintenance log indicates the history of each piece of equipment. If repairs are needed for the equipment, notes can be added to the maintenance log. Quality control samples should be run on in-house laboratory equipment on a regular basis as well; a log is occasionally required by the company as evidence that regular quality control and maintenance procedures have been completed on machines.

Logs may be kept for incoming telephone calls for a veterinary practice. Notes from telephone calls and conversations with current clients should be kept in those clients' files so that all team members can be familiar with the conversation that occurred. Calls from potential clients can be logged in a telephone log book; if the potential client arrives for an appointment, the conversation can be added to the medical record at that time.

⚖ VETERINARY PRACTICE and the LAW

Although some logs are required to be kept and maintained by state veterinary boards, other logs that the practice implements may provide more of a protection for the practice. Surgery logs may be required, whereas radiology checkout logs may not be required. Many times, radiographs are given to an owner to take with them for a specialty consultation, or the practice may send them to a boarded radiologist for review. Numerous times, these radiographs are not returned, and the staff spends hours looking for the lost items. Not only is the practice liable because the radiographs are unaccounted for, but the owner becomes infuriated.

Radiology checkout logs can prevent a lawsuit by accounting for the radiographs; they were released to either the owner or another practice. Efficiency of these logs can show an investigator or judge that the practice is responsible for the radiographs that are taken in the practice and can prove their checkout status.

Date	Time	Owner's Name	Patient's Name	Procedure	Pre-Anesthetic	Anesthetic	Gas	Initials
12/2/13	8:15 am	Berry	Vicky	K-9 OVH	0.1 mL Morph, 0.03 mL Ace	0.03 mL Tel	Iso	CS
12/2/13	8:45 am	Congleton	Flower	K-9 Neuter	1.0 mL Morph, 0.1 mL Ace	0.2 mL Tel	Iso	CS
12/2/13	9:15 am	Larsen	Sadie	K-9 OVH	0.5 mL Ket, 0.5 mL Diaz	0	Iso	NS
12/3/13	8:20 am	Davis	Blue	Fe Neuter	0.01 mL Ace, 0.04 mL Torb	0.05 mL Tel	Iso	MB
12/3/13	2:00 pm	Lockridge	Brooke	Laceration	0.3 mL Morph, 0.1 mL Ace	0.1 mL Tel	Iso	CS
12/4/13	8:30 am	Patterson	Gia	Growth Removal	2.0 mL Morph, 0.1 mL Ace	0.2 mL Tel	Iso	MB
12/4/13	10:15 am	Verda	Kile	Dental	1.0 mL Ket, 1.0 mL Diaz	0	Iso	CS
12/4/13	10:45 am	Saete	Looney	Fe OVH	0.01 mL Ace, 0.04 mL Torb	0.05 mL Tel	Iso	NS

FIGURE 17-3 Sample surgery log.

Date	Owner's Name	Patient's Name	Test	Result	Initials
5/4/13	Dasher	Rambo	HW/E/L/A	(−) (−) (−) (−)	HP
5/4/13	Biel	Whitney	Parvo	(−)	DB
5/5/13	Venzie	Kim	Felv/FIV	(+) (−)	DB
5/5/13	Bates	Sadie	HW/E/L/A	(−) (+) (−) (−)	HP

FIGURE 17-4 Sample laboratory log.

REVIEW QUESTIONS

1. What log is required by the U.S. Drug Enforcement Administration?
2. Why would a radiograph log benefit the team?
3. Logs potentially required by law include:
   a. Anesthesia maintenance logs
   b. Laboratory logs
   c. Surgical logs
   d. All of the above
4. Controlled substance logs should be kept for _____ years beyond last recorded entry.
   a. 1
   b. 2
   c. 3
   d. 4

Recommended Reading

Heinke MM: *Practice made perfect: a guide to veterinary practice management*, ed 2, Lakewood, CO, 2012, AAHA Press.

McCurnin D, Bassert JA: *Clinical textbook for veterinary technicians*, ed 7, St Louis, MO, 2010, Saunders Elsevier.

U.S. Department of Justice: *Drug Enforcement Administration: Physicians manual: an information outline of the controlled substance act of 1970*, rev ed, (Web site): www.deadiversion.usdoj.gov/. Washington, DC, 1990, GPO.

Accounts Receivable

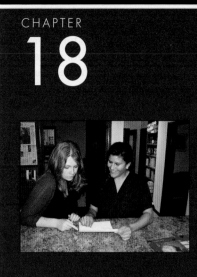

OUTLINE

Third Party Payment Plans, *308*
Delinquent Checks, *308*
Accepting Payment on Accounts
  Receivable, *309*
Instituting a No-Charge Policy, *309*
Monthly Statements, *310*
Collection Procedures for Outstanding
  Accounts, *311*

Fair Debt Collection Practices Act, *313*
Telephone Calls to Collect Outstanding
  Accounts, *313*
Collection Letters, *313*
Collections Agency, *314*
Employee Accounts Receivable, *315*

LEARNING OBJECTIVES

When you have completed this chapter, you should be able to:

1. Explain insufficient funds charges.
2. Describe the process used to accept payments on client accounts.
3. Define and enforce a no-charge policy.
4. Calculate finance charges.
5. Describe the process used to collect outstanding accounts receivable effectively.
6. Define the Fair Debt Collection Practices Act.
7. Develop effective collections letters.

CRITICAL COMPETENCIES

1. **Analytical Skills** - the ability to analyze information and use logic to address problems; the ability to quickly and accurately grasp complex information and concepts and to make correct inferences.
2. **Compliance** - being reliable, thorough, and conscientious in carrying out work assignments; has an appreciation for the importance of organizational rules and policies.
3. **Continuous Learning** - a curiosity for learning; actively seeks out new information, technologies, and methods; keep skills updated and applies new knowledge to the job.
4. **Critical and Strategic Thinking** - the ability to think critically about situations and to understand the relevance of information for different problems; use critical reasoning to generate and evaluate alternative courses of action or points of view relevant to an issue.
5. **Decision Making** - the ability to make good decisions, solve problems, and decide on important matters; the ability to gather and analyze relevant data and choose decisively between alternatives.

6. **Integrity** - honesty, trustworthiness, and adherence to high standards of ethical conduct.
7. **Leadership** - a willingness to lead and take charge; the ability to motivate others and mobilize group effort toward common goals.
8. **Oral Communication and Comprehension** - the ability to express one's thoughts verbally in a clear and understandable manner, and the ability to actively listen and attend to what others are saying; must have good group presentation skills.
9. **Persuasion** - the ability to change the attitudes and opinions of others and to persuade them to accept recommendations and change behavior.
10. **Planning and Prioritizing** - the ability to effectively manage time and work load to meet deadlines; the ability to organize work, set priorities, and establish plans for achieving goals.
11. **Writing and Verbal Skills** - ability to comprehend written material easily and accurately; ability to express thoughts clearly and succinctly in writing.

KEY TERMS

Accounts Receivable
Better Business Bureau
Billing Cycle
Collections Agency
Embezzlement
Fair Debt Collection
  Practices Act
Finance Charge
Interest
Ledger Cards
Monthly Statement
Post-dated Checks
Returned Checks
Statement

Accounts receivable is defined as the money owed to a business for services rendered or products that are sold and not paid for at the time of service. Each time clients are allowed to charge a service, profit for the veterinary practice decreases; essentially the practice has paid for the entire visit, receiving nothing in return. Every practice should institute a goal of not allowing accounts receivable to exceed 1.5% of the gross revenue. Amounts over 3% deserve the full attention of the entire team. A practice policy can be instituted, and all members of the team must follow the policy to *begin* to control the accounts receivable. If a client becomes upset that he or she cannot charge the services rendered, the team should discuss how valuable that client is. A bigger loss occurs to the practice from the collection process. Valuable time should be spent on clients who will pay for, and who value, the service they receive.

> **PRACTICE POINT** Accounts receivable should not be greater than 1.5% of gross revenue.

Discussing finances with a client can be emotional. It is important to discuss this sensitive issue in an exam room, away from other clients and team members. Clients may be embarrassed that they cannot afford the best care or are in a financial bind that is beyond their control. They can express anger, sadness, or fear toward the staff; team members should know not to take the expression personally. It is simply the responsibility of the team to offer the best medicine to every client regardless of finances. Conservative options can be presented as alternatives and should be documented in the record. This may alleviate some of the emotions of the client.

Compassion is an important aspect of the veterinary profession. The veterinary health care team loves animals, which is what makes team members enjoy their jobs. There will always be a charity case that a team member wants to help. Many veterinary practices have instituted a flex or indigent account. Some practices have given this account a special name and determine as a team which clients can use funds in this account. At times, wealthy clients want to donate money to help clients that cannot help their pets, and this is the perfect account to receive such donations. It allows the books to be balanced at the end of the day and generates a receipt for those who have donated. Clients must meet requirements for team members to consider the use of this account. Team members can develop guidelines, which may include such items as owner compassion, decreased finances, exceptional pet(s), and an intense owner-patient bond. These clients will truly appreciate the services and may eventually donate back to the fund once they are economically stable. Accounts of this nature must be discussed with a certified public accountant. State guidelines vary as to the setup and use of such accounts, and may require the filing of special documents for.

Third Party Payment Plans

With the economy being unstable, some clients are either reluctant to spend money on their pet, or do not have the money to spend on their pet. Practices should be proactive, trying to help the client before an accounts receivable is established.

First, practices may wish to establish wellness plans (see Chapter 19), which allow clients to make monthly payments for their pets care. The Bayer Veterinary Care Usage Study of 2011 indicated clients would like to have the ability to make monthly payments for their upcoming services.

Second, third party payment plans should be provided as an alternate for practices that will not extend credit to clients. CareCredit is a leading company in the veterinary industry, providing credit card services for clients. Clients simply fill out the application in the hospital (or at home on the Internet); team members either call in or enter client information on a secure Internet site, and the client is approved (or declined) within minutes of application submission.

Having options such as the two just mentioned allows the clinic to be perceived as *"working with all clients for all pets to receive the best care possible,"* instead of creating a negative response such as, *"all they care about is the money."*

> **PRACTICE POINT** Clients will also ask for payment plans to help pay for pet care; consider options that will be feasible for both the client and the practice.

Delinquent Checks

Checks returned for insufficient funds are a common problem for practices that do not use a check verification machine. Practices may try to collect these balances themselves or hire an outside collection agency to collect the funds. Returned check fees must be applied to the client account to recoup bank charges, lost time, and money (Figure 18-1). If a collection agency collects the delinquent amount, service fees will be deducted from the check total once it has been collected. Most companies add

---

Notice: By providing your check as payment, you authorize us to use information from your check to make a one-time electronic fund transfer from your account.

Funds may be drawn from your account the same day, and you will not receive your check back from your bank.

If payment is returned unpaid, you authorize ABC Veterinary Clinic to debit from your account a one-time electronic transfer fee of $30.00.

FIGURE 18-1 Sample insufficient funds notice.

a $30 service fee for returned checks. A notice indicating all fees that will be added to a client's account if a check is returned must be posted in a location that is clearly visible to clients.

An alternative to having checks returned for insufficient funds is to use a check machine that either verifies the account and funds available, or one that automatically debits the money from the clients account and deposits it into the practice account. Either of the two methods is acceptable; finance charges to the practice vary based on the service and company selected. Method two may be considered the most cost-effective, as this will eliminate the need to create a deposit slip at the end of the day, and it ensures money is electronically deposited.

Accepting Payment on Accounts Receivable

Two methods are available to record transactions when clients have paid on their account. Some clinics use a manual method of recording and tracking transactions, and others may use veterinary practice software.

Manual accounts receivable must be managed well to prevent internal embezzlement. All charges, statements, billing cycles, interest, account aging, and payments are calculated and recorded separately, generally on individual ledger cards. Aged accounts can be flagged with different colors, and appropriate notices can be sent to clients. When a payment is received, a receipt should be provided to the client, and a copy should be given to the accounts receivable manager, who will then update the ledger manually. This allows record keeping and payment handling to be separated.

A computerized accounts receivable management program has a large advantage over manual management. All calculations, interest, and statement fees are automatically calculated and added to the client's account. This eliminates errors associated with calculations and can decrease employee embezzlement. Clients simply pay on their accounts, a receipt is produced, and a new balance is listed.

Instituting a No-Charge Policy

Signs should be clearly posted for clients to see throughout the clinic regarding a no-charge policy. Signs should say, "Full payment is required at time of service" (Figure 18-2).

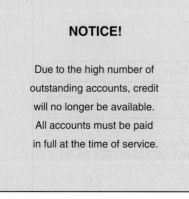

NOTICE!

Due to the high number of outstanding accounts, credit will no longer be available. All accounts must be paid in full at the time of service.

FIGURE 18-2 Sample "no charge" sign.

Although some practice owners believe this message is simple and to the point, it is unfortunately not adequate. Estimates (or treatment/medical plans) must be given to all clients, regardless of client "status," for all services that are expected to be rendered for that patient. Team members can print out an estimate, verbally review it with owners, and explain all procedures and medications the pet will be receiving. The client should sign the estimate; this gives the practice legal documentation that the client accepted the services that the veterinary team has recommended. Practices must collect a deposit of at least half (or more if the practice policy deems appropriate) at the time of client agreement; in addition, this must be communicated clearly to the client.

Every team member must understand and accept this policy, and it must be enforced consistently to be effective. A good policy can be both fair and compassionate.

Veterinary practice managers establish and enforce client credit policies.

Holding checks for clients is not recommended. A held check is defined as accepting a check with the current date that the check is written, but holding it for deposit until the client agrees on a date for it to be deposited. This adds another level of difficulty for the receptionist because held checks must be kept in a safe and secure place and deposited on the correct date. There is no guarantee that the funds will be available the day of deposit or that the client will not close the checking account. If a team member accidentally deposits the check early, the client will be unhappy with the practice and may try to collect returned check fees from the practice negligence. This creates a no-win situation, although the practice was trying to help the client.

PRACTICE POINT Review state laws regarding the acceptance of held checks and postdated checks; recent updates have been made in many states.

Accepting postdated checks is illegal in some states. A postdated check can be defined as a check that is written but dated at some point in the future. Some prosecutors will not pursue cases when a postdated check has been accepted. Check authorizing companies will not authorize or accept postdated checks.

Driver's license numbers should be documented for every client in case of nonpayment or a returned check. This allows practices to refer nonpaying clients to a collections agency to continue trying to collect the balance. The driver's license numbers can be collected from clients when they fill out the client/patient form. If a check machine is used, a driver's license number may be required to accept the check. If local district attorney's offices prosecute stolen check writers, a driver's license may be required for prosecution. Checking drivers licenses also follows the guideline's set forth in the red flags rule (see Chapter 20), verifying the presenter's identity (with the hopes of reducing fraud).

Monthly Statements

If clients are allowed to charge, there will be an accounts receivable collection. These clients have an outstanding balance and will have a statement generated monthly. A statement advises clients of their balance and indicates charges, payments, and the balance of their account for the month that has just concluded (Figure 18-3). Statements are also a request for money. Outstanding accounts can be difficult and time-consuming. Practice managers must remember to institute monthly statement fees. State laws vary regarding the amount of interest (if any) that can be added to an account. Laws should be verified before determining an interest rate. Adding interest fees to client accounts encourages quicker payoff because clients do not wish to pay additional fees.

Statement fees include time, paper, and postage along with any finance charges or interest rates the clinic feels are appropriate. Veterinary software systems allow a standard percentage to be added to each invoice, or a set dollar amount can be selected (Figure 18-4). One or two dollars is no longer an acceptable fee. Postage, paper, and the time it takes an employee to run statements far exceeds two dollars!

Statements should be printed on approximately the same day each month. Having one person in charge of accounts receivable will decrease mistakes and increase the efficiency of printing statements. This team member should indicate in the client's medical record the date, statement fee, new balance, and the team member's initials. This allows other team members to easily follow the billing fees if the client has any questions regarding the account.

<table>
<tr><td colspan="2">ABC Animal Clinic
555 Uptown Circle
Anytown, MN 89000
555-555-5555</td><td colspan="3" align="right">STATEMENT

Date 05/28/13
Page 1</td></tr>
</table>

Maria Rogers
6454 Downtown Circle
Anytown, MN 89001

Account # 21312

Date	Description/Patient	Invoice No.	Charges	Payments
04/28/13	Scruffy	1090	$398.34	$0.00

Current	30 Days	60 Days	90 Days	**Amount Due**
$398.34	0.00	0.00	0.00	**$398.34**

Payment is due upon receipt. For your convenience, we accept Visa, MasterCard, and Discover. PLEASE NOTE THAT A $5.00 MONTHLY STATEMENT FEE WILL BE ASSESSED TO ALL BALANCES OVER 30 DAYS PAST DUE.

FIGURE 18-3 Sample statement.

Collection Procedures for Outstanding Accounts

Although collection procedures can seem fairly simple, there are laws that protect the client. Accounts should be paid by clients within 30 days of charging. However, particular clients may have higher bills that will require longer collection times. Some veterinary software systems allow the practice to choose whether a statement fee and/or percentage of the balance should be added to those accounts less than 30 days old. The software will age accounts, generally 0 to 30 days, 31 to 60 days, 61 to 90 days, and over 90 days. This allows a practice manager to look at the status of accounts receivable with a more accurate prediction of

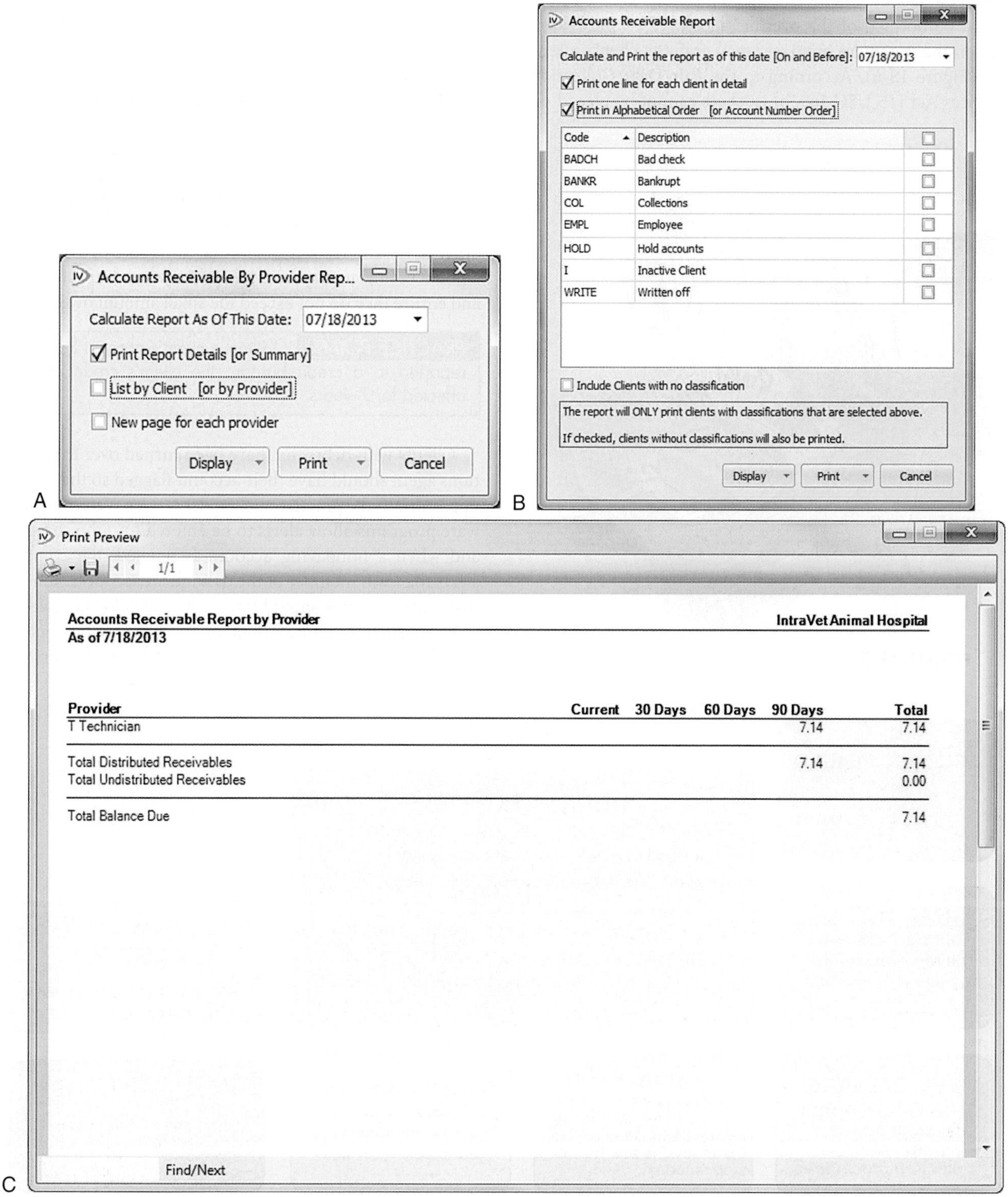

FIGURE 18-4 A to C, Sample accounts receivable report. (Courtesy IntraVet, Dublin, Ohio.)

payment. Accounts that are older than 90 days are very difficult to collect (Figure 18-5).

Clients should be sent a statement immediately after the service has been performed and medications have been dispensed. Clients are more willing to pay a balance while the treatment and procedures are still fresh in their minds.

If a client is making monthly payments, it is advisable to continue working with the client before turning accounts to a credit agency. Clients not making payments by 60 days should be notified of the overdue account. A handwritten note on the statement or sticker may grab the client's attention (Figure 18-6). According to the Fair Debt Collection Practices Act [15 USC 1692b], stickers cannot be placed on the outside of the envelope indicating a debt is trying to be collected.

Clients not making payments within 90 days can be notified that arrangements need to be made or the account will be turned over to a credit collection agency. Team members should try to call owners to discuss the account (see the next section on the Fair Debt Collection Practices Act), and try to make payment arrangements with the client. If contact has been made with the client, a summary of the conversation must be documented in the record. Once team members have exhausted all opportunities to collect the outstanding balance, accounts must be turned over to a collections agent. If the agent is unable to collect, the outstanding amount will be reported to a credit bureau or the consumer reporting agency. A credit bureau reports specific information about a person's previous payment history and provides information of public interest. A client's credit will be affected for the following 7 years. Practices may also wish to take the client to small claims court in order to try and recover owed money. Be sure to consider the amount of time to prepare for these cases and court filing costs, and ensure they do not exceed the small amount owed.

> **PRACTICE POINT**   When a client's account has been reported to a credit bureau, the client's credit can be affected for 7 years.

Clients with debts that have been turned over to a collections agent should have their account flagged so that they do not return to the practice and expect service. Veterinary software programs allow alerts to be entered into the computer, and when a nonpaying account is opened, the computer alerts the team member of the delinquent account. Noncomputerized practices should have a special color file folder to indicate uncollected accounts, or the file may be kept in a separate area. Some clients will return to a clinic years later,

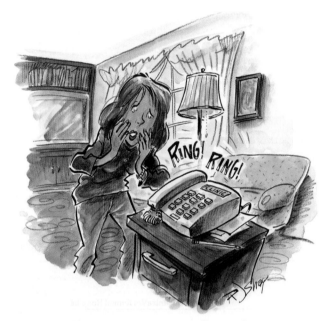

FIGURE 18-5 "Oh no! The vet's office is calling again!"

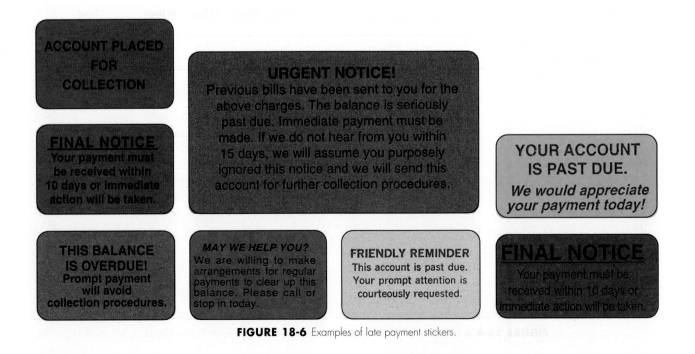

FIGURE 18-6 Examples of late payment stickers.

hoping that the staff will not remember the bad debt they once had. It is fair to ask the clients to pay the previous balance before any new services being rendered.

If a clinic decides not to turn an outstanding account over to a collection agent and is unable to collect the balance, it may be worthwhile to simply write off the account as bad debt. Again, the client record must be flagged so that all team members know of the account status. At the end of the day, time, money, and the effort spent collecting accounts receivable could be better spent on other areas of the practice. Speak with the practice's CPA to determine if the accounts being written off need to be reported on the yearly taxes (can depend on whether the practice reports as cash or accrual basis).

Fair Debt Collection Practices Act

The Fair Debt Collection Practices Act of 1996 regulates collection procedures of past due accounts. The act was passed to protect the public from unethical collection procedures and mainly applies to collection agencies. Debtors cannot be subjected to harassment, oppressive tactics, or abusive treatment. The law prohibits the collector from making any false statements to the client, such as claiming to be a lawyer or government agency. Clients may not be called at work if the employer or client objects or be called at inconvenient times or places, such as before 8 AM and after 9 PM. Delinquent payments can only be discussed with the clients themselves. These same regulations must be considered as the veterinary health care team attempts to collect outstanding accounts.

 Veterinary practice managers understand and ensure compliance with legal and ethical guidelines surrounding confidentiality of clients.

Telephone Calls to Collect Outstanding Accounts

Contact with clients can be made with a telephone call to try to determine the client's financial status. Team members may find it difficult to try to collect delinquent accounts over the phone and often find the client has a negative attitude once the phone call has been made. It should be remembered not to take the negative words personally; it is frustrating to everyone to be under financial strain. Team members should keep a friendly, helpful, and positive tone in their voices. Discussion of the animal should be avoided, keeping the conversation focused on the account collection. Clearly state the hospital policy regarding charging and set a date for when the account will be paid in full. Be prepared to offer the client a payment plan, and advise the client that interest charges will accrue each month.

Team members should remember not to call clients before 8 AM or after 9 PM, as stated by the Fair Debt Collection Practices Act. Team members must verify who they are speaking with, then identify themselves. "*Hello, is this Mr. Stone?*" Once the client has verified himself, the team member can

continue, "*This is Teresa with ABC Animal Clinic.*" The purpose of the phone call can then be established. Team members may act as if the client is going to pay the balance and that payment arrangements are simply being made. A specific date and amount of payment can be established and documented in the record. A written letter to follow up the details of the conversation can be sent to the client as a simple reminder. Clients should never be threatened, and the account should never be discussed with anyone other than the client. Messages should not be left regarding the delinquent balance; simply state the team member's name and a phone number where he or she can be reached.

Many clients have caller ID and will not answer the phone when an outstanding account or collections agent is calling. If possible, calls should be made on a blocked line eliminating the identification. Some clients still may not answer the phone, especially if they are in debt and have several businesses calling. All attempts to make contact with the client must be documented in the record. After several attempts have been made, a certified letter may have to be mailed. A certified letter requires that the recipient sign a card indicating receipt of the letter, and the card is then returned to the sender.

Collection Letters

A collection letter may be sent at the discretion of the veterinary practice along with a monthly statement. Veterinary software can generate a collection letter at any time management has specified in the setup program. A series of computer-generated letters can be sent at 30, 60, and/or 90 days after the account has become past due. Specified messages can be printed on each letter informing the client of the past due status of the account. Clients should be reminded that unpaid accounts will be sent to a collections agency and reported to credit bureaus. The last letter should include a deadline date of when the account will be turned over to collections if the recipient has not responded. Box 18-1 can be used as a guideline for developing a collection letter. Letters should be kept short and simple. Long, rambling letters will be ignored by the client and may inadvertently have words or

BOX 18-1	Guidelines for Developing an Effective Collection Letter

- Keep the letter short and brief.
- Make sure the date, amount, and client information are correct.
- Use simple words and phrases.
- Provide a specific date by which the client must respond.
- Provide a date for when a specific action will take place. For example, give the date when the account will be turned over to a collection agent.
- Be firm and polite.
- Include "thank you" at the end of the letter; this is a valuable tool in public relations.

ABC Animal Clinic
555 Uptown Circle
Anytown, MN 89000
555-555-5555

05/28/13

Maria Rogers
6454 Downtown Circle
Anytown, MN 89001

Dear Mrs. Rogers,

On April 28, 2013, you brought Scruffy into ABC Animal Clinic to be spayed. At the time of Scruffy's release, you notified the receptionist that you left your purse at home and asked if you could send a payment in the mail. The receptionist kindly extended credit to you, which was a rare circumstance.

It is against our policy at ABC Animal Clinic to extend credit. We have sent you several overdue notices but have received no response from you.

We have enclosed the original receipt with the total amount due of $398.94. If we do not hear from you by 06/15/13, we will be forced to turn your account over to our collections agency.

Please contact us immediately. Your prompt attention is greatly appreciated.

Thank you,

Melva Flowers
Practice Manager, ABC Animal Clinic

FIGURE 18-7 Sample collection letter.

phrases that will offend the client, ultimately delaying payment (Figure 18-7).

Studies show that clients pay outstanding balances for health care last, after paying rent, mortgage, and utilities, because of the fear of losing their homes. Team members can send a simple reminder to clients that a small payment each month will prevent the account from being sent to a collections agency.

Collections Agency

After every attempt has been made to collect the account, it may be necessary to appoint the services of a collection agency (Box 18-2). The longer an account is delinquent, the less likely it is the account will be collected on, regardless of

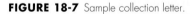

| BOX 18-2 | Vital Information to Provide to a Collection Agent |

- Client's full name, address, and all telephone numbers (including cell phone and work phone)
- Total balance due on account, including finance charges
- Client's occupation, if known
- Client's employment address, if known
- Client's driver's license number
- Copy of client information sheet and signature of client guaranteeing payment for services rendered

whether it is by the practice or a collection agent. Agencies will generally charge between 40% and 60% of the total balance that is being collected or may only charge the practice if they are able to collect (some agencies may charge an up-front, nonreturnable fees).

WHAT WOULD YOU DO/NOT DO?

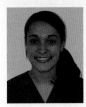

Linda, the office manager is in charge of accounts receivable and runs statements on a monthly basis. She notices that the employee accounts receivable is quite high, almost 20% of the accounts receivable total. Upon closer examination, she sees that several employees have not made a payment for several months. She realizes that the economy has been difficult for many, but does not know if she should verbally speak with the employees about their account balances.

What Should Linda Do?

Instead of speaking directly to the staff with past due accounts and possibly causing tension, she should discuss the situation with the owner and practice manager, allowing them to handle employees if (employees) become frustrated. Employees, like clients, can be embarrassed by their financial situation and become upset when addressed for lack of payments on their account. Leadership must also consider an employee accounts receivable policy, capping the amount allowed to be charged. Allowing team members to charge can create a negative cash flow, because the services and products are already being discounted, and the money is not being collected by the practice. Team members must understand how their accounts receivable can affect the practice in a negative manner.

Employee Accounts Receivable

Employees may accumulate a balance with a veterinary clinic as procedures and products are added to their accounts. If this is the case, it is important that each employee be mandated to make monthly payments. However, best practice is that employees are not allowed to charge.

> **PRACTICE POINT** An employee accounts receivable policy must be implemented and monitored; accounts should not be allowed to exceed $100.00.

Practices generally give employee discounts on services and products; therefore the veterinary practice is losing money by allowing employees to accumulate large balances. In addition, practices may be unable to collect on an account if the employee leaves. It can then be extremely difficult for the team to make phone calls and/or send the former employee to collections if he or she left the practice on good terms. It is in the best interest of the clinic to prevent employee balances from accumulating by mandating monthly payments or implementing a no charge policy.

Practices that withdraw money from employee paychecks must check state laws, because state regulations vary regarding this practice. Federal or state law may prevent money from being withheld that will exceed the employee receiving minimum wage on their paycheck. In addition, managers must have documentation that the employee authorizes the withholding from their check.

⚖ VETERINARY PRACTICE and the LAW

Collecting outstanding accounts can be a difficult and a time-consuming task. Team members must abide by the Fair Debt Collection Practices Act, which was passed to protect the public from unethical collection procedures. Those that do not follow the Fair Debt Collection Practices Act can be sued by clients in which any damage sustained by the client can be collected. A judge may determine the actual amount of damages, which cannot exceed $500,000 or a percentage of the total net worth of the debt collector. Collection procedures must be followed to prevent a lawsuit from occurring.

REVIEW QUESTIONS

1. What is the Fair Debt Collection Practices Act and why was it established?
2. What characteristics should be considered when choosing a collections agent?
3. What is an insufficient funds charge?
4. Why should a percentage of interest be added to outstanding client accounts?
5. What information is needed when reporting delinquent accounts to a credit bureau?
6. Why should postdated checks not be accepted?
7. What is a held check?
8. How often should statements be sent?
9. What percentage of gross profits should be allowed as accounts receivable?
10. If a practice generates a yearly gross income of $1,123,598.68, and accounts receivable is 1%, what is the total accounts receivable balance?
11. Accounts receivable should not exceed:
    a. 1.5% of Gross Revenue
    b. $2
    c. 5% of Gross Revenue
    d. 10% of Gross Revenue
12. Holding checks for clients is recommended when they cannot pay for services the day of.
    a. True
    b. False
13. Which of the following is a result of the Fair Debit Collection Act?
    a. Notification stickers can be placed on the outside of the envelope
    b. Conversations to collect outstanding AR can be held with any of the family members residing in the home
    c. Calls can be made between 8 AM and 9 PM
    d. Clients can be threatened that veterinary service will longer be available for them

14. Withdrawing the total amount due (for an employee accounts receivable) from employee checks is an acceptable form of payment.
    a. True
    b. False
15. Third party payment plans include:
    a. CareCredit
    b. Veterinary Pet Insurance
    c. PaymentBanc
    d. All of the above

Recommended Reading

Heinke MM: *Practice made perfect: a guide to veterinary practice management*, ed 2, Lakewood, CO, 2012, AAHA Press.

Pet Health Insurance and Wellness Plans

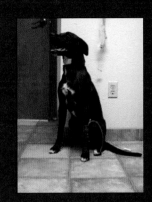

OUTLINE

Indemnity Insurance, *318*
  Premiums, *319*
  Deductibles, *319*
  Co-pay, *320*
  Annual Policy, Per-Incident, or Lifetime Limits, *320*
  Preexisting Health Conditions, *320*
  Waiting Period, *320*
  Hereditary and Congenital Conditions, *320*
  Chronic Conditions, *321*
  Exclusions, *321*

Benefits of Pet Health Insurance, *321*
Filing a Claim, *321*
Discount Clubs, *324*
Managed Care, *324*
Making Pet Health Insurance Work for the Practice, *324*
Recommendations to Clients, *325*
Offering Pet Health Insurance as a Benefit, *325*
Wellness Plans, *325*
  Components of a Wellness Plan, *325*
  Pricing, *326*

LEARNING OBJECTIVES

When you have completed this chapter, you should be able to:

1. Define and explain insurance policies to fellow team members and clients.
2. Identify the differences between hereditary and congenital conditions.
3. Clarify insurance claim forms.
4. Explain the disadvantages of third-party payment systems.
5. Define insurance plans to clients.

CRITICAL COMPETENCIES

1. **Adaptability** - being open to change and flexible work methods; the ability to adapt behavior to changing conditions or new information.
2. **Analytical Skills** - the ability to analyze information and use logic to address problems; the ability to quickly and accurately grasp complex information and concepts and to make correct inferences.
3. **Compliance** - being reliable, thorough, and conscientious in carrying out work assignments; has an appreciation for the importance of organizational rules and policies.
4. **Continuous Learning** - a curiosity for learning; actively seek out new information, technologies, and methods; keep skills updated and apply new knowledge to the job.
5. **Critical and Strategic Thinking** - the ability to think critically about situations and to understand the relevance of information for different problems; use critical reasoning to generate and

evaluate alternative courses of action or points of view relevant to an issue.
6. **Decision Making** - the ability to make good decisions, solve problems, and decide on important matters; the ability to gather and analyze relevant data and choose decisively between alternatives.
7. **Leadership** - a willingness to lead and take charge; the ability to motivate others and mobilize group effort toward common goals.
8. **Oral Communication and Comprehension** - the ability to express one's thoughts verbally in a clear and understandable manner, and the ability to actively listen and attend to what others are saying; must have good group presentation skills.
9. **Persuasion** - the ability to change the attitudes and opinions of others and to persuade them to accept recommendations and change behavior.
10. **Planning and Prioritizing** - the ability to effectively manage time and workload

KEY TERMS

Allowance
Annual Deductible
Annual Payout Limit
Benefit
Chronic Conditions
Claim
Congenital Conditions
Co-pay
Deductible
Exclusion
Hereditary Conditions
Incident
Indemnity Insurance
Lifetime Limit
Managed Care
National Commission on Veterinary Economic Issues (NCVEI)
Per-Incident Deductible
Per-Incident Limit
Preexisting Condition
Premium
Rider
Waiting Period

to meet deadlines; the ability to organize work, set priorities, and establish plans for achieving goals.

11. **Relationship Building** - the ability to develop constructive and cooperative working relationships with others and maintain them over time; must also be able to settle disputes, resolve grievances and conflicts, and negotiate with others.

12. **Writing and Verbal Skills** - ability to comprehend written material easily and accurately; ability to express thoughts clearly and succinctly in writing.

Pet health insurance has been available for more than 20 years but has not been a popular choice among owners until recently. Insurance is a method by which pet owners can manage the risks of expensive health care. Accidents and diseases are unexpected costs for owners, and insurance allows them to obtain the best treatment available. Many pet owners are forced to make treatment decisions based on cost alone. Insurance allows owners the financial resources they may need to provide lifesaving treatments they would otherwise not consider.

The cost of veterinary medicine has risen over the years, according to the American Veterinary Medical Association (AVMA), nearly 124% during the period of 1980 to 2005 (Wolf, et al., 2008). Several factors contribute to the increase, including better therapeutic options for pets, a stronger human-animal bond, and conscious effort for veterinary practices to align fees with services provided. Costs will continue to rise, furthering the need for pet health insurance for clients.

Pets are now living longer because veterinary health care has improved and clients are more willing to spend additional money to treat medical conditions (Box 19-1). Veterinary medicine has benefited from the progression of human medicine with regard to new pharmaceuticals, disease treatments, and diagnostic equipment such as computer-based imaging. These advancements have increased the quality,

quantity, and cost of veterinary care; with that, clients have also come to expect a higher level of service (Figure 19-1).

Owners that have pet health insurance are more likely to accept recommendations made by the veterinary team, because they are better able to handle emergency situations. A study released by Veterinary Pet Insurance in 2006 indicates that clients with insurance scheduled 40% more appointments, spent twice as much on veterinary care over the life of their pet, and had a 41% higher stop-treatment level than those without.

It is a false perception that pet health insurance is confusing. In fact, many practices do not offer insurance to clients

PRACTICE POINT   Owners that have pet health insurance are more likely to accept recommendations made by the veterinary team, because they are better able to handle emergency situations.

because they feel it could be difficult, time-consuming, and not worth the effort. Therefore clients are unaware of the benefits of such policies, and the practice is losing revenue. A brief overview is provided, to help team members become more familiar with the terms used in insurance policies (Box 19-2).

Indemnity Insurance

Indemnity insurance offers compensation for treatment of injured and sick pets. Owners purchase a policy directly from a pet health insurance company and are eligible for compensation based on the care provided and policy terms. Policies are available for comprehensive illness, standard care, and accident coverage and may cover species ranging from dogs and cats to exotics and birds.

Indemnity insurance is **different** from insurance available for people. Insurance on the human side is generally offered through health management organizations (HMOs) or preferred provider organizations (PPOs), which are managed organizations. Physicians are contracted to provide medical service at a set price and are then reimbursed directly by the insurance company.

Indemnity insurance is not managed care; indemnity insurance policies provide compensation for accidents and illnesses and are paid directly to the client. This leaves the

BOX 19-1	Most Common Reasons Pets Visit a Veterinarian
TOP 10 CANINE CLAIMS	**TOP 10 FELINE CLAIMS**
1. Ear infections	1. Lower urinary tract diseases
2. Skin allergies	2. Stomach upsets/gastritis
3. Pyoderma (hot spots)	3. Renal failure
4. Stomach upsets	4. Intestinal inflammation/ diarrhea
5. Intestinal inflammation/ diarrhea	5. Skin allergies
6. Bladder diseases	6. Diabetes
7. Eye infections	7. Colitis/constipation
8. Arthritis	8. Ear infections
9. Hypothyroidism	9. Upper respiratory virus
10. Sprains	10. Hyperthyroidism

veterinary practice out of the process because the client pays the veterinary practice when the service is rendered.

Premiums

A premium is defined as the amount an owner pays monthly or annually to maintain an insurance policy for a pet. Premium amounts are affected by a number of factors that

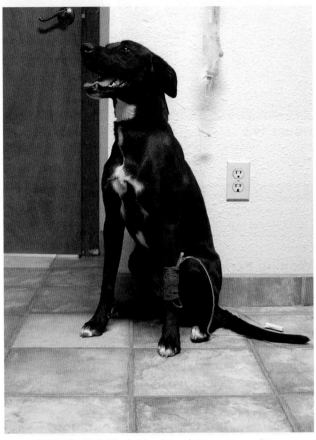

FIGURE 19-1 Black Labrador with intravenous catheter.

depend on the insurance provider, including the deductible; the co-pay; and the per-incident, annual, or lifetime payout limit. The cost of the premium is determined by several factors, including the species and breed of the animal, whether the pet is spayed or neutered, the age of the pet, and the geographic location of the owner in the United States. Cats tend to have lower premiums than dogs, and a Border Collie will have a lower premium than a Shar-Pei. Altered pets tend to have fewer behavioral issues and hormone-driven instincts and may have a decreased chance of developing hormone-related cancers; therefore a lower premium is likely. Owners living in rural Arizona will also have a lower premium than those who live in Los Angeles because the price of veterinary care is drastically different in these two locations.

> **PRACTICE POINT** Insurance rates can vary by species, age, breed, and client zip code, along with selected premium and deductibles.

Deductibles

A deductible is the amount an owner must pay before the insurance company will offer compensation. Insurance companies vary, offering either a per-incident deductible or an annual deductible. Per-incident deductibles refer to the owner paying the chosen deductible amount each time an incident occurs with the pet. An annual deductible refers to an owner paying the chosen deductible one time each year. Once the annual deductible amount has been met, the owner does not have to pay a deductible until the following year. For example, if a dog has an ear infection in March, a foreign body in June, and a fractured leg in November, and the owner chose a policy that was per-incident based, the owner would pay a deductible for each of the three claims. If the owner chose an annual deductible, he would pay the deductible amount once and would no longer be subject to a

---

BOX 19-2 | Helpful Terms

Allowance: The maximum amount available for a specific diagnosis.

Annual Deductible: The dollar amount the client chooses when signing up for an insurance plan. The client pays this amount before payout.

Annual Payout Limit: The maximum amount an insurance company will pay out on one policy, per year.

Benefit: The payment made for a specific diagnosis in accordance with an insurance plan.

Claim: A submission for a request for payment.

Co-pay: A specified dollar amount of covered services that is the policyholder's responsibility.

Deductible: The dollar amount an individual must pay for services before the insurance company will pay. Clients may have a choice of per-incident deductible or annual deductible.

Exclusion: A condition that is excluded from the coverage of a medical plan.

Incident: An individual accident, illness, or injury, including those that may require continual treatment until resolution.

Indemnity Insurance: A system of pet health insurance in which the client is reimbursed for services after they have been provided.

Lifetime Limit: The maximum dollar amount a company will pay out on one policy for the lifetime of the pet.

Per-Incident Deductible: The dollar amount that the policyholder is responsible for before the company will begin to pay out for each incident for which a claim form is submitted.

Per-Incident Limit: The maximum dollar amount an insurance company will pay out per incident filed.

Preexisting condition: Injury or illness contracted, manifested, or incurred before the policy effective date.

Premium: The amount paid annually or monthly for a policyholder to maintain an insurance policy.

Rider: An extension of coverage that can be purchased and added to a base medical policy.

deductible for the rest of the year. Lower deductibles increase the cost of the premium, just as higher deductibles lower the premium.

Co-pay

A co-pay is the percentage that the owner is responsible for after the deductible has been met. Lower co-pays increase the amount of the premium and generally range from 10% to 20%. As an example, if a client's policy includes a $100 deductible and a 10% co-pay and the invoice balance is $4500, the owner is responsible for $540. This is calculated as follows:

$$\$4500 - \$100\ \text{deductible} = \$4400 \times 10\%\ \text{co-pay} = \$440$$
$$\$440 + \$100 = \$540\ \ (\text{client responsibility})$$
$$\$4500 - \$540 = \$3960\ \ (\text{insurance responsibility})$$

Annual Policy, Per-Incident, or Lifetime Limits

Some insurance companies offer clients a choice of an annual policy or a per-incident limit; others offer one or the other. Annual limits refer to the maximum amount that the insurance company will pay for a condition or illness during the policy term. Per-incident limits refer to the maximum amount an insurance company will pay each time a new problem or disease occurs. Lifetime limits refer to the maximum amount an insurance company will pay during the pet's life.

Per-incident limits can range from $1500 to $6000, but some companies do not have a per-incident limit. Annual limits range from $8000 to $20,000, allowing a larger amount for serious conditions. If a pet has been diagnosed with cancer and must undergo surgery, chemotherapy, and radiation, the invoice will likely exceed the $6000 per-incident limit. Because the cancer is classified as one incident, the maximum amount paid to the client will be the per-incident limit established in the policy. If an annual limit was chosen, the total amount paid to the client will be higher, based on the annual maximum amount established in the insurance policy. Few companies offer a lifetime limit, but if they do, it may be as high as $100,000. Policies should be examined carefully to determine which limit would meet the client's needs.

Preexisting Health Conditions

A preexisting health condition is defined as any accident or illness contracted, manifested, or incurred before the policy effective date. The pet may be enrolled; however, any preexisting condition will be excluded from coverage. It is highly recommended to enroll puppies and kittens in an insurance plan before any medical conditions arise. Some insurance companies will review preexisting conditions; if a stated condition has been diagnosed and cured, the exclusion may be waived. An example is a puppy diagnosed with gastroenteritis. If it was a one-time gastrointestinal indiscretion that was cured, a company can remove the exclusion, allowing future indiscretions to be covered.

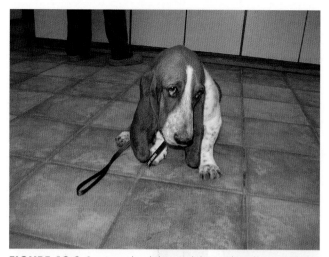

FIGURE 19-2 Some purebred dogs with known hereditary conditions may not be eligible for pet health insurance with certain companies.

PRACTICE POINT   Review a company's policy regarding preexisting conditions and hereditary defects before purchasing a policy.

Waiting Period

A waiting period is a period of time when coverage is not available and generally applies to the time between submission of the application and the date the policy becomes effective. Each company varies in the length of time between application acceptance and activation. Some companies may have a 48-hour waiting period for accidents and a 2- to 4-week waiting period for a condition or illness. Any condition that occurs during the waiting period is usually considered a preexisting condition.

Hereditary and Congenital Conditions

Purebred pets that are known to have congenital and hereditary conditions may, based on company policy, also be excluded from an insurance plan (Figure 19-2). Recent veterinary books, including *Current Veterinary Therapy, Medical and Genetic Aspects of Purebred Dogs,* and the *Textbook of Small Animal Internal Medicine,* reference common congenital and hereditary conditions. A congenital condition is generally defined as an abnormality present at birth, whether apparent or not, that can cause illness or disease.

Congenital defects may be caused by medications administered to the mother in utero. Examples of congenital defects may include an umbilical hernia, a cleft palate, or a portosystemic shunt. Presence of a shunt may not be known until the dog matures, whereas a cleft palate is obvious immediately after birth. A hereditary condition is an abnormality that is transmitted genetically from the parent to the offspring. Examples include hip dysplasia, luxating patella, or cardiomyopathy. Some companies may also argue that some congenital defects are hereditary, thereby excluding coverage of such conditions. A portosystemic shunt is an example of a condition that may be subject to such argument. Policies must be reviewed carefully for such exemptions.

Coverage of diseases may vary among insurance companies; therefore a list of excluded diseases and conditions should be requested. Some companies will cover congenital conditions if they have not been previously diagnosed; others will not cover them at all. Companies that offer coverage of hereditary diseases will have higher premiums.

WHAT WOULD YOU DO/NOT DO?

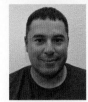

Ms. Luke, a longtime client has recently acquired a Great Dane puppy. Upon examination, Dr. Abbey tentatively diagnoses osteochondritis dissecans, a common skeletal growing abnormality in large breed puppies. However, to make a true diagnosis, Dr. Abbey recommends radiographs. Ms. Luke declines radiographs at this time for financial reasons. The team advises her that pet health insurance may be an option for her new puppy, and hand her a brochure discussing the benefits of health insurance.

The following month, Ms. Luke returns to the practice stating she has pet health insurance now, and would like the radiographs that were recommended last month. Alex, a longtime veterinary technician knows that preexisting health conditions are not covered by insurance, and because the pet had previously been seen for this condition, that they will likely not cover the costs of the radiographs. Alex advises the owner of this, who claims "they won't know the difference, they are only office workers!"

What Should Alex Do?
Alex should continue with the case, and take radiographs at the veterinarians' request. However, it is not his place to directly call the insurance company; this may create disloyalty of the client. He can however, offer to fill out the pet health insurance claim form for the owner, copy the medical records and send the claim for Ms. Luke. The insurance company will then be able to read the medical record and make a judgment based on the copies provided.

Chronic Conditions

Many diseases or conditions that are diagnosed will require years of care. Diabetes, Cushing disease, and Addison disease are just a few conditions that require care beyond the initial diagnosis and treatment (Figure 19-3). These conditions are known as *chronic conditions,* and some companies will only cover the initial diagnosis and treatment for the first year. Once it is time to reenroll the pet for the upcoming year, some insurance companies may consider the condition as a preexisting condition and exclude it from the policy.

Exclusions

Many companies have a list of exclusions: diseases, conditions, or treatments that are excluded from policies. Frequently, behavior counseling and medications are not covered, nor are compounded medications, nutraceuticals, or diets. Exclusions should be carefully reviewed before choosing a policy.

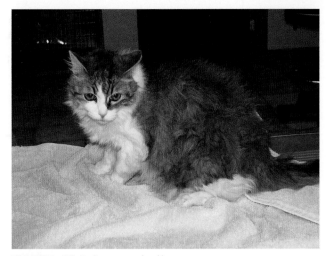

FIGURE 19-3 Some pet health insurance companies may cover chronic health conditions such as diabetes or renal failure.

Benefits of Pet Health Insurance

Pets can receive superior care with pet health insurance and can visit any hospital of the client's choice. If a client has an emergency at night, the client can visit the emergency hospital and have peace of mind that the expenses will be covered. If clients are traveling and need to see a veterinarian in another state, the insurance will still cover the cost of the veterinary service.

> *PRACTICE POINT* Clients with pet health insurance are more likely to follow recommended treatment plans than those who do not carry insurance policies.

Most pet insurance companies have streamlined the claims process, making it simple and hassle free. Clients simply fill out the pet and client information, and practices fill out the form indicating the diagnosis. The veterinarian signs the claim form and either the practice or client submits it to the company by fax, email, or mail. Clients receive reimbursement within a short period. Veterinarians can practice the medicine they want; clients can choose the best options available to them. The insurance companies do not make decisions for the doctor or client; medical decisions are made between the practice and client.

Filing a Claim

Depending on the specific insurance company, clients may be responsible for the full amount (paying the veterinary clinic at the time of service, and are then reimbursed immediately by insurances), or may be responsible for their portion (and the insurance company reimburses the practice immediately). Policyholders will receive several claims forms with their packet, or they can print forms from the insurance company's Web site (Figure 19-4). Clients simply fill out their information, policy number, and pet's information and sign the form. It is imperative that the team

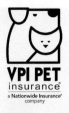

VPI®PET INSURANCE CLAIM FORM

Fill out one claim form per pet. Submit itemized, legible invoices. Incomplete claim submissions may delay claim processing.

VPI PET insurance® a Nationwide Insurance® company

No. of pages: _____

1 POLICYHOLDER INFORMATION

POLICY NUMBER:

PET NAME:

NAME:

ADDRESS:

CITY:

STATE: **ZIP:**

PHONE (H):   **PHONE (W):**

EMAIL:

NEW CONTACT INFORMATION? Write your new information here: _____

2 CLAIM DETAILS

REASON FOR VISIT (CHECK ALL THAT APPLY):

☐ **WELLNESS SERVICES**

☐ **INJURY OR ILLNESS** Write the diagnosis in the box below.

WHAT INJURY OR ILLNESS DID YOUR VETERINARIAN DIAGNOSE?

TREATMENT DATE(S):

FROM: /   /

TO: /   /

HOSPITAL/CLINIC NAME:

A diagnosis is the medical condition treated. Please do not list symptoms. For example, if your pet broke a bone, a symptom might be "limping," but the diagnosis would be "broken bone." Your veterinarian can help you with the diagnosis. Include a copy of your pet's treatment records and lab results for this visit if there is more than one condition being treated, your pet stayed at the hospital overnight or the diagnosis has not been determined. Please do not write "See Attached" or list the services shown on your invoice.

3 INVOICE(S) TOTAL

$

You must submit <u>itemized invoices</u> with your claim form.
Do not send estimates.

4 POLICYHOLDER SIGNATURE and DATE

X   /   /

By signing this claim form, I confirm that to the best of my knowledge the information I have provided is true and correct. I authorize my veterinarian to release medical records and give consent to Veterinary Pet Insurance Company in California and DVM Insurance Agency in all other states to communicate with my veterinarian or veterinarian's staff.

5 SUBMIT CLAIM FORM and INVOICE(S)

Please submit your claim by one method only.
Duplicate claim submissions will delay claim processing.

FAX   **(714) 989-5600** *No cover sheet necessary.*

-------------- **OR** --------------

MAIL   **VPI Claims Department**
PO Box 2344
Brea, CA 92822-2344

VPI CLAIMS DEPARTMENT NOTES ONLY

CF-1 (05-12)   ©2012 Veterinary Pet Insurance Company   12RET1882

FIGURE 19-4 Example of VPI's pet health insurance claim form. (Copyright Veterinary Pet Insurance Company.)

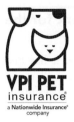

FAX ONLY THE FRONT PAGE OF THIS CLAIM FORM

DO NOT PAPERCLIP OR STAPLE ANYTHING THAT MAY COVER PART OF YOUR CLAIM FORM OR INVOICE

The VPI Policyholder Portal gives you 24/7 access to your policy. Log on at my.petinsurance.com.

Check Your Claim Status Online

Log on to the VPI Policyholder Portal at my.petinsurance.com and click on "View Claims History." The status of faxed or mailed claims will be available 72 hours after they are received.

Policyholder User Guide (PUG)

Find answers to common claims questions in the Policyholder User Guide (PUG for short). Each video addresses common claim-related policyholder questions, including:

- Where can I get claim forms?

- How do I file a claim?

- How do I avoid delays when filing a claim?

- What are medical records and what do they look like?

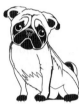

Log on to your VPI Policyholder Portal account at my.petinsurance.com or visit PUG directly at www.petinsurance.com/PUG.

Need Help?

Contact a Customer Care representative toll free at 800-540-2016, Mon-Fri from 5:00 a.m. to 7:00 p.m. or Sat from 7:00 a.m. to 3:30 p.m. (Pacific Time).

Fraud Warning: Any person who knowingly and with intent to defraud any insurance company or other person files an application for insurance or statement of claim containing any materially false information or conceals for the purpose of misleading, information concerning any fact material thereto commits a fraudulent insurance act, which is a crime and subjects such person to criminal and civil penalties. Not applicable in Nebraska, Oregon and Vermont.

FIGURE 19-4, cont'd

member helping the client with the claim form be knowledgeable about the pet's diagnosis. Incorrect wording and incomplete forms are the most common reason for claim payment delay. Some carriers offer a comprehensive list of diagnoses for team members to use when filling out forms. If a diagnosis has not been determined, some companies allow team members to include symptoms on the claim form; forms should be read for correct wording. If multiple diagnoses are made, then all diagnoses should be listed. For example, a dental prophylaxis may also find an abscessed tooth and periodontal disease; these must be written on the claim form so that the client is reimbursed for all three diseases, not just the dental procedure. Attaching a copy of the invoice and medical record will help insurance companies review the case more efficiently and will likely result in higher benefits payout. If a claim is denied, a request for review should be submitted as soon as possible. The request should provide additional information or clarification of a claim.

Discount Clubs

Discount clubs are member-driven organizations. Pet owners pay for a membership that allows access to a member veterinary practice. The practice agrees to provide discounted veterinary services and/or products to members. This may increase the awareness for veterinary services but decreases practice profitability because service relies mainly on discounts. Members are only allowed to visit a member veterinary practice, thereby limiting the discount to one hospital in a given area. These organizations may also offer discount plans. Clients should be warned against discount plans because these companies are not actual insurance companies; instead, pet owners pay a fee to receive a discounted service from participating veterinarians. These companies are not regulated as strictly as insurance companies are and can, at times, be fraudulent. Caution should be taken when dealing with companies of this sort. It should also be warned that veterinary clinics do not receive any benefit from these membership clubs, except a promise that it will bring more clients into the practice. Basically, the veterinarian is giving away services in exchange for the hope of receiving new clients.

Managed Care

Managed care allows veterinarians to join a network that may set fees for veterinarians. Veterinarians are then reimbursed in exchange for seeing patients that are part of the network. If patients go out of the network, they are penalized by fees. Managed veterinary care is similar to managed health care programs in human medicine, such as PPO and HMO organizations, and medical decisions tend to be made by the company instead of the veterinarian. Managed health care will probably never penetrate the pet health insurance industry because the market is too small.

Making Pet Health Insurance Work for the Practice

All parties benefit with pet health insurance. It has been demonstrated in the previous topics that pets will receive optimal, lifelong care, and veterinarians can practice cutting-edge medicine.

PRACTICE POINT   Improve client compliance rates and practice profits by recommending health insurance to every client.

To successfully implement insurance into a practice, place one person in charge of the program, and then choose a limited number (one or two) of insurance companies to recommend (this does not imply that the hospital will not accept other providers, it just simplifies the training for the team, and everyone understands the ins and outs of the company).

The training coordinator can then implement training programs for the staff, and also serves as a contact person for the pet insurance company. Every team member, including veterinarians, has to understand how insurance works, and how to educate clients about the benefit of it.

The training coordinator may place educational posters throughout the practice, brochures at the receptionist desk, and brochures in puppy and kitten kits. When clients call for appointments, team members may ask if they have pet health insurance. Although the majority will respond "no," the point is for the client to become familiar with the phrase "pet health insurance." Once clients become comfortable with the phrase, they may have interest in it and be ready to purchase a policy for their pets. They will look to the team for advice and recommendations, and because the team is well educated on the benefits of pet health insurance, any team member can make a helpful recommendation. Pet health insurance recommendations must also be placed on the practice's Web site.

Once policies are in use in the practice, a team member can fill out the diagnosis and simply have the veterinarian sign the claim form. The team member may want to copy the medical record for claim purposes to ensure that the client receives the largest benefit possible. The team member may want to continue to provide "wow" service to the client and place the claim form in the mail for the client. Clients appreciate this level of service.

In the future, claim forms may be available through computer software. Once team members click on a claim form, the client and patient information will be automatically populated onto the form. If the practice uses computerized medical records, the medical record will also be automatically uploaded with the form and sent electronically to the pet health insurance company. This will allow rapid claim processing, reimbursement of the client within a short time and, ultimately, an increase in client satisfaction.

Recommendations to Clients

In a study completed by Brakke Consulting in January 2008, 41% of owners surveyed said they would purchase insurance if it were recommended by their veterinary practice. A majority of the responders were younger, well educated, and more affluent urban/suburban pet owners. Veterinary practices may target owners of this class with materials for pet health insurance and explain the benefits associated with policies.

> **PRACTICE POINT**   A survey of owners revealed that 41% would purchase insurance if it was recommended by their veterinary practice.

Having brochures for recommended insurance companies at the counter for clients to see is an easy introduction to pet health insurance. Clients can ask questions about the insurance available, and team members can give them an estimate of how much they would receive if their pet was covered with insurance. Placing brochures in puppy and kitten kits as well as placing posters throughout the clinic in high traffic areas will also increase the awareness of insurance. Team members should remember the most important tip when discussing pet insurance: pet health insurance helps pay for unexpected accidents and/or illnesses. It is best for clients to enroll pets when they are young, before the manifestation of disease or illness. Once the pet ages and diagnoses are made, coverage may be limited.

Remember that 15% to 20% of the practice's active clientele account for 75% to 80% of the practice revenue. If clients with pet health insurance spend twice that of the uninsured, the practice volume, production, revenue, and quality of medicine will dramatically increase. More active clients will spend more money and opt for specialized services.

Offering Pet Health Insurance as a Benefit

Many companies offer pet health insurance as a benefit; veterinary clinics already discount services to team members. If pet health insurance is offered, the hospital receives full benefit. In addition, the team members understand in depth how insurance works, therefore making them an invaluable asset in client education. Many pet health insurance companies offer a discount to veterinary practices who wish to offer insurance as a benefit.

Wellness Plans

For many years, the veterinary industry relied on required vaccination protocols to bring clients into the hospital on a yearly basis. Unfortunately, as those vaccines were administered, the importance of preventive care was not relayed. The result was the decreased value of preventive care for pets. Now that vaccines in most areas are on a 3-year protocol, patient visits are declining, and pets are not receiving the preventive care they need to live long, healthy lives.

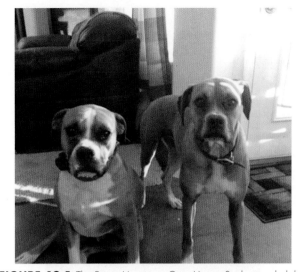

FIGURE 19-5 The Bayer Veterinary Care Usage Study revealed that 56% of cat owners and 59% of dog owners would take their pet to the veterinarian more often if they knew it would prevent problems and expensive treatments later.

The Bayer Veterinary Care Usage Study (BVCUS) of 2011 indicated that visits are decreasing for a number of reasons, including the fact that clients do not perceive the value of preventive care. In addition, the BVCUS indicated that 56% of cat owners and 59% of dog owners would take their pet to the veterinarian more often if they knew it would prevent problems and expensive treatments later (Figure 19-5). Further, 44% of cat owners and 46% of dog owners indicated that patient visits would increase if the veterinary office offered a wellness plan, in which they were billed monthly.

> **PRACTICE POINT**   The BVCUS revealed that 44% of cat owners and 46% of dog owners indicated patient visits would increase if the veterinary office could offer wellness plans, in which they were billed monthly.

Throughout the various chapters in this book, identifying and meeting the needs of customers has been discussed, and this is yet another method available to meet the client needs.

Wellness plans are defined exactly as stated: they incorporate all preventive recommendations that a patient would need for a 1-year period, then divide the cost into equal monthly installments.

Components of a Wellness Plan

A majority of patients that are seen in practice are dogs and cats, and at each visit, specific recommendations are made for those patients, based on their species and age group. Vaccine protocols may include assessment of their individual environmental exposure, but for the most part, recommendations are fairly consistent. With that in mind, wellness plans can be developed for each species and age group (Figure 19-6). A practice may consider groups for puppies, kittens, adult dogs, adult cats, senior dogs, and senior cats. Each age and species (in general) has different recommendations; in addition, as pets age, the cost of their care increases (Box 19-3).

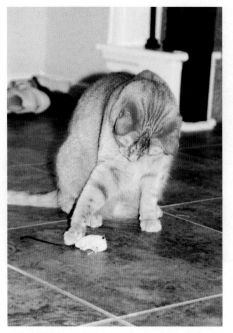

FIGURE 19-6 Wellness Plans must be developed for different species and age groups, because recommendations for each are slightly different.

BOX 19-3	Suggested Health Plans

- Puppy health plan
- Canine adult health plan
- Canine senior health plan
- Kitten health plan
- Feline adult health plan
- Feline senior health plan
  All of these can be further divided into basic, premium, and supreme plans to meet the financial needs of clients.

When creating wellness plans, the standards of care must be met; however, many clients have varying degrees of financial stability. Some clients may be able to afford the best of the best and can accept every recommendation made, whereas others want to provide the best, but can only afford a lesser amount. Once again, this is another area where a practice can identify and meet client needs, and create various levels of plans, allowing clients to accept what they can afford. Practices may consider a basic, premium, and supreme plan (with the basic plan offering the bare bones, and the supreme plan offering every service that is recommended, helping pets live longer, healthier lives).

Keep in mind, wellness plans are exactly that: they are used to promote the preventive care needed to maintain health. It is not used when the patient is sick. Plans should be kept simple, easy to explain for the staff, and easy to understand for the clients.

Pricing

A main reason for developing wellness plans is to help clients budget their money to afford the services that a practice recommends. However, some clients may look for additional incentive; if they choose to sign up for a plan, is there a discount involved?

> **PRACTICE POINT** Administrative costs cannot be forgotten when developing a pricing plan for wellness plans; development and management of such plans is time consuming.

Before any discounts can be considered, practices must determine what their costs are when developing a program. Practices may wish to enlist a third party to manage their wellness plans, or they may choose to develop and manage their own. Either way, an enrollment fee must be determined, because administration costs do accumulate with these plans.

Administration costs to consider in addition to plan development include how the plan will be implemented with the practice management software, how money will be collected from clients, how the team will be trained on the plans, how the plans will be promoted to clients, how doctors will be compensated, and how the program will be monitored for success (the following sections provide more detail on each of the mentioned topics).

In addition to administration costs, the absolute minimum of charges must be determined. In other words, if a practice wanted to offer a wellness plan at a deeply discounted price, what is the absolute minimum that could be charged while still producing a profit (use equations in Chapter 15 and Chapter 20 to help determine real costs associated with products and services). Compare this dollar amount to a standard invoice with current charges.

Plan Development – Factors associated with plan development include those mentioned previously and those that follow, and they must include an estimate of time for each factor. Practices must determine which services will be provided for each species, age group, and plan (basic, premium, or supreme) (Box 19-4).

Software Integration – Practices must consider how wellness plans will integrate with the current software. If using a third party company, contact them for specifics of software integration. Practices not using a third party system may create a code for each wellness plan developed, and an alert can be set in the client's account indicating they have purchased a wellness plan for the year.

Client Collection – Practices must consider how they will collect money on behalf of the client. Automatic debit or credit card charging is a must, as clients may not reliably make payments. A third party company can be used to manage the entire program or simply just to collect payments. The benefit of a third party collecting payments is that credit card numbers do not have to be kept on file in the practice, violating the red flags rule. In addition, if a credit or debit card has been canceled, they will work to collect the funds instead of hospital personnel. Money is then deposited into the practice account once monthly. If an account is uncollectible, the third party will notify the practice. Managers must then determine how they will manage accounts that have become uncollectible.

BOX 19-4 Examples of Potential Plans

Kitten Basic Plan
- Physical exam (2)
- All core vaccines
- Intestinal parasite exam
- Deworming
- Nail trim
- Nutritional counseling and BCS

Kitten Premium Plan
- Physical exam (4)
- All core vaccines
- FeLV/FIV/HWT
- Intestinal parasite exam
- Deworming
- Nail trim
- Flea/tick/HW prevention
- Nutritional counseling and BCS

Kitten Supreme Plan
- Physical exam (unlimited)
- All core vaccines
- FeLV/FIV/HWT
- Intestinal parasite exam
- Deworming
- Flea/tick/HW prevention
- CBC/comprehensive chemistry profile
- Nail trim
- Nutritional counseling and BCS

Feline Adult Basic Plan
- Physical exam (2)
- All core vaccines
- Intestinal parasite exam
- Deworming
- Nail trim
- Nutritional counseling and BCS

Feline Adult Premium Plan
- Physical exam (4)
- All core vaccines
- FeLV/FIV/HWT
- Intestinal parasite exam
- Deworming
- Nail trim
- Flea/tick/HW prevention
- Nutritional counseling and BCS
- Urinalysis
- Dental grade 1

Feline Adult Supreme Plan
- Physical exam (unlimited)
- All core vaccines
- FeLV/FIV/HWT
- Intestinal parasite exam
- Deworming
- Flea/tick/HW prevention
- Nail trim
- Nutritional counseling and BCS
- CBC/comprehensive chemistry profile
- Urinalysis
- Dental grade 2
- Thyroid screen
- Blood pressure

Feline Senior Basic Plan
- Physical exam (2)
- All core vaccines
- Intestinal parasite exam
- Deworming
- Nail trim
- Nutritional counseling and BCS
- Urinalysis
- Blood pressure
- Dental grade 1

Feline Senior Premium Plan
- Physical exam (4)
- All core vaccines
- FeLV/FIV/HWT
- Intestinal parasite exam
- Deworming
- Nail trim
- Flea/tick/HW prevention
- Nutritional counseling and BCS
- Urinalysis
- Blood pressure
- Thyroid screen
- Dental grade 2

Feline Senior Supreme Plan
- Physical exam (unlimited)
- All core vaccines
- FeLV/FIV/HWT
- Intestinal parasite exam
- Deworming
- Flea/tick/HW prevention
- Nail trim
- Nutritional counseling and BCS
- CBC/comprehensive chemistry profile
- Urinalysis
- Thyroid screen
- Blood pressure
- Radiographs
- Dental grade 2

BCS, Body condition score; *CBC*, complete blood count; *FeLV*, feline leukemia virus; *FIV*, feline immunodeficiency virus; *HW*, heartworm; *HWT*, heartworm test.

Educating Team Members – Team members must understand the benefit of such programs, before client education can begin. Wellness plans promote the best possible care for all patients, all year long. Wellness plans drive compliance, build relationships, and encourage clients to purchase all services and products at the hospital, not at competitive locations. One thing is certain: clients that can provide the best care for their pets directly decreases the compassion fatigue experienced by team members.

Educating Clients – Clients will learn of the program through team members, the Web site, and social media. Materials should be printed explaining the program, including the benefits of purchasing the program, including a lower cost of veterinary care.

Doctor Compensation – Determining how doctors are compensated with such programs can be a challenge, especially when they are paid on a production basis. This is an area that can increase the plan development and management costs, and becomes very time-consuming during payroll periods. When managed by a third party system, reports can be generated, reducing the amount of in-house hours used to determine compensation.

Managing and Improving – Once programs have been implemented, they must be monitored, always looking for methods of improvement. What is the compliance rate? Which team member has the best acceptance rate? What does she do that can help other team members improve? Can marketing techniques be changed or improved? Every profit center (this has to be looked at as a profit center) must be managed and scrutinized regularly, ensuring the money it is producing is covering the costs associated with developing, implementing, and managing it.

VETERINARY PRACTICE and the LAW

Because veterinary practices do not file insurance claims, they are rarely implicated in insurance fraud schemes. However, some clients will certainly try to defraud the system. Some clients will purchase an insurance policy and declare that there are no preexisting conditions; once the policy has been accepted, they will immediately file a claim for a preexisting lameness or abnormal blood work. Once this occurs, many insurance companies will call the practice and ask for a copy of the medical records. The medical records from practices indicate the true dates of the examinations and claim information, allowing insurance companies to identify fraudulent cases.

REVIEW QUESTIONS

1. Define an annual deductible.
2. What is a co-pay?
3. What is an annual premium?
4. What are the three most common canine conditions?
5. What are the three most common feline conditions?
6. What is the benefit of an annual deductible versus a per-incident deductible?
7. What is considered a hereditary condition?
8. What is considered a congenital condition?
9. What is a lifetime limit?
10. Why should wellness plans be available for clients?
11. Pet health insurance:
    a. Improves patient care
    b. Increases patient examinations
    c. Decreases stop treatment threshold
    d. A and B
12. Indemnity insurance is also known as:
    a. Managed care
    b. HMO delivered
    c. PPO delivered
    d. None of the above
13. An amount an owner pays on a monthly basis is known as a:
    a. Premium
    b. Deductible
    c. Co-pay
    d. All of the above
14. Wellness plans should be developed by:
    a. Species
    b. Age group
    c. Client preferences
    d. A and B
15. The purpose of Wellness Plans is to:
    a. Promote preventive care
    b. Promote all-inclusive care
    c. Promote pet health insurance
    d. None of the above

Recommended Reading

Ackerman LJ: *Blackwell's five-minute veterinary practice management consult*, Ames, IA, 2007, Blackwell Publishing.

Kenney D: *The complete guide to understanding pet health insurance*, 2008, Doug Kenney.

Volk J, Merle C: *A veterinarians guide to pet health insurance, National Commission of Veterinary Economic Issues*, January 2009.

References

Bayer Veterinary Usage Study, 2011; Bayer Healthcare, LLC Animal Health Division, http://www.ncvei.org/articles/FINAL_BAYER_VETERINARY_CARE_USAGE_STUDY.pdf; Accessed 8/11/13.

Wolf CA, Lloyd KW, Black JR: An examination of US Consumer pet-related and veterinary service expenditures, 1980-2006, *J Am Vet Med Assoc* 233:404–413, 2008.

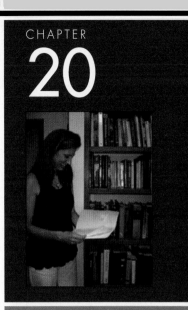

Finance Management

OUTLINE

Accounting and Bookkeeping, *330*
  Certified Public Accountant, *331*
Accounting Basics, *331*
  Cash-Basis and Accrual-Basis
    Accounting, *331*
  Key Performance Indicators, *332*
Benchmarking, *337*
Creating Financial Reports, *337*
  Balance Sheet, *338*
Profit and Loss Statements, *338*
  Chart of Accounts, *338*
  Income, *338*
  Expenses, *338*
  Net Income, *340*
  Producing Monthly Profit and Loss
    Statements, *340*
Troubleshooting Profit and Loss
  Statements, *340*
  Using KPIs to Help Analyze Data, *342*
  Comparing Income and Expense
    Centers, *342*
Maximizing Revenue, *343*

Fee Schedule, *343*
Missing Charges, *344*
Discounts, *344*
Standard of Care, *345*
Income Center Development and
  Management, *345*
Managing Client Visits, *346*
Customer Service, *346*
Key Performance Indicators, *346*
Reducing Expenses, *346*
Fraud and Embezzlement, *347*
  Decrease Practice Risk of Fraud
    or Embezzlement, *348*
Creating a Budget, *348*
  Steps of a Budget, *349*
  Areas of Expense, *352*
  Important Points to Remember, *354*
Cash Flow, *354*
Open-Book Management, *355*
Building Value in the Practice, *355*
Planning Retirement, *356*
Red Flags Rule, *356*

KEY TERMS

Accounts Payable
Accounts Receivable
Accrual Basis Accounting
Assets
Average Client
  Transaction
Balance Sheet
Benchmarking
Bookkeeper
Break-Even Analysis
Budget
Capital Inventory
Cash Basis Accounting
Cash Flow Statement
Certified Public Accountant
COGs
Compliance Rate
Direct Expense
Fixed Cost
General Administrative
  Expenses
Gross Income
Gross Profit
Income Statement
Indirect Expense
Intangible Property
Key Performance Indicators
Liabilities
Net Income
Net Profit
Owner Equity
Principle Cost
Profit and Loss Statement
Return on Investment
Revenue Centers
Tangible Property
Transaction
Variable Cost

LEARNING OBJECTIVES

When you have completed this chapter, you should be able to:

1. Identify the differences between book-keepers, accountants, public accountants, and certified public accountants.
2. Define the basics of accounting.
3. Correlate effective key performance indicators.
4. Develop a budget.
5. Develop a payroll budget.
6. Develop an equipment budget.
7. Describe methods used to purchase equipment.
8. Identify profits and profit centers.
9. Identify effective goals with the teams

CRITICAL COMPETENCIES

1. **Adaptability** - being open to change and flexible work methods; the ability to adapt behavior to changing conditions or new information.
2. **Analytical Skills** - the ability to analyze information and use logic to address problems; the ability to quickly and accurately grasp complex information and concepts and to make correct inferences.
3. **Compliance** - being reliable, thorough, and conscientious in carrying out work assignments; has an appreciation for the importance of organizational rules and policies.
4. **Continuous Learning** - a curiosity for learning; actively seeks out new information, technologies, and methods; keep skills updated and apply new knowledge to the job.

5. **Creativity** - the ability to think creatively about situations, to see things in new and different ways; use imagination and creativity to develop innovative solutions to problems.

6. **Critical and Strategic Thinking** - the ability to think critically about situations and to understand the relevance of information for different problems; use critical reasoning to generate and evaluate alternative courses of action or points of view relevant to an issue.

7. **Decision Making** - the ability to make good decisions, solve problems, and decide on important matters; the ability to gather and analyze relevant data and choose decisively between alternatives.

8. **Integrity** - honesty, trustworthiness, and adherence to high standards of ethical conduct.

9. **Leadership** - a willingness to lead and take charge; the ability to motivate others and mobilize group effort toward common goals.

10. **Oral Communication and Comprehension** - the ability to express one's thoughts verbally in a clear and understandable manner, and the ability to actively listen and attend to what others are saying; must have good group presentation skills.

11. **Persuasion** - the ability to change the attitudes and opinions of others and to persuade them to accept recommendations and change behavior.

12. **Planning and Prioritizing** - the ability to effectively manage time and work load to meet deadlines; the ability to organize work, set priorities, and establish plans for achieving goals.

13. **Relationship Building** - the ability to develop constructive and cooperative working relationships with others and maintain them over time; must also be able to settle disputes, resolve grievances and conflicts, and negotiate with others.

14. **Resilience** - the ability to cope effectively with pressure and setbacks; the ability to handle crisis situations effectively and remain undeterred by obstacles or failure.

15. **Resourcefulness** - the ability to understand what it takes to complete the job; apply knowledge, skills, and expertise to perform tasks quickly and efficiently.

16. **Writing and Verbal Skills** - ability to comprehend written material easily and accurately; ability to express thoughts clearly and succinctly in writing.

In the financial management domain, the veterinary practice manager analyzes financial reports for the practice, maintains practice financial accounts, oversees banking procedures, establishes client credit policies, conducts fee analyses, and manages the practice's payroll. In consultation with practice owner, the manager also monitors financial trends and projections and prepares budgets.

Knowledge Requirements

This domain requires knowledge of basic principles of financial accounting and forecasting. The manager must understand components of a balance sheet, profit/loss accounts, and financial ratios. Knowledge of current taxation law is also needed.

The lack of financial management can be detrimental to a practice. Unfortunately, many owners lack the confidence and knowledge to manage finances efficiently.

The recession hurt many practices. In fact, many that lacked appropriate plans or had poor management structure shut their doors. Those lucky to remain open squeaked by, learning a valuable lesson: without planning, this business could fail.

The basics of business/financial management must be covered first, enabling a budget to be developed. Budgeting allows planning to occur, with the goal of having a profit at the end of the year. At least 10% of the profit must be reinvested back into the practice, either in equipment, continuing education for the team, building maintenance and improvements, or staff compensation.

Accounting and Bookkeeping

Accounting and bookkeeping are closely related activities. The accounting process depends on the information produced by bookkeepers. A bookkeeper may be responsible for accounts payable, accounts receivable, and payroll. One

---

BOX 20-1 | Accounting Terms

Accrual basis method: A system that recognizes income as it is earned and expenses as they are incurred rather than when the actual cash transaction occurs.

Asset: Any property owned by a business or individual. Cash, accounts receivable, inventory, land, buildings, leasehold improvements, and tangible property are examples of assets.

Balance sheet: A financial report detailing practice assets, liabilities, and owner's equity.

Budget: An estimate of revenues and expenses for a given period.

Cash basis method: A system that recognizes income as it is received and expenses as they are paid, rather than when the income was earned or the expense was acquired.

Cash flow statement: Report on the sources and uses of cash during a given period of time.

Equity: The rights or claims to properties; Assets = Equities + Liabilities.

Fixed cost: A cost that does not change with the variation in business. Rent, mortgage, and utility costs remain the same regardless of how busy the practice is.

Income statement: Report on financial performance that covers a period of time and reports incomes and expenses during

that period. Income statements are also known as *profit and loss statements*.

Intangible property: Nonphysical property that has value; franchises, copyrights, client lists, goodwill, and noncompete agreements are examples of intangible property.

Key performance indicators: Statistics that can be generated from client transaction data and reviewed for performance data.

Liabilities: Obligations resulting from past transactions that require the practice to pay money or provide service. Accounts payable and taxes are examples of current liabilities.

Owner's equity: Owner's interest or claim in the practice assets.

Principal cost: Initial cost of equipment when purchased.

Profit and loss statement: Summary of the practice's income, expenses, and resulting profit or loss for a specified period of time (also known as the *income statement*).

Tangible property: Physical property, such as desks, chairs, equipment, computers, software, and vehicles that has value.

Transaction: A purchase that must be recorded.

Variable cost: Any cost that varies with the volume of business for the practice. The costs of medical supplies and drugs increase or decrease depending on the volume of business.

---

or more team members may actually share the duties of a bookkeeper yet never be defined as one. Bookkeepers may be employed by an accounting firm to aid in the practice's tax preparation, payroll, or benefit plans. An accountant is a professional that specializes in producing and interpreting financial statements, tax planning, cash flow projections, and estate planning. The use of an accounting firm may depend on the size of the practice and the experience of the managers. Some practices may use an accountant only once a year to help prepare year-end statements and tax documents; others may use an accountant on a monthly basis.

Certified Public Accountant

A certified public accountant (CPA) should be the first choice of a practice when looking to hire a professional accountant. CPAs have extensive experience and have passed a comprehensive exam that tests their knowledge of accounting and tax principles, auditing standards, and business law. They must attend yearly classes to maintain continuing education requirements and comply with a strict code of ethics. Bookkeepers may give themselves the self-designation as accountants, although they may not have attended college. Public accountants (PAs) may have attended college and completed a degree in accounting but have not taken the CPA exam. CPAs are held to the highest standard; a CPA should be a practice's chosen accountant.

A CPA's responsibility it to produce reports for the practice; however, unless the CPA is involved in the veterinary industry, he or she cannot determine how or where the business can make improvements. If a practice has the opportunity to contract with a veterinary industry CPA, it

is advised to do so. Investing in a professional that understands the veterinary profession will help determine areas of improvement and make recommendations that apply to the practice.

Accounting Basics

To help understand financial management, a few accounting terms must first be reviewed. This will help in the creation and understanding of profit and loss statements, balance sheets, and budgeting. Review Box 20-1 to gain an understanding of accounting terminology.

Cash-Basis and Accrual-Basis Accounting

Income and expenses can be recorded by two different methods: cash or accrual. Which method a practice chooses is usually dictated by the need for federal or state income tax reporting. If income is measured when cash is received and expenses are measured when cash is spent, then a practice uses cash-basis accounting. In practice, only fees paid by clients are recognized in cash-basis accounting; therefore accounts receivable are not included. Those fees have yet to be paid by clients. Accounts payable transactions are only recorded when they have been paid, not when they occurred.

> **PRACTICE POINT** A cash-basis reporting system records when cash is received, and when expenses are paid. An accrual-basis system reports when the income and expense occurred.

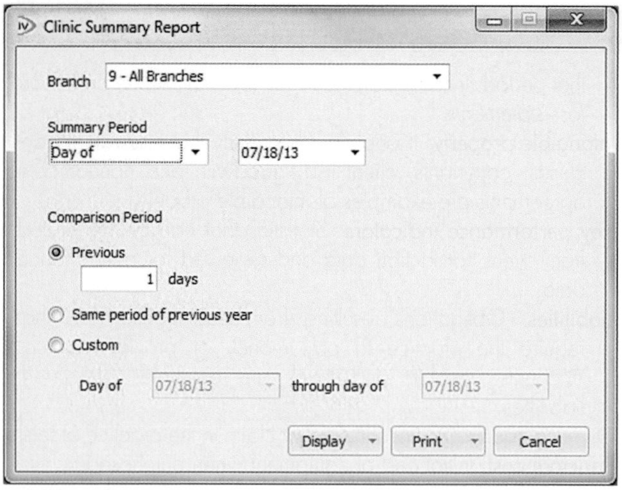

FIGURE 20-1 Sample clinic summary report (screen shot and report). IntraVet. (Courtesy IntraVet, Dublin, Ohio.)

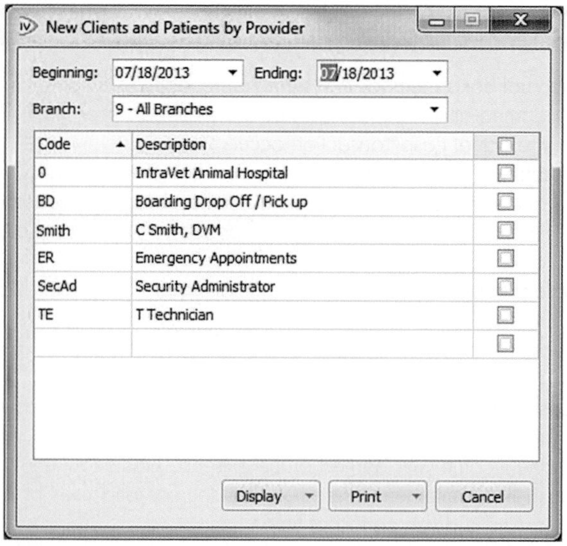

FIGURE 20-2 Sample new clients and patients report (screen shot and report). (Courtesy IntraVet, Dublin, Ohio.)

If a practice is recording income and expenses as they occur, then the practice uses an accrual-basis accounting system. Practices that use an accrual basis record fees as they are earned, therefore including accounts receivable. Accounts payable are recorded at the time of accrual, not at the time of payment.

Historically, practices have used a cash-basis method because it is easier to maintain and understand. When comparing the methods (cash and accrual basis), the reports will give two different pictures of the financial status of the hospital. Comparison of cash reports can provide varied results from month to month, especially when a practice has a large accounts receivable balance.

In 1998, the Internal Revenue Service (IRS) deemed many practices ineligible to use cash-basis accounting for taxation purposes because of the mixed sales of products and services. Therefore many practices have switched accounting methods. Consultation with the practice CPA is essential for determining which method a practice should use to prevent any wrongdoing in the eyes of the IRS.

Key Performance Indicators

A variety of basic information is needed when compiling reports for a veterinary hospital. These statistics are also known as *key performance indicators (KPIs)*, and should be used to monitor the practice on a monthly, quarterly, and yearly basis. KPIs can help explain changes in financial statements, and all contribute to the success of the hospital. Practices should take time to determine which KPIs are important to their particular hospital, and develop a spreadsheet to monitor for changes from month to month. If KPIs are monitored monthly, negative trends can be managed more effectively (Figures 20-1 and 20-2). The following are some examples of KPIs a practice may wish to follow:

- Accounts receivable summary
- Annual revenue per patient
- Average client transaction
- Average doctor transaction
- Cost of goods expenses, as a percent of gross income

BOX 20-2	Key Performance Indicators Adapted from Benchmarks 2013: A Study of Well-Managed Practices

KEY PERFORMANCE INDICATORS

# Active clients/FTE DVM/year	1990
# Active patients/FTE DVM/year	1445
# New patients/FTE DVM/year	381
Total # new clients/FTE DVM/year	221
Average DVM ADT	$173.00
Medical/product revenue/FTE DVM/year	$558,618
Medical transactions/FTE DVM/year	3082
All transactions/FTE DVM/year	5405

ADT, Average doctor transaction; *FTE DVM,* full-time equivalent veterinarian (based on 40 hours per week).

- Discounts per veterinarian
- DVM expenses, as a percent of gross income
- Income centers, as a percentage of gross income
- Number of active/new clients and patients
- Revenue and percent difference from previous period or year
- Staff expenses, as a percentage of gross income

Many benchmarks are available to use as comparisons when looking at KPIs (Box 20-2). However, KPIs can differ based on demographics, geographical location, urban versus rural setting, practice size and type, and hours of operation. External benchmarks (benchmarks made available by organizations) are great to help understand what is going on in the industry; internal benchmarks (benchmarks produced from in-house historical reports) are used to monitor trends within the practice. See the benchmarking section later in this chapter for more details.

Accounts Receivable Summary

Accounts receivable (AR) must be monitored on a monthly basis. A large AR can be detrimental to the practice. AR

```
┌─────────────────────────────────────────────────────────────────────────┐
│                        Accounts Receivable Report                         │
│                                                                           │
│      ABC Veterinary Hospital                          Accounts Receivable │
│                                                                           │
│      Total 30 days past due:      $1896.51                                │
│      Total 60 days past due:      $1455.07                                │
│      Total 90 days past due:      $3661.32                                │
│                                                                           │
│      Total past due:              $7012.90                                │
│      Total current balance:       $4652.79                                │
│      Total net receivables:       $11,665.69                              │
│                                                                           │
│      Total billing fees:            $78.00                                │
│      Total interest charges:       $125.49                                │
│      Total number of statements printed:  52                              │
│                                                                           │
│      Balance forward on transactions ON and BEFORE:  9/23/13              │
│      Printed statements as of:                      10/23/13              │
│                                                                           │
└─────────────────────────────────────────────────────────────────────────┘
```

FIGURE 20-3 Sample accounts receivable report.

reports should list the amounts due in current, 30-, 60-, and 90-day increments. Clients who owe practices money after 90 days not only are unlikely to pay, but also prevent practices from being able to pay their own accounts and employees. The practice must implement a no-charge policy to prevent AR from growing rapidly and hurting the practice's revenue. *Current AR should never be more than 1.5% of the gross revenue.*

 Veterinary practice managers manage accounts receivable and accounts payable.

Figure 20-3 is an AR report that shows that the largest balance of the accounts receivable is the current amount due, followed by the total of 90 days past due. The current balance must be monitored; if this balance does not decrease within 30 days, strategies must be implemented to prevent past due amounts from rolling over to 60 and 90 days past due. The sum of $3661.32 (90 days past due) is unlikely to be collected, and the AR manager must determine appropriate strategies to collect these funds as soon as possible. Chapter 18 discusses AR in more detail.

Annual Revenue Per Patient

Annual revenue per patient (ARPP) is a new KPI that has been developed, and it analyzes the revenue generated by a patient during an entire year. The benefit of this KPI is to manage client compliance for the entire year instead of focusing on the average client transaction of one visit. Managing ARPP can increase client compliance, and it enhances the potential to provide all services for a patient in-house (preventive medications, ancillary services such as grooming, nail trims, anal gland expressions, and nutrition). Consider services that are not being offered but could increase

the ARPP. Benchmarks are not yet available for ARPP; however, internal benchmarks can be created from internal historical data.

Average Client Transactions

Average client transactions (ACTs) include all transactions a client makes in the hospital: exams, diagnostics, diets, and medication refills. When a client returns for a recheck, diet, or medication refill, it causes the ACT to drop; unless each transaction is monitored, managers may become alerted to a declining ACT. When transactions are investigated, managers can see client follow-up is the cause, and the alert is justified.

Historically, the average client transaction has been a key KPI. It was monitored to ensure that team members were making recommendations, and clients were accepting them. If the average client transaction was consistently low, leaders should have determined why and developed a solution to increase the low figure.

Recently, ACTs have fallen out of favor, because practices have consistently increased ACTs without increasing the value to client. As a result, the veterinary industry has created "sticker shock" and decreased the consumer confidence in veterinary medicine. In addition, ACTs can vary tremendously when compared to external benchmarks, because of practice size, age, demographics, and management philosophies.

Internal benchmarks and ACTs are still important, because practice managers and owners know what is occurring in their hospital. If an ACT is declining, an investigation may be warranted; however, if the ACT is dropping because clients are following up as recommended, the investigation can cease. If the ACT is high and clients are not following up, then again, an investigation may be warranted, looking for opportunities to increase compliance.

Average Doctor Transaction

The average doctor transaction is perhaps a better KPI than an ACT, as it removes all refills, diets, and so on, from the equation. Average doctor transactions only consider charges that occurred during a patient visit.

Cost of Goods Expenses, as a Percent of Gross Revenue

Cost of goods (COGs) should be placed in a percentage and compared to that of gross revenue. Comparing COGs to external benchmarks is a good idea, helping practices determine where they can improve costs. Variable costs will rise and fall with the production of business; therefore percentages are imperative for comparison purposes. It is also important to compare this percentage with internal historical data, because dramatic increases or decreases warrant an investigation (described further in P&L).

Discounts per Veterinarian

This is a very important number to track. Discounting, which is described later in detail, has significant impact on the profits of the hospital. Tracking discounts by DVM can put this number into perspective. It helps manage who is responsible for discounting and what is being given away.

> **PRACTICE POINT** Every team member, not just DVMs, should be held accountable for unplanned discounts given to clients.

DVM Expenses, as a Percent of Gross Income

It is important to know how much a veterinarian is costing the hospital, especially in relation to how much they are producing. On average, a veterinarian should be producing five times (5×) the amount of his or her salary. If the expense is higher than what is being produced, alternative pay strategies may be considered.

Income Centers, as a Percentage of Gross Income

Income center management is imperative. Goals must be created and obtained. Showing these percentages will put these numbers into perspective, and gives the manager the tools to identify which income centers need further development, equipment, or training to increase profits.

Number of Active/New Clients and Patients

The number of active clients and patients in a practice is a benchmark number and allows comparison with other practices in the region. The definition of *active* can vary from practice to practice; therefore it is much more effective to measure from year to year for the same practice. If the number of active clients or patients is low, this may indicate the need for further internal and external marketing techniques. Internal techniques such as reminder systems should be evaluated for effectiveness, and external techniques may be developed. See Chapter 10 for more internal and external marketing tips.

 Veterinary practice managers develop and manage new client programs.

Revenue and Percent Difference from Previous Period or Year

These numbers are produced from the practice management software and allow managers to monitor trends that may be occurring. It is important to be able to further analyze where the revenue is being generated from (income centers) and the difference from previous periods.

Additional Reports to Consider

In addition to the KPIs listed previously, the following reports aid in managing the finances of the practice.

Accounts Payable

Accounts payable should be monitored on a monthly basis to ensure that there is not more spending than receiving. If the practice spends more money than it takes in, the practice will be in serious financial deficit in the upcoming months. Small practices that are relatively new may experience months that produce less than others, and a plan should be implemented in case this occurs. Spending must decrease, practice income must increase, and the practice employees should be held accountable for wastage. The fee structure may be re-evaluated, and practice managers should ensure charges are not being missed. If a line of credit is needed to keep the practice floating during the slow months, then a plan must be implemented to pay back the loan as soon as possible.

Client Surveys

Client surveys are an easy monitoring solution to understand the satisfaction and level of client comfort with the services the practice provides (Figure 20-4). Clients maintain the business; therefore it is imperative to make sure they are satisfied and perceive the value of the service provided. If clients are unsatisfied, practices want to be notified and given the opportunity to address the problem. Hospitals do not want to lose clients or have negative comments made about them throughout the community. It is very important to strive for a high level of satisfaction from every client.

 Veterinary practice managers obtain and report client feedback on services.

> **PRACTICE POINT** Every client should receive a survey after a visit; this allows managers to ensure client satisfaction.

Compliance Rates

Monitoring client compliance rates is useful in many ways. If clients are accepting recommendations, then the staff is doing an excellent job of educating clients and clients

Client Survey

We appreciate your business at ABC Veterinary Clinic and value your suggestions for improvement. Please take a few moments to fill out our survey and return it to the hospital.

Please rate the following questions from 1 (superior) to 5 (unacceptable).

I received an appointment that was convenient for me.	1 2 3 4 5
The hospital was clean when I arrived.	1 2 3 4 5
The receptionist acknowledged me immediately.	1 2 3 4 5
The veterinary technician was friendly.	1 2 3 4 5
The veterinary technician was knowledgeable.	1 2 3 4 5
The veterinarian was friendly.	1 2 3 4 5
The veterinarian was knowledgeable.	1 2 3 4 5
I received materials to take home and review.	1 2 3 4 5
My pet received exceptional care.	1 2 3 4 5
The staff cares about my pet.	1 2 3 4 5
The services are reasonably priced.	1 2 3 4 5

What can we do to improve our services for you? _____

_____

_____

_____

If one of our team members provided exceptional care today, please let us know so that we may recognize that person: _____

_____

_____

_____

FIGURE 20-4 Sample client survey.

perceive the value in the services that are being offered. Second, client compliance drives profits. The client relationship has already been established, and it is essential to maintain that relationship. It is easier (and cheaper) to maintain relationships than to build new ones. Compliance reports should include reminder compliance as well as the profit centers the practice has chosen to monitor (Figure 20-5). Client compliance is discussed in detail in Chapter 11.

Inventory of Equipment

It is very important to keep a list of equipment owned by the practice along with its purchase date and original purchase price. This is excellent for taxation purposes and also aids the practice if the equipment is stolen or damaged by fire or other natural causes. Serial numbers and model numbers may also be added for security, and they act as a quick reference when looking up information for warranty purposes.

Figure 20-6 lists equipment that was purchased before and after the practice manager began a capital inventory list. Anesthesia machine #1 was purchased before the list was developed. However, the model number and serial number are available for reference in case a fire or theft occurs. Anesthesia machine #2 was purchased in December 2003 for $400 as one unit. This is valuable information, along with the name of the manufacturer, in case a machine malfunction occurs and warranty dates come into question. A column could be added for warranty expiration dates, which would also help the practice manager.

Recommendation and Compliance Report			ABC Animal Hospital

For Period 1/1/13 - 12/31/13

Code	Description	# of Recommendations	# of Compliance (%)
R001	Vaccinations	1265	965 (76)
R002	Heartworm Test	1600	1500 (94)
R003	Heartworm Prevention	1600	1000 (63)
R004	Dental Prophylaxis	1456	920 (63)
R005	Pre-Anesthetic Profiles	1500	880 (59)

FIGURE 20-5 Sample compliance report.

Product	Name	Manufacturer	Purchase Date/Price	Model Number	Serial Number
Anal Gland Excision Kit		Jorgenson		J-101	
Anesthesia Machine #1	Anesthesia Machine #1	Matrix		VMS	6380
Anesthesia Vaporizer #1	Anesthesia Vaporizer #1	Cyprane LTD			300437
Anesthesia Machine #2	Anesthesia Machine #2	Matrix	12/24/2010		SN14989
Anesthesia Vaporizer #2	Anesthesia Vaporizer #2	Vet Tech 4	12/24/10, $400 for both	100F	SN BASPOX7
Aspirator	Schuco Vac	Schuco		130	49500008498
Autoclave	Tuttanauer Autoclave	Tuttanauer	04/02/09, $2600	2340M	2110582
Bird Scale		Pelouze		PE5	
Camera	Digital Camera	HP	Aug 2010, $177.52	Photosmart 320	CN318111DG
Cast Cutter		Stryker		9002-210	8H8
Cautery Unit	AA Cautery	Jorgenson		J313	
Centrifuge	MS Centrifuge MicroHCT	Damon/IEC Division		MB	2513
Centrifuge	Sta-o-Spin	Stat-o-Spin	3/14/13, $1026.83 Butler	V0901.22	607V90111962
Centrifuge (lab)	Cinaseal	Vulcon Tech		C56C	6840
Clippers	Speed Feed	DVM	12/15/11, $91		
Clippers Cordless	Oaster	Butler		78400-01A	
Clippers Cordless	Oaster	Butler		78400-01A	
Clippers Cordless	Oaster	Butler		78400-01A	
Credit Card Terminal					
Credit Card Terminal	Care Credit				SN 207-397-407
Copier	Cannon			PC 940	NVX37080
Dental Machine	Ultrasonic Scaler/Motor Pack	Delmarva			C028-647
Doppler, BP	Mini Dop ES 100VX	Hadeco	11/2008, $800		SN-00090054
Doppler Probe		Jorgenson			
Doppler Ultrasound	Grafco Mini Doppler			4070	
Dremel Unit		Craftsman		5 Speed	
ECG PAM	VM8000PAM Cardiac Monitor	Technology Transfer	12/10/08, $2775	VM8000	SN V04408
ECG Printer PAM		Technology Transfer	12/10/2008	930	1029
ECG Biolog		QRS Diagnostic	9/2013 DVM Solutions $2735		2004-054237
ECG Printer Biolog			Came with Biolog	Brother HL-2070	U61230M5J5
Glucometer	One Touch Ultra	Walgreens			RHW4E23Ft
Home Again Scanner		Schering Plough			SN 070535
Hair Dryer					
ECG Surgery	KENZ ECG 103	KENZ	GW Gift		9509-2815
IDEXX Electrolytes	VET LYTE	IDEXX	Aug. 2008		U15.9976
IDEXX Lasercyte	Lasercyte	IDEXX	Jun. 2013	93-30002-01	DXBP005586
IDEXX Vet Test	Vet Test 8000	IDEXX	08/01/08, $2700		OA26949
IDEXX Server				PCNE	H1BFQ91
IDEXX Printer				HP Deskjet 5650	MY45F4NOHI

FIGURE 20-6 Sample capital inventory report.

Inventory on Hand

Current inventory reports should be accessible at any time. Inventory is recorded as an asset and contributes to factors included on financial reports.

Inventory Sold Within a Given Period

Sales of products and services may need to be reported on a monthly basis for sales tax purposes.

Taxes Owed

Taxes must be paid on a monthly and/or quarterly basis, depending on what type of tax is due. Amounts should be calculated at the first of each month, with the scheduled dates of payment. Tax ledgers can be beneficial when paying monthly bills, preventing overspending. Quarterly taxes can be shockingly high and must be budgeted for when paying current accounts payable.

Benchmarking

Benchmarking is the process by which a practice compares its own data to others in the industry: locally, statewide, regionally, or nationally (external benchmarking). Benchmarking can also be taken from the practice's historical financial information (internal benchmarking). Both types of benchmarking must be considered when analyzing and making decisions for the practice. Benchmarking can be beneficial when determining what policies and procedures need to be implemented to take the practice to the next level.

> **PRACTICE POINT** Internal and external benchmarks must be evaluated together, looking for areas of improvement in the hospital.

Areas of desired improvement must be determined before steps can be taken. Common areas to analyze may include customer service, productivity, and profitability. Information should be collected regarding the practice's financial history, current practice data, and benchmark numbers, which are available from American Veterinary Medical Association (AVMA), Veterinary Hospital Managers Association (VHMA), American Animal Hospital Association (AAHA), and Well-Managed Practices (WMPs) (Figure 20-7). Comparison of numbers can be completed, analyzing differences and developing an explanation of why the difference(s) have occurred. National benchmarking numbers may not be in line with current practice figures because of differences in the economic status of the city or state, or it may be simply that the practice is not charging enough for inventory and services. Other factors that may affect differences include the size of the practice, type of practice, services offered, length of time the practice has been in business, and the location of the practice. Team members can then develop a plan to determine which factors they can improve and which changes can be implemented. A target date can then be set by the team in which a follow-up analysis can occur to determine whether the changes have been successful and if goals have been met. Once the issue has been resolved, another area can be targeted. Benchmarking is a continuous process that increases the practice's success while maintaining a high level of commitment and care to the clients and patients. Clients expect premier service, and they deserve to have the best available.

Creating Financial Reports

AAHA has an excellent chart of accounts that is highly recommended when creating financial reports. A chart of accounts is an organized listing of all income, expense, asset, liability, and equity categories used in the business, leading to the ultimate goal of creating a picture of the practice's operations on a daily, monthly, and/or yearly basis. AAHA's chart of accounts is detailed, yet flexible, and designed so that every veterinary practice can implement it.

Adapted from Benchmarks 2013; A Study of Well Managed Practices	
Income	
Exam	14.0%
Professional Services	3.6%
Laboratory	18.8%
Imaging	4.9%
Dentistry	2.5%
Vaccines	6.8%
Hospitalization	2.4%
Surgery	5.5%
Anesthesia	3.7%
Pharmacy	13.7%
Flea, Tick & HW	7.9%
Diets	4.2%
OTC/Retail	1.0%
Boarding	3.0%
Bathing & Grooming	1.2%
Expenses	
Non-DVM Wages	21.6%
Retirement	0.6%
Benefits	2.2%
Continuing Education	0.4%
Worker's Compensation	0.4%
TOTAL STAFF NON-DVM COSTS:	**25.2%**
Drugs & Medical Supplies	9.8%
Imaging	*incl. in above*
Flea/Heartworm/Tick Products	3.9%
Retail / OTC	0.4%
Diets	2.9%
Laboratory	4.0%
TOTAL COST-OF-GOODS:	**21.0%**
Rent	5.4%
Utilities *(Water, Gas, Electricity)*	0.8%
Facility Repair & Maintenance	0.6%
Equipment Repair/Maint./Support Contracts	0.4%
Janitorial; housekeeping; sanitation	0.4%
Property Insurance	0.2%
Real Estate Taxes	0.5%
TOTAL FACILITY COSTS:	**8.3%**
Office Supplies	0.7%
Credit Card processing	1.5%
Bad Debt/Collection fees	0.1%
Sales/Use Tax	0.7%
Postage/Shipping	0.2%
Advertising/Promotion/Marketing	0.8%
Cremation/After-life body care	0.6%
Professional Fees	1.2%
Communications (Phone & Internet)	0.5%
Technical Support Contracts (IT)	0.3%
Liability Insurance	0.2%
Licenses/Permits	0.1%
Entertainment	0.1%
Business/Staff Meetings	0.1%
Charitable Contributions	0.1%
Payroll Services/Benefits Administration	0.2%
Printing/Copies/Duplication	0.2%
Professional Dues/Subscriptions	0.2%
Other/Uncategorized	0.2%
TOTAL ADMINISTRATIVE COSTS:	**8.0%**

FIGURE 20-7 Expense benchmarks from *Benchmarks 2013: A Study of Well-Managed Practices*. (Adapted from *Benchmarks 2013: A Study of Well-Managed Practices*, Wutchiett Tumblin and Associates, Columbus, Ohio.)

PRACTICE POINT Financial reports must be generated and analyzed on a monthly basis.

Creating reports allows the comparison of the practice on a monthly, quarterly, or yearly basis. It also enables comparison with other practices industry-wide. Owners and practice managers can see the impact every decision has made throughout the year. The financial status of the practice must be made clear to help owners and managers make financially sound decisions.

 Veterinary practice managers analyze practice and financial reports.

Financial reports contribute to the understanding of the practice and allow a manager to recognize current problems and prevent further financial problems from occurring. By recognizing issues early, troubleshooting and repair can resolve problems before they become a financial nightmare for the practice. It is essential to develop a balance sheet and profit and loss statement monthly, to keep the snapshot of the practice's finances in clear view.

Balance Sheet

A balance sheet is referred to as the *statement of financial condition of the practice*. It summarizes the assets, liabilities, and equities of the practice. Balance sheets represent the basic accounting equation: Assets = Liabilities + Owner Equity. Assets include all things of value that the practice owns, including property, equipment, inventory, building, land, and goodwill. Liabilities include accounts payable and loans. Balance sheets may require the assistance of an accountant to complete. Discrepancies in amounts and percentages should be investigated to determine if a problem or opportunity exists. Problems should be resolved and opportunities capitalized on.

Profit and Loss Statements

A profit and loss statement (P&L) is a financial statement that summarizes income, expenses, and profits for a specific period, such as monthly, quarterly, or annually. These records provide information that shows the ability of a practice to generate a profit by analyzing and maximizing income, while trying to reduce expenses. P&Ls are also known as income statements, or income and expense statements.

P&Ls are started with the entry of the income, entry of the expenses (which are then subtracted from the income) resulting in a profit at the end of the statement. Entries are made in the checkbook ledger of QuickBooks (or whichever accounting software a practice uses). Entries must be entered in the correct category (detailed later) in order to produce accurate reports. Categories can also be referred to as a chart of accounts.

P&Ls are extremely important to a manager. Having the ability to develop these in-house enables the manager to evaluate them on a monthly basis and make changes when needed, before the negative trend has a severe impact on the practice. P&Ls must be established and analyzed before a budget can be put in place. When a manager can pick out red flags on a P&L, investigate the problem and implement change, a budget is then ready to be created. Until then, managers must focus on fine-tuning the skills needed to analyze profit and loss sheets.

QuickBooks is one of the most popular accounting software programs used in the veterinary profession (although others are available, which can complete the same tasks). For the sake of simplicity in this chapter, QuickBooks will be referred to.

It is very important to make sure that the profit and loss sheet is as detailed as possible, and that the proper chart of accounts is used. This allows managers to determine where inconsistencies may lie by comparing benchmarks, and gives a better direction on how to correct any inconsistencies.

Chart of Accounts

A chart of accounts is a list of created categories used to define each class of items for which money is spent or received. It arranges the finances of the practice in a manner to develop a better understanding, and creates an organizational structure to the income, expense, and profits. AAHA has an excellent chart of accounts that helps practices categorize income and expenses correctly, which also correlates with IRS tax forms. This helps simplify the year-end process when CPAs are filing business taxes (Figure 20-8).

 Veterinary practice managers maintain a chart of accounts.

Income

Income, which is generated through the deposits made to the practice on a daily basis (Figure 20-9), is entered into QuickBooks. Managers may wish to further break down this income, determining which income center the money is generated from (Figure 20-10). Income centers are known as the categories that generate income for the hospital: surgery center, dental center, pharmacy, laboratory, diets, grooming, and so on. When income centers are entered, they can be compared to the expenses associated with that center (covered in detail later in this chapter), ensuring that they are producing a profit and are not losing money for the practice.

PRACTICE POINT Detailed income centers on a profit and loss sheet allow easier compassion of expenses that are associated with each individual income center.

Expenses

Any outflow of money that is owed to another company to pay for a service or product is known as an expense. Expenses must be placed in the proper category or chart of accounts in order for accurate reports to be generated.

Administrative	Facility	Cost of Goods

Advertising/Promotion/Marketing
    Bad Debt/Collection Fees
    Bank/CC Fees
    Business/Staff Meetings
    Charitable Contributions
    Communications (Phone and Internet)
    Credit Card Processing
    Cremations
    Entertainment
    Insurance
        Business
        Liability
        Life
    Licenses/permits
    Office Supplies
    Payroll Services/Benefits Admin
    Printing/Copies
    Professional Dues/Subscriptions
    Professional Fees
        Accounting
        Consulting
        Legal
    Sales/Use Tax
    Travel
    Technical Support
        Software Support
	Biomedical Waste
	Contract Labor
	Equipment
	    Lease
	    Maintenance
	    Repair
	    Support Contracts
	Facility
	    Decorations
	    Maintenance
	    Repair
	    Security
	Janitorial/Housekeeping
	Property Insurance
	Real Estate Taxes
	Rent
	Utilities
	    Water
	    Gas
	    Electricity
		Diets
		Drugs and Medical Supplies
		    Injections
		    Rx Meds
		    Vaccines
		    Imaging
		    Surgical Supplies
		    Hospital Supplies
		    Boarding Supplies
		    Grooming Supplies
		HW/Flea/Tick
		Laboratory
		    Inside
		    Outside
		Retail/OTC

FIGURE 20-8 Chart of accounts.

Continued

Expenses are classified as either a fixed or variable expense. These classifications have categories associated with each. Fixed expenses include administrative expenses, facility expenses, and veterinary expenses (if they are paid on salary). Boxes 20-3 to 20-5 provide examples of fixed expenses common for veterinary practices. Variable expenses include COGs, staff expenses, and veterinary-related expenses (when paid on production) (Boxes 20-6 to 20-8).

Fixed Expenses

Fixed expenses are in general a set cost to the hospital; they do not change with the amount of business produced by the hospital. Regardless of the number of clients seen, the electricity use will be the same; rent will always be the same dollar amount, and the telephone bill will remain constant.

> **PRACTICE POINT**   Fixed expenses will remain stable, regardless of practice income.

If veterinarians are paid a salary only (no production) they are classified as a fixed expense (regardless of the number of clients seen, they will still receive the same paycheck). Medical insurance, retirement, and continuing education can either be placed within this category, or administrative (depends on practice preference). When comparing benchmarks, make sure to note where these expenses are placed in the benchmarks, so that they do not throw off the analysis. Some benchmarks are placed in administrative, whereas others are placed under veterinarians.

Variable Expenses

Variable expenses change with the amount of business produced by a practice. Cost of goods (COGs) is defined as the products used to produce a service for a client, or products sold to a client. If a practice sees 125 dogs for vaccinations in 1 month, but only 85 dogs the following month, the amount of vaccines ordered will vary.

Staff payroll can also be variable, especially in seasonal practices, hence the placement in the variable expense category. It can be argued in some practices that the staff expenses are relatively fixed; however, for comparison and analysis with benchmarks, it is referred to as a variable expense.

Veterinarians that are paid on production will be a variable expense, because the amount of money they receive in a paycheck will depend on the amount of business produced in a specified period. Just as with veterinarians paid on salary, production veterinarians and staff members may have medical insurance, retirement, and continuing education that can either be placed within this category or administrative (depends on practice preference).

Non DVM Expenses	DVM Expenses
Managers	Owner Veterinarian
Payroll	Payroll
Taxes	Taxes
Workers Comp	Workers Comp
Health Insurance	Health Insurance
Retirement	Retirement
CE	CE
Uniforms	Uniforms
Technicians	License and Fees
Payroll	Reimbursed Expenses
Taxes	Associate Veterinarians
Workers Comp	Payroll
Health Insurance	Taxes
Retirement	Workers Comp
CE	Health Insurance
Uniforms	Retirement
Assistants	CE
Payroll	Uniforms
Taxes	License and Fees
Workers Comp	Reimbursed Expenses
Health Insurance	Relief Veterinarian
Retirement	
CE	
Uniforms	
Receptionists	
Payroll	
Taxes	
Workers Comp	
Health Insurance	
Retirement	
CE	
Uniforms	

FIGURE 20-8, cont'd

Net Income

Net income is determined when the expenses are subtracted from the income, with the desire of having a positive number. If more money was spent than the income received, a negative amount will result. According to AVMA, the average net income (profit) a general practice produces in a given year is 10% to 12%. Each practice should implement procedures to maximize income and manage expenses to achieve these goals.

> **PRACTICE POINT** According to AVMA, average practice profit is 10% to 12%.

Producing Monthly Profit and Loss Statements

Now that income and expenses have been entered in the correct categories, profit and loss statements can be printed.

ABC Veterinary Hospital Profit and Loss Standard January through December 2013		
Ordinary Income/Expense	Jan-Dec 2013	% of Income
Income	$1,500,000	100%
Total Income	**$1,500,000**	**100%**

FIGURE 20-9 Income summary on profit and loss sheet.

As stated earlier, P&Ls should be produced in-house every month to help managers better manage the hospital.

In QuickBooks, the Profit and Loss Statement should be selected from the Reports menu. A detailed or summarized report can be chosen. The summarized report is recommended for analysis; when looking for discrepancies, a detailed report can be referred to.

When analyzing P&Ls, one should analyze percentages of gross revenue, not necessarily dollar figures. Expenses may increase or decrease with revenue, making it hard to compare. Percentages will give a more accurate picture than exact dollar amounts (Figure 20-11).

Practices may use external benchmarks to determine how well their practice is doing, and where improvements can be made. Internal benchmarks from historical figures should be considered as well, watching trends that may occur because of the seasonality of business in some parts of the country.

Troubleshooting Profit and Loss Statements

When percentages in a specific category are off, a red flag should be raised for managers. This is an indicator that an investigation into the discrepancy is warranted.

When managers first start to analyze data, percentages may be higher than benchmarks that are referred to. This is to be expected, and it allows managers to look for changes that can be implemented to bring the percentages into a normal level. Three steps must be taken when analyzing P&Ls. First, look at the percentages and compare. Then ask questions of the percentages; and finally, implement change.

Owners and managers must understand that income is the first area that must be addressed and is the *easiest* to manage (review the section, Maximizing Revenue, later in the chapter). Many expenses are set, and minimal changes that can be made may not have a severe impact on the percentages. The biggest area of expenses managers can have an effect on however, is cost of goods (review the section, Reducing Expenses, later in the chapter).

The following are examples of red flags that owners and managers should investigate:

During the month of January, utilities were 1.3%, and for the month of February, utilities were 5%. Benchmarks show utilities should be approximately 1% (see Figure 20-7). Historically, the utilities for this practice average 1.2%. One might assume the winter weather has increased the cost of utilities,

```
                    ABC Veterinary Hospital
                    Profit and Loss Standard
                  January through December 2013

Ordinary Income/Expense          Jan-Dec 2013      % of Income
     Income
          Exams                    $225,000            15%
          Professional Services    $64,500             4.3%
          Laboratory               $297,000            19.8%
          Imaging                  $64,5000            4.3%
          Dentistry                $72,000             4.8%
          Vaccines                 $103,500            6.9%
          Hospitalization          $39,000             2.6%
          Surgery                  $84,000             5.6%
          Anesthesia               $58,500             3.9%
          Pharmacy                 $228,000            15.2%
          Flea, Tick and HWP       $142,500            9.5%
          Diets                    $76,500             5.1%
          OTC/Retail               $22,0500            1.5%
          Boarding                 $22,500             1.5%
     Total Income                  $1,500,000          100%
```

FIGURE 20-10 Income detail on profit and loss sheet.

BOX 20-3 | Administrative Expenses

- Business licenses/permits
- Business meetings
- Advertising/marketing
- Copies/printing
- Office supplies
- Journals/library
- Postage
- Professional fees (legal, CPA)
- Software
- Bank/credit card fees*
- Travel
- Collection costs
- Communications
- Insurance (business, life)
- Payroll fees

*Bank credit card fees are often associated as a variable expense, because they rise and fall with business. However, for classification purposes, they are listed as a fixed expense in the administrative chart of accounts.

BOX 20-4 | Facility Expenses

- Equipment
- Building
- Property
- Utilities
- Rent
- Biomedical waste
- Contract labor

BOX 20-5 | Veterinary Related Expenses (When Paid on Salary)

- Payroll
- Taxes/workers' compensation
- Medical insurance, retirement*
- Continuing education*

*Can also be categorized into administrative costs.

BOX 20-6 | Cost of Goods (COGs) Expenses

- Drugs and medical supplies
- Heartworm/flea/tick
- Laboratory
- Diets
- Retail/OTC

BOX 20-7 | Staff Expenses

- Payroll
- Taxes
- Workers' compensation
- Medical insurance, retirement*
- Continuing education*

*Can also be categorized into administrative costs.

but when looked at in a dollar amount, it would be too large of an increase. Therefore the following would be investigated:

- Were some utility bills paid late (from January), thereby increasing February percentages?
- Did income drop significantly to cause this increase?
- Are more than just the practice's utility bills being paid?
- Are there maintenance issues occurring within the practice resulting in higher percentages?
- Was an expense misclassified?

> *PRACTICE POINT* Becoming familiar with the practices profit and loss sheet percentages will help identify areas that need immediate investigation.

A practice may also see that their COG percentage is higher (30%) than that of benchmarks (21%). To help determine why this percentage is high, a practice may look at *(this is not a complete list of reasons, but rather ideas to spark the investigation):*
- The amount of inventory sitting on the shelves
- Potential shrinkage
- Pricing model of inventory
- Misclassified expenses
- Significant income drop

Using KPIs to Help Analyze Data

KPIs are useful in helping to explain discrepancies or improvements that may be occurring. For example, there may be a decrease in the number of clients in one month, but

BOX 20-8	Veterinary Related Expenses (When Paid on Production)

- Payroll
- Taxes
- Workers' compensation
- Medical insurance, retirement*
- Continuing education*

*Can also be categorized into administrative costs.

an increase in the ADT. The increase in gross revenue and ADT may be explained if customer service initiatives were implement, and the practice started focusing on developing relationships with clients.

Managers and owners are trained to constantly improve numbers; however, it cannot be forgotten that when numbers are good, determine why. This allows one to capitalize on the successes and implement the strategy elsewhere within the business model.

Comparing Income and Expense Centers

It is important to be able to compare income and expense centers. As defined previously, income centers are those that produce revenue (or income) for the hospital. Expense centers are those expenses associated with that particular center. For example, a dental income center includes all money generated from dental prophylaxes, extractions, and dental radiographs. The dental expense center encompasses all inventoried items, staff time, and DVM time to produce the service. If it is costing more to generate a service than the income produced, the center must be re-evaluated for profitability.

If a center is not managed, it cannot be improved, and this is one area many managers neglect to evaluate or manage. The following information is required in order to evaluate the profitability of a service:
- Gross revenue per month (or year) for a specific service
- Square footage used by service
- Fixed costs per square foot (entire practice)
- Fixed costs per square foot for service
- Variable costs for service

Calculating the values in the previous list will determine if a profit is being generated. For example, consider the dental center presented in Box 20-9. The dental center produced $9889.45 and used 100 sq ft of the practices total space. Fixed costs have been determined (from P&L) to be $190.00 per square foot, equaling $19,000 per year ($1583.33 per month). Variable costs are determined to be $525.39 per month, allowing the center to produce a net income of $7880.32. This center is definitely profitable. Do not forget, equipment used to complete these services has been placed in the fixed costs category.

	April	%	May	%
Income - Total	$150,000.00	100.0%	$200,000.00	100.0
Expenses				
Admin	$12,600.00	8.4%	$16,800.00	8.4%
Facility	$14,100.00	9.4%	$18,800.00	9.4%
DVM Salary	$22,500.00	15.0%	$30,000.00	15.0%
COG	$33,150.00	22.1%	$44,200.00	22.1%
Non-DVM Wages	$42,000.00	28.0%	$56,000.00	28.0%
DVM Prod	$15,000.00	10.0%	$20,000.00	10.0%
Expenses - Total	$139,350.00	92.9%	$185,800	92.9%
Profit	$10,650.00	7.1%	$14,200.00	7.1%

FIGURE 20-11 Comparisons of dollars and percentages when gross revenue increases.

BOX 20-9	Dental Income Profitability Example	
Dental center gross income per month		$9989.45
Dental center, square feet used for center		100 sq ft
Annual fixed costs/sq ft (determined from P&L fixed costs: administrative, facility, and veterinary)		$190.00
Annual dental center fixed costs (100 sq ft × $190.00)		$19,000.00
Monthly dental center fixed costs (Annual costs ÷ 12)		$1583.33
Dental center variable costs		$525.39
Dental center net income ($9989.45 − $1583.33 − $525.39)		$7880.32

If a service is not profitable, managers may consider evaluating the client's cost for services and if the service is being used to its fullest potential.

> **PRACTICE POINT** Profit centers must be analyzed for both income and expenses.

Maximizing Revenue

A manager is most efficacious (when working with finances) by finding methods to maximize revenue. As stated previously, many expenses are fixed; therefore reducing them can be quite difficult. There are many facets to maximizing revenue; each is complex and takes time to see improvements. However, when a manager involves the entire team in the process, income becomes simpler to maximize and is very rewarding for the entire team.

Fee Schedule

Often, practices do not know how to price their services or their inventory, both of which have significant impact on the bottom line. Many times, the service pricing came with the practice when it was purchased and has taken incremental pricing increases over the years. However, as the practice has grown and more overhead has been added to the practice, owners and managers must ensure they are collecting fees appropriately.

 Veterinary practice managers conduct fee analysis, and monitor and update fee schedules.

To determine how much a service costs a practice to produce, several key points must be known:
- Fixed costs of hospital per minute
- Direct costs used to produce service (inventory)
- Staff costs per minute
- Veterinary costs per minute
- Number of staff minutes used to complete service
- Number of doctor minutes used to complete the service
- Desired profit

Equation to Obtain Service Pricing

(Fixed costs/minute + Staff costs/minute) × (length of procedure in staff minutes)
+ (DVM costs/minute) × (length of procedure in DVM minutes)
+ (Direct costs × 2)
+ Profit

Fixed Costs per Minute

Fixed costs per minute are determined from the profit and loss statement (administrative, facility, and DVM when paid on salary), along with the number of billable minutes the hospital is open.
- For example, if the hospital is open from 8 AM to 6 PM and does not close for lunch, it is available to produce services for 600 minutes per day (10 hours × 60 minutes per hour). That same practice is open Monday through Friday; therefore it is available to produce services for 3000 minutes per week (600 minutes × 5 days per week), which equals 12,000 minutes per month (3000 minutes per week × 4 weeks per month).

If the profit and loss statements states that the fixed costs for the practice are $20,000 for the month, then $20,000 ÷ 12,000 minutes per month = $1.67. *Fixed costs for the practice are $1.67 per minute.*

Staff Costs per Minute

Staff costs per minute are determined by calculating all costs associated with paying all non-DVM staff members. This number is then divided by the billable minutes the practice is open. Taking this equation one step further, the staff costs per minute are then multiplied by the number of non-DVM team members used to complete the procedure, along with the number of minutes it takes to complete the task.
- For example, the P&L indicates staff costs per month are $17,000. As indicated previously, the practice is available to produce services 12,000 minutes per month; therefore, $17,000 ÷ 12,000 minutes per month = $1.42. *Staff costs are $1.42 per minute per staff member.*
- If more than one staff member participates in the procedure, costs per minute can be multiplied by the number of staff members.

It can be estimated that it takes one veterinary technician 10 minutes to collect the cytology sample, stain the slide, and read the sample.

DVM Costs per Minute

Veterinary costs per minute are also determined from the profit and loss statement. P&Ls should be detailed enough to determine how much it costs to pay the veterinarian on a monthly basis. If the DVM is paid a salary, the costs should have been figured in the fixed costs; if DVMs are paid production, that cost will be added here. (For calculation purposes, if several DVMs are on staff, determine the average pay of all DVMs.) That total is then divided by the number of billable minutes the hospital is open. In our earlier example, the hospital is open 12,000 minutes per month, and the profit and loss sheet indicates that DVM costs are $7102.00

per month. Therefore $7102.00 is divided by 12,000 (billable minutes), resulting in $0.59 per minute.

Next, one would estimate how long it would take the DVM to diagnose the case based on this service. For this example, we will use 5 minutes (review and confirm results of cytologic analysis); $0.59 × 5 = $2.95. *DVM cost for this procedure is $2.95.*

Direct Costs

Direct costs are used to produce a cytologic analysis of an ear sample would include a cotton swab, microscope slide, stain, and mineral oil. For this example we will estimate that these inventoried items cost the hospital $1.23. Therefore *direct costs × 2 = $2.46.*

Profit

Profit can be determined based on the service, practice profit goals, or if the service is a shopped or nonshopped service. Cytologic analysis of an ear sample is generally not a shopped service and will have a higher profit. For this example, we will use 20% profit.

> **PRACTICE POINT** Profit percentages will vary when pricing services; shopped services will have a lower percentage than nonshopped services.

Putting It All Together

Fixed costs per minute + Staff costs per minute
× length of procedure
($1.67 + $1.42) × 10 minutes = $30.90

DVM costs per minute × length of procedure
= $0.59 × 5 minutes = $2.95

(Direct costs × 2) = $1.23 × 2 = $2.46

Profit = 20%

$30.90 + $2.95 + 2.46 = $36.31
$36.31 × 0.20 = $7.26
$36.31 + $7.26 = $43.57

This service should cost clients $43.57

Spot-check all services and adjust as needed. Remember, some services will take a higher profit than others.

One must remember that they cannot suddenly increase the price of services. Doing so will instill sticker shock, as indicated by the Bayer Veterinary Care Usage Study. Clients must receive value for the service they are paying; if they do not perceive the value, they will decline recommendations and find a cheaper hospital. Implementing value added services and developing relationships with clients can prevent this scenario from occurring. Review the section of customer service, later in this chapter, as well as Chapter 11 for more successful ideas.

Charging for inventory items are discussed at length in Chapter 15. Do not forget that holding and ordering costs

must be assessed to prevent the practice from losing money. Also, shopped and nonshopped items must be considered. Shopped items will have less of a markup than nonshopped items. For example, heartworm preventive will have perhaps a 50% mark up, whereas an injection may have a 200% mark up. Managers must consider what products the practice is taking a loss on, and make up for the loss in other products.

Missing Charges

On average, a single veterinarian misses $64,000 in fees per year (Opperman, 2010). This number can be difficult to average, because many practices do not know they are even missing charges. Medical record audits must be completed on a daily basis to determine what has left the practice uncharged. Chapter 14 discusses medical record audits in length. If a hospital produces $1,500,000.00 a year, and 10% of services and inventoried items go uncharged, the practice has lost $150,000! If medical record audits are not performed, a manager or owner will never know this money was lost.

Training is critical for team members, and managers must identify why charges are being missed. Is the team understaffed? Does a team member lack focus? Do all team members understand the financial impact of missed charges?

To help reduce missed charges, managers may implement several items or tasks. Travel sheets (review Chapter 3) may be implemented for paper and paper-light practices; electronic medical records that invoice automatically should help reduce missed charges; however, if the medical record is left incomplete, charges will be missed. Managers may need to implement procedures indicating medical records must be complete before client checkout.

When analyzing profit and loss statements, a loss of $200,000 can alter the percentages significantly. All managers must investigate this area when trying to maximize revenue (Figure 20-12).

Discounts

Many practices do not manage the total dollars in discounts that are given to clients, nor review any return on investments (ROIs) from these discounts. Discounts come in two forms: managed and unmanaged. Managed discounts are those that are planned (however, rarely are these reports analyzed). For example, a managed discount would be: buy 11 doses and get one free, or giving a free bottle of shampoo with every exam.

Unmanaged discounts are those that are unplanned, and given out of guilt or because the practice has failed the client in some way. For example, a veterinarian may want to continue providing the best care for a patient, but the client can no longer afford the service; the DVM continues the treatment regardless. Another example: the team failed to communicate an increase in the treatment plan (estimate); the client is angry, therefore a discount is applied to the client's account to satisfy (and maintain) the client.

Unfortunately, these discounts add up. If a practice is already losing 10% (of gross revenue) in missed charges, how much additional is provided in discounts? Every product that is given away as a planned discount must have a code. This allows managers to track these discounts. In addition, the client needs

Income	$1,600,000.00	100.0%	$1,400,000.00	100.0%
Expenses				
Admin	$134,400.00	8.40%	$134,400.00	9.60%
Facility	$150,400.00	9.40%	$150,400.00	10.74%
DVM Salary	$240,000.00	15.00%	$240,000.00	17.14%
COG	$353,600.00	22.10%	$353,600.00	25.26%
Non-DVM Wages	$448,000.00	28.00%	$448,000.00	32.00%
DVM Prod	$160,000.00	10.00%	$160,000.00	11.43%
Total	$1,486,400.00	92.90%	$1,486,400.00	106.17%
Profit	**$113,600.00**	**7.10%**	**($86,400.00)**	**-6.17%**

FIGURE 20-12 Missing charges of $200,000 has significant impact on the profits of the hospital, in addition to affecting the percentages, based on gross revenue.

to know how much that product costs (the invoice unit price must be listed); if the client does not know the costs, they cannot associate a value for it. Third, managers must track these codes and watch the ROI. Is the client returning for future services when discounts of this magnitude are occurring?

> **PRACTICE POINT** Missed charges account for the loss of approximately 10% of gross revenue. For a practice that generates $1.5 million dollars, $150,000.00 is lost annually.

Unmanaged discounts devalue the practice. Continuing care beyond the client's financial ability teaches clients to expect this service in the future; when the free service is not received in the future, they are angry and leave the practice. Many team members find this concept hard to relate to, because *"we love the animals and want to do what is best for the patient."* Unfortunately, when this occurs, we cannot provide better wages for the team or purchase higher quality equipment to continue providing the best quality of medicine. When team members make mistakes, each should be held accountable, and a learning process should entail. In scenarios such as this one, managers should implement a plan to become proactive instead of reactive, because the latter devalues the practice.

A potential solution for discounting in the hospital is to allot a budget; each doctor receives an annual budget for the amount of discounts they wish to give (discounts are going to be given; therefore, instead of battling the concept on a daily basis, a solution should be considered). When a DVM runs out of "discount dollars" for the year, they can no longer discount. The first year, the discount dollars will be used rapidly. The second year, they learn to be more conservative.

Standard of Care

To help increase and promote revenue on all levels, teams should be dedicated to promoting excellent veterinary medicine. This includes diagnostics, treatments, and preventive medicine. A case should be completely worked up with diagnostic tests before a diagnosis is given. Assuming an animal has pancreatitis according to clinical signs is not working up a case. Blood work, such as the Spec cPL test, and radiographs may be indicated to complete the diagnosis.

Complete treatment for pancreatitis should also be initiated; conservative treatment of sending the pet home on a bland diet is unacceptable. Pets should have the comprehensive care they deserve to improve their painful condition.

Standards of care (SOCs) can be created by veterinarians when the patient and client are not in front of them to change their diagnostic approach to a case. This allows every patient to receive the same recommendations, regardless of the financial status. When SOCs are developed, the entire team is on the same page, delivering a consistent message to the client. Review Chapter 11 for more helpful ideas of establishing SOCs.

Preventive medicine must be offered and encouraged to all clients, regardless of the perceived client economic factor. Excellent quality of care must be offered across the board.

> **PRACTICE POINT** Create standards of care (SOCs) to improve client communication and compliance, and to offer every client and patient the same high-quality medicine.

Income Center Development and Management

Income centers were defined earlier, and each practice has its own set of centers. Practices may consider which income centers they do not have and investigate what could be implemented (Box 20-10). One may determine that the veterinarians are recommending a particular service on a regular basis, but cannot provide that service within the hospital. This would then be a service worth considering.

Once a service has been developed, it must be managed. Goals must be set and training must occur; without these two items, profits will be limited, if the program succeeds (if a service is not managed, it cannot be improved). If goals are not being obtained, managers should investigate why this is happening. Is the service being recommended? Is the price set to high? Are clients receiving the proper education regarding the service? If recommendations are being declined, is the team following up? Once an answer has been determined, steps must be taken to implement actions in order to achieve these goals.

BOX 20-10	Potential Income Centers

- Anesthesia
- Boarding
- Dentals
- Diets
- Examinations
- Grooming
- Hospitalization
- Laboratory
- Pharmacy
- Radiology
- Retail/OTC
- Surgery

Income services must also be maximized. For example, a dental prophylaxis machine and digital radiograph machine have been purchased by the hospital. How many hours out of the day are these two pieces of equipment being used? Maximizing their use on a daily basis decreases the cost per use associated with the machines and increases profits for the hospital. The dental center is traditionally the lowest producing income center of the hospital, and should be reviewed on a yearly basis.

Managing Client Visits

Managers must analyze the client visit, from the very beginning of the client calling to make an appointment, until the client leaves the hospital. When the client called the hospital to make an appointment, what did the client experience? Did the client feel welcome? Did the team member answering the phone identify himself or herself? (Review Chapter 2.) Was the client able to make an appointment that was convenient, or is there a lengthy waiting period?

When the client enters the practice property, what do they experience? Is it clean? Does it have a professional appearance and an easy entry? When the client enters the practice, what do they feel and smell? These questions must be asked at every point the client interacts with the practice. Further, medical records must be analyzed for recommendations. When medical records are reviewed and prepared before the appointment, it is less likely that the team will miss recommendations.

How long does the client have to wait to be seen? If appointments are running behind, how is the client notified? Review Chapter 13 for more details on appointment management. Clients that experience delayed appointments will have lower compliance. Every manager must manage this time and adjust appointment schedulers if this is a constant issue.

> **PRACTICE POINT**   Clients experiencing delays will have lower compliance rates. Monitor appointment times, and ensure clients are seen on time.

How are treatment plans presented to the clients? Numerous studies indicate veterinarians should not be responsible for the presentation of treatment plans, and team members should be knowledgeable in order to have the best client acceptance. Verbal and nonverbal skills of every team member should be optimized to help increase compliance rates (review Chapter 11).

How are clients invoiced out? Clients should receive a detailed, line-by-line invoice that they can understand (abbreviations are not acceptable). Receptionists must explain each line to the client before reaching the final amount due. Clients must understand the value they are receiving for the price they are paying (review Chapter 2).

Customer Service

Excellent customer service keeps clients returning; it also keeps clients referring their friends and family to the practice. Excellent customer service builds relationships, thus enhancing compliance. Without outstanding customer service, revenue will not be maximized. Review Chapters 2 and 11 for client service tips.

Key Performance Indicators

To better understand income, KPIs must be analyzed. New client and patient numbers, active client and patient numbers, ACT, ADT, and ARPP are especially helpful. Compliance with preventive products and income centers should also be analyzed. Training, customer service, and marketing techniques should result in better KPIs for the practice.

Reducing Expenses

Expenses should be monitored on a monthly basis, reducing where possible. However, as stated previously, an extensive amount of time should not be dedicated to reducing expenses; income should receive this attention. The few areas that do require attention are mentioned next.

Credit cards charges: Processing fees seem to creep up every few months, contracts are amended or additional charges are added to the practices account. Due diligence of the manager includes consulting with the current company asking where fees can be decreased, while shopping around for reduced merchant fees. Although it is a hassle to change companies every few years, it can save the practice money over the course of the year. Benchmarks show credit card fees average 1.5% of gross revenue.

Health insurance: Health insurance premiums for employees increase on a yearly basis. Insurance policies should be shopped every few years, keeping in mind preventative health care coverage, prescriptions, and deductibles. Having an insurance agent that represents multiple companies can aid in this search.

Communications: Communications include telephone, Internet, and cable. Many practices have bundled services, yet many of these bundled services are not fully utilized. Review contracts and determined if all of the services are being used; consider accepting unbundled packages for a reduced price.

Professional fees: Consider contract negotiation for payroll services, accounting, and attorney fees.

Cost of goods fees: Inventory is the second largest expense of the hospital. Shopping for inventory is not a good use of time, because most manufactures have set costs, meaning

whichever distributor is chosen, the price will remain the relatively the same. Therefore shopping for products will increase ordering costs. A more effective use of time is to develop effective turnover rates, reorder quantities, and reorder points. This will significantly reduce soft costs (known as holding and ordering costs) as well as shrinkage that are associated with inventory management. Managers must also consider product consolidation and effective pricing when reviewing effective inventory policies. Review Chapter 15 for further details.

> **PRACTICE POINT**   Reduce COG expenses by implementing effective turnover rates, reorder quantities, and reorder points.

Equipment is different than inventory items and must be shopped. However, one must not forget the following key components when shopping for equipment: product, warranty, installation, available technical service if equipment needs servicing, and training. Many companies offer a nice product, but do not include any training for team members, installation, or servicing should the unit need it. Just because a piece of equipment is cheaper up front does not mean it is the best piece of equipment to suit all of the hospital's needs.

Payroll: The first area many managers want to cut is payroll. It seems to be the magic place everyone wants to start with. However, this can also be the practices biggest mistake. Let's not forget that overtime must be managed; however, if overtime is being achieved by many team members, then it must be considered that the practice is short-staffed. Short-staffing leads to employee burnout, resulting in decreased production by the entire team. If overtime is significant, consider hiring more team members or restructuring the schedule to accommodate busy times/days in the practice.

Having a lean payroll hurts customer service. Veterinary medicine is a service-based industry, and if practices are not providing that superior service, clients will go elsewhere. When team members are working at a quick pace, they do not have the time to spend developing relationships with clients (resulting in decreased client compliance, both with preventive and emergency care).

Payroll must be the last area that is cut, because it will most significantly affect the profits of the hospital. To help maximize payroll, managers may wish to review training policies and staff leveraging. Are team members being used to their fullest potential? If not, could team training be implemented to make this happen? Consider having every team member write down the duties they accomplish on a daily basis for 5 consecutive days (veterinarians included). Managers can then compile the lists and determine how to more effectively use the staff. Increased staff utilization prevents burnout, creates accountability, increases client compliance, and decreases staff turnover.

Analyzing KPIs with payroll is useful. If the client retention and bonding rates are high, this can be attributed to an excellent team. Lower retention and compliance rates (along with new and active clients) can indicate customer service issues, resulting from a lean payroll.

Team wages must be analyzed on a yearly basis. Good team members cost money, and good team members produce money. Employees with high wages should be performing to expectations, and constantly striving to reach the next level. Review Chapter 3 on employee expectations, performance reviews and coaching, along with Chapter 5 on the development of employee job descriptions.

Veterinarian salary and/or production must also be analyzed. Many practices wish to pay DVMs strictly on salary because it is easy to calculate and owners feel that it decreases the potential for competition between associates and charging clients for unneeded services. However, it can also cause veterinarians to "just show up to work" and not put forth 100% and promote the best medicine. Comments such as, "*It doesn't matter to me, I get paid the same amount whether they take it or not*" must be managed ASAP. Managers and owners may discuss a bonus or production program that facilitates the best medicine approach and also breeds positive culture within the practice. Good attitudes start at the top and trickle down to team members. Doctors with a negative attitude affect the entire team.

Fraud and Embezzlement

Fraud occurs in small businesses globally. In fact, more than 5% of gross revenue is lost to fraud and embezzlement on a yearly basis. Unfortunately in veterinary medicine, many owners and managers are in denial that fraud and/or embezzlement occur in their practice. Traditionally, practices are "family oriented" and the thought is that "family would not steal from me." In an independent study completed by Marsha Henike, DVM, CVPM, CPA, 67.8% of practices had been a victim of fraud or embezzlement. It is not a matter of *if* it occurs; it is a matter of *when* it will occur to each practice.

> **PRACTICE POINT**   Fraud and embezzlement occur in more than 5% of small businsses per year.

Theft includes inventoried items, equipment, and cleaning and office supplies. In addition, time theft (employees clocking in for work, but eating breakfast first) and cash theft (petty cash drawer, padding payroll) must be considered.

Team members that steal from practices have opportunities presented to them; it is the managers' responsibility to decrease these opportunities. A checks and balances system must be implemented for every area of the practice.

End-of-day reconciliation: The person taking in the payments throughout the day should not be the person to reconcile at the end of the day. Having this duty assigned to the same person allows one to alter the books and pocket cash. In addition, the employee responsible for accepting payments should not be the person making bank

deposits. Last, practice managers must oversee all daily and monthly banking procedures, making sure to investigate any discrepancies.

 Veterinary practice managers oversee daily and monthly banking procedures

Check machine: Consider using check machines that will automatically deposit funds into the practices account, eliminating the potential for stolen checks.

Password protection of veterinary management software: Only management is allowed to delete invoices, or change codes or prices.

Client credit cards: Do not retain client credit card numbers in the files. Many embezzlement cases are the result of stolen credit card numbers. Follow the red flags rule, as outlined later in this chapter.

Employee accounts: Treat employee accounts as you would a client account. A member of management must enter all products and services obtained by a team member. This prevents missed charges and/or the reduction of costs associated with the invoice.

Inventory: Implement spot-checking and comparison of physical and computer inventories, as outlined in Chapter 15. A large percentage of fraud cases occur when employees are stealing products (and tests) to sell to their friends and family, or on eBay and craigslist. Discrepancies must be investigated; when they are not and a checks and balances system is not in place, the door is wide open for employee theft.

Security cameras: Many owners and team members are discouraged by having security cameras in the hospital, because they fear it will decrease team morale. However, the benefit far outweighs the risk of a potentially negative culture. Positive cultural builders can be implemented to overcome the fear, and security cameras can reduce theft. Simply place a sign in the lobby for clients to know security cameras are in use. Also post warnings in the break room and the employee manual, so the team remembers.

Controlled substances: Veterinary practices have drugs that are commonly abused by people, and employees may want some for themselves or to sell. Outsiders may also want controlled substances, and it is up to the practice to ensure these drugs are kept in a secure location, with limited access (see Chapter 16). Place security cameras over these secure locations and implement a Drug-Free Workplace Program, with random drug testing (see Chapter 5).

Key access: Limit the number of team members that have access to the hospital after hours. Owners may wish to implement a personal security code system that tracks when employees enter and exit the building. Unlimited, unmanaged access invites employee theft.

Profit and loss statement: Know your percentages: If a practice does not have a monthly P&L, it can be hard to track percentages. However, managers that analyze these reports monthly will immediately notice when a percentage is "out of whack." These percentages can be a red flag, and an investigation into the abnormal percentage is launched. It is much easier to detect a problem that has recently risen, rather than finding out after thousands of dollars are missing.

Decrease Practice Risk of Fraud or Embezzlement

Along with checks and balances for each area of the practice mentioned earlier, positive cultural builders can be implemented, which can initiate employee accountability, enhance a team environment, and increase staff morale (thus resulting in decreased employee turnover).

Owners and managers may want to consider including pet health insurance in an employee benefits package. This will ensure that all employees receive the same discount (see Chapter 19), preventing the perception of favoritism.

Practices may also refer to staff feeding programs that are offered by the various nutrition companies. Reduced costs for team member pets may decrease the temptation to steal food for their pet. Manufacturers also have sampling programs for team members. Relationships must be developed with manufacture representatives, and the product must be sold within the hospital; however, a win-win situation is produced when these programs are used. All team members are treated equally, and again, the temptation to steal products for their own pet(s) is less.

Consider having an open-book management system. Sharing the financials with team members helps them understand where all the money goes (covered in further detailed in the section titled, Open-Book Management. Often, receptionists see that the practice has produced nearly $10,000 for the day. To them, that is a large amount of money; but they do not understand where all of the money goes.

> **PRACTICE POINT**   Open-book management facilitates employee accountability and understanding of practice finances. It also helps team members achieve practice goals.

Creating a fair and positive work culture will help reduce the threat of fraud. Review Chapter 3 for many ideas of implementing positive cultures.

Creating a Budget

A budget is a critical management tool that can be used for strategic planning. For many people, the word *budget* carries a negative connotation and indicates that it is just a number-crunching game. Instead, a budget should be considered a useful planning tool that helps ensure practice success. Budgets should be created for both income and expenses; income budgets are developed to reach strategically planned goals, whereas expense budgets are used to determine where the cash went and to create goals to reduce costs where possible.

WHAT WOULD YOU DO/NOT DO?

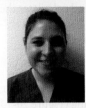

Shelly, a long time office manager, has recently attended continuing education classes and has learned the importance of creating and maintaining a budget for the practice. She has never created a budget, because the owners of the practice (in business for 20 years) have never needed one. The practice has "functioned fine" without one, so why start now? After attending the continuing education, Shelly feels that she can make a drastic impact on the practice if a budget was created and maintained.

What Should Shelly Do?

First, Shelly should develop a proposal stating how she feels the budget could make a change for the practice, and how it is worth her time to develop one. Shelly may need to attend further classes on the development of a budget before making the recommendation. She should not make the recommendation if she cannot follow through with the proposal. A practice budget may be developed, allowing her to outline her weakness and learn how to correct them before creating a permanent budget for the practice.

Veterinary practice managers prepare budgets and long-range fiscal planning.

Steps of a Budget

First, it is important to ensure that the practice has an adequate program to help with the budget process. QuickBooks has an excellent program that includes a preestablished budgeting program. Microsoft Excel spreadsheets also allow data to be exported into tables to create a budget. Creating a budget by hand can be overwhelming because subcategories can fill as many as 30 to 40 line items; therefore an effective software program must be implemented. In a software spreadsheet model, a 1% increase in projected gross income flows through the entire expense categories, and changes them automatically while providing a new calculation of the estimated net profit. This will take much less time in QuickBooks or a spreadsheet as opposed to completing the calculations by hand. Although a basic budget could be prepared by hand, making adjustments to the budget or preparing a breakdown of a yearly projection into monthly or quarterly mini-budgets can become unreasonable. Computerized spreadsheets make it easy to visualize the results of countless changes, assumptions, and trials.

Second, take a closer look at the relation of specific expenses to gross income. By having a few years of data, what is normal for the practice can be compared with benchmark data. The previous year's complete financial statements plus any results from the current year of operations will be needed. If financial statements are not available, reconciled checkbook registers will suffice for the expense portion of the budget. Reports will need to be generated from the practice management software to help create the revenue budget.

It is critical that expenses are listed in the correct chart of accounts when they are entered. Occasionally there are inconsistencies as to how an expense is entered. Perhaps the purchase of computer-generated reminder cards were classified as office supplies one month, computer supplies another month, and nonmedical supplies in a third month. A decision should be made in cases such as this to allow each expense to be consistently classified into the same account.

Computerized check-writing programs help provide consistent classification of expenses because they retain the specific transaction. When a recurring payee is used, the computer automatically classifies that payee to a specific account based on the previous transaction. Such programs quickly and easily provide profit and loss reports, the underlying data for the budget, after the end-of-month and checkbook reconciliation. An in-house profit and loss report is more than adequate for providing the historical information that forms the basis of the budget. The annual financial statements provided by an accountant are also useful but will never be as quickly available and do not allow the monthly assessment needed to successfully manage a budget.

Third, budgeting requires the reassessment of the present fee structure, evaluation of the total gross practice income, and a plan of how to achieve the necessary growth to result in adequate profits. There are many methods for establishing budgets. Budgets can be established for the entire practice or for small segments of the practice. For example, where staffing costs have historically been higher than normal in the practice, a budget for different segments of support staff, including receptionists, technicians, and veterinarians, may be established. Likewise, mixed practices may benefit from budgeting for the different segments of the practice, which likely have different profit margins.

Expenses

There are several budgeting methods that work in veterinary practice; the "top-down" method appears to be used the most. Expenses from the previous year's budget are forwarded to the following year's budget, allowing the input of changes needed to reach the goals established for the following year. For example, if the cost of goods (COGs) in Figure 20-13 is 15.6% (column 4) of the gross revenue ($1.5 million) for 2013, 15.6% will then be forwarded to the projected 2014 budget. It is at this time that the percentage can be changed based on the goals established for the following year's budget. It should be remembered that gross revenue is the total money received before expenses or taxes.

The cost of supplies will increase in the new year; therefore the increase needs to be projected and budgeted. An average increase of 4.8% will cover the increase for most variable costs (fixed costs will remain relatively constant). Figure 20-14 highlights the 4.8% projected increase in variable expenses for the 2014 fiscal year. If a payroll budget has been created, projected values for payroll, payroll tax, and benefit contributions may be added for a more accurate projection.

2013 Expenses
EXPENSES Jan-Dec 2013 ABC Animal Hospital

Revenue Jan-Dec		$ 1,500,000.00	%
Column1	Column 2	Column 3	Col 4
COGs	Medical Supplies	$ 98,874.32	6.6
	Pharmacy	$ 101,189.23	6.7
	Radiology	$ 1,890.43	0.1
	Surgery	$ 2,298.94	0.2
	Dentals	$ 1,384.05	0.1
	Foods	$ 19,897.43	1.3
	Retail/OTC	$ 8,987.43	0.6
		$ 234,521.83	15.6
Administrative	Accountant	$ 7,441.82	0.5
	Advertising	$ 9,874.09	0.7
	Check Machine Fee's	$ 2,477.28	0.2
	Communications	$ 5,768.78	0.4
	Credit Card Fee's	$ 5,600.00	0.4
	Charitable Contribution	$ 3,564.60	0.2
	Client Care (Flowers)	$ 3,694.34	0.2
	Insurance - Liability	$ 6,598.00	0.4
	License	$ 2,356.03	0.2
	Office Supplies	$ 5,678.99	0.4
	Shipping	$ 2,767.34	0.2
	Taxes -Sales	$ 62,500.00	4.2
		$ 118,321.27	7.9
Facility	Cable/Satellite Television	$ 600.00	0.0
	Cell Phone	$ 2,456.87	0.2
	Electricity	$ 5,115.85	0.3
	Natural Gas/Water/Sew	$ 3,657.98	0.2
	Building Maintenance	$ 2,398.09	0.2
	Equipment Maint.	$ 1,529.88	0.1
	Equipment Purchase	$ 4,800.00	0.3
	Equipment Lease	$ 6,720.97	0.4
	Insurance- Property	$ 2,987.34	0.2
	Rent	$ 54,698.30	3.6
		$ 84,965.28	5.7
DVM	Payroll-DVM-Owner	$ 125,000.00	8.3
	Cont Ed	$ 1,427.88	0.1
	Insurance Health	$ 4,800.00	0.3
	Insurance Workers Comp	$ -	0.0
	sIRA	$ -	0.0
	Taxes-Payroll	$ 8,750.00	0.6
	Unemployment	$ 1,250.00	0.1
DVM	Payroll-DVM-Assoc	$ 202,403.24	13.5
	Cont Ed	$ 3,450.00	0.2
	Insurance Health	$ 9,600.00	0.6
	Insurance Workers Comp	$ 234.10	0.0
	sIRA	$ 2,622.40	0.2
	Taxes-Payroll	$ 8,986.76	0.6
	Unemployment	$ 1,650.87	0.1
		$ 370,175.25	24.7
Non DVM	Payroll-Non-DVM	$ 190,987.54	12.7
	Insurance-Health	$ 3,600.00	0.2
	Insurance- Workers Comp	$ 2,106.90	0.1
	sIRA	$ 7,756.45	0.5
	Taxes- Payroll	$ 6,678.90	0.4
	Unemployment	$ 7,176.00	0.5
		$ 218,305.79	14.6
	Total Expenses	$ 1,026,289.42	68.4
	Revenue-Expenses=PROFIT	$ 473,710.58	15.9

FIGURE 20-13 Expenses for 2013.

The green column in Figure 20-14 demonstrates actual expenses incurred in 2013. The blue column adds 4.8% to account for increased expenses (column 5) and calculates the new, predicted expense (c olumn 6 and 7). The orange column gives the monthly projected value (column 8).

Creating a Spreadsheet

If an accounting software such as QuickBooks is not being used, creating a spreadsheet is easy and exciting (Figure 20-13 shows columns 1 through 4). The first column refers to the type of expense. The second column is the subcategory, based on the chart of accounts. The third column lists dollar amounts associated with each expense category, which is linked to a formula, allowing expenses to be shown as a percentage of the total practice gross revenue (column 4).

The cost of goods is shown as a percentage of gross revenue by creating a mathematical formula representing total dollars expensed, divided by total dollars of gross revenue. For example, the cost of medical supplies is $98,874.32. This figure, divided by $1.5 million = 0.066 × 100 = 6.6% (rounded up to 7%). Remember, to express a value as a percentage, the equation must be multiplied by 100.

The reason for this approach is to create a spreadsheet that will automatically update the percentages whenever changes are made to the absolute values for income and expense. Next year, when the budget spreadsheet is updated, new data will be added. All related percentages will be calculated by the spreadsheet because of the preestablished formulas.

Income

The next step is to begin a projection forward to the next financial period. An expected rate of growth is projected for the hospital based on historical gross revenue increases. Figure 20-15 lists the revenue centers for 2013 (column 1), along with the practice's predicted 10% growth (column 5) for the 2014 fiscal year. ABC Animal Hospital historically has a 10% increase each year. Each revenue center's income is multiplied by 10% to predict the 2014 revenue.

At the top of the revenue spreadsheet, enter a description, "Projected Rate of Growth." In the cell adjacent to the description, insert a percentage increase such as 5% or 10%. This number can be changed as assumptions are made regarding growth of the practice.

Gross revenue is projected for the following year as a formula, multiplying the current gross income (column 2) by the projected rate of growth of 10% resulting in column 4. If the cells are referenced correctly, any change in the percentage growth rate changes the gross income projected for the upcoming year. Column 5 is the estimated total gross revenue based off of a 10% increase in business.

When revenue centers have been established, changes can be identified, and it can be determined whether intervention is needed to prevent loss or if an area needs to be capitalized on (comparing income to expense centers). For example, dentistry is a common revenue center in veterinary practice. To determine the percentage of profit that the dental center is contributing to the overall gross revenue, a simple equation

ABC Animal Hospital

Projected Revenue Jan-Dec = $1,650,000.00 %   4.8% Increase in Expenses   Per Month

Projected Increase of Expenses = 4.8%

Column1	Column 2	2013 Actual Column 3	% Col 4		Column 5	Total Column 6	% Col 7		Total Column 8
COGs	Medical Supplies	$ 98,874.32	6.6		$ 4,745.97	$ 103,620.29	6.3		$ 8,635.02
	Pharmacy	$ 101,189.23	6.7		$ 4,857.08	$ 106,046.31	6.4		$ 8,837.19
	Radiology	$ 1,890.43	0.1		$ 90.74	$ 1,981.17	0.1		$ 165.10
	Surgery	$ 2,298.94	0.2		$ 110.35	$ 2,409.29	0.1		$ 200.77
	Dentals	$ 1,384.05	0.1		$ 66.43	$ 1,450.48	0.1		$ 120.87
	Foods	$ 19,897.43	1.3		$ 955.08	$ 20,852.51	1.3		$ 1,737.71
	Retail/OTC	$ 8,987.43	0.6		$ 431.40	$ 9,418.83	0.6		$ 784.90
		$ 234,521.83	15.6		$ 11,257.05	$ 245,778.88	14.9		$ 20,481.57
Administrative	Accountant	$ 7,441.82	0.5		$ -	$ 7,441.82	0.5		$ 620.15
	Advertising	$ 9,874.09	0.7		$ -	$ 9,874.09	0.6		$ 822.84
	Check Machine Fee's	$ 2,477.28	0.2		$ -	$ 2,477.28	0.2		$ 206.44
	Communications	$ 5,768.78	0.4		$ -	$ 5,768.78	0.3		$ 480.73
	Credit Card Fee's	$ 5,600.00	0.4		$ -	$ 5,600.00	0.3		$ 466.67
	Charitable Contribution	$ 3,564.60	0.2		$ -	$ 3,564.60	0.2		$ 297.05
	Client Care (Flowers)	$ 3,694.34	0.2		$ -	$ 3,694.34	0.2		$ 307.86
	Insurance - Liability	$ 6,598.00	0.4		$ -	$ 6,598.00	0.4		$ 549.83
	License	$ 2,356.03	0.2		$ -	$ 2,356.03	0.1		$ 196.34
	Office Supplies	$ 5,678.99	0.4		$ -	$ 5,678.99	0.3		$ 473.25
	Shipping	$ 2,767.34	0.2		$ -	$ 2,767.34	0.2		$ 230.61
	Taxes -Sales	$ 62,500.00	4.2		$ 3,000.00	$ 65,500.00	4.0		$ 5,458.33
		$ 118,321.27	7.9		$ 5,679.42	$ 124,000.69	7.5		$ 10,333.39
Facility	Cable/Satellite Television	$ 600.00	0.0		$ -	$ 600.00	0.0		$ 50.00
	Cell Phone	$ 2,456.87	0.2		$ -	$ 2,456.87	0.1		$ 204.74
	Electricity	$ 5,115.85	0.3		$ -	$ 5,115.85	0.3		$ 426.32
	Natural Gas/Water/Sew	$ 3,657.98	0.2		$ -	$ 3,657.98	0.2		$ 304.83
	Building Maintenance	$ 2,398.09	0.2		$ -	$ 2,398.09	0.1		$ 199.84
	Equipment Maint.	$ 1,529.88	0.1		$ -	$ 1,529.88	0.1		$ 127.49
	Equipment Purchase	$ 4,800.00	0.3		$ -	$ 4,800.00	0.3		$ 400.00
	Equipment Lease	$ 6,720.97	0.4		$ -	$ 6,720.97	0.4		$ 560.08
	Insurance- Property	$ 2,987.34	0.2		$ -	$ 2,987.34	0.2		$ 248.95
	Rent	$ 54,698.30	3.6		$ -	$ 54,698.30	3.3		$ 4,558.19
		$ 84,965.28	5.7		$ -	$ 84,965.28	5.1		$ 7,080.44
DVM	Payroll-DVM-Owner	$ 125,000.00	8.3		$ 6,000.00	$ 131,000.00	7.9		$ 10,916.67
	Cont Ed	$ 1,427.88	0.1		$ -	$ 1,427.88	0.1		$ 118.99
	Insurance Health	$ 4,800.00	0.3		$ 230.40	$ 5,030.40	0.3		$ 419.20
	Insurance Workers Comp	$ -	0.0		$ -	$ -	0.0		$ -
	sIRA	$ -	0.0		$ -	$ -	0.0		$ -
	Taxes-Payroll	$ 8,750.00	0.6		$ -	$ 8,750.00	0.5		$ 729.17
	Unemployment	$ 1,250.00	0.1		$ -	$ 1,250.00	0.1		$ 104.17
			0.0						

FIGURE 20-14 Budget for 2014.

Continued

can be used. The total amount of the dental revenue divided by the total gross revenue and multiplied by 100 gives the percentage needed for comparison purposes.

Figure 20-15 lists dental services as producing $45,000 for the 2013 fiscal year. Gross revenue produced $1.5 million. The sum of $45,000 divided by $1.5 million equals 0.03. To express this number as a percentage, $0.03 \times 100 = 3\%$. Therefore 3% of gross revenue is contributed by the dental revenue center. The practice can then set goals to increase this number the following year. If this number is lower than the previous year, management can implement changes to prevent this number from decreasing further.

DVM	Payroll-DVM-Assoc	$	202,403.24	13.5	$	9,715.36	$	212,118.60	12.9		$	16,676.55
	Cont Ed	$	3,450.00	0.2	$	-	$	3,450.00	0.2		$	287.50
	Insurance Health	$	9,600.00	0.6	$	460.80	$	10,060.80	0.6		$	838.40
	Insurance Workers Comp	$	234.10	0.0	$	-	$	234.10	0.0		$	19.51
	sIRA	$	2,622.40	0.2	$	-	$	2,622.40	0.2		$	218.53
	Taxes- Payroll	$	8,986.76	0.6	$	-	$	8,986.76	0.5		$	748.90
	Unemployment	$	1,650.87	0.1	$	-	$	1,650.87	0.1		$	137.57
		$	**370,175.25**	**24.7**	**$**	**17,768.41**	**$**	**387,943.66**	**23.5**		**$**	**32,328.64**
Non DVM	Payroll-Non-DVM	$	190,987.54	12.7	$	9,167.40	$	200,154.94	12.1		$	16,679.58
	Insurance-Health	$	3,600.00	0.2	$	172.80	$	3,772.80	0.2		$	314.40
	Insurance- Workers Comp	$	2,106.90	0.1	$	-	$	2,106.90	0.1		$	175.58
	sIRA	$	7,756.45	0.5	$	-	$	7,756.45	0.5		$	646.37
	Taxes- Payroll	$	6,678.90	0.4	$	-	$	6,678.90	0.4		$	556.58
	Unemployment	$	7,176.00	0.5	$	-	$	7,176.00	0.4		$	598.00
		$	**218,305.79**	**14.6**	**$**	**10,478.68**	**$**	**228,784.47**	**13.9**		**$**	**19,065.37**
	Total Expenses	$	1,026,289.42	**68.4**	$	49,261.89	$	1,075,551.31	65.2		$	89,629.28
	Revenue-Expenses=PROFIT	$	623,710.58	**15.9**	$	29,938.11	$	653,648.69	39.6		$	54,470.72

FIGURE 20-14, cont'd

Revenue Centers 2013 ABC Animal Hospital

Projected Rate of Growth   10%   2014

10% = $1,650,000.00

Column 1	Column 2	Column 3	Column 4	Column 5	Column 6
Examination	$ 240,000.00	16.0%	$ 24,000.00	$ 264,000.00	16%
Professional Service	$ 60,000.00	4.0%	$ 6,000.00	$ 66,000.00	4%
Laboratory Fees	$ 270,000.00	18.0%	$ 27,000.00	$ 297,000.00	18%
Imaging	$ 67,500.00	4.5%	$ 6,750.00	$ 74,250.00	5%
Dentistry	$ 45,000.00	3.0%	$ 4,500.00	$ 49,500.00	3%
Vaccines	$ 105,000.00	7.0%	$ 10,500.00	$ 115,500.00	7%
Hospitalization	$ 45,000.00	3.0%	$ 4,500.00	$ 49,500.00	3%
Surgery	$ 90,000.00	6.0%	$ 9,000.00	$ 99,000.00	6%
Anesthesia	$ 60,000.00	4.0%	$ 6,000.00	$ 66,000.00	4%
Pharmacy	$ 210,000.00	14.0%	$ 21,000.00	$ 231,000.00	14%
Flea, Tick and HW	$ 135,000.00	9.0%	$ 13,500.00	$ 148,500.00	9%
Diets	$ 75,000.00	5.0%	$ 7,500.00	$ 82,500.00	5%
OTC/Retail	$ 30,000.00	2.0%	$ 3,000.00	$ 33,000.00	2%
Boarding	$ 37,500.00	2.5%	$ 3,750.00	$ 41,250.00	3%
Bathing/Grooming	$ 30,000.00	2.0%	$ 3,000.00	$ 33,000.00	2%
	$ 1,500,000.00	100.0%	$ 150,000.00	$ 1,650,000.00	100%

FIGURE 20-15 Example of predicted revenue centers for 2014.

Denise Tumblin (Wutchiett Tumblin and Associates) has created a chart that highlights the average percentages produced by ideal income centers. The goal is to achieve these percentages; it is important to remember that many factors contribute to revenue, and not all practices may be able to meet these percentages, but they can strive to get as close as possible (Box 20-11).

Profits

Last but not least, profits must also be budgeted. Remaining profits may also use the top-down approach, using previous percentages in the future budget. If profits are inadequate to achieve goals, additional assessments are needed and a price increase for professional services may be warranted. The goal is to obtain the necessary profit to allow adequate return on investment and reinvestment to the practice. See the section "Analyzing Profits" later in this chapter for additional information.

PRACTICE POINT   Profits must also be budgeted, just as income and expenses are.

Areas of Expense

Equipment Budget

When creating a budget for equipment, two topics need to be kept in mind: the maintenance of existing equipment and the

BOX 20-11	Average Benchmark Income Percentages, Adapted from Benchmarks 2013: A Study of Well-Managed Practices
Exam	14.0%
Professional services	3.8%
Laboratory	18.8%
Imaging	4.9%
Dentistry	2.5%
Vaccines	6.8%
Hospitalization	2.4%
Surgery	5.5%
Anesthesia	3.7%
Pharmacy	13.7%
Flea, tick, and heartworm	7.9%
Diets	4.2%
OTC/retail	1.0%
Boarding	3.0%
Bathing & grooming	1.2%

BOX 20-12	Break-Even Analysis

Price of equipment ÷ (Client cost − cost to produce service)

$$\frac{\$11,000}{\$88 - \$22} = \frac{\$11,000}{\$66} = 167 \text{ views to break even}$$

purchase of new equipment. Existing equipment may need repairs, or there may be maintenance agreements that must be kept. When purchasing new equipment, several issues must be addressed:

• Is the equipment completely new, or is it replacing an existing piece of equipment?
• Is the new piece of equipment going to provide improved, more accurate results compared with the piece it is replacing?
• Is the money used to purchase the new equipment being used in the most efficient manner?
• How will the equipment be paid for? Cash? Leasing? Financing?
• If the practice is going to finance the capital, what is the interest rate? Can a better rate be found elsewhere? How much are the doctors going to use this piece of equipment?
• What will the client charge be?
• How long will it take to achieve the payback period?
• How long will it take to make a profit on the equipment?

If a budget has been created in advance, cash should be set aside for an equipment purchase. This is the smartest, most economical way to pay for equipment because practices will not accumulate application fees, finance charges, or late penalties if a late payment is sent.

Equipment leasing should be used with caution because finance charges are built into the payment. Interest rates tend to be higher for leases, and a balloon payment may be due at the end of the lease period if the practice wants to keep the equipment. Other options include returning the equipment at the end of the lease, which leaves the practice without any equipment. This may be of benefit to some practices if they want to purchase a new and updated piece of equipment at the end of the lease. If a piece of equipment has a short life and is replaced with an update quickly, leasing may be the best option. However, most pieces of equipment in veterinary medicine hold value and provide service for a

long period, especially when correct maintenance and repair schedules are followed. Companies offer low payments that entice practices to lease equipment; however, all options should be examined before making a decision.

When borrowing money, practices must consider the financing rate and the length of time the money will be borrowed. Cash flow projections of revenue and expenses should be developed as well as a payback plan. Credit lines should not be used for equipment purchases because they generally have to be fully paid within a year and are better to leave for emergency withdrawals if needed. Equipment loan lengths should not exceed the expected life of the piece of equipment, normally 5 to 7 years.

A break-even analysis should be completed before purchasing the equipment. The break-even point is the point at which the sales of the service will cover all costs related to the equipment, including maintenance, supplies, and the capital itself. A break-even point can be determined by dividing the total cost of the equipment by the cost to the client. The resulting number gives the number of times the service must be performed to break even (Box 20-12). For example, a practice wants to purchase a digital dental radiograph unit. The unit originally costs $11,000. The practice will charge the client $88 for a set of radiographs. The cost associated with taking the radiographs is $22; this includes the technician's time to take the views and the veterinarian's time to interpret the views. $88 − $22 = $66. $11,000 divided by $66 equals 166.67 views; therefore 167 views must be taken to break even with a digital dental radiograph unit. If two dentals are completed on a daily basis, and both dentals have radiographs completed, it will take 83 business days to recover the cost of the equipment.

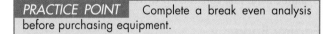

PRACTICE POINT Complete a break even analysis before purchasing equipment.

Payroll Budget

Payroll is the largest expense in the operating budget and, depending on the practice, can be considered a variable or fixed expense. Practices that are busy year-round and have a similar payroll each period can consider payroll a fixed expense. Practices that are busy in the summer and slow in the winter should consider payroll a variable expense because it changes with the revenue of the practice (however, for benchmarking purposes, staff payroll is considered a variable expense).

Veterinary practice managers manage payroll.

To help with budget estimations, a weighted hourly wage may be used for each employee. A weighted hourly wage takes the average of a team member's pay when a raise will be expected later in the fiscal year. The original pay plus the new pay divided by two gives the weighted hourly wage.

When developing a payroll budget, it should be remembered that not every employee would receive a raise each year. Raises should be based on team member skills, assets and meeting of performance expectations, not on length of employment. Some practices may give a cost-of-living raise; those team members who have achieved new skills and have proven competency should receive more.

A maximum amount should be determined each year for payroll, allowing for raises, bonuses, and an allocation for new team members if needed. If the practice does not hire a new team member, the funds can be disbursed as a bonus to all employees. Team members can be ranked from most valuable to least valuable. Raises can be disbursed as management feels appropriate, reaching the amount set aside for the payroll budget. When estimating projected gross income increases, consider which individuals will help produce that gross, and determine raises or bonuses accordingly.

Remember to review employees who receive minimum wage, and keep abreast of the changes in minimum wage at both the federal and state levels. Both federal and state minimum wages can change at any time.

Overtime eats practice profits. Team members' schedules should be created with the intent to decrease the amount of overtime the practice has to pay.

If payroll costs are more than anticipated, the answer may be to improve scheduling to make better use of staff time. Another solution is to increase revenues so that support staff cost, as a percentage of gross, stays in line with practice health.

Do not forget that the staff is the center of the client's customer service experience. Thinning staff hours to meet a budgeted payroll could be detrimental to income generation. The budget and customer service must be balanced—a great manager can make this occur with a positive culture and a dynamic team that consistently drives revenue.

Facility Budget

The practice structure and property must be maintained; however, improvements will need to be made at some point. Just as with equipment, paying cash instead of obtaining a loan for such improvements is better for cash flow. In addition, emergencies can occur (leaky roof, natural disaster, etc.), and money should be available to tend to emergencies when needed.

> **PRACTICE POINT** | Create a budget for facility maintenance and enhancement. Modernized facilities bring value to the practice.

Analyzing Profits

The bottom line should be the remaining profits after expenses have been subtracted from the revenue. If this profit number is not high enough, adjustments must be made to both revenue and expense categories.

In Figure 20-13, the profits for ABC Animal Hospital during 2013 were $473,710.58, or 15.9%. This is an excellent percentage and a goal that each practice should strive for. It is advised to reinvest at least 10% of the profits back into the practice on an annual basis. This allows the budgeting of equipment, building maintenance and upgrades, team incentives, and an owner's return on investment for the 2013 fiscal year. To maintain this profit for 2014, a budget must be created and implemented.

Important Points to Remember

Creating budgets is a trial and error process. It is based on assumptions, and mistakes will occur. Future, unpredictable events can occur and will affect projections in ways beyond the practice's control. Natural disasters such as hurricanes or tornados can affect the practice as well as the economy surrounding the practice. Therefore it can be detrimental to project more than 3 years in advance.

Creating a budget also has a learning curve. Effectively collecting and adding data occurs during year one. Tweaks will have to be made, and investigations into discrepancies will help the owner/manager understand what worked and what did not work. Year two will be more successful, with fewer tweaks needed and more goals achieved. By year three, owners/managers must hold themselves accountable for meeting budgeted goals. The learning curve must be surmounted; expecting 100% success the first year is detrimental and will cause an owner/manager to give up. Budgeting is a highly powerful tool that every practice MUST implement.

Once a budget has been created, teams can effectively look at subcategories, determine what areas are controllable, and make an impact on those areas. It is essential to communicate the budget to the staff. Numbers, projections, and goals should be posted for the team to share. Goals should be celebrated when they have been achieved, and brainstorming sessions should be held when they have not been met. The team environment goes beyond working together and satisfying clients; it is also about helping and contributing to the success of the practice. Increased profits lead to increased salaries for team members, allow greater reinvestment into the practice, and increase the owner's profits. These lead to a satisfied team that will work efficiently, intelligently, and happily, because an exceptional place of employment has been created.

Cash Flow

Cash flow is defined as the movement of money into and out of a business, usually during a specified period of time. Many managers are under the perception that the bottom line on a profit and loss statement should equal the balance in the

checking account. However, this is untrue, as several discrepancies do exist:

- Inventory purchased is sitting on shelves and has not sold
- Accounts receivable have not been settled
- Bills have been paid, but have not yet cleared checking account

A cash flow statement will give a snapshot of the checking account, with the net income for the period being analyzed as stated.

Unfortunately, many practices have cash flow issues; cash is not available to pay accounts payable. Several reasons exist for cash flow crunches, including:

- Mismanaged inventory (excess product sitting on shelves)
- Mismanaged payroll (excess overtime)
- Embezzlement
- Large dividends paid to owner(s) when income is low or nonexistent

Cash flow issues must be addressed and corrected as soon as possible to keep the practice doors open.

Open-Book Management

Sharing the finances with the team will create accountability. It was stated earlier that the team only sees the cash coming into the practice in a daily basis; they do not see the costs associated with maintaining the business. Team members often compare their paycheck to the daily totals (and do not know all of the additional taxes a practice pays on individual employees).

Team members want to know how to contribute to the practice; keeping the finances a secret prevents employees from having a full understanding of the business. Owners and managers may start with sharing KPIs and benchmarks, slowly moving into a summarized P&L. By showing team members how the dots are connected, they will buy into practice recommendations, which results in less resistance when policies are implemented. If they do not understand the *why* and the *how,* team members will continue with old habits, preventing the practice from moving forward.

Developing goals and budgets as a team contributes to an overall positive culture within the practice, increasing accountability, productivity, and team morale.

Building Value in the Practice

There are many factors that contribute to the value of a practice. It is advisable to have the practice valued every few years, to ensure the value is continuously increasing. Industry trends are showing that for many years, practices have "flown by the seat of their pants," and profitability has been at a standstill. When these practices wish to sell, there is little to no value in the hospital. For years, owners planned that when they sold their practice, it would be their retirement. Unfortunately, this is not the case. Visit www.vetpartners.com for more detailed information on obtaining a practice valuation from a professional. Consider building value in the hospital now, before plans for selling come into play.

> **PRACTICE POINT** Medical records, client retention, team member retention, building appearance, modern equipment, and financial records all contribute to the value of a practice.

Factors to help build value include (but are not limited to):

Medical records: Are recommendations being made? Are medical records complete and legible? If recommendations are not being made (or they are, but client compliance rates are low), the practice value is decreased. Why would a perspective buyer purchase a practice that has low client compliance and poor record keeping?

Clients: Obviously, clients fall into the category of goodwill, but what is being done to increase the goodwill value? Goodwill is driven by reputation. Are clients recommending friends and family? Is that being tracked? What is the client compliance rate? Are they accepting the recommendations being made? What is the practice doing to build and maintain the reputation of the hospital? Client feedback should be mandatory: listening to clients, identifying their needs, and meeting their needs will drive goodwill. This will keep clients coming back, and referring new clients to the practice. In addition, goodwill must be able to be transferred to a new owner. For example, if Smith Veterinary Hospital is strictly built around Dr. Smith (and not the team), can the goodwill be transferred? Probably not; it will, therefore lower the value. However, if Apple Orchard Veterinary Hospital has built the reputation on Apple Orchard, the team, and all of the associates (not just Dr. Smith), a higher value will transfer to the new owner.

Team members: Employee retention rates say a lot about a hospital. If a team has been with a practice for a long time, the value can increase. High turnover rate leads to decreased client compliance and loyalty. Consider investing in the staff through continuous team training; creating and sharing the mission, visions, and values of the hospital; and creating an organizational structure. Mismanaged teams reduce the value of the practice.

Building: Buildings must look appealing to draw new clients and keep clients returning. Old buildings that do not have curb appeal significantly decrease the practice value (Figure 20-16). Buildings must be maintained and updated frequently (interior and exterior). Consider the reception and exam rooms. What do they look and smell like? Claustrophobic, dark, and smelling of urine? Or, clean, light, and airy?

Equipment: Equipment must be modern and suitable for producing an income.

Financial records: Creating, maintaining, and analyzing financial data is critical. Simply reviewing data on a monthly basis can increase profits; imagine what creating a budget can do?

Revenue: Continuously plan how to increase the income produced by the hospital. Making a profit is impossible without revenue. Do not plan on annual price increases to do the trick.

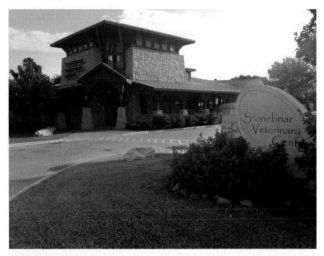

FIGURE 20-16 Modern and updated buildings bring value to the practice. (Photo courtesy Stanton Foster, Stonebriar Veterinary Centre, and Dr. Jennifer Wilcox.)

Profits: Continuously increase profits. Hospitals must look to meet and exceed the profits of previous years. In addition, reinvest a minimum of 10% of the year's profits into something that brings income back into the hospital. Consider team training, profit centers, equipment, building maintenance or upgrades, and marketing.

Planning Retirement

Because the value of practices is much less than owners usually estimate, retirement planning outside of the practice must be considered. It is highly advised to visit with a retirement specialist to start this plan early. Many owners work hard (80 hours a week, with emergencies) for 20 to 30 years to find out their practice is worth a quarter of what they planned for. Start increasing the value of the hospital, and create a proper exit strategy, preventing the hospital from simply closing the doors when an owner is ready to retire.

Red Flags Rule

Managers must be familiar with the Red Flags Rule developed by the Federal Trade Commission (FTC) in 2010. The Red Flags Rule was established to protect against identity theft. It requires many businesses and organizations to establish an identity theft prevention program to detect the warning signs, or red flags, of identity theft in their daily operations. By identifying red flags in advance, businesses will be better equipped to spot suspicious patterns that may arise and take steps to prevent a red flag from escalating into a costly episode of identity theft.

> **PRACTICE POINT**   Red Flags Rule should be recognized in every practice, helping to decrease fraud and identity theft.

Veterinary practices have been released from being held to standards of the Red Flags Rule (as of September 2013),

however, it should be a top priority of every manager to prevent identify theft from occurring within the hospital. Consider the following guidelines to prevent identity theft in the practice:

- Do not maintain client credit numbers in files
- Do not ask for/maintain client social security numbers in files
- Verify identity of client when payment is accepted by checks or credit cards
- Confidential employee information must be secured in a locked cabinet
- Consider how to safely accept credit card payments over the phone, ensuring the person providing the information has the authority to authorize the transaction

Many cases of identity theft occur when employees steal credit card numbers and personal information from clients. Prevent security issues from affecting the hospital by implementing safe and secure policies.

⚖ VETERINARY PRACTICE and the LAW

Although veterinary practices have been exempt from the Red Flags Rule, there is no reason every person on the team should not be accountable for reducing the number of fraud cases and stolen identities. Identity theft is growing, and it's a very lucrative crime. Unlike stolen cash, stereos, or drugs, identities can be sold over and over again. People whose identities are stolen spend countless hours and dollars trying to fix their credit rating and reestablishing their reputations. Often, irreparable damage is done to the victim's identity. Many people believe identity theft is only financial in nature, but this is not true. It actually can include any aspect of one's identity, including medical, driver's license, Social Security, professional, criminal, and financial identities.

As a respected member of the veterinary community, each team member has ethical and legal responsibilities to protect clients' and employees' personal information as much as possible. Team members do not want it to happen to them, nor do they wish to carry the blame for the theft of a client's identity.

REVIEW QUESTIONS

1. Define benchmarking, and describe the difference between internal and external benchmarks.
2. What is the difference between a CPA and a bookkeeper?
3. What is the purpose of a client survey?
4. What is a key performance indicator and why are they important to track?
5. Why should a budget be created?
6. What is a variable expense? Give some examples.
7. What is a fixed cost? Give some examples.
8. Define some areas that could cause a cash flow crunch.
9. How can a manager increase the value of a hospital?
10. Define the Red Flags Rule, and discuss why it should be implemented by the veterinary practice.

11. If a practice reports services when they are invoiced, they are said to report by which standard?
    a. Cash basis
    b. Accrual basis
12. Current accounts receivable percentages should not exceed:
    a. 1.5%
    b. 2.5%
    c. 3%
    d. 4.5%
13. Staff payroll is considered a _____ expense for benchmarking purposes.
    a. Fixed
    b. Variable
14. Approximately what percentage of gross revenue is lost because of missed charges?
    a. 1%
    b. 5%
    c. 10%
    d. 20%

15. In order to maximize revenue, a practice manager may:
    a. Cut payroll
    b. Negotiate contracts
    c. Analyze fee schedules
    d. Shop for lower credit card finance fees

Recommended Reading

AAHA: *Financial and productivity pulsepoints*, ed 7, Lakewood, CO, 2012, AAHA Press.

Chamblee J, Reiboldt M: *Financial management of the veterinary practice*, Lakewood, CO, 2010, AAHA Press.

National Commission of Veterinary Economic Issues: A service of AVMA, (Web site): www.ncvei.org. Accessed August 15, 2013.

Opperman M: *Veterinary practices miss $64,000 in fees each year*, 2010; Veterinary Economics. http://veterinarybusiness.dvm360.com/vetec/article/articleDetail.jsp?id=685134.

Wutchiett Tumblin and Associates: *Benchmarks 2013: a study of well-managed practices*, 2013, Veterinary Economics.

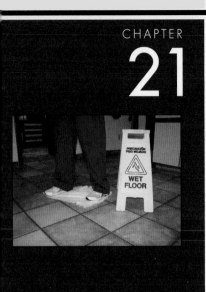

Safety in the Veterinary Practice

Zoonotic Diseases, *359*
  Disease Transmission, *362*
  Control of Zoonotic Diseases, *362*
Occupational Safety and Health
  Administration, *362*
  Employer Responsibilities, *363*
  Employee Responsibilities, *363*
  Administrative Tasks, *363*
  Inspections, *363*
  Hazard Communication: The Right to
    Know, *363*
  Physical Hazards in the Veterinary
    Practice, *368*

Chemical Hazards in the Veterinary
  Practice, *373*
  Diamond Labeling System, *378*
  Biohazards in the Veterinary Practice, *381*
  Radiation Safety, *382*
  Laser Safety, *383*
  Accident Reporting and Investigation, *384*
  Documentation, *387*
Developing and Implementing Safety
  Protocols, *387*
  Implementation, *390*
  The Hospital Safety Manual, *390*

KEY TERMS

Biohazard
Carcinogen
First Notice of Accident
Hospital Safety Manual
Occupational Safety and
  Health Administration
  (OSHA)
OSHA 300
OSHA 300A
Permissible Exposure
  Limits
Personal Protective
  Equipment (PPE)
Safety Data Sheet (SDS)
Scavenger System
The Right to Know
Waste Anesthetic Gases
Zoonotic Disease

LEARNING OBJECTIVES

When you have completed this chapter, you should be able to:

1. Identify zoonotic diseases.
2. Describe methods used to prevent the transmission of zoonotic diseases.
3. Identify the hazards associated with veterinary medicine.
4. List methods used to lift equipment and animals appropriately.
5. Define the role of the Occupational Safety and Health Administration.
6. Develop safety protocols.
7. Define the right to know.

8. Define employer and employee rights and responsibilities as outlined by OSHA.
9. Develop and implement a hospital safety manual.
10. Discuss and implement a training program.
11. Describe how to prevent fires and promote a safe working environment.
12. Interpret Safety Data Sheets (SDS).
13. Discuss methods used to prevent the escape of animals.

CRITICAL COMPETENCIES

1. **Adaptability** - being open to change and flexible work methods; the ability to adapt behavior to changing conditions or new information.
2. **Analytical Skills** - the ability to analyze information and use logic to address problems; the ability to quickly and accurately grasp complex information and concepts and to make correct inferences.
3. **Compliance** - being reliable, thorough, and conscientious in carrying out work assignments; has an appreciation for the importance of organizational rules and policies.
4. **Continuous Learning** - a curiosity for learning; actively seek out new

information, technologies, and methods; keep skills updated and apply new knowledge to the job.
5. **Critical and Strategic Thinking** - the ability to think critically about situations and to understand the relevance of information for different problems; use critical reasoning to generate and evaluate alternative courses of action or points of view relevant to an issue.
6. **Decision Making** - the ability to make good decisions, solve problems, and decide on important matters; the ability to gather and analyze relevant data and choose decisively between alternatives.

7. **Integrity** - honesty, trustworthiness, and adherence to high standards of ethical conduct.
8. **Leadership** - a willingness to lead and take charge; the ability to motivate others and mobilize group effort toward common goals.
9. **Oral Communication and Comprehension** - the ability to express one's thoughts verbally in a clear and understandable manner, and the ability to actively listen and attend to what others are saying; must have good group presentation skills.
10. **Persuasion** - the ability to change the attitudes and opinions of others and to persuade them to accept recommendations and change behavior.
11. **Planning and Prioritizing** - the ability to effectively manage time and work load to meet deadlines; the ability to organize work, set priorities, and establish plans for achieving goals.
12. **Resourcefulness** - the ability to understand what it takes to complete the job; apply knowledge, skills, and expertise to perform tasks quickly and efficiently.
13. **Writing and Verbal Skills** - ability to comprehend written material easily and accurately; ability to express thoughts clearly and succinctly in writing.

In the law and ethics domain, the veterinary practice manager monitors the procedures and policies of the practice to determine whether events and processes comply with laws, regulations, or standards.

Knowledge Requirements

The tasks related to legal and ethical standards require knowledge of state/provincial and federal laws, legal codes, government regulations, professional standards, and agency rules.

Many hazards exist in a veterinary practice, and each team member must be aware of all hazards. Every employee must be proactive and prevent hazards from occurring, keeping the facility safe for all team members, patients, and clients.

It is essential to prevent the transmission of zoonotic diseases, which can spread from animal to human and may spread by different methods depending on the disease. Team members must be made aware of diseases that are transmissible to them and take all precautions necessary to prevent transmission. Some diseases can be treated, whereas others may be fatal.

The Occupational Safety and Health Administration (OSHA) was developed in 1970 to ensure employee safety. Every employer must provide a safe working environment for all team members, and OSHA will severely penalize those that do not follow regulations. OSHA oversees all workplace hazards, including the safe use and disposal of chemicals. Each practice must have Safety Data Sheets (SDSs) available for quick reference in case any team member is exposed to a chemical hazard. SDSs provide information regarding the chemical, specifications for cleanup and exposure, as well as any special properties the chemical possesses. SDSs were originally called MSDSs, Material Safety Data Sheets. In order to become compliant with worldwide standards, the term SDS became effective in 2014. The impact on the conversion will be minimal for veterinary hospitals and must be done to stay compliant with OSHA standards.

> **PRACTICE POINT** SDSs (Safety Data Sheets) have replaced the term MSDS, effective 2014.

Safety manuals should be developed by veterinary hospitals for team members. Often, a safety officer is appointed, who is in charge of developing, implementing, and maintaining safety manuals, allowing the practice to remain compliant with OSHA standards. Safety manuals aid in the creation and implementation of a safe working environment and serve as a training tool for team members. These are required by OSHA and must include safety plans. Hazards and emergencies will happen in the veterinary practice, and team members must be prepared to handle them.

Zoonotic Diseases

Zoonosis is defined as a disease that may be directly or indirectly transmitted to humans from wild or domesticated animals. More than 1400 diseases are currently known to be zoonotic, of which 60% are caused by pathogens known to cross species lines. The need to educate the public and veterinary practice team members is imperative, because veterinarians may be held liable for the transmission of such diseases. Veterinarians play a vital role in public health and control of zoonotic diseases (Table 21-1).

TABLE 21-1	Zoonotic Diseases				
	CAUSATIVE ORGANISM	**SMALL-ANIMAL HOST**	**LIVESTOCK HOST**	**WILDLIFE HOST**	**MODE OF TRANSMISSION**
Bacterial Infection					
Anthrax	*Bacillus anthracis*	Dogs	Cattle, sheep, horses, goats	Most except primates	Contact
Brucellosis	*Brucella melitensis*	Dogs	Cattle, pigs, sheep, goats	All except primates	Contact, inhalation, ingestion
Campylobacteriosis	*Campylobacter fetus*	Dogs, cats	Cattle, poultry, sheep, pigs	Rodents, birds	Ingestion, contact
Capnocytophaga infection	*Capnocytophaga canimorsus*	Dogs, cats			Bite wound
Cat scratch disease	*Bartonella henselae*	Cats		Cats	Cat bite, scratch
Erysipelas	*Erysipelothrix rhusiopathiae*		Pigs, sheep, cattle, horses, poultry	Rodents	Contact
Leptospirosis	*Leptospira* spp.	All	All	Rats, raccoons	Contact with urine or birthing fluids
Lyme disease	*Borrelia burgdorferi*	Dogs, cats	Cattle, horses	Deer, birds, rodents	Tick bite
Pasteurellosis	*Pasteurella multocida*	Dogs, cats		Bite wound	
Plague	*Yersinia pestis*	Cats		Rodents, rabbits	Flea bite
Q fever	*Coxiella burnetii*		Cattle, sheep, goats	Birds, rabbits, rodents	Inhalation, milk ingestion, contact
Rat bite fever	*Streptobacillus moniliformis*			Rats	Rat bite
Salmonellosis	*Salmonella* spp.	All	All	Rodents, reptiles	Ingestion
Tetanus	*Clostridium tetani*		Horses	Reptiles	Wound
Tuberculosis	*Mycobacterium tuberculosis*	Dogs, cats	Cattle, pigs, sheep, goats, poultry	All except rodents and monkeys	Ingestion, inhalation
Tularemia	*Francisella tularensis*	All	All except horses	Rodents, rabbits	Tick bite, contact with tissue
Fungal Diseases					
Cryptococcosis	*Cryptococcus neoformans*			Birds	Contact
Ringworm	*Trichophyton* spp.	Dogs, cats	Cattle, horses, pigs, sheep	Rodents	Contact
Parasitic Infection					
Cryptosporidiosis	*Cryptosporidium parvum*		Cattle		Ingestion
Hydatid disease	Echinococcus	Dogs	Herbivores	Wolves	Ingestion
Larva migrans	*Toxocara, Ancylostoma, Strongyloides* spp.	Dogs, cats	Pigs, cattle	Raccoons	Ingestion
Scabies	*Sarcoptes scabiei*	Dogs, cats, rodents	Horses	Primates	Contact
Schistosomiasis	*Schistosoma*	Dogs, cats	Pigs, cattle, horses	Rodents	Contact
Taeniasis cysticercosis	*Taenia*		Pigs, cattle	Boars	Ingestion
Toxoplasmosis	*Toxoplasma gondii*	Cats	Pigs, sheep, goats		Ingestion
Trichinosis	*Trichinella spiralis*		Pigs	Rats, bears, carnivores	Ingestion

TABLE 21-1	Zoonotic Diseases—cont'd				
	CAUSATIVE ORGANISM	SMALL-ANIMAL HOST	LIVESTOCK HOST	WILDLIFE HOST	MODE OF TRANSMISSION
Rickettsial Diseases					
Psittacosis	*Chlamydophila psittaci*	Psittacine birds	Ducks, turkeys	Birds	Inhalation
Rocky Mountain spotted fever	*Rickettsia rickettsii*	Dogs		Rodents, rabbits	Tick bite
Viral Diseases					
Contagious ecthyma (orf)	Poxvirus	Dogs	Sheep, goats		Contact
Encephalitis (EEE, WEE)	Togavirus		Horses, poultry	Birds, rodents	Mosquito bite
Hantavirus	Hantavirus			Rodents	Contact
Lymphocytic choriomeningitis	Arenavirus	Mice			Varied
Monkeypox	Orthopoxvirus			Rodents	Contact
Newcastle disease	Paramyxovirus	Domestic birds	Poultry	Wild fowl	Contact, inhalation
Rabies	Rhabdovirus, togavirus	Almost all	Most	Most	Animal bite
Simian herpes	Herpesvirus simiae			Primates	Animal bite, direct contact
Yellow fever	Togavirus			Primates	Mosquito bite
Protozoal Infection					
Balantidiasis	*Balantidium coli*		Pigs	Rats, primates	Ingestion
Cryptosporidiosis	*Cryptosporidium* spp.	Most	Calves, sheep	Birds	Ingestion
Giardiasis	*Giardia lamblia*	Dogs, cats	Pigs, cattle	Beavers, zoo monkeys	Ingestion
Sarcocystosis	*Sarcocystis*	Dogs, cats	Pigs, cattle		Ingestion
Toxoplasmosis	*Toxoplasma gondii*	Cats, rabbits, Guinea pigs	Pigs, sheep, cattle, horses	Cats	Ingestion

EEE, Eastern equine encephalitis; *WEE,* Western equine encephalitis.

Veterinarians are ethically required to educate the public about zoonotic diseases. Because public health has been addressed in the American Veterinary Medical Association (AVMA) Code of Ethics, many state boards and regulatory agencies have mandated such education, which can leave many veterinarians liable for a malpractice suit. To present a claim for malpractice, four elements must be proven: existence of a valid client-patient relationship, failure to practice the standard level of care, proximate cause, and harm that occurred to the patient as a result of substandard care. For more information on malpractice, see Chapter 4.

Once a patient has been presented to a practice for treatment, a client-patient relationship has been established. Because veterinarians have been trained in the risks and transmission of zoonotic diseases, it has become the standard of care for team members to educate the public. Therefore if a patient with a zoonotic disease is presented for treatment, it is the obligation of the veterinary practice not only to diagnose and treat it, but to also educate the client regarding the disease and to recommend that the client visit a physician to seek medical attention. If a patient has not been diagnosed with a zoonotic disease, it is standard of care to educate clients about potential zoonotic diseases that are present in the environmental area and advise methods of prevention, if available.

It is recommended that any new puppy or kitten brought to the practice be dewormed on the first visit. Puppies and kittens can easily transmit intestinal parasites, and this is the best opportunity to educate clients about these potential risks. If the veterinary practice initiates deworming protocols, sends clients home with material to read, and documents the procedure in the record, it has taken the initial steps to protect itself from a lawsuit.

If a practice educates a client about the risk of contracting a zoonotic disease and advises a treatment protocol to reduce the risk of contracting that disease and the client refuses the treatment, it must be documented in the record.

Team members should receive extensive training on zoonotic diseases and the precautions to take to decrease

the possibility of transmission. Employees should sign a statement indicating that they have received prevention training. General cleanliness, handwashing, and the use of disinfectants are essential and must be implemented in every practice's protocol to reduce transmission of disease.

Disease Transmission

The mode of disease transmission is important to understand when implementing a prevention program. Reservoirs and hosts must also be considered, as these are necessary in the transmission of infectious diseases. A *reservoir* is a place where an infectious organism survives and replicates, such a within an animal or the soil. A *host* is a living organism that offers an environment for maintenance of the organism but that may not be required for the organism's survival. Depending on the disease, the organism may be transmitted to more than one host or reservoir. Programs are generally aimed at reservoirs and hosts of diseases when control methods are being implemented.

Direct transmission of diseases requires close contact between the reservoir of the disease and the susceptible host. Contact with infected skin, mucous membranes, or droplets from the infected animal or human can cause disease. Soil or vegetation that is contaminated also serves as a method of direct transmission. *Indirect transmission* of diseases is more complex and involves intermediaries that carry the agent of disease from one source to another. A *vector* is a living organism that transports infectious agents. A *vehicle* is a mode of transmission of an infectious agent from the reservoir to the host. Airborne transmission involves spread of the agent through dust particles or droplet particles over long distances.

Arthropods, such as fleas, ticks, and mosquitoes, are considered vectors. They can carry an infectious agent to a susceptible host as well as be involved in the multiplication of organisms. They can also assist in a specific stage of development of the organism.

Food and water are vehicles of indirect transmission of disease; both may be sources of bacterial, viral, and parasitic diseases. Foodborne diseases are acquired by the consumption of contaminated food or water and may be caused by toxins released by bacteria that are contained in the food. Parasites can also be transmitted through food, either through the ingestion of eggs or undercooked meat that contains cysts.

Control of Zoonotic Diseases

Because of the contact veterinarians and veterinary technicians have with potentially infected pets, they may be the first to notice symptoms. It is important to recognize the most common diseases seen in a practice's local area and be knowledgeable about their symptoms, treatments, and prevention. Prevention programs require complete knowledge of the disease and how it is maintained to break the cycle of the disease. Prevention of disease may be aided by a vaccination for such diseases, water filtration, and excellent hygiene skills.

PRACTICE POINT Pregnant or immunocompromised individuals must take extra precautions and protect themselves against zoonotic diseases.

People at particular risk of zoonotic disease are those with compromised immune systems, such as those undergoing chemotherapy and/or treatment for HIV or AIDS. Pregnant women and individuals who have had their spleens removed are also immunocompromised and should use extra precaution when working with or around animals with zoonotic potential. Children may also be at a higher risk because they come into contact with contaminants in the outdoor environment.

Animal Bites

Animal bites can be a source of infection, trauma, and zoonotic diseases. An animal bite is defined as a bite wound that penetrates the skin, causing bleeding and swelling at the area. *Pasteurella* species are the most common bacteria present in both dog and cat bites (Talan, et al., 1999). Other bacteria that may be present in animal bites include *Staphylococcus aureus, Staphylococcus epidermidis, Streptococcus* spp., *Bacteroides* spp., *Fusobacterium* spp., and other gram-negative bacteria. In people, these bacteria can cause fever, septicemia, meningitis, endocarditis, and septic arthritis. Any team member who is bitten by a patient should wash the area well with warm, soapy water for at least 5 minutes, apply a dilute povidone-iodine (Betadine) solution, and then rinse with a strong stream of water. The team member should consider seeking medical attention, taking into account the potential risk for infection. If a team member declines to seek medical treatment, a form should be signed and placed in the employee's medical file. This is necessary for protecting the practice in a workers' compensation case.

Occupational Safety and Health Administration

It is the responsibility of every veterinary practice to remain in compliance with safety regulations at the local, state, and federal levels. The Occupational Safety and Health Administration (OSHA) enforces federal laws to ensure a safe workplace environment. These laws require employers to have a safety program that includes the training of employees.

Veterinary practice managers understand and ensure compliance with appropriate regulations at all government levels, including the OSHA Hazard Communication Standard, and state and local safety regulations.

Many states also have a state mandated OSHA program that is more stringent than federal programs. The practice should abide by whichever program is more strict.

Employer Responsibilities

- Provide a safe working environment
- Set and enforce safety rules
- Inform employees about the inherent risks associated with their jobs
- Provide and train on the proper use of personal protective equipment (PPE)

Employee Responsibilities

- Read the workplace rights poster (OSHA poster #3165) (Figure 21-1)
- Comply with safety standards determined by the hospital
- Use PPE that has been provided
- Report hazardous conditions to management
- Report any injuries received and seek immediate treatment for them

Penalties and fines exist for those who break the law. For example, not displaying the OSHA Job Safety and Health: It's the Law poster carries a $1000 fine. Other willful violations can exceed $70,000.

PRACTICE POINT Severe penalties exist for not complying with OSHA's safety program.

There are four sections to fulfilling OSHA's compliance and safety program:

1. Administrative tasks
2. Evaluation of the facility (hazard analysis)
3. PPE
4. Training program

Administrative Tasks

Administrative tasks include the posting of signs and information, along with training and documentation. The safety program must be in writing and placed in a central location. It should be available to all team members at all times.

Veterinary practice managers develop and manage personnel training programs and developmental programs (including safety training).

An evacuation plan should be displayed for clients and employees to see. A diagram of the practice should list potential hazards and safety equipment in each room. The diagram should include exits, circuit breakers, compressed gas cylinders, hazardous materials, and fire extinguishers. A fire evacuation plan is required for practices with 10 or more employees.

Inspections

OSHA has the right to inspect any veterinary practice. Every veterinary practice owner and or safety officer has the right to be present for an OSHA inspection. When developing the safety manual, practice owners/managers should appoint a specific person that is to be present, should an OSHA inspector arrive at the hospital. This document should be kept in the front of the safety manual, and all team members should be well aware of the inspection procedure. If the owner is not present and a representative has not been appointed, OSHA can be denied the opportunity to inspect the premises. If OSHA has a court order, however, it must be allowed in to inspect the premises. Arrangements must be made, and an inspection must occur within 72 hours of the initial visit. Safety officers and/or owners should walk through the premises with the inspection officer; never allow an untrained team member to act as escort.

The inspection notice must be posted on the staff bulletin board for all team members to see until the inspection has been completed. Copies of violations must be posted for at least 3 days or until the violation is corrected, whichever is longer. OSHA often returns, following up on violations that were noted on the initial inspection.

OSHA does not endorse products. Many companies use marketing tactics to say that their product is "OSHA approved" when, in reality, the product only meets OSHA standards.

Hazard Communication: The Right to Know

OSHA's Hazard Communication Standard requires that all team members who come in contact with hazards in the practice be aware of those hazards and instructed on how to protect themselves from those hazards (Table 21-2). This applies to all chemicals, including anesthetic gases, radiology chemicals, alcohol, and formalin. To establish compliance, a practice must have:

- A designated safety manager; this employee is responsible for training all team members and ensuring the safety program meets standard requirements
- A written safety plan
- A summary of all hazardous chemicals available, including injectable medications, pesticides, antiseptics/disinfectants, and laboratory agents, as well as those listed previously
- SDSs available at all times
- All chemical containers accurately labeled with descriptions and potential hazards, including when chemicals are transferred to other containers; an example is disinfectants that are transferred to a spray bottle to clean exam room tables
- An explanation of the labeling system
- A protocol for emergency evacuation
- A training program implementing the use of PPE and monitoring devices as well as the hazards of the practice; this is required for all practices with 11 or more employees

PRACTICE POINT SDSs must be available to any team member, at any time.

Hazard Analysis

When evaluating the facility, all potential hazards should be analyzed. Doors should have one-way locks, which allow clients and team members to escape from the inside at any time. Emergency lighting must be available to help

Job Safety and Health

It's the law!

OSHA®

Occupational Safety and Health Administration U.S. Department of Labor

EMPLOYEES:

· You have the right to notify your employer or OSHA about workplace hazards. You may ask OSHA to keep your name confidential.

· You have the right to request an OSHA inspection if you believe that there are unsafe and unhealthful conditions in your workplace. You or your representative may participate in that inspection.

· You can file a complaint with OSHA within 30 days of retaliation or discrimination by your employer for making safety and health complaints or for exercising your rights under the *OSH Act*.

· You have the right to see OSHA citations issued to your employer. Your employer must post the citations at or near the place of the alleged violations.

· Your employer must correct workplace hazards by the date indicated on the citation and must certify that these hazards have been reduced or eliminated.

· You have the right to copies of your medical records and records of your exposures to toxic and harmful substances or conditions.

· Your employer must post this notice in your workplace.

· You must comply with all occupational safety and health standards issued under the *OSH Act* that apply to your own actions and conduct on the job.

EMPLOYERS:

· You must furnish your employees a place of employment free from recognized hazards.

· You must comply with the occupational safety and health standards issued under the *OSH Act*.

*This free poster available from OSHA –
The Best Resource for Safety and Health*

Free assistance in identifying and correcting hazards or complying with standards is available to employers, without citation or penalty, through OSHA-supported consultation programs in each state.

1-800-321-OSHA (6742)
www.osha.gov

OSHA 3165-02 2012R

FIGURE 21-1 OSHA's Job Safety and Health – It's the Law poster.

TABLE 21-2	Occupational Hazards	
HAZARD	**ASSOCIATED PROBLEMS**	**COMMON SOLUTIONS**
Animal handling	Animal bites, zoonotic disease transmission	Proper restraint devices
Ethylene oxide	Spills, improper use	Proper safety training
Ergonomics	Back injuries	Proper lifting techniques
Facility hazards	Old lead paint, slippery tile	Update facility; nonskid shoes
Fire	Exiting facility promptly and safely	Fire evacuation plan, accessible extinguishers, emergency lighting
Food	Ingestion of toxic chemicals and organisms	Separate refrigerator; no food in working areas
Housekeeping	Chemical mixing and toxicities	Do not mix cleaning products
Medical waste	Poking or cutting self with needles, glass, or blades	Appropriate use of biohazard containers
Radiology	Radiation exposure, toxic chemicals	Safety training, use of personal protective equipment; ventilate room; do not mix chemicals
Violence	Disgruntled clients or employees, angry family members, thieves	Listen to comments made by team members and clients

guide clients and team members to exits in the event of an emergency or a power outage. Areas that should not be overlooked when evaluating the practice include but are not limited to:

- Air quality (good flow? even heating and cooling distribution?)
- Damaged equipment (broken rollers, exposed electrical wire, etc.)
- Distance between fire extinguishers
- Emergency lighting
- Ergonomics
- Fire alarms
- Lighting
- Proper lighting in all rooms
- Smoke alarms
- The use of extension cords
- Walking surfaces (smooth or uneven?)

 Veterinary practice managers monitor hospital violations and dangerous situations.

This hazard evaluation must be completed when the safety manual is being developed (Figure 21-2). It is also advised to complete an analysis each year, looking for any changes that may have occurred on the premises throughout the year. It is also recommended to have the entire team participate in a hazard analysis. More eyes will pick up hazards that are present, and help keep the team accountable when hazards do rise. Place this analysis in the binder documentation area.

PRACTICE POINT Complete a hazard analysis of the practice on a yearly basis.

Evaluation of Personal Protective Equipment

Under OSHA guidelines, PPE must be used (where available) at all times. This includes (but is not limited to) protective equipment for radiology, surgery, dentistry, and laboratory

Job Title:	Job Location:	Analyst	Date
Task #	Task Description:		
Hazard Type:	Hazard Description:		
Consequence:	Hazard Controls:		
Rational or Comment:			

FIGURE 21-2 Example of a hazard analysis that should be completed on an annual basis. (Courtesy Safety and Health Administration, Department of Labor, Washington, DC.)

functions. Eyewear must be worn when performing tasks that could inflict injury to the eye, and eyewash stations must be available for team members and clients to use in case of emergency. Review all areas of the hospital; list the PPE that is available, how to use it, and when it should be used (Figure 21-3). Train employees on each piece of PPE, then document the training with signature verification from each team member.

PPE HAZARD ASSESSMENT FORM

I am reviewing (check the appropriate box):	◉ A worksite	Specify location:	
		Name of employee:	
	☐ A single employee's job description	Position Title:	
	☐ A job description for a class of employees	Position Titles:	
		Location:	
Your Name:		**Department/Division:**	**Date:**

EYE HAZARDS: Tasks that can cause eye injury include: working with chemicals or acids; UV lights; chipping, sanding, or grinding; welding; furnace operations; and metal and wood working.

Check the appropriate box for each hazard:		Description of hazard(s):	Required PPE
Chemical Exposure	☐		
High Heat/Cold	☐		
Dust/Flying Debris	☐		
Impact	☐		
UV/IR Radiation	☐		
Other:			

HEAD/NECK/FACE HAZARDS: Tasks that can cause head/neck/face injury include: working below other workers who are using tools or materials that could fall, working on energized electrical equipment or utilities, and working in trenches or confined spaces.

Check the appropriate box for each hazard:		Description of hazard(s):	Required PPE
Chemical Exposure	☐		
Dust/Flying Debris	☐		
Impact	☐		
UV/IR Radiation	☐		
Electrical Shock	☐		
Other:			

FOOT HAZARDS: Tasks that can cause foot injury include: exposure to chemicals or acids, welding or cutting, materials handling, renovation or construction, and electrical work.

Check the appropriate box for each hazard:		Description of hazard(s):	Required PPE
Chemical Exposure	☐		
High Heat/Cold	☐		
Impact/Compression	☐		
Electrical	☐		
Puncture	☐		
Slippery/Wet Surfaces	☐		
Other:			

FIGURE 21-3 Example of a personal protective equipment assessment form used to evaluate available and needed PPE for the premises. (Courtesy Occupational Safety and Health Administration, Department of Labor, Washington, DC.)

Team Training

Staff training is imperative; without training, safety programs are useless. It is advisable to videotape training sessions; this not only provides training as new team members are added to the practice, but it also provides proof that a safety program exists if a complaint is ever filed against the practice.

All team members must be trained on the use of the safety manual and the right-to-know standards. Further training can be tailored to the particular job duties assigned to each position. For example, if the bookkeeper does not restrain pets, he or she does not need to receive training on proper method of animal restraint. However, if the receptionist occasionally restrains a patient, he or she must have the training, and the practice must document that training occurred.

When safety meetings begin, it is wise to cover the most serious hazards first while team members are paying attention. Less severe hazards can follow. Several training topics are required by OSHA, and each is covered in detail in the following sections (Box 21-1).

HAND HAZARDS: Hand injury can be caused by: work with chemicals or acids, exposure to cut or abrasion hazards (for example, during demolition, renovation, woodworking, or food service preparation), work with very hot or cold objects or materials, and exposure to sharps.

Check the appropriate box for each hazard:	Description of hazard(s):	Required PPE
Chemical Exposure ☐		
High Heat/Cold ☐		
UV/IR Radiation ☐		
Electrical Shock ☐		
Puncture ☐		
Cuts/Abrasion ☐		
Other:		

BODY HAZARDS: Injury of the body (torso, arms, or legs) can occur during: exposure to chemicals, acids, or other hazardous materials; abrasive blasting; welding, cutting, or brazing; chipping, sanding, or grinding; use of chainsaws or similar equipment; and work around electrical arcs.

Check the appropriate box for each hazard:	Description of hazard(s):	Required PPE
Chemical Exposure ☐		
High Heat/Cold ☐		
Impact/Compression ☐		
Electrical Arc ☐		
Cuts/Abrasion ☐		
Other:		

FALL HAZARDS: Personnel may be exposed to fall hazards when performing work on a surface with an unprotected side or edge that is 4 feet or more above a lower level, or 10 feet or more on scaffolds. Fall protection may also be required when using vehicle man lifts, elevated platforms, tree trimming, performing work on poles, roofs, or fixed ladders.

Check the appropriate box for each hazard:	Description of hazard(s):	Required PPE
Fall hazard ☐		

NOISE HAZARDS: Personnel may be exposed to noise hazards when working in mechanical rooms; machining; grinding; sanding; cage washing; dish washing; working around pneumatic equipment, grounds equipment, generators, chillers, motors, saws, jackhammers, or similar equipment.

Check the appropriate box for each hazard:	Description of hazard(s):	Required PPE
Noise hazard ☐		

RESPIRATORY HAZARDS: Personnel may be exposed to respiratory hazards that require the use of respirators: during emergency response, when using certain chemicals outside of a chemical fume hood; when working with hazardous powders; when entering fume hood plenums, when working with animals; when applying paints or chemicals in confined spaces; when welding, cutting, or brazing on certain metals; and when disturbing asbestos, lead, silica, or other particulate hazards.

Check the appropriate box for each hazard:	Description of hazard(s):	Required PPE
Chemical exposure		
Particulate exposure		
Other:		

I certify that the above hazard assessment was performed to the best of my knowledge and ability, based on the hazards present on this date.

_____ (signature)

FIGURE 21-3, cont'd

BOX 21-1 | Safety Topics

- Anesthetic gas safety
- Bite injuries
- Diamond labels and pictograms listing hazards associated with chemicals
- Emergency prevention plans
- Employees' rights and responsibilities
- Ethylene oxide
- Evacuating animals
- Formaldehyde
- Handling chemical spills
- Handling human blood
- How to use a fire extinguisher
- Location of SDSs and how to use and interpret
- Occupational noise exposure
- Personal protective equipment; use and location
- Proper lifting techniques
- Proper restraint
- Radiation safety
- Rendering first aid to humans

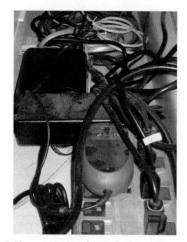

FIGURE 21-4 This is an extremely unsafe electrical box with six electrical plugs.

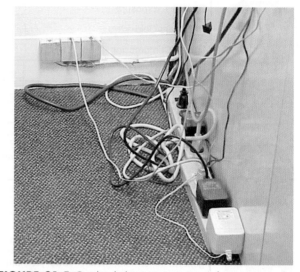

FIGURE 21-5 Overloaded surge suppressors of extension cords can start a fire. (From Bassert JM, McCurnin DM: *McCurnin's clinical textbook for veterinary technicians,* ed 7, St Louis, 2010, Saunders Elsevier.)

Physical Hazards in the Veterinary Practice

Each team member must practice safety while working in the practice. Many hazards exist, and everyone must be responsible for his or her own safety and prevention of injury. Moving equipment, slips, and lifting are a few causes of injuries that can be prevented. Team members should become diligent about washing their hands to prevent accidental ingestion of toxic substances as well as the spread of zoonotic diseases. Safety protocols must be developed and enforced; fire prevention, response, and rescues should be discussed among team members. Each person contributes a significant amount of time and energy to each practice, and each practice must protect these valuable team members.

> *PRACTICE POINT* Every team member must know what hazards exist with their job duties, and they should be outlined in the safety manual.

Animal Behavior and Restraint

There are a number of safety issues that are unique to veterinary hospitals, but none so much as animal behavior. Team member training should focus on animal psychology and restraint.

- Watch animal's body language
- Listen to the animal

Determine the types of restraint available, and outline how to use each. Restraint options fall into three categories: physical restraint (holding), chemical restraint (tranquilizers), and mechanical restraint (muzzles, poles, ropes, bags, or blankets).

Keep in mind that pain can cause a friendly dog to act out, and fear can cause a "good dog" to bite.

Electrical Safety

Electrical safety in the veterinary practice generally focuses on outlets and power cords. Overloaded circuits or faulty

wiring causes most fires in the veterinary practices (Figure 21-4). Therefore team members should frequently check cords for wear and tear, especially when cords are kept near patient cages. Check for crimps or breaks in the wires, either from cage doors or animal chewing.

Extension cords should only be used temporarily. If more outlets are needed, contact a certified electrician. Overloaded circuits should not be allowed. Receptacles, extension cords, surge protectors, or any plug multipliers must handle only the load they are meant to handle. Check the amperage of the equipment being used as well as the cord rating to be certain that it is not overloaded. Symptoms of electrical problems include frequently tripping circuits and lights that dim when large pieces of equipment are used.

Reviewing electrical safety should be a part of the hazard analysis completed each year (Figure 21-5).

Emergency Action Plan

OSHA requires an emergency action plan (EAP) to be written and placed in the safety manual. The EAP must list

potential reasons for an evacuation to occur and how the evacuation will be carried out. Consider the following conditions that *can* occur:

- Tornadoes
- Hurricanes
- Blizzards
- Floods
- Earthquakes
- Criminal activity
- Fire
- Explosion
- Medical emergencies (consider a client or team member having a stroke or heart attack)

> **PRACTICE POINT** Emergency action plans (EAPs) are a required part of a safety program, and they prepare the team for fires, tornados, blizzards, floods or any emergency that can happen to a practice.

The basic evacuation procedures should include how employees will be notified, how the emergency will be reported, where and how to exit the building, where the designated meeting place is outside of the building, and how to check in with the safety coordinator. Although not required by OSHA, EAPs should also include an evacuation plan for clients, especially those that may be visually or hearing impaired.

Patient evacuation is also important; however, team member safety cannot be compromised when there is risk. Always leave rescues to the properly trained professionals.

Safety coordinators should also be aware of where the emergency shutoff valves are located for gas, water, and electricity (where applicable).

Ergonomics

Ergonomics refers to reducing operator fatigue and discomfort through proper equipment use and the way we use our bodies. Although there are no OSHA standards regarding ergonomics, safety officers should consider any and all situations that may contribute to injuries. Employees suffering from the following conditions have a higher rate of absenteeism, lower work performance, and a poor attitude, due to the discomfort.

> **PRACTICE POINT** Ergonomic injuries decrease team member productivity, accountability, and morale.

The main concern with ergonomics is back injury, though carpal tunnel syndrome is a problem for small animal surgeons and technologists who perform dental prophylaxes all day. In large animal work, the number one ergonomic injury is rotator cuff injury. Many people only think of computer workstations when they think of ergonomics, and veterinary hospitals have that concern as well.

Escaping Animals

Every measure must be taken to prevent the escape of an animal. Many reasons exist for a patient to become scared

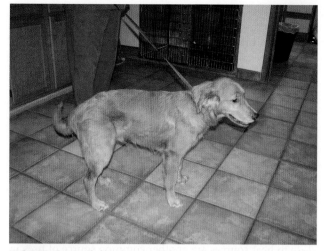

FIGURE 21-6 Slip leashes should be used anytime a patient is transferred from one area of the hospital to another.

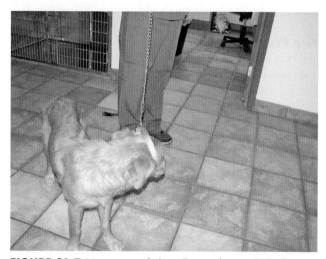

FIGURE 21-7 Many owners fit the collars too loose, which allows an animal to escape from team members.

and try to escape, and the practice can be held liable for the escape of an animal. Windows should never be left open, regardless of whether there is a screen on the window. Cats can claw through screens. Doors should never be left open; dogs may escape from restraint or slip a leash. Dogs are also great at being able to escape from kennels without the knowledge of team members. Any dog that is being removed from a cage or kennel should have a slip leash applied (Figure 21-6), not the owner's collar and leash. Many times, the owner's collar and leash are very loose and the animal can pull right out (Figure 21-7). A slip leash tightens around the neck, preventing the dog from slipping away.

Feral animals should be handled with caution at all times. If an examination is necessary, they should be placed in a quiet room that does not have any other animals in it. The desired room should have minimal shelving and breakable items if the animal escapes from restraint. Some feral animals can be examined with mild restraint; slow and cautious movements should be used to prevent startling the animal. If the animal escapes, it should be given some time to calm

down. If this is not possible, then capture techniques will need to be used. A fish net may help capture a feral cat; a rabies pole may be needed for an aggressive dog. All caution must be taken to prevent being bitten. Feral animals may need sedation before any exam for the safety of the staff.

All caution must be used when walking dogs outdoors. Ideally, practices should have a fenced-in area to walk dogs to help prevent an escape. Again, slip leashes should be used at all times; specific dogs may be denied walks based on the likelihood of them becoming scared and trying to escape while outside. In situations such as this, the owner may be asked to come and walk the dog during the day.

Fire Safety

Along with overloaded electrical circuits, items stored too close to heat sources are another common source of fires in the veterinary practice. Newspapers, blankets, files, and supplies must not be stored near a furnace, water heater, or heat source, and portable heaters should never be left unattended.

Fire Prevention

Practices with 10 or more employees must have a fire prevention and response plan, which must be included in the safety manual. Fire prevention measures include a monthly walk-through of the facility. Smoke and fire alarms should be tested; if the building is equipped with a sprinkler system that should be evaluated as well. Fire extinguishers should be checked monthly for any damage or evidence of tampering. Walk-through inspections and equipment checks should be documented.

Fire Codes and Inspections

Fire codes vary by location, so each practice should become familiar with codes in its geographic area. In general, the fire department is responsible for inspections of businesses and for ensuring that they are compliant with regulations established. Requirements may exist regarding exit signs and emergency lighting. Fire extinguishers are required, as are smoke detectors.

Exit Signs and Lighting

Signs must indicate where the exit is located (Figure 21-8). If a door looks like an exit but is not, it must be labeled "Not an Exit."

> **PRACTICE POINT** Doors that are not an exit must be indicated as such with a sign reading "NOT AN EXIT."

Emergency lights are required and must be tested on a yearly basis to ensure that they are working properly. Lights should be installed in locations that light the pathway to the exit, as well as in locations where team members might be performing duties that could result in injury if the lighting system fails (Figure 21-9).

Fire Extinguishers

Fire extinguishers must be located no more than 75 feet from any distance within the practice and placed 32 to 48 inches

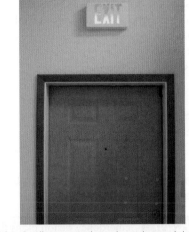

FIGURE 21-8 All exits must be indicated as such by an exit sign.

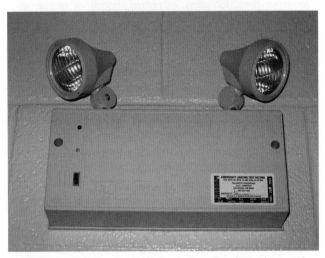

FIGURE 21-9 Emergency lighting is required and must be tested on a yearly basis.

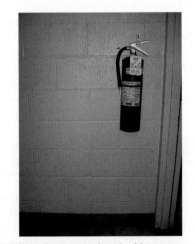

FIGURE 21-10 Each team member should receive training in the use of a fire extinguisher.

above the ground surface. Along with being placed in a central location of the clinic, extinguishers should be placed near the exit doors of the practice (Figure 21-10).

All employees must be trained in the use of a fire extinguisher. If a training facility is available, team members

should practice using extinguishers because common sense often disappears during an emergency. Practicing will help instill automatic reactions. Team members can remember the word "pass" to help initiate the use of an extinguisher when needed:

P = **P**ull the pin.

A = **A**im low. Point the extinguisher to the bottom of the fire.

S = **S**queeze the handle.

S = **S**weep from side to side at the base of the fire until it appears to be out.

Before fire extinguishers are used, employees should make sure that the fire alarm has been sounded. Team members should never attempt to fight a fire that is larger than the immediate area, and if it is spreading, they must exit the building.

Smoke Detectors

Batteries should be replaced on a yearly basis whether a change is needed or not. Monthly testing will ensure the product is in working condition.

Blocked Entries/Exits

Entries and exits must not be blocked with anything, not even for a few minutes. In the event of a fire, anything that might prevent emergency exiting could have devastating effects.

Fire Response

The response portion of the plan should include the evacuation of employees and clients, escape routes and procedures, a procedure to account for all team members, and a method to report the fire. The name of the safety officer should be included as well. A fire could happen to any practice at any time. It could occur with no one in the building or during the busiest time of the day.

> **PRACTICE POINT** A fire can occur during the busiest time of the day, and a plan must be in place to safely evacuate clients and team members (and patients if the opportunity is available).

Fire escape drills should be a part of regular team training. At minimum, they should be conducted once a year. The goal is to have a plan that supports order and control during this emergency process.

Indoor Air Quality

Good indoor air quality is important to keep employees safe—especially those with respiratory conditions like asthma. Every employee should know to report any fumes or chemical odors immediately, and to let the safety officer know if they have experienced any sensitivity to fumes or odors, such as irritated nasal passages or headache. Masks, respirators, and fume hoods should be used as needed.

The number one fume hazard in veterinary practices comes from radiologic processing chemicals. The exhaust fan should always be on when these are in use. Anesthetic

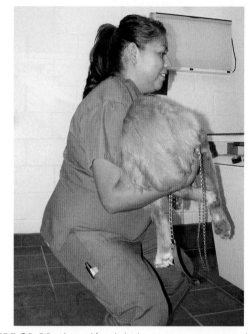

FIGURE 21-11 Always lift with the legs to prevent injuries to the back.

gases are another safety issue. Employees need to check tubing and fittings for leaks before each use. Laboratory chemicals are a third source of potential air quality problems and team members should be instructed to use a fume hood when appropriate.

Lifting

Team members must learn how to lift properly to prevent back injuries. These are the second most common job-related injury in veterinary medicine, and they often result from repeated trauma and micro tears to the tissues and supporting structures in the back. Injuries can be chronic or acute; whichever the case, both can be debilitating for life. All employees must use the proper techniques to prevent injuries from occurring.

Lifting must always be done with the legs rather than the back; women are especially prone to using their backs (Figure 21-11). Team members should watch out for each other and guide others when lifting objects to ensure the back is kept straight and the legs are used to the maximum potential. The hospital policy should be that animals over 40 lb must be lifted by two team members to prevent back injuries. It is also advised to obtain tables that can be raised to a variable height, either by hydraulic control or with the use of a foot pump (Figure 21-12).

Moving Equipment

When moving equipment, multiple employees should be involved. If the equipment is heavy, more than one person must be responsible for the lifting. Another team member should ensure the entryway is clear of clutter and debris that would trip the team members. One team member should be allowed to lift up to 40 lb if he or she is able. Anything over 40 lb should require additional team members.

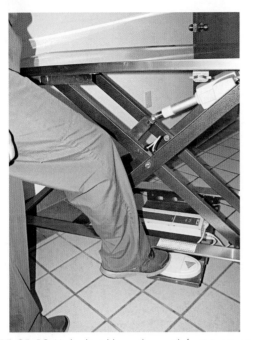

FIGURE 21-12 Hydraulic tables or those with foot pumps are excellent for lifting large breed dogs.

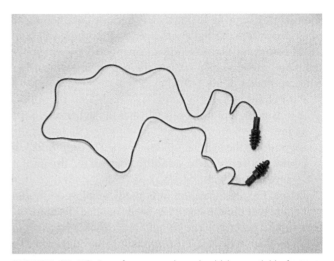

FIGURE 21-13 Form fitting ear plugs should be available for team members to wear in kennel areas when sound exceeds 85 dB.

Noise Hazards

Loud noises occur in many hospitals, especially those that also house boarding facilities. Hearing must be protected, and OSHA has standard guidelines in place to do so.

Employee exposure to excessive noise depends upon a number of factors, including:

- The loudness of the noise as measured in decibels (dB)
- The duration of each employee's exposure to the noise
- Whether employees move between work areas with different noise levels
- Whether noise is generated from one or multiple sources

Generally, the louder the noise, the shorter the exposure time before hearing protection is required. Some kennels will exceed the noise level that is considered to be safe for short-term and long-term hearing of employees who are exposed. Exposure to high levels of noise can lead to hearing deficiencies and hearing loss. OSHA Standard 1910.95 requires noise measurement, noise protection, and hearing testing when noise measurement exceeds 85 dB. Noise measurement can be completed with a decibel meter and should be done at least annually, or at times when the noise level has raised.

> **PRACTICE POINT** Hearing protection should be available for team members when the noise level is above 85 dB.

Hearing protection should be provided when exposure to noise occurs for prolonged periods of time. Single use earplugs made of cotton, foam, silicone, or rubber work well when properly inserted. Preformed earplugs (Figure 21-13) can be fitted for each individual, or earmuffs can be provided.

Noise hazard areas should be identified with a sign, notifying team members that hearing protection is required for prolonged exposure.

Running

Team members should not be allowed to run through the practice, regardless of how busy the practice is. Running increases the risk of slipping, especially on wet surfaces. An employee may have finished mopping the floor and just be setting the signs out; if a team member is running through the area at the same time, he or she will not know the floor is wet. The same applies to horseplay while at work. Both should be forbidden and outlined in the safety manual.

Toxicities

There are many possibilities for toxic exposures in veterinary medicine. Chemical exposure can come in the form of cleaning supplies, chemotherapy agents, x-ray developer solutions, and medications that are dispensed or used in the hospital for patients.

The mixing of two or more chemicals can create caustic fumes that are harmful to both team members and patients. The fumes may not seem harmful, and at times may even smell good, such as those produced when bleach and a lemon disinfectant are combined; however, prolonged exposure may be dangerous and can cause respiratory irritation.

Every team member is exposed to chemotherapy agents (discussed in further detail later in this chapter) if they are administered in the veterinary practice. Many chemotherapeutic agents are expelled in the urine and feces of pets; therefore each time the animal eliminates in the cage, some of the drug is left behind. Therefore team members may be exposed to the drug unknowingly.

Radiology developer rooms should be ventilated to the outdoors because the chemicals used to develop radiographs are strong and harmful. If the developer and fixative mix for some reason, the odor released can be caustic. The chemical used to develop radiographs can be poured down the drain, but the fixing solution must be collected by a specialized company, because it is damaging to the environment. This applies to both used and unused fix solutions.

It is often forgotten that when handling medication, excess drug powder and residual collects on the team members' hands. Various types of medications are handled as team members' count and dispense medications for owners or pull medications to treat patients. If team members do not wash their hands immediately after handling medications, they may ingest the substance or wipe it onto their faces. Many drugs appear to be safe, but repeated ingestion is not. Some drugs are known to have side effects. Chloramphenicol, for example, may suppress bone marrow production in individuals who have a reaction to it. Unfortunately, this reaction is not known for months, or even years, after exposure to the drug. It is essential that all team members wash their hands immediately after handling medication, just as hands are washed immediately after handling an animal, to prevent the accidental ingestion of medications.

> **PRACTICE POINT** Wash hands after counting medication (or wear gloves) to prevent accidental ingestion of drugs.

Workplace Violence

Workplace violence is not unique to a veterinary practice, and OSHA includes it as a general safety topic to be addressed in the safety manual and with employees. Clients, co-workers, family, friends, drug seekers, and thieves are all potential candidates for causing violence in the workplace.

During the hazard assessment of the facility, do not forget to include potential situations that could expose team members to violence. Safety plans should identify potential threats as well as prevention and response measures.

A zero tolerance policy (for workplace violence) should be developed for the protection of all team members (see Chapter 5).

Wet Floors

When floors are being mopped, they can become extremely slippery. Signs that indicate a wet floor should be posted around the wet area, and team members should dry the wet area as soon as possible with a towel. Team members and clients should be encouraged to walk around the wet area. However, the sooner it is dry, the less likely it is that a slip or fall will occur (Figure 21-14). Team members are encouraged to wear nonskid shoes to help prevent slips in the veterinary practice.

Chemical Hazards in the Veterinary Practice

The work involved in documenting chemical hazards in the workplace can be substantial, especially when one considers the number of chemicals that OSHA categorizes as hazardous. Veterinarians and team members are exposed to many chemicals with a wide range of health hazards (irritating, sensitizing, carcinogenic, etc.) and physical hazards (flammable, reactive, corrosive). Often team members take these chemicals for granted, dismissing the possibility of harm to themselves and thinking only of getting their jobs done, in other words, taking care of patients.

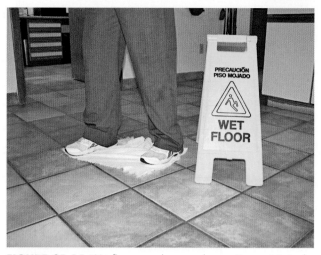

FIGURE 21-14 Wet floors are always a danger. Prevent injuries by drying the floor with a towel (while a wet floor sign is posted).

Hazardous chemicals are not limited to laboratory reagents or to liquids, and may include cleaning products, clerical products, or pharmaceuticals. They take many forms: liquids, solids, gases, vapors, fumes, and mists. Common chemicals used in the veterinary facility include (but are not limited to) the following:

- Alcohol (isopropyl)
- Anesthetic gases
- Antineoplastic drugs
- Povidone-iodine (Betadine)
- Bleach
- Formalin
- Glass cleaners
- Glutaraldehyde
- Room deodorizer
- Wite-Out
- X-ray fixer and developer

> **PRACTICE POINT** Room deodorizer (although often not thought of in this manner) is a chemical agent that team members are exposed to.

As stated in the hazard communications section, each employee must be familiar with all chemicals on the premises, know the hazards of these chemicals, and know how to protect himself or herself from each hazard. Two ways to ensure this occurs are to create and maintain a chemical inventory list, and create and maintain Safety Data Sheets (SDSs).

Chemical Inventory List

A chemical inventory list should be completed on an annual basis (Figure 21-15). Anytime a new product is brought into the hospital, it should be added to this list and an SDS obtained. The new SDS sheet must also be posted in an area visible for all team members to view for 2 weeks.

Veterinary practices also have chemicals that can be extremely dangerous to employees, and team members should pay special attention to these substances. Many of these chemicals are listed on OSHA's IDLH list, or Immediately

Sample - Hazardous Chemicals Inventory List

Hazardous Chemical Name	Operation/Area Used	Date Brought to Site	Date Removed From Site

In accordance with 29 CFR 1910.1020(d)(1)(ii)(B), this form shall be retained for 30 years after the chemical has left the premises.

Sample Hazard Communication Program   12

FIGURE 21-15 Example of a chemical inventory list that should be completed once a year in the veterinary practice. (Courtesy Occupational Safety and Health Administration, Department of Labor, Washington, DC.)

Dangerous to Life or Health. Chemicals in this classification include (and are not limited to) ethylene oxide, formaldehyde, chemotherapy agents, and anesthetic gases. View a full list of IDLH chemicals at www.cdc.gov/niosh/idlh/intridl4.html.

Safety Data Sheets

SDSs are fact lists for chemicals and provide important information related to hazards (Figure 21-16). Information included on SDSs is as follows:

- The identity of the chemical
- Physical and chemical characteristics
- Health hazards
- Permissible exposure limits
- Whether the product is a carcinogen (cancer producing)
- Emergency first aid procedures
- Specific hazards

SDSs must be maintained for every hazardous chemical kept in the practice. Sheets must be kept current within 3 years of the date printed on the sheet. Manufacturers and distributors have SDSs on hand; many are available on a CD or their Web site for easy referencing and printing.

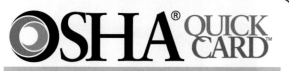

Hazard Communication Safety Data Sheets

The Hazard Communication Standard (HCS) requires chemical manufacturers, distributors, or importers to provide Safety Data Sheets (SDSs) (formerly known as Material Safety Data Sheets or MSDSs) to communicate the hazards of hazardous chemical products. As of June 1, 2015, the HCS will require new SDSs to be in a uniform format, and include the section numbers, the headings, and associated information under the headings below:

Section 1, Identification includes product identifier; manufacturer or distributor name, address, phone number; emergency phone number; recommended use; restrictions on use.

Section 2, Hazard(s) identification includes all hazards regarding the chemical; required label elements.

Section 3, Composition/information on ingredients includes information on chemical ingredients; trade secret claims.

Section 4, First-aid measures includes important symptoms/effects, acute, delayed; required treatment.

Section 5, Fire-fighting measures lists suitable extinguishing techniques, equipment; chemical hazards from fire.

Section 6, Accidental release measures lists emergency procedures; protective equipment; proper methods of containment and cleanup.

Section 7, Handling and storage lists precautions for safe handling and storage, including incompatibilities.

(Continued on other side)

For more information:

OSHA® Occupational Safety and Health Administration
U.S. Department of Labor
www.osha.gov (800) 321-OSHA (6742)

OSHA 3493-02 2012

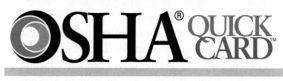

Hazard Communication Safety Data Sheets

Section 8, Exposure controls/personal protection lists OSHA's Permissible Exposure Limits (PELs); Threshold Limit Values (TLVs); appropriate engineering controls; personal protective equipment (PPE).

Section 9, Physical and chemical properties lists the chemical's characteristics.

Section 10, Stability and reactivity lists chemical stability and possibility of hazardous reactions.

Section 11, Toxicological information includes routes of exposure; related symptoms, acute and chronic effects; numerical measures of toxicity.

Section 12, Ecological information*
Section 13, Disposal considerations*
Section 14, Transport information*
Section 15, Regulatory information*

Section 16, Other information, includes the date of preparation or last revision.

*Note: Since other Agencies regulate this information, OSHA will not be enforcing Sections 12 through 15 (29 CFR 1910.1200(g)(2)).

Employers must ensure that SDSs are readily accessible to employees.
See Appendix D of 29 CFR 1910.1200 for a detailed description of SDS contents.

For more information:

OSHA® Occupational Safety and Health Administration
U.S. Department of Labor
www.osha.gov (800) 321-OSHA (6742)

OSHA 3493-02 2012

FIGURE 21-16 SDS descriptions. (Courtesy Occupational Safety and Health Administration, Department of Labor, Washington, DC.)

OSHA allows a few SDS exemptions (meaning an SDS is not required). This includes many articles used by the practice; for example, tape, hematocrit sealer, and pens do not require SDSs. Food and nutritional products, common household cleaning items, and drugs sold in tablet form are also exempt.

PRACTICE POINT Nutritional products are exempt and do not require an SDS.

To be exempt, cleaning items must be used in the same format that a household would use them. To clarify this exemption further, consider Windex, which is commonly

used to clean windows. A practice probably washes their windows with the same frequency as a homeowner would. Now, consider rubbing alcohol, also commonly used in households and veterinary practices. The amount of alcohol used in practice is much greater than a household would use. Therefore this chemical is not exempt, and an SDS must be maintained.

If tablets can be directed to be crushed or made into a dissolving solution, then an SDS must be kept on-site. Capsules, gels, and solutions are not exempt from SDS requirements.

If a chemical is no longer carried by a hospital, an SDS sheet must be maintained for 30 years beyond the date it is discontinued. These SDSs can be kept in a separate binder. OSHA mandates that each SDS for a discontinued substance contains a summary of how the product was used, where it was stored, and how long it was supplied. The reason for this mandate is that it can take up to 30 years for personnel to see side effects from particular chemicals. This ensures the practice has reference material available in case this situation should arise.

Special Chemicals

Chemicals that require special attention include ethylene oxide, formaldehyde, glutaraldehyde, chemotherapeutic agents, and anesthetic gases.

Ethylene oxide is a carcinogen that is used for gas sterilization procedures. It is extremely important to have a safe handling protocol when this product is used. Only approved sterilization devices must be used with ethylene oxide, and levels should be monitored to ensure team member safety (Figure 21-17). This chemical is very flammable and must be used with caution.

Formaldehyde, which is used to fix tissue samples, is also a carcinogen. Vapors can be extremely dangerous and are known to cause cancer and abortion. Practices should order biopsy jars that are prefilled with formalin. This prevents unnecessary exposure to team members. If gallon containers of formalin are used, the chemical should be poured into smaller containers under a fume hood that will capture the vapors. Goggles and gloves should also be worn when

> **PRACTICE POINT** Formaldehyde is a known carcinogen; take all necessary precautions to prevent skin contact and inhalation of vapors.

handling the chemical to prevent any contact.

Glutaraldehyde is a chemical used to disinfect instruments, generally in cold trays. It is an excellent fungicide and virucide but can be extremely traumatic to tissue. If glutaraldehyde is not diluted properly, it can cause tissue damage to both team members and patients. Many other disinfectants provide superior protection and are much safer to use in the veterinary practice.

Radiology chemicals are among the most common chemicals found in animal and veterinary facilities. Although suppliers now do most of the mixing and pouring, accidents can occur. Hazards from x-ray fixer are almost nonexistent. The use of personal protective equipment (gloves and eye shields) with good ventilation should prevent problems. Should exposure occur, wash the affected area thoroughly with soap

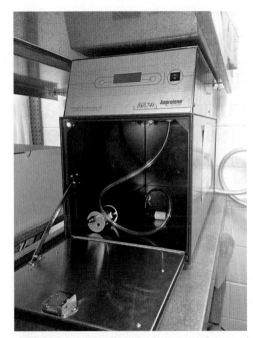

FIGURE 21-17 Ethylene oxide is used in gas sterilizers and must be used with caution. (Photo courtesy Brenda Rasmussen.)

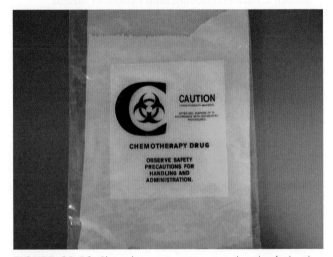

FIGURE 21-18 Chemotherapeutic agents must be identified with a bright yellow label.

and water. If the eyes are exposed, use an eyewash station. The x-ray developer, on the other hand, can cause kidney damage, skin and eye irritation, and allergic skin reactions.

Personal protective equipment should be worn when handling x-ray developer and should include, minimally, heavy-duty utility gloves and eye protection. X-ray developer should be handled only in well-ventilated areas.

Chemotherapeutic Agents

Every team member is exposed to chemotherapeutic agents if they are being administered in the practice. Chemotherapy is composed of chemicals used to kill tumor cells; these chemicals inadvertently affect healthy cells as well. Therefore all precautions must be taken when working with these drugs (Figure 21-18). Patients' bodily

excretions, including vomitus, urine, and feces, will contain the drugs in both metabolized and unmetabolized forms.

When prepping such drugs for administration, PPE must be worn. This includes a mask, eye protection, a disposable gown, and thick, unpowdered gloves. Chemicals can be easily inhaled, and a fume hood with a vent must be used during the mixing process. A mask provides minimal protection, but the fume hood will remove the excess aerosolized chemical. Contact lenses should not be worn at any time during the mixing and or administration of chemotherapy agents, regardless of eye protection. A disposable gown should be used and disposed of when the mixing and administration processes have been completed. Cuffs should be tucked inside gloves. Thick, unpowdered gloves are the only acceptable glove type. Thin latex gloves protect the team member to a lesser degree; powdered gloves tend to attract drug residue.

Once the entire mixing and administration process has been completed, all gloves, gowns, needles, and items used must be disposed of in a yellow biohazardous waste container. The yellow container indicates that chemotherapeutic agents are inside; these containers will be incinerated separately from other biohazard containers.

Bedding used for animals receiving chemotherapy should be handled with gloves; the team member should also wear a disposable gown for protection. Bedding must be washed separately from other bedding. It must also be washed twice with laundry detergent. Chemotherapeutic agents are released in the urine and bowel movements of patients. Anytime the bedding or kennel is contaminated, it must be treated as such, and appropriate measures must be taken to clean the area.

If a chemotherapeutic agent is spilled, team members and patients must evacuate the area. One team member should double glove and place an absorbable material over the spill. Once the agent has been completely absorbed, all material must be placed in a yellow biohazardous waste container. The area must be washed with 70% alcohol twice before the area can be declared safe.

Practices that provide chemotherapeutic treatments to patients should strongly consider meeting the minimum standards (ventilation, isolation, PPE) before the implementation of any protocols. Safety of the team members should be the number one priority.

> **PRACTICE POINT** When chemotherapy is administered in the practice, a majority of team members are exposed to the drugs when precautions are not taken. Drugs are eliminated in the urine and feces, and these must be cleaned up with caution.

Clients must also be considered when patients are receiving chemotherapy. If clients have pets at home, and the pet urinates and defecates, the children may be at risk, along with their parents. Client education materials must clearly indicate the precautions that should be taken, based on the drug administered for that particular patient.

Anesthetic Gases

Because of their proximity to the source, veterinarians and veterinary surgical technicians are at the highest risk for overexposure to gases. Other operating room employees in the veterinary clinic are also at risk. The primary hazardous gases are nitrous oxide and halothane, which can cuase congenital birth defects, abortions, cancer, irritability, depression, and headaches.

> **PRACTICE POINT** Inspect anesthetic machines for leaks EVERY DAY before any anesthetic procedures.

Inhaled anesthetic agents include two different classes of chemicals: nitrous oxide and halogenated agents. Halogenated agents currently in use include halothane, enflurane, isoflurane, desflurane, and sevoflurane.

Every team member that is monitoring an anesthetized patient, whether perioperative or postoperative, must receive proper training. Team members must be able to respond to emergencies that occur at any time, dealing with hypoxia, hypothermia, hyperthermia, a sudden decrease in blood pressure, or an abnormal ECG.

Anesthesia-related training topics should include:
- Depth and planes of anesthesia
- Medication's mechanism of action, side effects, and contraindications
- Proper anesthetic hose size
- Correct endotracheal tube size and proper inflation
- Anesthesia machine maintenance
- Scavenging systems
- Cleanup of liquid anesthesia spills
- Leak-checking machine

Anesthesia safety meetings should occur regularly to remind team members of the risks of anesthesia. New team members must be fully trained and made aware of the risks involved while working with anesthesia and anesthetized patients.

Some common reasons for exposure to anesthetic gases and potential preventative measures are as follows:

Improperly functioning scavenging systems: The reservoir bag should be fully collapsed to half full. If it is underfilled or overfilled, the system will not function optimally. Several scavengers exist; the practice should use the one that works best in that individual practice. Active scavengers provide the best protection; however, passive exhaust and adsorption scavenging systems are also effective means of removing gases.

The active system has some means of energetic collection. This is usually a fan enclosed in a box that creates a vacuum through a series of tubes that are connected to the patient or machine. Active scavengers may also attach directly to the machine and push the waste anesthetic gases through the system instead of producing a vacuum. Active scavengers are best for practices that handle a large volume of procedures requiring anesthesia or that perform them at various locations throughout the practice. The main disadvantage to an active scavenger system is cost. Systems can range in price from $400 to $4000, depending on the complexity of

the system. Other lesser disadvantages include maintenance of the machine and manual activation. Team members must turn on a switch to activate the scavenger; many forget until the patient's breathing bag fails to work properly.

The passive exhaust system channels waste anesthetic gases through a tube to an acceptable location for evacuation. This system is only good for short distances because the only means of expelling the gas is the patient's lung pressure and the flow rate of gas. Therefore small and weak animals may not be able to expel gases efficiently.

The adsorption scavenger uses charcoal to remove all halogenated gases. It does not adsorb nitrous oxide. Charcoal canisters must be replaced after 20 g of adsorption; therefore canisters must be monitored for replacement. If canisters are not replaced, waste anesthetic gases will overflow into the room.

For the safety of both the patient and team members, anesthetic machines must have adequate scavenging systems.

Improperly fitted endotracheal tubes with cuffs inadequately inflated: Ensure that the correct size of endotracheal tube is selected for the patient and that the cuff is filled to an appropriate level.

Not flushing the system with oxygen before removing patient from machine: To help decrease waste anesthetic gases, team members should turn off the anesthesia to the patient (upon completion of a procedure), allowing the continued flow and intake of oxygen. This allows the patient to breath off excess anesthetic gas, which circulates through the system instead of in the operating room for team members to inhale. Once the patient has received approximately 5 to 10 minutes of oxygen, it can be moved to the recovery area of the practice. "Boxing-down" patients (placing them in a sealed container with direct administration of oxygen and anesthesia) also creates waste anesthetic gases that the team inhales. Every effort should be made to use an injectable means of anesthetic induction until the patient is ready for an endotracheal tube. If the box or mask is needed, proper ventilation in the room should be mandatory.

> **PRACTICE POINT** Allow patients to breath in oxygen for 5 to 10 minutes before removing from anesthetic machines; this allows anesthetic vapors to be exhaled into the machine, not into the room.

Equipment leaks: Machines should be inspected daily for leaks. A pressure test should be performed indicating that the machine holds pressure without leaks, the vaporizer refill lid is secure, all hoses are attached properly, and the bag does not contain a hole. Hoses and gaskets should be replaced yearly as part of an anesthetic maintenance plan, which helps prevent small, undetectable leaks. OSHA expects that practices will have a professional service maintain their anesthetic machines every 3 to 12 months. Some state veterinary medical boards require a professional, annual inspection of all anesthetic machines.

When team members change soda lime granules on anesthetic machines, gloves should be worn. Used soda lime can be caustic to tissues.

Team members who are pregnant and required to work around anesthetic gases should wear an anesthetic monitoring badge along with proper PPE for their own safety. OSHA's exposure limit for halogenated gases (e.g., halothane, isoflurane, sevoflurane) is 2 ppm/year. Nitrous oxide's maximum exposure limit is 25 ppm/year.

If a spill of liquid anesthesia occurs, all other team members should be evacuated from the area. Windows should be opened and exhaust fans turned on. Cat litter can be poured over the spill. Once it has been absorbed, the litter can be swept up and disposed of. Spills may occur when the machine is being refilled or as bottles are being unpacked from a received order. All caution should be taken to prevent the inhalation of gases.

Diamond Labeling System

The National Fire Protection Association (NFPA) uses colored diamond labels to indicate the risks associated with health, fire, reactivity, and special hazards of specific chemicals. These diamond stickers are placed at the entry point of the practice (Figure 21-19), along with the room the hazard is located in. These are not only important for team members, but also for emergency personnel if they need to enter the practice; the stickers allow them to quickly determine what hazards are in the practice and their location. These labels must also be placed on chemicals that are transferred from their original bottle (disinfectants placed in spray bottles for cleaning). HMIS II (hazardous materials identification system) and NFPA labels are two types of labels that are commonly used. HMIS II labels have colored bars, whereas NFPA labels have colored diamonds (Figure 21-20). Transferring contents from one bottle to another and labeling appropriately is known as secondary labeling.

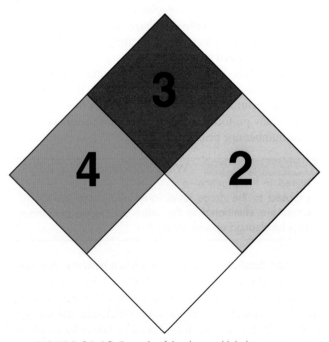

FIGURE 21-19 Example of the diamond labeling system.

> **PRACTICE POINT** ALWAYS label secondary bottles with proper labels. If emergency personal entered the clinic, they should be able to immediately determine whether the chemical within the bottle is hazardous.

NFPA Label

Numbers, colors, and letters are all ways in which chemicals are labeled on an NFPA label. Colors are used to identify the hazards of chemicals; red indicating fire, blue indicating health, and yellow signifying reactivity with other chemicals. Numbers 0 to 4 are placed in the sections, indicating the level of danger. The white diamond indicates that PPE is required (Figure 21-21).

Common items that tend to be overlooked when labeling and storing hazardous chemicals used in the practice include alcohol, cold sterilants, disinfectants (especially diluted bleach or chlorhexidine solutions), instrument soaks (enzymatic, ultrasonic, lubricant), and x-ray developer and fixative solutions. These chemicals are often placed into secondary containers and do not get labeled.

With the updated Hazard Communication Standard that will occur through the year 2016, label requirements will also change; however, OSHA will allow continued use of the NFPA and HMIS II labels in the workplace, as long as team members understand both systems. Labels can include pictograms (which will be required when products are shipped to the veterinary practice) (Figure 21-22). The major changes to labels will not affect veterinary practices, except that team members must be able to interpret them.

Chemical Spills

Spills can occur in any situation; accidents happen. A preparedness plan will help facilitate easy cleanup and prevent unnecessary exposure. A spill kit should be developed and maintained, and each team member must know where the kit is located. A safety program should instill role playing so each member knows how to use the kit in case of emergency.

When developing a spill kit, hazardous chemicals that are kept inside the practice need to be identified. SDSs indicate the best cleanup method if a spill occurs. The information should be consolidated into an information sheet that is easy to understand. The sheet can then be laminated for protection.

A spill kit should include a large plastic container to keep contents together. Contents include cat litter, a dustpan and broom, a pair of nitrile gloves, eye protection, and a

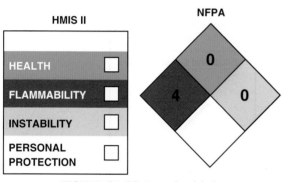

FIGURE 21-20 Secondary labels.

RATING NUMBER	HEALTH HAZARD	FLAMMABILITY HAZARD	INSTABILITY HAZARD	RATING SYMBOL	SPECIAL HAZARD
4	Can be lethal	Will vaporize and readily burn at normal temperatures	May explode at normal temperatures and pressures	ALK	Alkaline
3	Can cause serious or permanent injury	Can be ignited under almost all ambient temperatures	May explode at high temperature or shock	ACID	Acidic
				COR	Corrosive
2	Can cause temporary incapacitation or residual injury	Must be heated or high ambient temperature to burn	Violent chemical change at high temperatures or pressures	OX	Oxidizing
				☢	Radioactive
1	Can cause significant irritation	Must be preheated before ignition can occur	Normally stable. High temperatures make unstable	₩	Reacts violently or explosively with water
0	No hazard	Will not burn	Stable	₩OX	Reacts violently or explosively with water and oxidizing

NFPA Rating Explanation Guide

FIGURE 21-21 National Fire Protection Association Rating Explanation Guide. (Courtesy of ComplianceSigns.com.)

HCS Pictograms and Hazards

Health Hazard	Flame	Exclamation Mark
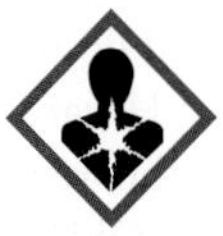	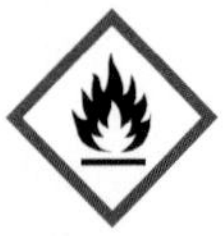	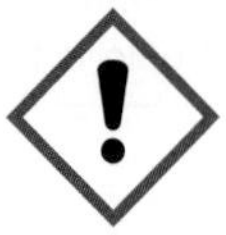
• Carcinogen • Mutagenicity • Reproductive Toxicity • Respiratory Sensitizer • Target Organ Toxicity • Aspiration Toxicity	• Flammables • Pyrophorics • Self-Heating • Emits Flammable Gas • Self-Reactives • Organic Peroxides	• Irritant (skin and eye) • Skin Sensitizer • Acute Toxicity (harmful) • Narcotic Effects • Respiratory Tract Irritant • Hazardous to Ozone Layer (Non-Mandatory)
Gas Cylinder	Corrosion	Exploding Bomb
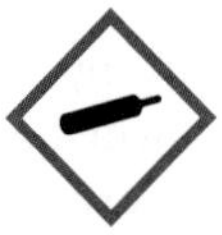	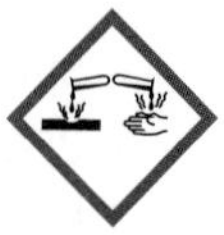	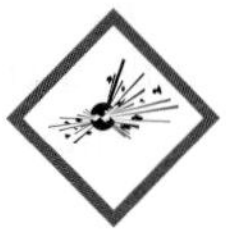
• Gases Under Pressure	• Skin Corrosion/Burns • Eye Damage • Corrosive to Metals	• Explosives • Self-Reactives • Organic Peroxides
Flame Over Circle	Environment (Non-Mandatory)	Skull and Crossbones
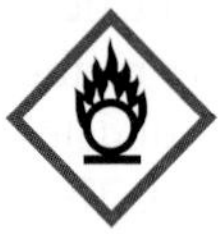	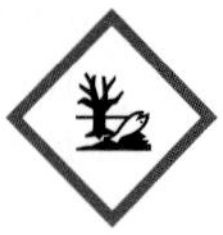	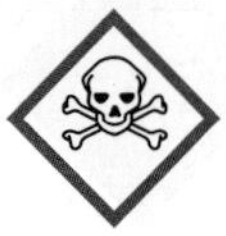
• Oxidizers	• Aquatic Toxicity	• Acute Toxicity (fatal or toxic)

FIGURE 21-22 Pictograms will be part of the new labeling system effective in the year 2014.

laminated copy of cleanup procedures. The spill kit should be centrally located and easy to access (Figure 21-23).

Chemical Spill Cleanup Procedures
- Remove unnecessary people and pets from the area to prevent spreading and exposure to chemical
- Increase ventilation to the area; open windows and turn on exhaust fans and vents
- Put on protective gloves; put on gown if needed
- Cover spill with absorbable material, either cat litter or paper towels
- Clean up saturated absorbent material
- Place chemical in trash bag and dispose of it properly
- Wash area with plain water and allow it to dry
- Wash hands
- Replace materials used in spill kit

Eyewash Stations
Eyewash stations are required of every safety program and must be available if a team member or client gets a chemical or foreign object in the eye. Affected team members must be able to walk to an eyewash station within 10 seconds of being exposed to a chemical; therefore large practices must have more than one eyewash station.

> **PRACTICE POINT**   Eyewash stations should be centrally located and easy to access at any time.

A variety of eyewash stations are available, ranging from handheld bottles to stations connected to a consistent water supply. The most common are the eyewash stations that simply attach to the top of a water faucet spout and are capped until needed. If the station is needed, a lever on the station is turned to allow water pressure to dispense; water is squirted upward, allowing the employee to place his or her eyes in direct contact with pressurized water (Figure 21-24). This allows the flushing of any chemical that entered the eye. Most chemicals require flushing for 5 to 10 minutes; this information can be obtained from the SDS. Water feels uncomfortable when flushing first begins because it is not the same pH as the eye and does not have the same salt content; however, team members must understand flushing is essential to remove potentially harmful substances and objects.

Eyewash stations that are connected to a consistent water supply are ideal because they apply the same amount of pressure to the eye for a period of time. Handheld bottles (Figure 21-25) run out of water and do not supply constant pressure. If a faucet-mounted station is used, the hot water should be

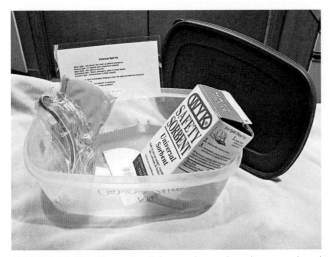

FIGURE 21-23 Chemical spills kits can be purchased or created, and should be located centrally within the veterinary hospital.

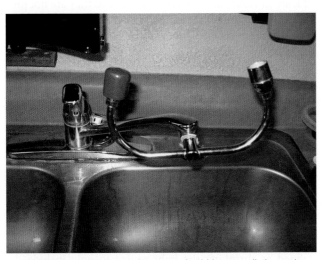

FIGURE 21-24 Eyewash stations should be centrally located.

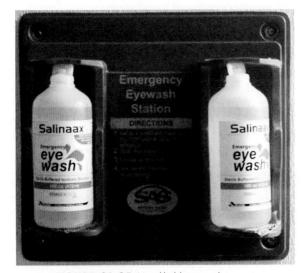

FIGURE 21-25 Hand-held eyewash station.

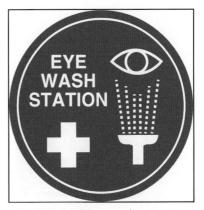

FIGURE 21-26 Eyewash station sign.

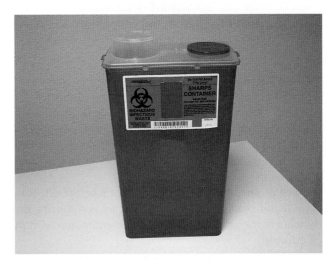

FIGURE 21-27 Biohazardous waste container.

disconnected to prevent further injury to the eye. Each team member should practice using the eyewash station so that all are familiar with it in the event of an emergency. Eyewash stations should be marked with a sticker or sign indicating equipment location (Figure 21-26).

The process of maintaining the eyewash station or stations will vary slightly depending on the type of unit; however, a log documenting the performance of weekly maintenance checks must be maintained. The American National Standards Institute (ANSI) requires 3-minute flushing weekly.

Biohazards in the Veterinary Practice

Needles, glass, slides, surgical blades, and coverslips are all considered sharps and must be discarded in a biohazard or sharps container. Containers must be puncture resistant and sealable once the container is full. Milk jugs are unacceptable. Biohazard containers (Figure 21-27) are red and come in a variety of sizes depending on the needs of the practice. A specialized company that incinerates the contents should pick up these containers on a regular basis. Some states may require proof of biohazard incineration; be sure to keep all receipts indicating when the biohazard container was picked up, as well as the date of incineration.

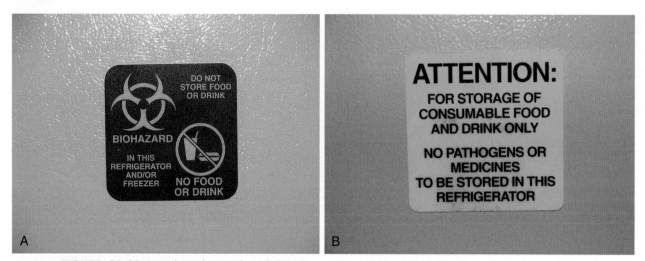

FIGURE 21-28 A, Biohazard materials, including vaccinations and tests, should never be stored with human food intended for consumptions. **B,** Consumable food should never be stored with biohazard materials. Magnets can be placed on refrigerators to indicate contents.

Team members must take every precaution when handling biohazard material to prevent poking themselves or exposing themselves to unnecessary disease and injury. Containers cannot be opened once the cap has been applied unless the plastic tabs are broken. If this happens, the container is regarded as unusable and must be emptied and discarded.

Needles should not be cut off at the tip before disposal, because this practice increases the risk for aerosolizing the contents of the needle and syringe. The entire needle must be discarded.

Practices should have two separate refrigerators; one for human food and the other for biologics, laboratory tests, and drugs (Figure 21-28). This prevents the contamination and ingestion of products used to practice medicine. Team members should be encouraged to keep food, coffee, and drinks in break rooms or lounges instead of on hospital counters or exam tables. Bacteria, dirt, and residual medications reside on counters and can be easily ingested when food is placed on them.

> **PRACTICE POINT**   If team members are allowed to consume food on the premises, a safe environment (break room) must be provided for them to do so. This safe environment must be free of chemical and physical hazards that exist throughout the hospital (OSHA's general duty clause).

Frequent handwashing with antiseptic soap must be done between patients and when counting medication, cleaning, or maintaining equipment.

Radiation Safety

Radiation exposure in a practice must be taken seriously. Excess radiation causes birth defects, decreased fertility, and cancer; therefore every precaution must be taken when exposed. Team members must wear PPE at all times when taking radiographs. Employers who do not provide proper PPE are in violation of OSHA standards, as they are not providing a safe work environment. OSHA states that if PPE is provided, team members must be trained on proper use and therefore must use it when needed. Practices can include a section in their employee and safety manual that states if employees do not abide by the requirements set forth by the hospital, they can be terminated immediately for lack of or improper use of protective equipment.

Lead gloves, gown, and thyroid collars comprise the minimum PPE that must be worn to take radiographs. If at all possible, team members should leave the room for best protection. If an animal is sedated, rice bags, sand bags, ties, and tape can be used to position the animal for the desired view, allowing the team members to leave.

Radiographs should be collimated, preventing excess radiation exposure to team members. **Collimation** can be defined as shrinking the light source to only include the patient; this light source indicates where the radiation beam will penetrate. If excess beams miss the patient and bounce off the table, this is termed scatter radiation, which increases a team member's exposure to radiation.

Gloves should never be in the direct x-ray beam because radiation can penetrate lead that is cracked and/or broken. Full gloves are the only gloves that can provide protection for team members' hands. Partial gloves may make it easier to restrain pets, but the exposure to radiation increases dramatically (Figure 21-29). In addition, partial gloves do not meet OSHA standards (many team members prefer partial gloves over full gloves, because it is easier to restrain patients). Never compromise team member safety for convenience.

> **PRACTICE POINT**   Never compromise team member safety by using partial gloves for radiographs (as a convenience to the patient).

All PPE should be x-rayed on a yearly basis to look for cracks that may have occurred. Cracks develop when team members fold the gowns, gloves, or thyroid collars instead

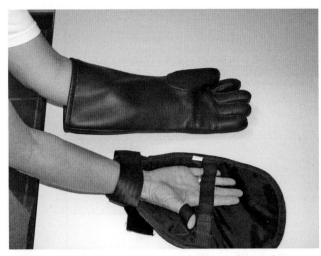

FIGURE 21-29 Full x-ray gloves (top glove) provide complete protection, whereas partial gloves (bottom glove) provide minimal protection against radiation exposure.

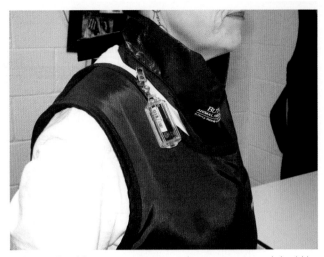

FIGURE 21-30 Dosimeters monitor radiation exposure and should be worn outside of PPE.

of hanging or laying them on a flat surface. If any cracks or holes have developed, the PPE device must be replaced immediately. Radiographs should be kept for comparison from year to year.

Portable units are often found in large animal practices, and can be dangerous because the x-ray beam can be pointed in any direction. A cassette-holding pole should be used to hold the cassette during the x-ray process. A gloved hand should never hold the cassette. Team members should also make sure there is not another person in the direct line of the beam, even at a distance.

Some hospitals may have their x-ray machine located in the main treatment room. Although this is not ideal, some hospitals may not be able to relocate the machine, because of structural or design challenges. It should be practice policy that unprotected team members must leave the room until the radiograph images have been captured. Scatter radiation puts unprotected team members at risk.

A dosimeter, used to measure radiation exposure, must be worn every time an x-ray is taken. The badges should be stored outside the room to prevent scatter radiation from affecting the badges. Badges should be worn at collar level, outside of the PPE (Figure 21-30). Dosimeters indicate the amount of exposure the team member is receiving. Badges should be sent to a monitoring company on a monthly or quarterly basis, where a report will be generated and returned to the practice. These reports must be monitored and reviewed upon their return to check for any significant change in exposure readings. If a badge reads high, this could indicate that the x-ray machine is functioning improperly and emitting excess radiation. This is detrimental to employee safety and must be corrected immediately.

Dosimetry reports must be kept on hand for 30 years, as mandated by OSHA. Team members should always have access to data regarding the amount of radiation that they have been exposed to while employed at the practice (Figure 21-31).

Veterinary staff members are allowed a maximum exposure of 5 rem/year of radiation, whereas the general public is only allowed a maximum exposure of 0.5 rem/year.

> **PRACTICE POINT** Damage to human body parts after excessive exposure to radiation is real. ALWAYS wear PPE as designated to prevent long-term health risks.

Machines may need to be registered with the appropriate state agencies on a yearly basis. Most state agencies will inspect the machine(s), ensure the paperwork matches in serial and model numbers, and conduct individual tests. These tests indicate the safety of the machine and that it is working properly and in an acceptable condition. Inspection reports may be required to be posted in the x-ray room, pending state regulations.

Appropriate signage must be posted outside radiology rooms.

Some states also require rights and responsibilities of both employers and employees to be posted, along with a written protocol of how to take and process a radiograph.

Dental x-ray machines also emit radiation, although at smaller doses. Safety must still be top priority. Team members should always be at least 6 feet away from the head of the x-ray unit, with attention being paid to the direction in which the head is pointed (stay out of the direct line of the beam). Dosimetry badges help detect inadvertent exposure, and dental film should never be held in the patients mouth. Gauze and positioning aids must be available to aid in obtaining dental radiographs.

Laser Safety

The human eye is vulnerable to damage when exposed to lasers. Laser therapy is now being introduced into veterinary practices, and a safety program must come with it to protect team member's eyes.

Lasers are classified into various levels, and include Class 1, Class 1M, Class 2, Class 2M, Class 3, and Class 4.

Account Number: 0000976

Report Date: 02/13/2013

Wear Period: 01/09/2013 to 02/07/2013

ANNUAL RADIATION EXPOSURE LIMITS:
Whole body, blood forming organs   5,000 mrem/yr
Lens of eye   15,000 mrem/yr
Extremeties and skin   50,000 mrem/yr
Fetal   500 mrem/gestation period
General public   100 mrem/yr

These limits are based on USNRC Regulation Title 10, Part 20.

DOSAGE LEGEND

curr - current badge reading
ytd - year-to-date accumulated dosage
life - lifetime accumulated storage

View your dosage report online & provide feedback at http://myTLDaccount.PLMedical.com

	Name	Employee ID / DOB	Type	Badge #	Dose Equivalents (in millirem)			Comments
						Deep	Eye	Shallow	

OCCUPATIONAL RADIATION DOSE RECORD — Page 1 of 1

	Name	Employee ID / DOB	Type	Badge #		Deep	Eye	Shallow	Comments
1	Control	-----	T		curr				
					ytd				
					life				
2	Bevery Rains	001 -----	T	0049402	curr	18	18	18	
					ytd	18	18	18	
					life	421	421	409	
3	Bernice Kim	002 -----	T	0103557	curr	11	11	11	
					ytd	11	11	11	
					life	292	292	282	
4	Alice Lynch	003 -----	T	0104208	curr	25	32	21	
					ytd	25	32	21	
					life	264	264	258	
5	Nicole Allen	004 -----	T	0041925	curr	MR	MR	MR	
					ytd	MR	MR	MR	
					life	284	284	275	
6	Margaret Moss	005 -----	T	0052765	curr	45	43	45	
					ytd	45	43	45	
					life	280	280	270	
7	Mary Williams	006 -----	T	0042873	curr	MR	MR	MR	
					ytd	MR	MR	MR	
					life	315	315	301	
8	Jeffrey Dodson	007 -----	T	0034456	curr	MR	MR	MR	
					ytd	MR	MR	MR	
					life	252	252	245	
9	Roy Robinson	008 -----	T	0044819	curr	101	97	98	
					ytd	101	97	98	
					life	255	255	246	
10	Christopher Gagne	009 -----	T	0083207	curr	MR	MR	MR	
					ytd	MR	MR	MR	
					life	242	242	234	

This report must not be used to claim product certification, approval, or endorsement by NVLAP, NIST, or any agency of the Federal Government. A copy of the PL Medical Co., LLC NVLAP certificate and scope of accreditation can be found on http://www.plmedical.com/public/Accreditation.htm.

FIGURE 21-31 Example of a dosimetry report.

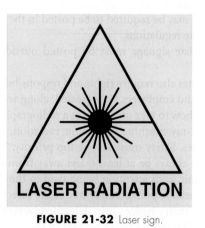

LASER RADIATION

FIGURE 21-32 Laser sign.

Each class has its own restrictions and protection; therefore it is imperative to determine the type of laser a practice owns, and develop a plan based on those risks. Protective equipment includes skin protection, protective eyewear and laser warning signs (Figure 21-32).

Accident Reporting and Investigation

Every accident that occurs in the practice must be reported to the safety manager and/or practice manager and owner. If medical treatment is needed, appropriate paperwork should be available for the employee to take to the doctor or hospital. Paperwork may include the First Notice of Accident or Injury and Illness Incident Report and/or a Workers' Compensation Insurance Claim Form. This will ensure that the employer's insurance is charged for the visit, not the team member's. When the employee returns from the medical visit, paperwork should be sent to the appropriate companies, state, or local authorities. Since workers' compensation varies by state, each practice must have a full understanding of the required filing procedures.

 Veterinary practice managers document and report accidents and file appropriate reports

Practices with 11 or more employees must record all accidents on an OSHA Form 300. Only injuries resulting in death or the hospitalization of five or more employees must be reported to OSHA. OSHA Form 300 (Figure 21-33) must be kept for 5 years. Because this form contains personal employee information, it should be kept in a locked cabinet.

All accidents and injuries that occur while on the job must be investigated and documented by leadership; however, only fatalities must be reported to OSHA.

How to Fill Out the Log

The *Log of Work-Related Injuries and Illnesses* is used to classify work-related injuries and illnesses and to note the extent and severity of each case. When an incident occurs, use the *Log* to record specific details about what happened and how it happened.

If your company has more than one establishment or site, you must keep separate records for each physical location that is expected to remain in operation for one year or longer.

We have given you several copies of the *Log* in this package. If you need more than we provided, you may photocopy and use as many as you need.

The *Summary* — a separate form — shows the work-related injury and illness totals for the year in each category. At the end of the year, count the number of incidents in each category and transfer the totals from the *Log* to the *Summary*. Then post the *Summary* in a visible location so that your employees are aware of injuries and illnesses occurring in their workplace. **You don't post the *Log*. You post only the *Summary* at the end of the year.**

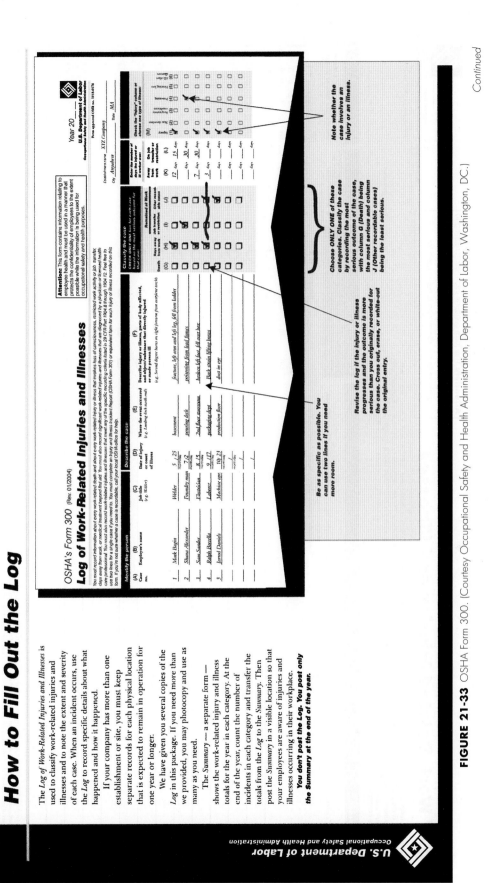

FIGURE 21-33 OSHA Form 300. (Courtesy Occupational Safety and Health Administration, Department of Labor, Washington, DC.)

Continued

OSHA's Form 300 (Rev. 01/2004)

Log of Work-Related Injuries and Illnesses

Year 20___

U.S. Department of Labor
Occupational Safety and Health Administration

Form approved OMB no. 1218-0176

Attention: This form contains information relating to employee health and must be used in a manner that protects the confidentiality of employees to the extent possible while the information is being used for occupational safety and health purposes.

You must record information about every work-related death and about every work-related injury or illness that involves loss of consciousness, restricted work activity or job transfer, days away from work, or medical treatment beyond first aid. You must also record significant work-related injuries and illnesses that are diagnosed by a physician or licensed health care professional. You must also record work-related injuries and illnesses that meet any of the specific recording criteria listed in 29 CFR Part 1904.8 through 1904.12. Feel free to use two lines for a single case if you need to. You must complete an Injury and Illness Incident Report (OSHA Form 301) or equivalent form for each injury or illness recorded on this form. If you're not sure whether a case is recordable, call your local OSHA office for help.

Establishment name _____

City _____ State _____

Identify the person

(A) Case no.	(B) Employee's name	(C) Job title (e.g., Welder)

Describe the case

(D) Date of injury or onset of illness	(E) Where the event occurred (e.g., Loading dock north end)	(F) Describe injury or illness, parts of body affected, and object/substance that directly injured or made person ill (e.g., Second degree burns on right forearm from acetylene torch)

month/day

Classify the case

CHECK ONLY ONE box for each case based on the most serious outcome for that case:

Death (G)	Days away from work (H)	Remained at Work — Job transfer or restriction (I)	Remained at Work — Other recordable cases (J)

Enter the number of days the injured or ill worker was:

Away from work (K)	On job transfer or restriction (L)
___ days	___ days

Check the "Injury" column or choose one type of illness:

(M)

Injury (1)	Skin disorder (2)	Respiratory condition (3)	Poisoning (4)	Hearing loss (5)	All other illnesses (6)

Page totals ▶

Be sure to transfer these totals to the Summary page (Form 300A) before you post it.

Injury (1)	Skin disorder (2)	Respiratory condition (3)	Poisoning (4)	Hearing loss (5)	All other illnesses (6)

Public reporting burden for this collection of information is estimated to average 14 minutes per response, including time to review the instructions, search and gather the data needed, and complete and review the collection of information. Persons are not required to respond to the collection of information unless it displays a currently valid OMB control number. If you have any comments about these estimates or any other aspects of this data collection, contact: US Department of Labor, OSHA Office of Statistical Analysis, Room N-3644, 200 Constitution Avenue, NW, Washington, DC 20210. Do not send the completed forms to this office.

Page ___ of ___

FIGURE 21-33, cont'd

It is imperative to investigate accidents that occur and document all information that is obtained. OSHA inspectors may ask for this (along with any other investigator) obtaining information for a worker's compensation claim. This information should be contained in OSHA Form 301 (Figure 21-34).

OSHA requires form 300A to be posted in a conspicuous place for all team members to view from February 1 to April 30 of each year. Form 300A (Figure 21-35) summarizes all injuries and illnesses from form 300, removing all confidential information.

Documentation

Documentation of the safety program must exist. Outlines of training programs, attendees, dates, and signatures should be kept on file. A summary of all hazardous chemicals, a workplace safety manual, and any workplace injuries and illnesses must be kept together.

Developing and Implementing Safety Protocols

Now that safety hazards have been addressed, it is time to develop and implement protocol. All team members should role-play the protocols to be comfortable if an emergency situation ever arises. All common sense may be lost in the event of an emergency; the more the hospital implements role-playing, the safer the practice will be. Safety must be addressed at every meeting; it is taken for granted in many situations and needs to be discussed frequently.

Common sense can be applied to many safety procedures and protocols, and should be used when storing supplies. Heavy items must be placed on the lower shelves, along with chemicals and liquids. All chemicals must be stored in tightly sealed containers and be placed below eye level in case they are spilled. Shelves should never be overweighed with products, causing them to fall on team members. If a product on an upper shelf is needed, a step stool should be used; never climb on countertops or shelves to get products.

Autoclaves produce intense heat and should always be properly vented before opening the door. Steam should be allowed to dissipate slowly and completely before fully opening the door. The face and hands should be kept away from both the vent and door when venting and opening the autoclave.

Team members must always use caution when working with large animals and chutes. A team member's body must never be placed in a chute with an animal. The animal can be led into the chute with a rope from the outside; large animals can injure team members when there is nowhere to escape. Large animal stalls may also need to be locked, preventing the theft of patients. Large, durable locks that cannot be cut off must be used.

Bathing and dipping patients can create a hazard; eye protection should be worn each time a bath or dip is performed. Pets tend to shake when they get wet; chemicals still present on the pet when it shakes could splash into a team member's eye, causing damage. If this should occur, team members should not rub the eye(s), but rather find the nearest eyewash station and rinse the eyes for the amount of time suggested by the SDS. Dipping areas should also be well ventilated, as the fumes from many dips can be caustic.

Compressed oxygen tanks must be secured in an upright position with a chain. Team members that are walking by can bump into unsecured tanks and cause them to fall on a team member or to the floor (Figure 21-36). Tanks may explode on impact; therefore securing tanks is essential. All tanks should be kept away from heat sources such as furnaces, water heaters, and direct sunlight.

Team members must dress appropriately for the job, as outlined in employee manuals. For safety purposes, open-toed shoes are not allowed; if team members will be working with large animals, steel-toed boots may be required. Jewelry should be kept to a minimum, because long earrings and bracelets could get tangled up in pets, causing injury to both team members and patients.

WHAT WOULD YOU DO/NOT DO?

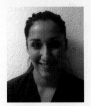

Mr. Yazzi, a long-time client, has come into the practice with Taco, a small Pomeranian. Upon walking to the counter to check out, Mr. Yazzi trips on the weight scale, which has recently been moved to the hallway between the examination rooms. He is able to catch himself and not fall; however, he twists his back, sending it into muscle spasms. He states that he is fine; it was his fault for not looking down and seeing the scale on the floor. Ashleigh, the receptionist that saw the incident offers him a chair to sit on, and rest until his back relaxes. He declines to sit down, stating he just needs to get home and lay down on the bed.

Ashleigh is afraid that the client may sue the practice.

What Should Ashleigh Do?

Ashleigh should first notify the owner and practice manager of the incident and write down the entire incident, before fine details are forgotten. Pictures should be taken of the scale, and how the client tripped. If the client calls and threatens the practice, the professional liability company should be called and informed of the incident.

Second, the practice should invest in some large protective barriers that clients can see, preventing them from tripping on the low lying scale. Pictures of the barriers should also be taken, indicating the corrective action the practice has taken, to prevent incidents such as this from occurring again. If it is feasible, the practice can sink the scale into the floor creating a flat surface (simply cut a space out of the concrete that will tightly fit the scale). Place a mat or rug over the scale for a nice appearance.

OSHA's Form 301
Injury and Illness Incident Report

U.S. Department of Labor
Occupational Safety and Health Administration

Form approved OMB no. 1218-0176

Attention: This form contains information relating to employee health and must be used in a manner that protects the confidentiality of employees to the extent possible while the information is being used for occupational safety and health purposes.

This *Injury and Illness Incident Report* is one of the first forms you must fill out when a recordable work-related injury or illness has occurred. Together with the *Log of Work-Related Injuries and Illnesses* and the accompanying *Summary*, these forms help the employer and OSHA develop a picture of the extent and severity of work-related incidents.

Within 7 calendar days after you receive information that a recordable work-related injury or illness has occurred, you must fill out this form or an equivalent. Some state workers' compensation, insurance, or other reports may be acceptable substitutes. To be considered an equivalent form, any substitute must contain all the information asked for on this form.

According to Public Law 91-596 and 29 CFR 1904, OSHA's recordkeeping rule, you must keep this form on file for 5 years following the year to which it pertains.

If you need additional copies of this form, you may photocopy and use as many as you need.

Completed by _____

Title _____

Phone (_____) _____ - _____   Date ___/___/___

Information about the employee

1) Full name _____

2) Street _____
   City _____ State ____ ZIP _____

3) Date of birth ___/___/___

4) Date hired ___/___/___

5) ☐ Male
   ☐ Female

Information about the physician or other health care professional

6) Name of physician or other health care professional _____

7) If treatment was given away from the worksite, where was it given?
   Facility _____
   Street _____
   City _____ State ____ ZIP _____

8) Was employee treated in an emergency room?
   ☐ Yes
   ☐ No

9) Was employee hospitalized overnight as an in-patient?
   ☐ Yes
   ☐ No

Information about the case

10) Case number from the *Log* _____ (Transfer the case number from the Log after you record the case.)

11) Date of injury or illness ___/___/___

12) Time employee began work _____ AM / PM

13) Time of event _____ AM / PM ☐ Check if time cannot be determined

14) *What was the employee doing just before the incident occurred?* Describe the activity, as well as the tools, equipment, or material the employee was using. Be specific. *Examples:* "climbing a ladder while carrying roofing materials"; "spraying chlorine from hand sprayer"; "daily computer key-entry."

15) *What happened?* Tell us how the injury occurred. *Examples:* "When ladder slipped on wet floor, worker fell 20 feet"; "Worker was sprayed with chlorine when gasket broke during replacement"; "Worker developed soreness in wrist over time."

16) *What was the injury or illness?* Tell us the part of the body that was affected and how it was affected; be more specific than "hurt," "pain," or sore." *Examples:* "strained back"; "chemical burn, hand"; "carpal tunnel syndrome."

17) *What object or substance directly harmed the employee? Examples:* "concrete floor"; "chlorine"; "radial arm saw." *If this question does not apply to the incident, leave it blank.*

18) *If the employee died, when did death occur?* Date of death ___/___/___

Public reporting burden for this collection of information is estimated to average 22 minutes per response, including time for reviewing instructions, searching existing data sources, gathering and maintaining the data needed, and completing and reviewing the collection of information. Persons are not required to respond to the collection of information unless it displays a current valid OMB control number. If you have any comments about this estimate or any other aspects of this data collection, including suggestions for reducing this burden, contact: US Department of Labor, OSHA Office of Statistical Analysis, Room N-3644, 200 Constitution Avenue, NW, Washington, DC 20210. Do not send the completed forms to this office.

FIGURE 21-34 OSHA Log 301. (Courtesy Occupational Safety and Health Administration, Department of Labor, Washington, DC.)

OSHA's Form 300A (Rev. 01/2004)

Summary of Work-Related Injuries and Illnesses

Year 20____

U.S. Department of Labor
Occupational Safety and Health Administration

Form approved OMB no. 1218-0176

All establishments covered by Part 1904 must complete this Summary page, even if no work-related injuries or illnesses occurred during the year. Remember to review the Log to verify that the entries are complete and accurate before completing this summary.

Using the Log, count the individual entries you made for each category. Then write the totals below, making sure you've added the entries from every page of the Log. If you had no cases, write "0."

Employees, former employees, and their representatives have the right to review the OSHA Form 300 in its entirety. They also have limited access to the OSHA Form 301 or its equivalent. See 29 CFR Part 1904.35, in OSHA's recordkeeping rule, for further details on the access provisions for these forms.

Number of Cases

Total number of deaths	Total number of cases with days away from work	Total number of cases with job transfer or restriction	Total number of other recordable cases
_____ (G)	_____ (H)	_____ (I)	_____ (J)

Number of Days

Total number of days away from work	Total number of days of job transfer or restriction
_____ (K)	_____ (L)

Injury and Illness Types

Total number of . . .
(M)

(1) Injuries _____
(2) Skin disorders _____
(3) Respiratory conditions _____

(4) Poisonings _____
(5) Hearing loss _____
(6) All other Illnesses _____

Post this Summary page from February 1 to April 30 of the year following the year covered by the form.

Public reporting burden for this collection of information is estimated to average 58 minutes per response, including time to review the instructions, search and gather the data needed, and complete and review the collection of information. Persons are not required to respond to the collection of information unless it displays a currently valid OMB control number. If you have any comments about these estimates or any other aspects of this data collection, contact: US Department of Labor, OSHA Office of Statistical Analysis, Room N-3644, 200 Constitution Avenue, NW, Washington, DC 20210. Do not send the completed forms to this office.

Establishment information

Your establishment name _____

Street _____

City _____ State _____ ZIP _____

Industry description (e.g., Manufacture of motor truck trailers) _____

Standard Industrial Classification (SIC), if known (e.g., 3715) __ __ __ __

OR

North American Industrial Classification (NAICS), if known (e.g., 336212) __ __ __ __ __ __

Employment information (If you don't have these figures, see the Worksheet on the back of this page to estimate.)

Annual average number of employees _____

Total hours worked by all employees last year _____

Sign here

Knowingly falsifying this document may result in a fine.

I certify that I have examined this document and that to the best of my knowledge the entries are true, accurate, and complete.

_____   _____
Company executive   Title

_____   _____
Phone   Date

FIGURE 21-35 OSHA Form 300A. (Courtesy Occupational Safety and Health Administration, Department of Labor, Washington, DC.)

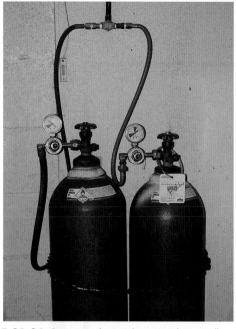

FIGURE 21-36 Oxygen tanks must be secured to a wall at all times.

PRACTICE POINT For safety purposes, open-toed shoes are not allowed on the veterinary practice floor.

Implementation

Four easy steps will help implement any safety plan within a practice. Gathering information is the first step, followed by delegating and preparing, training, and finally implementation.

When gathering information for the safety plan, a safety officer must be designated. This individual, who is in charge of several administrative duties (Box 21-2), must be highly motivated and task oriented. The safety officer should evaluate the entire facility annually and list any item that is a hazard or could be one in the future. Hazards include slippery floors, sharp corners, damaged radiology shielding, chemicals, and biohazard containers. Many more topics can be added to the lists of both administrative duties and hazards to inspect for; these are only examples.

The safety officer should have a meeting with the entire team to discuss the importance of the safety plan, review the Hazard Communication Standard as well as the rights of the practice and as those of the employees. Information should be gathered from team members of hazards they have recognized in the practice that may have been overlooked during the safety officer's walk-through inspection.

During the delegation and preparation phase, hazards can be identified, analyzed for ways to correct and stabilize the hazard, determine what PPE would be needed for the hazard, and order PPE and/or other materials as needed.

The third phase includes training on each hazard and the use of PPE for those hazards. Implementing the program is now easy to accomplish because the practice has the proper materials needed, and the staff has been trained. When an

BOX 21-2 | Safety Officer Responsibilities

- Ensuring that the radiograph machines are registered with the correct state department
- Inspections are posted
- Drug Enforcement Agency registration is current for the practice and for all doctors
- Job safety poster is visible to all team members
- Post OSHA Form 300A of employee injuries every February
- Develop and maintain hospital safety manual
- Evaluate hospital yearly for potential hazards

emergency occurs, the staff will know the proper response to accommodate that emergency.

The Hospital Safety Manual

A hospital safety manual (HSM) should include an overview of all materials previously covered. It should include the hazardous communication plan, the SDS filing system, and an explanation of secondary container labeling systems. An HSM can be created for each individual clinic or ordered. Tabs can be used to separate topics and allow easy identification.

VETERINARY PRACTICE and the LAW

It is the responsibility of the employer to inform all employees or volunteers regarding the job hazards that may affect the health of employees or volunteers in the veterinary practice in which they are employed. Those hazards are listed as physical, chemical, and biological. Federal law requires that each veterinary practice design and implement a written plan that describes how each workplace complies with the OSHA Hazard Communication Standard. Veterinary employers should also become familiar with the occupational hazard laws of their own state, understand the Pregnancy Discrimination Act, Title VII, and state statutes, which specifically regulate maternity leave policies.

It is essential for employers to conduct and document training at the time of hiring, annually, and anytime a hazard has occurred.

REVIEW QUESTIONS

1. What is a zoonotic disease?
2. How should an animal heavier than 40 lb be lifted onto a table?
3. What is OSHA?
4. What is the Right to Know poster?
5. What is an SDS?
6. What is the purpose of PPE?
7. When does OSHA Form 300A have to be posted?
8. What is an eyewash station?
9. What is a biohazard material?
10. What are some hazardous chemicals used in veterinary practice?

11. Under OSHA guidelines, employees are responsible for which of the following:
    a. Read the Right to Know Poster
    b. Order PPE for the practice
    c. Train fellow team members on the use of PPE
    d. Document conditions in which PPE must be used
12. If an OSHA inspector arrives at the hospital, which of the following options should be exercised?
    a. Introduce the inspector to the safety officer
    b. Allow the inspection to proceed without a team member
    c. Hide violations from the staff
13. Which of the following contribute to the majority of fires in the veterinary practice?
    a. Paper files stacked up to the ceiling
    b. Blankets next to a furnace
    c. Overloaded electrical outlets
    d. Heating units left unattended
14. Back injuries can be classified as which type of injury?
    a. Physical
    b. Biohazard
    c. Caustic
    d. Ergonomic

15. Noise protection should be provided for employees when noise levels reach which decibel level?
    a. 75 dB
    b. 85 dB
    c. 95 dB
    d. Ear protection is not required

Recommended Reading

Lappin M: General concepts in zoonotic disease control, *Vet Clin North Am* 35:1, 2005.
OSHA: *Employee workplace rights*, Washington, DC, 1994, OSHA Publications Office.
Seibert PJ: *Be safe! A managers guide to hazardous substances*, Lakewood, CO, 2008, AAHA Press.
Seibert PJ: *Be safe! A managers guide to radiation and waste anesthetic gases*, Lakewood, CO, 2008, AAHA Press.
Seibert PJ: *Be safe! A managers guide to veterinary workplace safety*, Lakewood, CO, 2007, AAHA Press.
Veterinary safety: workplace topics for your veterinary practice, Schaumburg, IL, 2003, American Veterinary Medical Association Professional Liability Trust.

Reference

Talan DA, Citron DM, Abrahamian FM, et al.: Bacteriologic analysis of dog and cat bites, *New England Journal of Medicine* 340:85–92, 1999.

Security

KEY TERMS

Computer Hacker
One-Way Door Locks
Perimeter Lighting
Personal Protection
  Device
Security System

OUTLINE

Computer System, *393*
Theft, *393*
Security System, *394*
Cameras and Recording Devices, *395*
Perimeter Lighting, *395*

Emergency Calls, *395*
Mobile Practices, *395*
Methods of Defense, *396*
  Personal Protection Devices, *396*
Safety of Hospitalized Patients, *396*

LEARNING OBJECTIVES

When you have finished this chapter, you should be able to:

1. Define the importance of one-way door locks.
2. Describe methods used to protect a computer system against embezzlement and hackers.
3. Describe methods used to protect the practice against theft from both employees and thieves.
4. Identify an effective security system for the practice.
5. Define perimeter lighting.
6. Define personal protection devices.

 ## CRITICAL COMPETENCIES

1. **Adaptability** - being open to change and flexible work methods; the ability to adapt behavior to changing conditions or new information.
2. **Analytical Skills** - the ability to analyze information and use logic to address problems; the ability to quickly and accurately grasp complex information and concepts and to make correct inferences.
3. **Continuous Learning** - a curiosity for learning; actively seek out new information, technologies, and methods; keep skills updated and apply new knowledge to the job.
4. **Creativity** - the ability to think creatively about situations, to see things in

new and different ways; use imagination and creativity to develop innovative solutions to problems.
5. **Critical and Strategic Thinking** - the ability to think critically about situations and to understand the relevance of information for different problems; use critical reasoning to generate and evaluate alternative courses of action or points of view relevant to an issue.
6. **Planning and Prioritizing** - the ability to effectively manage time and workload to meet deadlines; the ability to organize work, set priorities, and establish plans for achieving goals.

Security for team members and the practice must be considered a top priority. Practices have an ethical obligation to provide a safe and secure working environment for employees as well as a safe and secure hospital for clients and their pets. Safety goes beyond the standard preventions for slips and falls; security must be included and viewed from several aspects. Computer systems must be protected from employees, clients, the general public, and especially hackers. The practice must be protected from robbers and thieves, and clients and patients must be protected from harm and danger.

Practices should use deadbolts on all doors and one-way locks on all doors except the client entrance. When the business is open, the deadbolts must remain unlocked. The one-way door lock only allows access into the building with a key, but clients and employees can exit anytime. The client entrance door must let clients enter and exit as needed; therefore a standard door lock can be installed. All doors must be locked before the last team member leaves the premises to ensure the safety of the practice.

Entrances must be protected and monitored for those who enter. Any door other than the one clients enter must be locked at all times. A person could enter through any unlocked door in the rear of the practice and hide until the practice closes. He or she could harm employees quickly and force them into inconceivable actions. It is imperative to secure doors, and they must remain locked from the outside at all times. One-way door locks allow employees and clients to escape if an emergency occurs.

Computer System

The computer system is a valuable asset to the practice and must be protected from hackers, employees, and clients. A computer hacker is an individual or group or individuals who attempt to break into programs or networks that are restricted. Once they gain access to the restricted program, the hackers can cause damage to the program or network. This damage can range from changing prices to deleting transactions as well as installing viruses that can cripple the system. Chapter 8 describes several products that can be used to protect a system from hackers. Antivirus software, firewalls, and antispyware should be installed on each computer that is linked to the system to aid in the protection.

Practices should ensure that the system is backed up on a nightly basis, either to an off-premises location or onto a CD that is removed from the system. If a thief breaks into the practice at night and steals the computer or severely damages it, information can be fully reinstalled onto a new computer immediately.

 Veterinary practice managers maintain protocols for hospital procedures and risk management plans.

It is terrible to assume that computers must be protected from employees; however, employees will, on occasion, steal client mailing lists and sell them, either to a competing veterinarian or to a mail order company that is willing to pay for the names and addresses.

> **PRACTICE POINT** Veterinary computer software should be password protected for specific procedures.

Passwords should be put in place on a computer system, allowing only certain individuals access to financial reports, mailing lists, and deletion codes. Office managers should be the only employees allowed to delete transactions, and practice managers and owners should be the only team members allowed to change or delete product and service codes. Managers should also be the only authority to change and/or override prices of products and services. Managers should review the audit trail daily looking for any signs of embezzlement or theft.

If computers are located in exam rooms, a password-protected screen saver should be enabled. Clients waiting to be seen may try to access the Internet or their record. These clients may obtain confidential information if they access the practice management system.

Theft

Theft can occur at any time, either by an employee or by a person who enters the building with the intent to commit a crime. Employee theft can range from embezzling cash to stealing products and/or food. Procedures must be implemented to prevent either situation from occurring. Cash transactions must be recorded immediately, both in the computer and in the client's record. Receipts must be produced for clients indicating their account has been paid with cash. End-of-day totals must match the cash in the drawer, along with all credit card and check transactions. The deposit must then be double-checked by the practice manager, ensuring that the deposit made to the bank at the end of the day matches the end-of-day deposit in the computer. If any discrepancy exists, it must be investigated immediately. Review Chapter 2 for more information on end-of-day reconciliation security features.

Team members purchasing products should always have the designated office manager enter the products or services into the computer. This ensures consistency in entering codes and allows someone other than the team member purchasing the product to determine the total. If owners, associates, or practice managers see an employee taking a product that has not been charged for out of the building, the employee should be questioned immediately, not days later.

Practices must always be prepared for criminal intent. Practices are the target for theft of both drugs and cash. Many practices do not keep a large amount of cash on hand, especially since the payment trend has shifted to debit cards instead of cash for payment of services. However, thieves continue to believe that veterinary practices

WHAT WOULD YOU DO/NOT DO?

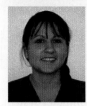

Chade, a new veterinary assistant, observed a long-term associate place a box of Heartgard in her purse and leave the practice. She does not know yet what the procedures are for charging employees for products, and assumes that the associate has been charged for the product. Two months later, she sees the same associate place cephalexin capsules in a pill vial, but did not create a label for the medication. Chade has learned that labels are created once a product is entered into the computer, which charges appropriately. Chade is unsure about the process but feels that the associate may be taking product from the clinic. She is unsure if she should talk to the owner about the associate. She feels that because she is the new employee, that the owner or practice manager may not believe her.

What Should Chade Do?

The practice should have an open-door policy regarding communication, making it easy for Chade to talk with her superiors about the possible employee theft. She should talk with the owner or practice manager when other employees are not around and address her concerns. She should detail both incidents and explain that she is not trying to get anyone in trouble; rather, she wants to protect the practice from loss associated with shrinkage. She may suggest the installation of a video camera system to help deter employee theft, and offer to find a variety of systems for the practice to consider.

hold a large amount of cash on premises. Individuals also want controlled substances, which have a large dollar value on the streets. It is imperative that all drugs be locked in a safe that cannot be moved. Review Chapter 16 for information on safes approved by the U.S. Drug Enforcement Administration.

If a person with criminal intent enters the practice, all money should be given to him or her from the cash drawer. Team members should not risk injury or death to themselves, clients, or other team members to protect the small amount of money that the practice has on premises. If the thieves request drugs, give them what they want; the sooner they leave the practice, the safer the team members and clients will be. All doors should be locked and police should be called immediately.

> **PRACTICE POINT** Remaining calm during a robbery is essential to help prevent team members from being injured by thieves.

If the team is able to get a description of the thieves, it will be helpful to police, along with a description of the vehicle used to get away. Details can be hard to obtain in a stressful situation such as this.

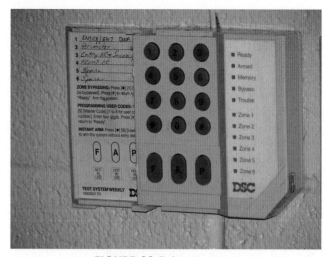

FIGURE 22-1 Security system.

Security System

Security systems should be installed to protect the premises while the practice is closed. Sensory devices should be placed on all windows and doors; if any window or door is broken or opened after the system as been activated, an alarm will sound. Systems may also have a motion detector; once the alarm has been activated, any motion that is detected inside the building will trigger the alarm (Figure 22-1). Many security systems are connected to a monitoring system, which will automatically place a call to police if the alarm is triggered. Many practices have keypads at the employee entrance, allowing the alarm to be set or deactivated. Others have a badge reader; employees must swipe their badges to gain access to the building. This also allows employee monitoring during closed hours. Both devices can prevent entry if an employee is terminated and tries to reenter the building after the practice has closed.

Many security devices have the ability to send text messages or alerts to owners and practice managers regarding who has activated and deactivated the system and when. This allows the monitoring of the practice over the weekend, if and when employees are on the premises when they should not be. Unfortunately, some robberies are the result of an inside job or tip-off; all perimeters must be monitored closely to protect the business in all fashions.

Some security systems have the option of installing panic buttons. These buttons are excellent in the event of a robbery or assault and should be placed in the front office in a convenient, yet hidden, location. If an emergency occurs, team members can hit the panic button to automatically call 911.

Emergency and specialty clinics often install buzzers at their front doors, adding a second level of protection for team members. When clients arrive, they push a buzzer; the receptionist can verify the clients and allow access.

Emergency clinics must take special precautions for safety because they are open throughout the night and weekend. This is a particularly easy time for criminals to target the business. Many emergency clinics have fewer employees at night, and there are fewer witnesses to observe unlawful actions.

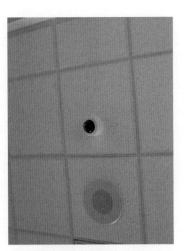

FIGURE 22-2 Camera.

Some practices may also install security devices on pharmacy doors, allowing the monitoring of team members who enter and exit the pharmacy room. This can decrease shrinkage (i.e., employee theft).

Cameras and Recording Devices

Cameras can be placed at all entrances and exits, allowing recording of all employees and clients as they enter and leave the premises (Figure 22-2). Cameras and monitoring systems should be of high quality, allowing replication of images if needed. Action can be recorded on DVD-R, which allows more information to be stored than a CD, and can be written over with the permission of the operator. Cameras can be linked through the server, allowing an owner to view actions occurring through a home computer. If the alarm was triggered by a loose animal, the police can be notified of the false alarm.

Cameras can also be placed over cash drawers, near controlled substance locations, and within the pharmacy location to thwart potential employee embezzlement.

Perimeter Lighting

The practice must have excellent lighting on the outside of the building and parking lot for the protection of clients and employees (Figure 22-3). Potential criminals may find a dark corner and wait for an employee to leave the building alone at night. They may either attack the employee in the parking lot or follow the person to another location. The same can occur for clients, who are less observant when leaving practices; they are generally preoccupied with their pets and loading them safely into the vehicle. Bright lights act as a deterrent to criminals and provide a safer environment.

> **PRACTICE POINT** Parking lots and the perimeter of the building must be lit well for the protection of both team members and clients.

When team members are leaving a practice, they should use the buddy system, with a minimum of two employees

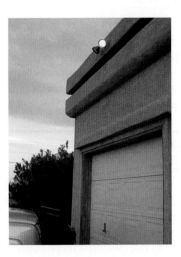

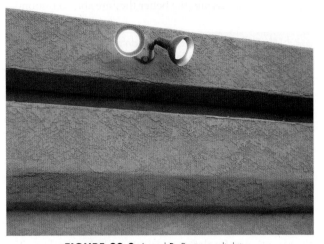

FIGURE 22-3 A and B, Perimeter lighting.

leaving together. If only one employee needs to leave, two others should walk the team member to his or her car, then return to the practice as the car is leaving. If team members must be at a practice alone (weekend treatments, etc.) they should be instructed never to answer the door. Thieves are creative at being able to get into a business after hours, especially if they see a lone employee inside. Team members should always inspect the outside premises before leaving to ensure no one is lingering in the parking lot.

Emergency Calls

Many practices in small communities are on call for emergencies. In such situations, veterinarians are at an increased risk for attempted assaults, and all precautions should be taken when meeting clients. Calls should not be taken alone; a technician should arrive with the doctor, regardless of the time or day. Clients should be viewed through the peephole in the door to visualize the pet and ensure that the client has an actual emergency.

Mobile Practices

Mobile practices are at an increased risk for robbery and assault because they do not have the same security options

that are available within a building. Mobile veterinarians may carry drugs with them, along with cash, making them excellent targets for assailants. Veterinarians should always carry cell phones with emergency numbers programmed for quick access. Carrying some type of device for personal protection is recommended.

Methods of Defense

A recommendation for a monthly meeting topic is methods of defense in case any violent crime or assault occurs. It is also advisable to have a local defense expert provide valuable training for the staff. Experts can locate areas of weakness in safety in and around the practice and can create scenarios for team members to role play. The more aware team members are of a possible assault, the better they are able to respond.

> *PRACTICE POINT* Personal defense courses are recommended for all team members and can be implemented into a continuing education seminar.

Personal Protection Devices

The ASP Tactical Baton is the most tactically sophisticated impact weapon currently available (Figure 22-4). Easily carried and readily available, ASP batons have an incredible psychological deterrence and control potential. ASP batons are small to carry, but once swung to open, the baton extends immediately, providing excellent protection for an individual. ASP batons can be kept in the front office with the receptionist for defense against would-be attackers. The receptionist would be able to swing the baton open in the event of an attack. ASP batons are also ideal for mobile veterinarians.

Mace is a brand of tear gas that is often used by police to deter potential attackers. Mace must be sprayed directly at the attacker and creates an intense burning sensation in the eyes and lungs. Mace can be extremely effective when used correctly.

Tasers are often thought of as weapons used by law enforcement to subdue those who are apprehended. Fortunately, models are also available for personal protection. A Taser is an electroshock weapon that uses electrical current to disrupt voluntary control of muscles, resulting in muscle contractions.

Both ASP batons and Tasers may require training in some states. Practices and mobile veterinarians should inquire with the local police department about the use and regulations of such devices. The manufacturers of both products offer courses with certified trainers to allow individuals to become comfortable with the use of such items. Both personal protection devices can cause great harm to another individual and should never be used carelessly.

Safety of Hospitalized Patients

Patients that are hospitalized must be protected at all times. It has been reported that criminals sometimes break into a

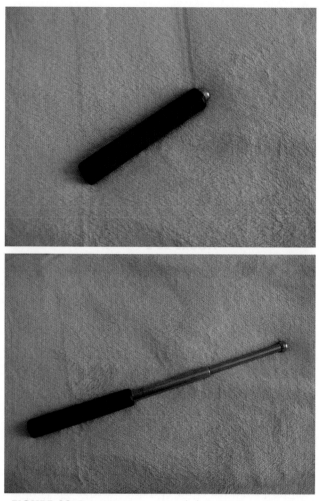

FIGURE 22-4 A, ASP Baton unextended. B, ASP Baton extended.

practice, steal a few items, and release all the animals that are hospitalized or being boarded. If it is possible to lock doorways between the practice and cages, patients are at less of a risk of being targeted. However, if a fire occurs in the building after hours, this may hamper rescue efforts.

⚖ VETERINARY PRACTICE and the LAW

One function of the veterinary practice that has been affected by the Privacy Act is patient check-in. Clients that sign in may do so on a sheet with adhesive pull off strips for each line so that clients cannot read names of those that have signed in before them. The Privacy Act does permit incidental disclosures as long as the practice has reasonable guards against disclosure of personal information. Clients may be called to the examination room by their pet's name, protecting the privacy of their last name. Silent pagers can also be used, paging clients as a room becomes available.

It is also important to protect the computer screen from clients; personal information should not be viewable to clients as they check in or out. Screen privacy protectors can be applied to monitors, preventing the viewing of documents from an angle. A shredder should also be available to shred documents as needed, protecting clients from criminal activity.

REVIEW QUESTIONS

1. Why should computer systems be backed up at the end of every shift?
2. Why should computer software be password protected?
3. What is the purpose of one-way door locks?
4. What should team members do if an armed individual enters the practice and demands money or drugs?
5. How can security systems provide practice protection?
6. Why is exterior perimeter lighting so critical?
7. What is an ASP baton?
8. Computers systems should be backed up:
   a. Every 24 hours
   b. On a CD or DVD
   c. Off-site
   d. All of the above

9. Personal protective devices available to the general public include all of the following except:
   a. Tactical batons
   b. Mace
   c. Tasers
   d. Personal hand guns
10. Security systems may include:
    a. Window alarms
    b. Doorway alarms
    c. Video camera
    d. All of the above

## PART IV

Clinical Assisting in the Veterinary Practice

Veterinary assistants and technicians play a vital role in the success of the practice, especially when it comes to clinical assisting. The veterinarian(s) must be able to depend on the assistants to obtain accurate histories of the patient, restrain animals properly for examination, and perform diagnostic procedures efficiently and correctly. Procedures completed incorrectly or by cutting corners can yield unreliable and false results and therefore poor patient care. Procedures completed incorrectly also result in lost income for the practice, as tests must be repeated, at no charge to the client.

It is imperative for veterinary assistants and technicians to understand the risks associated with anesthesia and surgery, and relay the information to the clients. Many clients do not understand that such risks are present and may become extremely upset if a tragic event occurs while their pet is in the hospital. Not only do the medications present a risk for surgery, but the surgical packs, equipment, and room must be prepared correctly to prevent nosocomial infections, which can also present risk for the patient. Correct instrument cleaning procedures, autoclaving techniques, and pack preparation must be initiated and enforced.

Anesthesia machine maintenance and administration of gases fall in the hands of assistants and technicians, who must be able to troubleshoot and correct problems within minutes. A machine working at optimum levels and a machine that is barely functioning can mean life or death of a patient, and the assistant and technician must be able to prevent death from occurring (because of machine error). Autoclaves must also be maintained, allowing packs to be sterilized correctly, killing any and all infectious agents that may lie within.

All equipment must be maintained in some fashion within the practice; properly maintained equipment lasts longer and provides optimal results for the life of the equipment. Properly maintained equipment increases efficiency of the team, provides superior service to the clients, and causes less stress on the patient.

Pharmacology is another important topic for veterinary assistants and technicians. Team members must become familiar with products that are carried in the practice, drug dosages, and routes of administration. This helps prevent mistakes from occurring, should a direction be misinterpreted. Many times, the veterinarian or credentialed technician make mistakes unintentionally, and assistants or other technicians may catch the mistake. This is why teamwork is so important; members of the team help each other out while providing exceptional patient care. Knowledge of drugs is also important so that clients can be educated on the side effects of products as well as the interaction with other drugs. Client education is essential.

Practices see many puppies and kittens and provide care through the pets' senior years. Often, clients ask nutritional advice of the team. Assistants must be familiar with the nutritional needs of patients and be able to recommend appropriate diets. Many therapeutic diets are available, and team members should be familiar with those carried by the practice. Parasite prevention and education is essential for owners of puppies and kittens as well as owners of adults that live in highly endemic areas. Warm and humid climates attract a variety of parasites, and it is the responsibility of the practice to educate the clients of the risks associated with those parasites. Programs should be implemented to control and prevent diseases associated with these parasites.

Emergencies may come at any time during open office hours. Team members must be familiar with common emergencies and have supplies prepared in case the emergency is real and severe. Many conditions occur to animals that may not be an emergency; however, being prepared for the worst case is best. The same applies to common disorders seen by the practice; the more informed the team members are about diseases or conditions, the more information can be relayed to owners.

With all of the knowledge that is gained through practice, school, and real-life experiences, professional development occurs on a daily basis. It is important to continuing developing skills in case one ever wishes to switch careers. Many self-assessment tests can be completed indicating strengths and weaknesses of an individual, allowing oneself to continuously improve the weaknesses. Employment opportunities go far beyond a veterinary practice, allowing the skills obtained in practice to be used in other areas of the industry. All members of the team must be prepared to market themselves in a professional and diligent manner; the first impression is a lasting impression. If career change is necessary, one must consider retirement. It is never too early or too late for retirement planning; as the cost of living increases, so does the cost of retirement. One must learn to save money for the future, because Social Security retirement benefits may not be available when you need them.

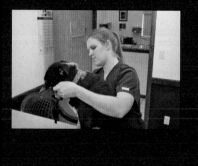

O U T L I N E

Examinations, *401*
   Taking a History, *401*
   Restraint, *401*
Lifetime Care and Disease Prevention, *402*
   Vaccinations and Diseases, *402*
   Common Diseases, *403*
   Wellness Exams and
      Recommendations, *404*
   Puppies and Kittens, *404*
   Adults, *406*
   Seniors, *406*
Diagnostics, *407*
   Blood Work, *407*
   Cytology, *407*
   Urinalysis, *407*
   Fecal Analysis, *408*
   Electrocardiogram, *408*
   Blood Pressure, *408*
Diagnostic Imaging, *408*
   Safety, *408*
   Guidelines, *409*
   Digital Radiographs, *410*
   Fluoroscopy, *410*
   Ultrasound, *410*
   Computed Tomographic Scanning, *410*
   Magnetic Resonance Imaging, *410*
Surgery, *411*
   Preanesthetic Documentation, *411*
   Anesthesia, *411*
   Endotracheal Tubes, *411*
Pharmacology, *412*
   Chemical, Nonproprietary, and Propri-
      etary Names, *412*
   Prescriptions, *412*
   Dispensing Medications, *413*
   Calculations and Conversions, *413*
   Administration of Medications, *413*
   Expired Medications, *413*
   Over-the-Counter Pharmaceuticals, *413*
   Labels, *414*
   Drugs, *414*
Therapeutic Diets, *416*
   AAFCO, *416*
   Puppies, *419*
   Large-Breed Puppies, *420*
   Kittens, *420*
   Adults, *422*
   Seniors, *422*
   Conditions that can be Treated
      or Maintained by Diet, *422*

Parasites, *425*
Common Small Animal Emergencies, *425*
   Anaphylactic Reaction, *425*
   Antifreeze Ingestion, *425*
   Bleeding, *425*
   Blocked Cat, *425*
   Cardiopulmonary Resuscitation, *425*
   Dyspneic Animal, *425*
   Dystocia, *426*
   Gastric Torsion, *426*
   Car Accident, *426*
   Heatstroke, *426*
   Proptosed Eye, *426*
   Seizure, *426*
   Toxicities, *426*
Common Equine Emergencies, *427*
   Colic, *427*
   Laceration, *427*
Common Bovine Emergencies, *427*
   Down Cow, *427*
   Dystocia, *427*
   Uterine Prolapse, *427*
**Common Ovine and Caprine
   Emergencies,** *427*
   Pregnancy Toxemia, *427*
Common Canine Disorders, *427*
   Allergies, *427*
   Anal Gland Impaction and/or
      Infection, *428*
   Ear Infection, *428*
   Gingivitis, *428*
   Hypothyroidism, *428*
   Kennel Cough, *428*
   Ocular Discharge, *429*
   Skin Diseases, *429*
   Obesity, *429*
   Tumors, *429*
Common Feline Disorders, *429*
   Abscesses, *429*
   Asthma, *430*
   Feline Lower Urinary Tract
      Disease, *430*
   Hyperthyroidism, *430*
   Megacolon, *430*
   Ringworm, *430*
Housekeeping, *430*
Boarding, *431*
   Admitting, *431*
   Nail Trims, *431*
Condo Facilities, *432*

KEY TERMS

Adjuvant
Anesthesia
Anorexia
Carnivore
Electrocardiogram
Enucleated
Fomites
General Anesthesia
Gingivitis
Hypothyroidism
Injection Site Sarcoma
Killed Vaccine
Kilocalorie
Lethargy
Local Anesthesia
Modified Live Vaccine
Omnivore
Recombinant Vaccine

409

LEARNING OBJECTIVES

When you have completed this chapter, you should be able to:

1. Identify common diseases and vaccinations.
2. Define diagnostic equipment and procedures.
3. Explain the importance of preanesthetic procedures.
4. Calculate medication doses.
5. Explain the importance of labeling medications.
6. Explain to owners how to administer medications.
7. Define the nutritional needs of puppies and kittens.
8. Differentiate therapeutic diets based on characteristics.
9. Define common emergencies.
10. Explain the most common diseases of animals.

There are many facets involved with assisting veterinarians and veterinary technicians. There are excellent books (referenced at the end of the chapter) available that give greater detail for the topics listed below. This chapter is intended to provide brief information for the new student and team member. Once these basic skills have been mastered, a review of the books referenced will help develop more advanced skills.

Examinations

Taking a History

It is the responsibility of all team members, but especially veterinary assistants and technicians, to check the patient into a room and obtain a complete history from the client. Chapter 14 provides detailed instructions on how to take an accurate history. It is very important to know if a pet has been vomiting or has diarrhea, how long it has had the presenting symptoms, and whether the owner can correlate any symptoms with abnormal events. The history taker must write down all the information provided by the owner; the details may provide a valuable tool for the doctor as an attempt is made to determine a diagnosis. A good history taker is a valuable asset to the practice.

Vital signs are completed at the same time the history is being obtained. Five vital signs are now recognized by the American Animal Hospital Association (AAHA): weight, temperature, heart rate, respiratory rate, pain and body condition score.

Restraint

It is the duty of the team to prevent the veterinarian or veterinary technician from being bitten by the patient. Restraint is one of the most important tasks that must be learned and mastered. Patients can be wiggly and excited. All patients have their own emotions and deal with stress differently. They may be scared and may bite out of fear; others will bite because they are in pain or are aggressive. Every animal should be treated as if it could bite, puppies and kittens

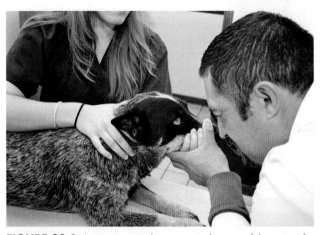

FIGURE 23-1 Assistants must always secure the nose of the patient for veterinarians and veterinary technicians completing an ophthalmic exam.

included. When doctors look into the patients' eyes and ears, they may become scared and bite out of fear. Dogs and cats can bite the tip of the doctor's nose when they are looking in a patient's eyes. Cats are quick with their forefeet and will strike with no warning (Figure 23-1).

Time and experience will teach new team members the best way to restrain animals and how much restraint is needed for each individual. Some cats may react best with little restraint; when the scruff is grabbed for restraint, they begin to object.

All animals should be observed while being restrained. The patient should remain pink and able to breathe well. If the patient's mucous membranes become blue (cyanotic) at any time, the animal should be given a break.

If a muzzle is needed at any time, team members should not hesitate to use it (Figure 23-2). Muzzles are made to protect team members from being bitten! Some owners may argue that their pet does not need a muzzle; however, for everyone's safety, including the owner's, muzzles should be used. Both dog and cat muzzles are available and come in a variety of sizes. Muzzles should fit snugly on a dog's nose. If the dog can open its mouth, the muzzle is too large, and the purpose of the muzzle is defeated. Cat muzzles

should fit snugly over the entire head. Cat bags and towels may also be helpful to prevent team members from becoming scratched (Figure 23-3). The full cat body is placed inside the bag with only the head exposed. Most bags have two small openings that will allow front legs to be pulled through if needed.

> **PRACTICE POINT** A muzzle should never be left on an unattended pet because it may vomit and aspirate stomach contents.

WHAT WOULD YOU DO/NOT DO?

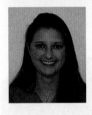

Sami Yung has brought Spot into the practice for her annual examination. Because there is a large Asian population in the area, the veterinary practice has learned two things about the Asian culture; they are brought up to respect elders and have a great a great respect for harmony. If they do not understand something, they may not admit it to avoid disrupting harmony. Mrs. Yung speaks a moderate amount of English, but previously she has not administered medications as directed. The team feels that it may due to a misunderstanding. Spot is 7 years old now and is advised to have a senior wellness exam, including blood work, urinalysis and an ECG. Mrs. Yung approves the estimate for the senior wellness exam, which reveals a urinary tract infection. Teresa, the veterinary technician working with Mrs. Yung feels that Mrs. Yung may not understand the recommendations, although she signed the estimate. Dr. Dreamer examines Spot and explains to Mrs. Yung that a urinary tract infection has been diagnosed, and a further work up is recommended to determine the cause. Mrs. Yung only nods her head, but never asks any questions or states the words "yes or no" when asked specific questions.

What Should Teresa Do?
Because Teresa always has concern for clients and their understanding, she has determined that Mrs. Yung may not understand everything that is being stated to her. Teresa should create another estimate for a further work up. She should be able to find printed information regarding the workup for urinary tract infections, including radiographs to rule out stones and a culture to rule out a bacterial infection. Teresa should be able to advise Mrs. Yung to find a family member or friend to review the information with her, and schedule a follow-up visit in 2 days to determine what the next step will be, or if conservative treatment will be the only option. It is imperative to understand the cultural diversity and actions of clients that do not fully understand veterinary procedures, and take into consideration their lack of understanding.

Lifetime Care and Disease Prevention

Veterinary technicians and team members are responsible for educating clients about the care of their pets, from neonatal through geriatric stages of their lives. Preventative care promotes improved health, longevity, and patient happiness.

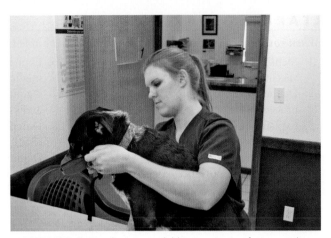
FIGURE 23-2 Muzzles are available in a variety of sizes, and must fit the patient snugly.

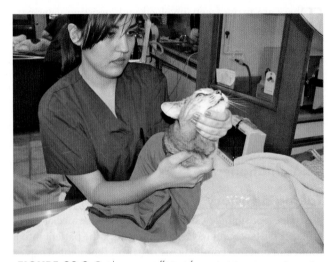
FIGURE 23-3 Cat bags are efficient for restraining aggressive cats.

When clients perceive their pet is happy, their compliance increases.

Team members must educate clients about vaccinations, disease prevention, nutrition, obesity prevention, and dental care, at minimum.

Vaccinations and Diseases

Pets are exposed to a variety of diseases throughout their lifetime and should receive vaccinations to protect against potential disease or infection. Vaccination protocols can vary with the age of the animal, location within the United States, colostral antibodies, vaccine type and route, nutritional status of the patient, and whether any other medications are being administered. Vaccine manufacturers print protocol guidelines on the product information insert to help veterinarians develop protocols for each species.

Vaccines are available in three types: modified live, killed, or recombinant. Modified live vaccines use a virus or bacteria that has been passed through a culture to reduce its virulence, whereas a killed vaccine introduces an inactivated virus into the body. Recombinant vaccines are available in two types.

The first is the subunit vaccine, produced by a microorganism that has been engineered to make a protein, which then elicits an immune response in a target host. Another is the recombinant vector type, in which harmless genetic material from a disease-causing organism is inserted into a weakened virus or bacterium (the vector). When the vector organism replicates, the genetic material that was inserted elicits the desired immune response.

The animal generates an immune response to antigens in the vaccine, thus providing protection from disease. Killed vaccines use an adjuvant to enhance an immune response to the vaccine; vaccines made with modified live viruses do not need an adjuvant because viral antigens alone can induce a strong enough response to provide protection. Recombinant vaccines provide superior, faster, and safer protection than modified live or killed vaccines. However, at present only a few vaccines use recombinant technology.

Most vaccinations are given subcutaneously (under the skin) and take several weeks to reach optimal immunity levels. Vaccines must be shipped on ice and kept cool until the pet receives them. Warm temperatures will deactivate vaccines; it is therefore imperative that they remain refrigerated until used. Some vaccines are only in liquid form; others require reconstitution with a sterile diluent before use. For those that require reconstitution, a sterile syringe and needle are aseptically inserted into the bottle of sterile diluent and the entire milliliter of diluent is removed. The needle is then inserted into the powder vial and the diluent is injected.

The syringe and needle can be removed and kept clean. The vial can be mixed by rotating it back and forth. Once all the powder has dissolved, the needle can be reinserted into the vial and the contents removed. It is important to remember that the needle should not touch anything except the rubber stopper; fingers must stay away from the needle! Sterile syringes should always be used. Never use resterilized syringes for vaccines; the process from the autoclave will deactivate the vaccination.

> *PRACTICE POINT*   Vaccine reactions can occur at any time, and every client must be advised of the risks associated with the administration of vaccines.

A variety of combinations of vaccinations are available on the market; the preference rests with the veterinarian as to which combination to order. It is highly recommended to indicate in the medical record where on the body the vaccine was given. Some vaccines may cause localized reactions, and if the location of administration has been documented in the record, vaccine reaction can be ruled in or ruled out. Stamps are available to chart the location easily (Figure 23-4).

Common Diseases

Boxes 23-1 to 23-3 are not a complete list of diseases, but rather a summary of diseases for which there are vaccines. A brief description of the disease and symptoms is also included. Some tests are available for in-house diagnostics to

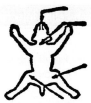

FIGURE 23-4 Utilizing a stamp in the medical record allows the staff to record where a vaccination was administered.

BOX 23-1 | Common Canine Infectious Diseases

Coronavirus
A contagious viral infection of the gastrointestinal tract that causes vomiting and diarrhea. Symptoms are similar to those of parvovirus, but the virus is not as hardy as the parvovirus, nor is the disease as life threatening.

Distemper (CDV)
A widespread and often fatal disease that can cause vomiting, diarrhea, pneumonia, and neurologic problems. The disease is transmitted by aerosol droplets from all body excretions of infected animals. Death is common with distemper, and recovery is rare.

Hepatitis
A viral disease that targets the liver. When infected, adult dogs may recover; however, it is often fatal in puppies.

Kennel Cough
An extremely contagious infection of the upper respiratory tract that is characterized by a persistent dry, hacking cough. The infection is transmitted by aerosol droplets. Contributing infections include adenovirus (CAV-2), CDV, and the bacteria *Bordetella bronchiseptica*, as well as the parainfluenza virus.

Leptospirosis
A bacterial infection that may lead to permanent kidney and liver damage. It is contagious to humans and is spread through contact with infected urine or contaminated soil or water.

Lyme Disease
A disease transmitted by ticks that infects both humans and animals. The disease can affect the joints, kidneys, and other tissues. This disease is common in the southern and eastern United States.

Parvovirus (CPV)
A highly contagious and potentially fatal disease that causes severe vomiting and bloody diarrhea. It is especially dangerous in young dogs, but all unvaccinated dogs are at risk of contracting this severe disease. This disease attacks all rapidly dividing cells, including those of the intestinal tract and the bone marrow. The disease is transmitted by contact with contaminated feces and vomit. This virus can stay in the ground for 2 years; therefore contaminated areas should be disinfected well. The best treatment available is to hospitalize the pet and treat it with intravenous fluids and antibiotics.

Rabies
A fatal viral infection of the central nervous system that can affect all mammals, including humans. The virus is transmitted through the bite of an infected animal. Routine vaccination is the key to controlling this deadly disease.

BOX 23-2 | Common Feline Infectious Diseases

Calicivirus (FCV)

An upper respiratory infection of cats with signs similar to those of feline rhinotracheitis. In addition, ulcers may be seen on the tongue and in the mouth. FCV also has a carrier state, in which healthy-looking cats are carriers of the virus. Infection is acquired by ingestion or inhalation of infectious virus present in saliva, secretions, or excretions from infected cats.

Feline Infectious Peritonitis (FIP)

This viral disease is most often seen in young adult cats. Once clinical signs are exhibited, the disease is progressive and leads to death. There are two types of clinical disease: the wet form and the dry form. In the wet form, large amounts of fluid buildup in the body cavities, especially the abdominal cavity. In the dry form, the clinical signs are variable depending on the organ systems that are affected, such as the intestines, kidneys, liver, lungs, nervous system, or eyes. The dry form usually has a longer clinical course and death may not occur for a year or more. The virus may be contracted by ingesting infected feces.

Feline Immunodeficiency Virus (FIV)

This is a retrovirus that causes immunodeficiency in cats. It is in the same subfamily as human immunodeficiency virus, the causative agent of human AIDS. Stomatitis, upper respiratory infection, recurrent infections, persistent diarrhea, fever, and wasting are common signs of FIV. Transmission occurs through saliva.

Feline Leukemia Virus (FeLV)

Infection with this virus can cause serious disease and death in cats. The virus decreases the ability of the immune system to respond to infection and may lead to the development of different types of cancer. FeLV is passed from cat to cat by direct contact (saliva). It is not contagious to people. FeLV is the leading cause of death in cats.

Panleukopenia (FPV)

A widespread and potentially fatal disease that may cause a sudden onset of severe vomiting and diarrhea, fever, and loss of appetite. It is extremely dangerous in kittens but can also be fatal in adults. Even when recovery occurs, a normal-looking kitten may shed the virus for up to 6 weeks. The virus is shed in secretions and excretions from infected animals.

Feline Pneumonitis Chlamydia

This is another common respiratory infection in cats producing sneezing, fever, and a thick discharge from the eyes. Chlamydial infection may be associated with the development of more serious bacterial complications.

Rabies

A fatal viral infection of the central nervous system that can affect all mammals, including humans. The virus is transmitted through the bite of an infected animal. Routine vaccination is the key to controlling this deadly disease.

Feline Viral Rhinotracheitis (FVR)

A common respiratory infection of cats, which can be fatal in kittens. Sneezing, decreased appetite, and fever, followed by a thick discharge from the eyes and nose are often observed. FVR also has a chronic state, in which recovered cats become carriers for life. These carriers may or may not experience signs of the disease and will shed the virus intermittently. Transmission of the virus requires direct contact with infectious secretions or excretions.

---

determine if a pet has a disease, whereas other tests need to be submitted to an outside laboratory for diagnostics. Table 23-1 summarizes tests available for diagnostics.

Wellness Exams and Recommendations

Regular patient examinations build client relationships and improve the pets' disposition when entering the hospital. Pets that experience happy visits will enjoy returning to the hospital; whereas stressed pets are less likely to return (the clients perception is the pet is stressed; therefore, they do not like coming to the vet, and will only come when required).

It is through these regular visits that team members can educate clients about the lifetime care of their best friend. Each species and age group have different recommendations, with the same goal in mind: developing happy, healthy patients.

Wellness plans, which focus on client "needs and wants," are an excellent program for practices to provide. Client compliance is driven by these plans, while providing budgeting assistance for each client (payment for 1 year of care is divided over a 12-month pay plan). Review Chapter 19 for more information.

Puppies and Kittens

Practices see a high number of puppies and kittens on a daily basis. Crate training, litter box training, and nutrition are the issues that clients most frequently ask about. Team members must remember every other topic to train the client on!

Team members must provide clients with written documentation to help them remember all of the key points, and remind them crate training takes time and patience. Client handouts can be obtained through outside sources, or they can be created by team members.

Discussions about nutrition are an absolute requirement. Pets depend on nutrition to live their lives. Nutrition is covered in detail later in this chapter; however, we must remember a few important points. Growing puppies and kittens need more calories at this point in their life than any other time. As they age, the caloric needs will decrease. If the intake is not reduced, an obese animal will result.

Fat cells can always be added by excess intake, but they will never die off. Therefore clients should prevent obesity while the patients are young.

Feeding high-quality food that is easily digested is important. The higher the digestibility of the nutrients, the more

BOX 23-3	Common Large Animal Diseases

The following infectious viruses have vaccinations available for protection.

Equine

Encephalomyelitis (Eastern, Western, and Venezuelan Equine Encephalomyelitis)

The virus is commonly carried by mosquitoes, birds, and rodents and can result in moderate to high mortality rates (within 2 to 3 days after signs begin). Symptoms include fever (106° F), hypersensitivity to sound, excitement, and restlessness. Shortly thereafter, the signs associated with brain lesions appear: drowsiness, drooping ears, and abnormal gait. The last stage is paralysis, and then death. Venezuelan equine encephalitis is a foreign animal disease and is reportable.

Influenza

This is the most common respiratory virus, and outbreaks spread rapidly (incubation of 1 to 3 days). Symptoms include fever, cough, and upper respiratory signs.

Potomac Horse Fever (Ehrlichiosis)

Unknown transmission, but multiple vectors are suspected, including the American dog tick. Symptoms include depression, high fever (107° F), profuse watery diarrhea, and colic. Concurrent laminitis may also occur.

Rhinopneumonitis (EHV-1)

Caused by several herpes viruses; can induce a fever of 106° F for several days. Presenting symptoms include clear nasal discharge and coughing that may last for several weeks. Mares may abort fetuses 3 to 4 months after infection. Antibiotics are used to treat secondary infections.

"Strangles" or Distemper (Streptococcus equi Infection)

Submandibular and retropharyngeal lymph node swelling and fever are often seen, often accompanied by coughing and nasal discharge. Lymph nodes often rupture, and the contents are extremely contagious.

Tetanus

A clostridial disease also known as *lockjaw*. Spores are introduced through a break in the skin and are often associated with lacerations from fence wounds. Symptoms of tetanus include muscle rigidity and spasms; if left untreated, it will result in death. Success of treatment depends on how far the disease has progressed.

Rabies

A fatal viral infection of the central nervous system that can affect all mammals, including humans. The virus is transmitted through the bite of an infected animal. Routine vaccination is the key to controlling this deadly disease.

Cattle

Bovine Viral Diarrhea (BVD)

BVD is a multisystemic viral disease. Classic symptoms of BVD include diarrhea, depression, anorexia, dehydration, and oral erosions. Chronic BVD is known as *mucosal disease* and is 100% fatal. Persistent infections may occur.

Brucellosis (Bang's Disease)

Brucellosis is caused by *Brucella abortus*, which is a coccobacillus. Transmission occurs via ingestion of organisms that are shed in milk and uterine discharges. Symptoms include abortions in healthy cows. *Brucella* is a zoonotic disease and is therefore reportable.

Clostridial Infection

Clostridia spores live in the soil and may be ingested while eating, or they enter the body through an open wound. Various clostridia forms exist, which can cause severe enteritis and dysentery (with high mortality rates) in young calves, lambs, and pigs. Clostridia can cause sudden death.

Infectious Bovine Rhinotracheitis (IBR)

Contagious; carriers can be seen. IBR causes upper respiratory signs, especially during times of stress (shipping); therefore it is also known as *shipping fever*. Symptoms may also include secondary bronchopneumonia, diarrhea (enteric form), abortion, and severe hyperemia of the muzzle (commonly referred to as *red nose*).

Moraxella bovis Infection (Pinkeye)

Contagious pinkeye is especially common in Herefords. Symptoms include conjunctivitis, corneal edema, and blindness.

Rabies

A fatal viral infection of the central nervous system that can affect all mammals, including humans. The virus is transmitted through the bite of an infected animal. Routine vaccination is the key to controlling this deadly disease.

Sheep and Goats

Clostridial Infection (Especially Type D)

Clostridium is a bacterium that grows best under anaerobic conditions and often comes from contaminated soil. Enterotoxemia is most likely to occur and is easily preventable with vaccination.

Tetanus

Same as in the horse.

---

the patient benefits. The lower the digestibility, the more the patient excretes.

Kittens should be fed a variety of foods that have different textures and tastes. Introducing kittens to canned and dry foods is important, as this is when they learn to develop preferences. If kittens are fed food with only one texture, they are more likely to reject other choices in the future. This causes problems if they ever need a special diet.

Spaying and neutering pets is another topic that should be discussed with owners. Most veterinarians recommend completing the procedure after the vaccine series is complete. Spaying and neutering decreases overpopulation and improves the health of the patient later in life. This is an excellent time to teach clients about anesthesia and the benefits of completing preoperative diagnostics, ensuring a safe surgical procedure. In addition, once pets are spayed or neutered, their food intake requirements decrease by 30%. Team

TABLE 23-1	Tests Available for Common Diseases	
DISEASE	**IN-HOUSE**	**LABORATORY**
Feline		
Calici		PCR
FIP		PCR, antibody
FIV	X	ELISA, Western blot
FeLV	X	ELISA, IFA
Panleukopenia		PCR
Pneumonitis, chlamydia		PCR
Herpesvirus		PCR
Rhinotracheitis		
Heartworm	X	ELISA
Canine		
Coronavirus		PCR
Distemper		PCR, conjunctival scrape
Adenovirus		PCR
Bordetella infection		PCR
Leptospira infection		PCR, antibody
Lyme disease	X	IFA, ELISA
Parvovirus	X	PCR, fecal antigen
Heartworm	X	ELISA
Herpesvirus		PCR
Equine		
Herpesvirus		PCR
Equine infectious anemia		AGID, cELISA
Equine influenza virus		PCR

AGID, Agar gel immunodiffusion; *ELISA,* enzyme-linked immunosorbent assay; *FeLV,* feline leukemia virus; *FIP,* feline infectious peritonitis; *FIV,* feline immunodeficiency virus; *IFA,* immunofluorescent assay; *PCR,* polymerase chain reaction.

members must advise clients to decrease caloric intake once the procedure has been completed.

Vaccine protocols are developed by each practice; however, team members must understand why boosters are critical. Most patients have a short immunity that they received from their mother; the effectiveness of the first vaccines may be slightly decreased because of this maternal antibody. Therefore additional vaccines are needed, ensuring the pet is completely protected. Most vaccines are first administered at about 6 weeks of age, and boosters are given every 3 to 4 weeks until 12 to 16 weeks of age. Rabies, by law, must be administered once the pet is 12 weeks of age; the rabies booster vaccine is then given at 1 year.

Parasite prevention varies depending on the geographical location of the practice. Many areas of North America are heavily infested with parasites, whereas other areas are dry and arid, decreasing the viability of such parasites. It is the ethical and legal obligation to inform clients of parasites that are prevalent in the area, potential zoonotic diseases carried by these parasites, and preventative measures that are available.

Behavior is a topic often left of the exam room table, especially with puppies and kittens. This is the age where they start to develop behavioral habits; therefore discipline and socialization during this life stage is critical. Practices strive to offer "cradle to grave" services; however, the most common reasons that pets are given up are behavioral issues (marking, aggression, anxiety). Take this opportunity to discuss behavioral traits with clients.

Dental disease is not common in puppies and kittens, but it is an ideal time to teach clients how to brush their pets' teeth. Pets think they are receiving attention, and will probably receive a treat once the procedure is completed. Getting a client on board with dental disease prevention early in their pet's life will help reduce dental disease in the future, and increase client compliance when a dental prophylaxis is recommended.

Adults

Adult patients have different needs than younger patients, and yearly exams are important at detecting diseases early. If a disease is detected early, it is often cheaper, and easier to treat. A detailed history should be obtained from clients, asking open-ended questions, to identify any underlying disease process that the owner may be unaware of.

Five vital signs should be obtained with every examination: weight, temperature, heart rate, respiratory rate, pain levels, and a body condition score. If these parameters are routinely monitored, a trend would be noted. Healthy animals should not have a pain score and should be an ideal body condition (5/9) (see Figures 23-14 and 23-15). If a pet is overweight, owners must be consulted about the effects of obesity in dogs and cats.

Vaccines for the first annual visit are routine; thereafter, the patient may be analyzed based on risk assessment and environmental exposure. Educate clients that a vaccine protocol is established for each individual patient, which further enhances the client relationship.

Behavior must be addressed in adults, just as in puppies and kittens. Often at this age, owners are embarrassed to talk about behavioral dispositions and are reluctant to bring up the subject. Be proactive and initiate the discussion. Separation anxiety and aggression are the most common behaviors in dogs; marking or spraying is a common behavior in cats.

Remind owners to continue brushing their pet's teeth. Provide a dental disease scorecard, and ask owners to score their pets teeth. Look for any signs of dental disease, including red and irritated gums, swelling or loose teeth. Start making recommendations now for dental care; treating stage 1 disease is a lot cheaper than treating stage 4.

Seniors

Many older patients start to experience age-related illnesses, therefore examination frequency may need to increase to every 6 months. Blood work, including a complete blood count (CBC), chemistry panel, electrolytes, and a urinalysis will need to be completed and evaluated at least yearly, if not more frequent, based on previous results.

Senior patients tend to exercise less and are overweight; therefore diet recommendations should be discussed again. Senior pets need a high protein diet to help maintain muscle mass, and may benefit from supplements such as omega-3 fatty acids, glucosamine, and chondroitin.

Vaccines, parasite prevention, and dental disease should be covered with senior patients, just as they are in puppies, kittens, and adults.

Diagnostics

Many factors are considered when determining a diagnosis. History, physical exam, and laboratory results all provide information to the veterinarian. Diagnostic testing can take hours to accomplish and can depend on the client's financial situation. Clients should be provided with estimates before starting any diagnostics, so that they may elect to proceed with one test at a time.

Laboratory tests may include in-house blood work or panels sent to an outside laboratory (see Chapter 9). In-house lab work may consist of a CBC and blood chemistry analysis (both abbreviated and complete panels are available), heartworm test, fecal analysis, urinalysis, cytologic analysis, combined feline leukemia virus (FeLV)/feline immunodeficiency virus (FIV)/heartworm (HWT) tests, and parvovirus test. A variety of companies produce a number of tests that are available for use in practice; the product insert should be used as a guide to completing each test correctly (see Table 23-1). Directions that are not followed correctly can yield inconclusive results, producing a false-positive or false-negative result. Not only does this provide substandard medicine, it decreases the profits of the veterinary practice. Any failed tests should be repeated and reported to the practice manager in case the tests are tracked.

Blood Work

It is imperative for the veterinary assistant and technician to become familiar with general tests that are run in-house. Clients will ask what test correlates with what bodily system, and these questions must be answered clearly and confidently. Table 23-2 lists the names of common tests and the system with which the test correlates.

Cytology

Samples for cytologic analyses are prepared for a number of reasons, the most common of which is to look at cells under the microscope. Cytology preparation can depend on the sample, the doctor, and the stain that will be used.

Different cells take up stain differently, which helps in diagnosis. Many veterinarians and technicians become proficient at reading cytologic preparations; however, a histopathologist that is employed by a laboratory can provide a more definitive diagnosis.

Urinalysis

Urine samples can provide a wealth of information for the veterinarian, and several tests can be performed on one

TABLE 23-2	Common Blood Work Tests
TEST	**ASSOCIATED WITH**
AST	Liver
ALT	Liver
Total bili	Liver
Alk phos	Liver
GGT	Liver
Total protein	Protein
Albumin	Protein
Globulin	Protein
A/G ratio	Protein
Cholesterol	Lipids
BUN	Kidney
Creatinine	Kidney
BUN/crea ratio	Kidney
Phosphorus	Mineral
Calcium	Mineral
Glucose	Diabetes
Amylase	Pancreas
Lipase	Pancreas
Sodium	Electrolytes
Phosphorus	Electrolytes
Na/K ratio	Electrolytes
Chloride	Electrolytes
Triglycerides	Lipids
Magnesium	Mineral
WBC	White blood cell count
RBC	Red blood cell count
HGB	Hemoglobin concentration
HCT	Hematocrit
MCV	Mean corpuscular volume
MCH	Mean cell hemoglobin
MCHC	Mean cell hemoglobin concentration
Total T-4	Thyroid
T-4 equil. dialysis	Thyroid
TSH	Thyroid
Bile acids	Liver

A/G, albumin/globulin; Alk phos, alkaline phosphatase; ALT, alanine aminotransferase; AST, aspartate aminotransferase; bili, bilirubin, BUN, blood urea nitrogen; crea, creatinine; equil., equilibrium; GGT, gamma-glutamyl transferase; Na/K, sodium/potassium; TSH, thyroid-stimulating hormone.

sample. Most urine samples are obtained by free catch; either the owner has obtained a sample or an assistant has walked the dog and caught a midstream urine sample (Figure 23-5). Other methods of collection include cystocentesis or catheterization. If a urine sample will be sent to the laboratory for culture, a sample acquired by cystocentesis is highly recommended because it is a sterile sample that is obtained without any contamination. Cystocentesis is the process of inserting a needle into the bladder and withdrawing a sample.

The tests that can be completed on urine are numerous; the most common tests completed in the hospital include

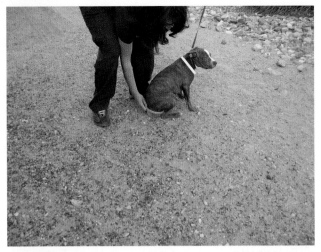

FIGURE 23-5 Urine may be caught by free catch when walking dogs.

BOX 23-4	Urine Dipstick Tests

- Leukocytes
- Blood
- pH
- Ketones

- Glucose
- Bilirubin
- Nitrates

BOX 23-5	Urine Sediment Evaluations

- White blood cells
- Red blood cells
- Epithelial cells

- Bacteria
- Casts
- Crystals

specific gravity, stick urinalysis, and sediment (Boxes 23-4 and 23-5). The specific gravity provides the concentration of the urine and is a key indicator of how well the kidneys can concentrate the urine. Certain disease processes can affect the concentration, including renal disease and diabetes.

A stick urinalysis is performed by dropping a small sample of urine onto each testing block (Figure 23-6). A sediment is then essential to verify the information provided by the stick.

Fecal Analysis

Fecal analysis is extremely important in puppies and kittens and in pets with diarrhea. A fecal analysis can diagnose internal parasites such as *Giardia,* coccidia, roundworms, hookworms, whipworms, or tapeworms.

It can also indicate severe bacterial overgrowth and determine if a sample should be sent to the laboratory for further diagnosis.

Electrocardiogram

Electrocardiograms, often referred to as EKGs or ECGs, are recordings of the heart's electrical activity. The recording traces the entire heartbeat process, through both the systolic and diastolic phases. Arrhythmias and conduction disturbances of the heart can be detected on ECGs, and an ECG

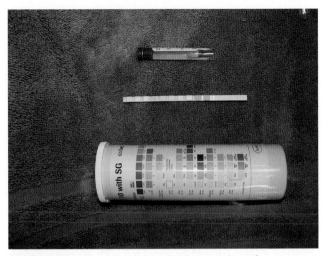

FIGURE 23-6 A stick urinalysis and sediment and specific gravity measurements should be done on every urine sample.

is highly recommended before administering anesthesia to patients.

Blood Pressure

Measurement of blood pressure is an underused tool in veterinary medicine. Variations in blood pressure are characteristic of a number of diseases. By definition, blood pressure is the pressure exerted by the blood on the wall of the vessel. The systolic pressure is the maximal force caused by the contraction of the left ventricle of the heart. The diastolic pressure is the minimal force during the relaxation phrase, when the aortic and pulmonic valves are closed. The mean arterial pressure is the average pressure of both.

Diagnostic Imaging

Most practices use a radiograph machine to produce high-quality x-rays. A radiograph is a visible record produced by x-rays penetrating an object. Radiographs can provide a great amount of detail in a short amount of time.

Safety

Care must be taken when taking radiographs. Safety cannot be emphasized enough. Studies indicate that excess radiation causes cancer, birth defects, a decreased life span, and fertility issues. Protection must be worn at all times while taking radiographs (Box 23-6 and Figure 23-7). Lead thyroid collars, gowns, and gloves are the absolute minimum that should be provided to all team members allowed to take radiographs. Eye goggles are also a good idea (eyes cannot be replaced!) to provide ultimate protection. Team members who are exposed to radiation on a daily basis have a higher incidence of reproductive, thyroid, and eye cancers.

> *PRACTICE POINT*   Team member safety must never be compromised for patient convenience. Always wear proper personal protective equipment (PPE) when taking radiographs.

BOX 23-6 | Minimum Radiology PPE

- Lead thyroid collar
- Lead gown
- Goggles
- Lead gloves
- Dosimeter badge

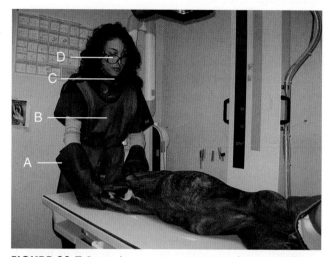

FIGURE 23-7 Personal protective equipment must be worn at all times when radiographing a pet. **A,** Lead gloves. **B,** Lead gown. **C,** Lead collar. **D,** Protective goggles.

Lead aprons, collars, and gloves should never be folded; any fold can crack the lead and allow radiation to penetrate the team member, decreasing safety (Figure 23-8). All apparel should be hung on a wall or laid flat on a table surface to prevent cracking. Aprons, collars, and gloves should be radiographed yearly to check for any cracks that may have appeared (Figure 23-9). Radiographs should be compared year to year, and safety equipment should be replaced as soon as visible cracks appear. Team member safety cannot be compromised.

Guidelines

Several regulations must be followed to comply with guidelines set for employee safety. All team members in the room during the radiograph process must be older than 18 years. Dosimeter badges must be worn at all times, and pregnant team members should especially avoid exposure to radiation. Personal protective equipment (PPE) must be worn. Employers must enforce the use of PPE, and employees must wear PPE. According to the Occupational Safety and Health Administration (OSHA), employers can be fined for not providing or enforcing the use of PPE, and employees can be terminated for not wearing PPE (when detailed in the employee manual). Excess radiation can have detrimental effects, and all protection must be used.

A dosimeter measures radiation exposure and should be worn on the collar at the thyroid gland level. The maximum permissible dose (MPD) is 5000 millirems per year (a millirem is 1/1000 rem), and it should be monitored closely. The average exposure is 5 rem per year for a small or mixed practice. The U.S. Nuclear Regulatory Commission

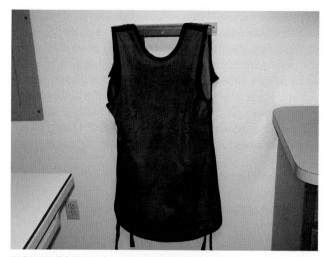

FIGURE 23-8 Lead aprons should be hung when not in use to prevent the lead from cracking.

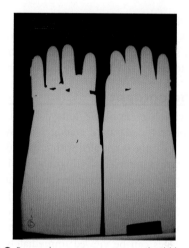

FIGURE 23-9 Personal protective equipment should be x-rayed yearly for cracked lead. This pair of gloves has several areas of damage and must be replaced.

has determined that the MPD is a dose that is unlikely to harm a person over a lifetime of taking radiographs. Every precaution should be taken to keep radiation exposure low by wearing all protective gear. If a practice manager notices high levels of exposure on a dosimetry report, an investigation should be launched to determine the source of radiation. Machines may malfunction, and this may be the only way to detect the excess radiation being emitted. Dosimetry reports should be kept for 30 years, in case any medical issues rise from a team member's exposure to radiation. It can take several years to see any effects of radiation on the human body system.

All radiograph machines must be registered, monitored, and inspected by a state official. The department that inspects radiology machines varies by state, as does the frequency of inspections. The certificate of inspection must be posted in the radiology room.

A radiology log can be helpful to team members when a digital system is not used. Figure 17-1 shows an example, listing the date, client and patient name, area being studied, position, and machine settings. This type of log allows team

members to retrieve settings used in previous radiographs in case repeat or follow-up radiographs are required. To compare radiographs, the same setting should be used on both. Different settings may produce slight differences in quality of images, thereby making comparison difficult. Digital radiographs have setting information stored with the image, allowing exact settings to be used. Films must be stored in a system that allows quick and easy retrieval. Digital radiographs are stored in the patient's file, allowing quick access at all times.

Regular films may be alphabetized by the client's last name or patient name, or numerically by client ID number. Whichever system is used, it must be simple and prevent loss of films. Lost films are the biggest hassle of film storage. Many clinics now use a scanner or digitizer to enter radiographs onto a CD for easy retrieval, freeing up storage space once taken by radiographs. This also eliminates lost radiographs.

Radiograph checkout logs should also be implemented when owners take x-rays for second opinions or when films are sent to a specialist. Figure 17-2 shows a log that allows radiographs to be traced if they have not been returned.

Digital Radiographs

With the technology available today, digital x-rays have begun to replace the standard analog x-ray systems. With digital x-rays, the tube is coupled with a specialized receiver that changes x-rays into electrical signals. The image is digitized and displayed on a computer screen, then stored on a DVD, CD, or magnetic optical disk (MOD). The advantages of a digital system are numerous. The processing time is reduced to seconds because film does not have to be processed. Images can be viewed immediately and can be manipulated with software to lighten, darken, or magnify the image. If a film needs to be repeated for positioning only, it can be done in a shorter amount of time. Views are stored within the computer system and/or disk, so images are never lost. Images can also be sent to a specialist for a second opinion by phone, DSL, or T1 cable line.

Fluoroscopy

Fluoroscopy involves projecting a continuous x-ray beam onto an image intensifier. Fluoroscopic units are suited for the study of moving structures and can provide the maximum information regarding the processes of the moving structures. Fluoroscopic studies are usually limited to gastrointestinal studies, myelography, and heart and vascular studies. They are rarely used in veterinary medicine for economic reasons.

Ultrasound

The use of ultrasound is becoming popular within veterinary practices, especially as the price of units decreases. Ultrasound is noninvasive and well tolerated by patients. A major disadvantage is the learning curve associated with using the unit. It takes practice and patience to master ultrasound imaging; the diagnosis is only as good as the diagnostician.

Ultrasound utilizes sound technology. The frequency of sound is computed into an image with an equation that involves wavelength and frequency. Sound reflection forms the basis of an ultrasound image. The thicker the tissue, the less sound is reflected, creating a darker image on the screen. The thinner the tissue, the more sound is reflected, creating a lighter image of the organ.

Ultrasound can be useful in diagnosing and evaluating tendon injuries, tendon sheath infections, adhesions, or foreign bodies. Joints can be evaluated for injury, neoplasia, or osteomyelitis. Abdominal cavities can be evaluated for fluid, cancer, or congenital defects. The list of uses for ultrasound is endless, making it a useful diagnostic tool when evaluating pets for disease.

Computed Tomographic Scanning

Computed tomographic (CT) scanning is performed by passing a thin x-ray beam through the patient and measuring the x-ray attenuation at multiple sites within a thin slice of a patient's anatomy. A computer then configures the data and provides a cross-sectional image on a video monitor. In veterinary medicine, a CT scan is generally used to diagnose neurologic disorders within the spinal column or brain. It can also be helpful to identify musculoskeletal, thoracic, and abdominal disorders.

Patients must be fully anesthetized to prevent movement within the machine. The patient is placed in a ventrodorsal position on a table that moves through the machine. As the table moves, the CT scanner obtains cross-sectional data. Two studies are generally performed: the first without any contrast media, the second after an intravenous injection of iodinated contrast. Contrast allows visualization of vascular structures.

Magnetic Resonance Imaging

Magnetic resonance imaging (MRI) is the newest imaging modality for veterinary medicine. MRI is similar to CT scanning in that it takes thin slices in cross-section and transfers the images to a video screen. MRI differs in that it does not use radiation to create the image; it uses radio wave signals in which hydrogen nuclei have been disturbed by a radiofrequency pulse. MRI produces superior results; clearer images and sensitivity to the composition of tissues are just two qualities worth mentioning. These qualities are excellent for diagnostics involving the brain and spinal cord.

Some veterinary teaching hospitals and veterinary specialty practices use MRIs; most animals are referred to a human hospital, imaging center, or a truck-based mobile MRI unit. Patients must be anesthetized for these centers; therefore the veterinarian must provide everything that would be needed for anesthesia, resuscitation (if needed), and recovery. The animal's bowels and bladder should be empty, and it should be parasite free.

Because MRIs use a strong magnetic field, anything metal must be removed from the room. The magnetic field will forcefully pull any metal object into the magnet, injuring anything in its path. Therefore animals must be anesthetized

with injectable anesthesia. This can be a disadvantage because it can be difficult to monitor patients while they are undergoing the procedure. MRIs generally take 45 to 60 minutes to complete. They can be done with and/or without contrast media.

Surgery

Surgery entails a wide variety of topics. Team members should familiarize themselves with the following summaries, then seek further training. A surgical procedure does not start in the operating room; it begins with client education. Clients must fully understand the procedure their pet will be receiving and understand the risks associated with anesthesia. With the appropriate drug choice, monitoring, and recovery, the anesthetic risk is decreased. Client communication and education is the No. 1 preoperative procedure.

> *PRACTICE POINT* Ensure the client has a full understanding of the procedure and risks associated with anesthesia before moving to the next step.

After clients have received all appropriate education regarding the procedure and the risk of anesthesia, they must sign an anesthetic release. Examples of anesthetic release forms are provided in Chapter 2. It is imperative that the client's phone number, cell phone, and/or pager be listed in case an emergency occurs and the client must be contacted during the procedure.

Clients must be informed of the risks and benefits the pet is subject to before the procedure is performed. Informed consent ensures that the client has been advised, understands the risks, and agrees to the procedures elected. Chapter 4 defines informed consent in more detail.

Preanesthetic Documentation

Preanesthetic questions MUST be addressed and documented. It should be confirmed that patients have been held off food and water (NPO) per practice instructions. Owners must be given the option (if it is not hospital policy) to have preoperative tests performed on their pet before anesthesia.

- Blood work: The very minimum that should be offered is blood work that evaluates the kidney and liver function, as well as red blood cells, white blood cells, and platelet function. Most manufacturers offer preoperative panels that include blood urea nitrogen, creatinine, alanine aminotransferase, alkaline phosphatase, glucose, total protein, and a complete blood count. Anesthesia is metabolized by the liver and kidneys; it is imperative to know if they are functioning correctly. If a patient is deficient in platelets, it is helpful to know this before surgery; a patient with a low platelet level could bleed to death.
- ECG: An ECG is an excellent indicator of heart disease. An ECG will detect premature ventricular contractions or other abnormalities that may necessitate postponement of surgery.

- IV catheter and fluids: If IV fluids are not a requirement of the practice, the owner should be strongly advised to permit them. IV fluids help maintain the patient's blood pressure while under anesthesia, help support the kidneys, and allow an access port to the vein in case of emergency. If a patient goes into cardiac arrest while under anesthesia, drugs can be administered much faster through an existing line versus placing a catheter in an emergency.
- Histopathology: If a patient is having a mass or growth removed, clients should be advised to send the growth to a pathologist to determine the correct pathology. Many cancerous tumors look benign but are not. A pathologist who reviews cytologies as a profession can make an informed diagnosis of masses submitted.

If a patient is going to be spayed or neutered, it should be checked for testicles. Owners cannot always tell the correct gender of an animal; therefore it must be verified before surgery (it is frustrating and wasted time when a veterinarian cuts into the abdomen of a patient looking for a uterus to find out it is a male!). If a mass will be removed from the patient, the hair should be clipped (before the owner leaves) to verify the mass or masses that the owner has agreed to remove. If any other masses are found on physical exam, the owner should be called for permission to remove the additional masses.

Each patient should receive a physical exam at least 12 hours before anesthesia. The heart and lungs should be evaluated with both heart rate and respiratory rate noted. The mucous membranes should be pink, and the capillary refill time should be within 2 seconds. The pulse should be strong; any pulse deficits should be noted. The abdomen should feel normal to palpation, as should the lymph nodes. The pet should be well hydrated and have a normal temperature, and a weight should be taken for the current visit.

Anesthesia

Once all the parameters are evaluated and the patient is deemed healthy enough for surgery, an anesthetic protocol will be developed. Each patient is unique, and consideration should be given to each patient regarding the anesthesia protocol.

Anesthesia is the loss of sensation that can be induced by a number of drugs. Local anesthesia deadens sensory nerves; an injection of lidocaine is given at the site of the procedure. General anesthesia influences and desensitizes the central nervous system; it produces unconsciousness. Spinal anesthesia interrupts the function of nerves.

Endotracheal Tubes

Patients that are undergoing anesthesia should always be intubated. Intubation prevents the patient from aspirating contents from the stomach if it vomits while under anesthesia. Intubation also prevents mucous and salivary secretions from entering the lung field. Intubation is extremely important during dental procedures. Excess water from the scaling instruments can pool in the lungs, causing severe complications for the patient. Along with these precautions, endotracheal tubes deliver anesthetic gases to the patient (Figure 23-10).

Pharmacology

Pharmacology is a very important topic, and one with which assistants and technicians must be familiar. Pharmacology not only deals with drugs that are dispensed, it also involves knowledge about the administration of drugs, drug interactions, and the amount of a drug that is to be given with each dose.

> *PRACTICE POINT*   Team members must become familiar with the drugs their practice carries, including side effects and potential drug interactions.

Chemical, Nonproprietary, and Proprietary Names

Drugs are also commonly referred to by three different names. The chemical name describes the chemical composition

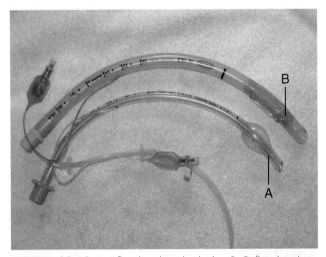

FIGURE 23-10 A, Inflated endotracheal tube. B, Deflated endotracheal tube.

of the product. The nonproprietary name, also referred to as the *generic name,* is a more concise name given to the chemical compound. Examples of nonproprietary names include aspirin, acetaminophen, and amoxicillin. The proprietary name, or trade name, is the name of the drug given by the manufacturer. Examples of proprietary names include Baytril, Tylenol, and Amoxi-Tabs. Because many manufacturers produce similar products, a single generic drug can be sold under several trade names. Amoxicillin is sold as Amoxi-Tabs, Robamox V, and Amoxil (among others).

Dosage forms include tablets, capsules, solutions, injectables, topical applications, and implants. Tablets or capsules can be given orally. Some suppositories are packaged in caplet form but are given rectally. Solutions can be given orally in a suspension or syrup; they can also be applied to the eye and/or ears. Injectables can be given under the skin, in the muscles, or in the vein. Topical applications are generally applied to the skin and can be manufactured in a solution, ointment, or cream base. Ointments can be applied topically or in the eye; paste is generally administered orally, and implants are placed under the skin for release of a drug over an extended period of time.

Prescriptions

A prescription is an order from a licensed veterinarian directing a pharmacist to prepare a drug for use by a client's animal (Figure 23-11). A valid veterinarian/patient/client relationship must exist for a veterinarian to write a prescription, and the drug must be meet proper requirements for labeling. Documentation must be kept in the pet's record regarding the prescription. Valid prescriptions must contain the following information: date, client's name, pet's name, and species; the drug name, concentration, and number of units to dispense; directions for the client treating the animal; the doctor's name, address, and

---

ABC Veterinary Clinic
1000 Anyroad, Anytown, PA 19874
555-555-5555

Client name_____ Patient _____ Species _____ Date_____

Address _____

Rx

Refills   0 1 2 3 4   _____ DVM

FIGURE 23-11 Sample prescription order form.

phone number; the abbreviation "Rx"; and the veterinarian's signature.

Dispensing Medications

Medications that are dispensed must be in childproof containers. If a child accesses a medication container and becomes poisoned, the veterinarian can be found liable. Many clients may request containers that are not childproof; pill vials and lids can be specially ordered that can be reversed, allowing the flip side of the lid to close the container without the use of the childproof side. It must be verified with the owner, however, that no children reside in the premises.

Calculations and Conversions

Calculating the dose of medication is easy, but calculations must be verified with the veterinarian before administration to ensure correct dosing. The following information is needed before the calculation procedure:

- Pet's weight
- Recommended dose of medication (milligrams per kilogram of body weight)
- Strength or concentration of medication supplied (e.g., milligrams of drug per milliliter or milligrams per tablet)

Chapter 24 covers the topics of conversions, equations, and examples of medication calculation in depth. Every team member must be familiar with common drugs and doses and double-check medications for errors. Mistakes are less likely to occur if more team members double-check medications before dispensing.

Administration of Medications

Medications can be given in a variety of methods. PO means per os, or by mouth. SQ refers to under the skin, or subcutaneous. IM is intramuscular, or in the muscle, whereas IV means in the vein, or intravenously. Medications given by mouth can be difficult to administer because many patients do not cooperate. If the pet is allowed to eat, the medication can be offered in food; the pet must be monitored to ensure it ingests the tablet. Many pets are creative and eat around the pill. If the pill is not taken in food form, the jaw must be opened and the pill must be placed in the rear of the mouth. It must be placed as far back on the tongue as possible because the animal can spit the pill out. Once it has been placed on the back of the tongue, the mouth should be closed and held shut immediately. The throat should be rubbed to induce swallowing. Water should then be given with a syringe, helping the pill slide into the stomach. Without water, many pills can lodge in the esophagus, causing ulcers and lesions when the pill begins to break down. This can be an extremely painful condition that will prevent the pet from eating and drinking for days. Pill poppers are also available to aid in the medication of pills.

> **PRACTICE POINT** Double-check every medication before administration, ensuring the correct drug, dose, route, and frequency.

One must use caution and double-check that the medication is being administered by the correct route. Many drugs have different effects if administered the wrong route. Not only can the medications have an adverse affect, the patients may be overdosed or underdosed if the drug is given improperly. Every veterinary assistant and technician must become familiar with the drugs supplied in the practice and the common routes of administration for each one. Assistants and technicians should also be familiar with common doses and be able to determine incorrect dosing or administration procedures. Assistants and technicians are the second eyes and ears for veterinarians and will frequently detect unintentional mistakes. It is always better to double-check than to administer a potentially fatal dose of medication.

Controlled substances are covered in Chapter 16 and should be reviewed carefully. Controlled substances must be logged correctly and balanced. Any significant discrepancy at the end of the year must be reported to the local police department, the U.S. Drug Enforcement Administration (DEA), and the state board of veterinary medicine. If theft occurs, the missing product must be reported immediately.

Expired Medications

Medications often expire in the veterinary practice. This can present a large loss for the business; therefore preventing drugs from expiring is essential. Inventory and inventory management are critical; by controlling the inventory, losses can be cut (see Chapter 15).

If a product expires, the manufacturer or distributor that the practice ordered the product from should be determined, and the return policy reviewed. Some companies will replace expired medication with later dating, preventing the practice from taking a loss. If they do not return the product, it will need to be disposed of properly. Expired medication cannot be sold. Not only is selling expired product against the law, the efficacy of the product has been determined to be less than what is deemed appropriate.

Expired tablets can be dissolved in water, poured over a small amount of cat litter, and then discarded. Injectables can be poured in cat litter as well. The U.S. Environmental Protection Agency (EPA) has advised against the practice of pouring expired medication down the drain or in the toilet because the possibility of contaminating water sources is high.

Controlled substances that expire must be sent to a return agency that certifies the destruction of drugs (see Chapter 16).

Over-the-Counter Pharmaceuticals

Over-the-counter (OTC) pharmaceuticals include products that are available at the pharmacy or grocery store without the need for a prescription. OTC drugs include Robitussin (dextromethorphan), Benadryl (diphenhydramine), Dramamine (dimenhydrinate), Chlor-Trimeton (chlorpheniramine), Tagamet (cimetidine), and Imodium (loperamide). The list is extensive because many products can be purchased OTC.

Labels

Every medication that is dispensed from a veterinary practice must have a label on it. Each label must state the client's name, pet's name, and date; the name, address, and phone number of the practice; the veterinarian prescribing the drug; the name of the drug, its strength, and expiration date; and the directions for the client. Each label must also read "Keep out of the reach of children."

Warning labels can be affixed to medication vials to catch the client's attention (Figure 23-12). ("Refrigerate and mix well before using," and "This prescription cannot be refilled without an examination," are examples of labels that can be generated.) Box 23-7 gives examples of common abbreviations used in making labels.

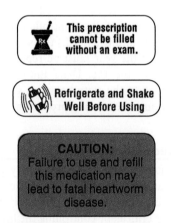

FIGURE 23-12 Example of labels.

BOX 23-7	Common Abbreviations

A complete list of abbreviations is available in the appendices.

SID	once daily
BID	twice daily
TID	three times daily
QID	four times daily
QOD	every other day
cc	cubic centimeter
g or gm	gram
hr	hour
s or sec	second
m or min	minute
lb or #	pound
mg	milligram
mL	milliliter
od	right eye
os	left eye
ou	both eyes
au	both ears
ad	right ear
as	left ear
PO	by mouth
prn	as needed
q	every
stat	immediately
t or tsp	teaspoon
T or tbl	tablespoon

Drugs

Drugs are placed into categories according to their function and the properties of the active ingredient. The active ingredient is defined as the main chemical that provides the desired result. Other chemicals may also be added to carry the drug, provide synergistic features, or provide a flavor.

Anti-Inflammatories

Drugs that reduce inflammation are called *anti-inflammatories.* They often reduce pain, and some reduce fever as well. There are two types of anti-inflammatories: steroidal and nonsteroidal. Steroidal anti-inflammatories are known as *glucocorticoids* and can be classified as short acting, intermediate, or long acting. Short-acting glucocorticoids generally relieve pain for less than 12 hours, whereas intermediate glucocorticoids relieve pain for 12 to 36 hours. Intermediate glucocorticoid examples include prednisone, prednisolone, triamcinolone, methylprednisolone, and isoflupredone. Long-acting glucocorticoids include dexamethasone, betamethasone, and flumethasone, which provide relief for more than 48 hours. Overuse of steroidal anti-inflammatories can result in Cushing syndrome; physical symptoms may not appear for weeks.

Nonsteroidal anti-inflammatory drugs (NSAIDs) are regarded as a safer class of drug for pain relief because their side effects are generally fewer and less severe than those of glucocorticoids. Aspirin, ibuprofen, ketoprofen, and naproxen are NSAIDs available OTC. Flunixin meglumine (Banamine), carprofen (Rimadyl), deracoxib (Deramaxx), and firocoxib (Previcox) are some NSAIDs commonly used in veterinary medicine. Dimethyl sulfoxide (DMSO) is applied topically, primarily in horses.

Antimicrobials

Antimicrobials are drugs used to kill or inhibit bacteria, protozoa, viruses, or fungi. Antibiotics include penicillins, cephalosporins, bacitracins, aminoglycosides, fluoroquinolones, tetracyclines, sulfonamides, lincosamides, macrolides, metronidazole, nitrofurans, chloramphenicols, and rifampin. Amphotericin, ketoconazole, itraconazole, and griseofulvin are antifungal drugs. Each type of antibiotic or fungal agent is chosen based on the particular type of bacteria or fungus for which the patient is being treated. Each class of antibiotics has a variety of drugs available within its class, each of which may also have different properties based on its chemical composition.

Antiparasitics

Anthelmintics are used to treat various types of internal parasites. Fenbendazole, thiabendazole, oxibendazole, and albendazole are examples of anthelmintics used in practice. Organophosphates are used for external parasites such as fleas, ticks, and flies. Pyrethrins and pyrethroids are the largest group of insecticides marketed in the United States. Insect growth regulators and sterilizers are also becoming popular and are very safe to use on pets.

Cardiac Drugs

Many drugs have effects on the cardiovascular system but are not classified as cardiac medications. Medications must be analyzed for interactions or enhancement with other drugs. Antiarrhythmic drugs are used to produce a normal conduction sequence. Lidocaine, procainamide, and quinidine reverse arrhythmias.

> PRACTICE POINT   Some drugs enhance the effects of others. Always check for potential drug interaction before dispensing a new drug to a patient.

Vasodilators open constricted valves, making it easier for the heart to pump blood to the vessels. Hydralazine, nitroglycerine, enalapril, and captopril are examples of vasodilators available.

Diuretics increase urine formation and promote water loss. Patients in cardiac failure tend to retain water and sodium, causing edema and ascites. Examples of diuretics include furosemide and spironolactone.

Disinfectants and Antiseptics

Disinfection is the destruction of pathogenic microorganisms or their toxins. Antiseptics are chemical agents that kill or prevent the growth of microorganisms on living tissues. Disinfectants are chemical agents that kill or prevent the growth of microorganisms on objects (surgical equipment, tables, floors, etc.). Alcohols are commonly used as antiseptics, but they are ineffective against bacterial spores and must remain in contact for several seconds to be effective against bacteria. Quaternary ammonium compounds are used to disinfect objects. They are generally safe and nonirritating to the skin and noncorrosive to objects but are ineffective against parvovirus. Clorox is an example of a chlorine compound; it is effective on fungi, algae, parvovirus, and vegetative forms of bacteria. It is not effective against bacterial spores. Betadine is an example of an iodophor and is used to disinfect tissue. Biguanides are commonly used to clean cages, surgical sites, and minor wounds. Chlorhexidine is the most common example; it may have residual activity when left in contact with the surface of the skin.

Endocrine Drugs

Hyperthyroidism, an increase in the production of the thyroid hormone, is common in cats. Methimazole is the most common treatment and can be supplied in tablet or topical form.

Hypothyroidism, a decrease in the production of the thyroid hormone, is more common in dogs. Levothyroxine is usually the drug of choice for this condition.

Insulin is responsible for the movement of glucose from the blood into the tissue cells. In diabetes mellitus, insufficient insulin is produced, resulting in high blood glucose levels. The treatment of choice is the administration of insulin, which is supplied in a variety of trade names, all of which are developed by different methods. Types of insulin currently available include NPH, glargine, and Vetsulin.

Gastric Drugs

Drugs that affect the gastrointestinal tract are called *gastric drugs*. They can be further described by their function within the gastrointestinal tract. Emetics are drugs that induce vomiting, whereas antiemetics prevent or decrease vomiting. Examples of emetics include apomorphine and ipecac, whereas examples of antiemetics include acepromazine, chlorpromazine, metoclopramide, and maropitant (Cerenia). Diphenhydramine, dimenhydrinate, and maropitant can also reduce vomiting associated with motion sickness.

Antidiarrheals combat diarrhea, whereas adsorbents and protectants prevent toxins from attaching to, or coming in contact with, the gastrointestinal wall. Examples of antidiarrheals include diphenoxylate (Lomotil), loperamide, aminopentamide (Centrine), and bismuth subsalicylate (Pepto-Bismol). Activated charcoal is an example of an adsorbent.

Laxatives and stool softeners facilitate evacuation of the bowels. Metamucil is an excellent source of indigestible fiber, which helps retain water in the feces. Milk of Magnesia and phosphate salts create a strong osmotic force and attract water into the bowel of the lumen. Lubricants include mineral oil or cod liver oil and make the stool more slippery.

Antacids and antiulcer drugs reduce acidity of the stomach or reduce acid production. Examples of drugs that reduce acidity include calcium carbonate (Tums, Maalox), Rolaids, and aluminum hydroxide gel (Amphojel). Drugs that reduce acid production include cimetidine (Tagamet), ranitidine hydrochloride (Zantac), and famotidine (Pepcid). Sucralfate (Carafate) treats ulcers by adhering to the ulcer site.

Nervous System

Anesthetics are a class of drug that affects the nervous system. Examples of injectable anesthetics include propofol, ketamine, and tiletamine with zolazepam (Telazol). Gas anesthetics include nitrous oxide, methoxyflurane, halothane, isoflurane, and sevoflurane.

Tranquilizers and sedatives reduce anxiety and produce a relaxed state. Acepromazine can be used alone to produce the desired effect. Diazepam, midazolam (Versed), and clonazepam are used in conjunction with other drugs as part of a preanesthetic plan. Xylazine and medetomidine (Domitor) produce a calming effect and decrease the ability to respond to stimuli.

Analgesics are drugs that reduce the perception to pain without affecting other sensations. Butorphanol (Torbugesic), oxymorphone (Numorphan), meperidine (Demerol), and buprenorphine (Buprenex) are examples of analgesics.

Anticonvulsants are drugs used to control seizures. Phenobarbital and diazepam are the most common choices of drugs used in veterinary medicine.

Stimulants are drugs used to stimulate the central nervous system. Doxapram (Dopram) is a stimulant used to increase respiration in animals with apnea.

Respiratory

Antitussives block the cough reflex, whereas mucolytics, expectorants, and decongestants are designed to break up mucus in the respiratory tract. Butorphanol, hydrocodone, codeine, and dextromethorphan are commonly used antitussives. Mucomyst is an example of a mucolytic, whereas guaifenesin is an expectorant.

Bronchodilators inhibit constriction of the smooth muscle surrounding the deep bronchioles. Terbutaline, albuterol, theophylline, and aminophylline are examples of bronchodilators used in veterinary medicine.

Therapeutic Diets

Often, the term *prescription diet* is thought of as requiring a prescription for the product to be sold. This is not true. Therapeutic diets, as they should be called, require a valid doctor/client/patient relationship as recommended by the manufacturer (Figure 23-13). These diets are recommended for certain diseases or conditions and may aid in the treatment of such disease; they should be fed at the recommendation of a veterinarian. For example, a diet high in protein to treat obesity, should not be fed to a cat with renal failure that would most benefit from a low-protein diet. Assistants and technicians should be familiar with diets available, the conditions they treat, and the benefits and risks of each. The following section on nutrition covers a wide range of therapeutic diets available, along with a description of diseases or conditions in which that they aid in the treatment.

> **PRACTICE POINT** Therapeutic diets do not require a prescription, however they must be sold within a veterinary practice.

Therapeutic diets have been developed to aid in the treatment of or maintenance plan for disease but do not cure the disease. Clients must understand that foods cannot cure diseases or conditions.

AAFCO

The Association of American Feed Control Officials (AAFCO) was established in response to the increasing number of diets available on the market, some of which did not meet the specific nutritional needs of animals. AAFCO is made up of a variety of individuals and is not regulated or managed by any pet food manufacturer. Any foods that are recommended should meet the expectations and testing of AAFCO.

A label that reads "complete and balanced" must either meet a nutrient profile or pass a feeding trial. The food must meet all nutrient minimum and maximum ranges that have been established by AAFCO as being safe.

Minimum level requirements were established for protein, fat, carbohydrate, and essential amino acids as diseases associated with nutrient deficiencies have become more prominent. Maximum level requirements were established for calcium, phosphorus, magnesium, fat, water-soluble vitamins, and trace

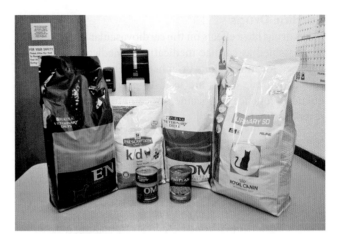

FIGURE 23-13 Example of therapeutic diets.

minerals to prevent nutrient excess, which has become a larger problem with the pet foods available in today's market.

Maximum levels for methionine, zinc, and vitamins A and D have been established for adult cat foods, reflecting current studies available on the toxic effect of these nutrients. Taurine levels have been established for both canned and dry cat food because the bioavailability of taurine is decreased in canned food.

All foods must either be categorized as growth and lactation or maintenance. Foods can state "for all life stages," which indicates the food has been able to meet stringent requirements for both categories. Canine growth and lactation nutrient requirements have higher levels of zinc, iron, and fat and decreased levels of calcium, phosphorus, and sodium.

To compare diets, food must be looked at on a "dry matter basis." AAFCO's definition of dry matter basis (DM) is the level of nutrients contained in a food. A "guaranteed analysis," or "as fed basis" must be converted to DM to effectively compare diets. For example, a canned diet contains approximately 75% moisture, whereas a dry diet contains approximately 10% moisture. To effectively compare the two products, the moisture content must be removed.

Ingredients are listed on the label by weight and can include moisture. Therefore some products may list chicken as the main ingredient, but the chicken may only weigh more than the corn or wheat products that follow because of its moisture content. Moisture is burned off during the cooking process; therefore it is important to look at the entire ingredient and nutrient profile when determining the appropriate diet for a patient.

The most commonly used unit of measurement is the kilocalorie (kcal), defined as the amount of heat necessary to raise the temperature of one kilogram (kg) of water by one degree Celsius. Calories are used to maintain physical activity, digestion, growth, and basal metabolism. Most foods are recommended in kcal/8 oz or kcal/can. Puppies and kittens require a larger amount of energy early in life and a lesser amount as they age. It is important to follow the feeding recommendations established by the pet food manufacturer because diets vary by company as well as within a specific product line.

Tables 23-3 and 23-4 list the AAFCO nutrient requirements for both puppies and kittens, respectively.

TABLE 23-3	AAFCO Recommendations for Puppies

NUTRIENT	UNITS DM BASIS	GROWTH AND REPRODUCTION MINIMUM	ADULT MAINTENANCE MINIMUM	MAXIMUM
Dog Food Nutrient Profiles*				
Protein	%	22.0	18.0	
Arginine	%	0.62	0.51	
Histidine	%	0.22	0.18	
Isoleucine	%	0.45	0.37	
Leucine	%	0.72	0.59	
Lysine	%	0.77	0.63	
Methionine-cystine	%	0.53	0.43	
Phenylalanine-tyrosine	%	0.89	0.73	
Threonine	%	0.58	0.48	
Tryptophan	%	0.20	0.16	
Valine	%	0.48	0.39	
Fat†	%	8.0	5.0	
Linoleic acid	%	1.0	1.0	
Minerals				
Calcium	%	1.0	0.6	2.5
Phosphorus	%	0.8	0.5	1.6
Calcium/phosphorus ratio		1:1	1:1	2:1
Potassium	%	0.6	0.6	
Sodium	%	0.3	0.06	
Chloride	%	0.45	0.09	
Magnesium	%	0.04	0.04	0.3
Iron‡	mg/kg	80.0	80.0	3000.0
Copper§	mg/kg	7.3	7.3	250.0
Manganese	mg/kg	5.0	5.0	
Zinc	mg/kg	120.0	120.0	1000.0
Iodine	mg/kg	1.5	1.5	50.0
Selenium	mg/kg	0.11	0.11	2.0
Vitamins				
A	IU/kg	5000.0	5000.0	250000.0
D	IU/kg	500.0	500.0	5000.0
E	IU/kg	50.0	50.0	1000.0
Thiamine¶	mg/kg	1.0	1.0	
Riboflavin	mg/kg	2.2	2.2	
Pantothenic acid	mg/kg	10.0	10.0	
Niacin	mg/kg	11.4	11.4	
Pyridoxine	mg/kg	1.0	1.0	
Folic acid	mg/kg	0.18	0.18	
B_{12}	mg/kg	0.022	0.022	
Choline	mg/kg	1200.0	1200.0	

DM, Dry matter; *ME*, metabolized energy.

*Presumes an energy density of 3.5 kcal ME/g DM, based on the modified Atwater values of 3.5, 8.5, and 3.5 kcal/g for protein, fat, and carbohydrate (nitrogen-free extract), respectively. Rations greater than 4.0 kcal/g should be corrected for energy density; rations less than 3.5 kcal/g should *not* be corrected for energy.

†Although a true requirement for fat per se has not been established, the minimum level was based on recognition of fat as a source of essential fatty acids, as a carrier of fat-soluble vitamins, to enhance palatability, and to supply an adequate caloric density.

‡Because of very poor bioavailability, iron from carbonate or oxide sources that is added to the diet should not be considered as a component in meeting the minimum nutrient level.

§Because of very poor bioavailability, copper from oxide sources that is added to the diet should not be considered as a component in meeting the minimum nutrient level.

¶Because processing may destroy up to 90% of the thiamine in the diet, allowance in formulation should be made to ensure the minimum nutrient level is met after processing.

TABLE 23-4	AAFCO Recommendations for Kittens			
NUTRIENT	UNITS DM BASIS	GROWTH AND REPRODUCTION MINIMUM	ADULT MAINTENANCE MINIMUM	MAXIMUM
Cat Food Nutrient Profiles*				
Protein	%	30.0	26.0	
Arginine	%	1.25	1.04	
Histidine	%	0.31	0.31	
Isoleucine	%	0.52	0.52	
Leucine	%	1.25	1.25	
Lysine	%	1.20	0.83	
Methionine-cystine	%	1.10	1.10	
Methionine	%	0.62	0.62	1.50
Phenylalanine-tyrosine	%	0.88	0.88	
Phenylalanine	%	0.42	0.42	
Threonine	%	0.73	0.73	
Tryptophan	%	0.25	0.16	
Valine	%	0.62	0.62	
Fat†	%	9.0	9.0	
Linoleic acid	%	0.5	0.5	
Arachidonic acid	%	0.02	0.02	
Minerals				
Calcium	%	1.0	0.6	
Phosphorus	%	0.8	0.5	
Potassium	%	0.6	0.6	
Sodium	%	0.2	0.2	
Chloride	%	0.3	0.3	
Magnesium‡	%	0.08	0.04	
Iron§	mg/kg	80.0	80.0	
Copper (extruded)¶	mg/kg	15.0	5.0	
Copper (canned)¶	mg/kg	5.0	5.0	
Manganese	mg/kg	7.5	7.5	
Zinc	mg/kg	75.0	75.0	2000.0
Iodine	mg/kg	0.35	0.35	
Selenium	mg/kg	0.1	0.1	

Nutrients are required for basic bodily function, including acting as structural components, enhancing chemical reactions, transporting substances throughout the body, maintaining temperature, and providing energy. Nutrients are divided into six categories:

1. **Water:** Water is the most important nutrient and has several functions. It helps regulate temperature, provides shape and resilience to the body, enhances chemical reactions, and transports substances through the body.
2. **Carbohydrates:** Carbohydrates include sugars, starches, and fiber, and they function primarily to provide energy.
3. **Protein:** Protein is composed of various amino acids and provides energy. Protein is the principle structural component of body tissues and organs.
4. **Fats:** Fats supply energy and essential fatty acids that the body cannot produce.
5. **Minerals:** Minerals comprise all inorganic elements in food. Minerals play a large role in enzyme and hormone systems.

6. **Vitamins:** Both water-soluble and fat-soluble vitamins are cofactors in enzyme reactions and play a role in DNA synthesis.

Homemade diets are generally incomplete and therefore are not recommended. When preparing meals, owners may omit ingredients because of a lack of money or inability to find a product, or they may change a product because of personal preference. Many homemade canine diets contain excessive protein but are deficient in calories, calcium, vitamins, and microminerals. Uncooked recipes may contain high levels of pathogenic bacteria that not only risk harm to the pet receiving the diet, but to the owner preparing the meal as well. If a homemade diet is preferred by the client, ensure that a boarded veterinary nutritionist has prepared a recipe for that particular patient.

> **PRACTICE POINT**   Ensure homemade recipes for patients have been prepared by a boarded veterinary nutritionist, preventing toxicities and deficiencies that commonly occur.

TABLE 23-4	AAFCO Recommendations for Kittens—cont'd			
NUTRIENT	UNITS DM BASIS	GROWTH AND REPRODUCTION MINIMUM	ADULT MAINTENANCE MINIMUM	MAXIMUM
Vitamins				
A	IU/kg	9000.0	5000.0	750000.0
D	IU/kg	750.0	500.0	10000.0
E‖	IU/kg	30.0	30.0	
K**	mg/kg	0.1	0.1	
Thiamine††	mg/kg	5.0	5.0	
Riboflavin	mg/kg	4.0	4.0	
Pantothenic acid	mg/kg	5.0	5.0	
Niacin	mg/kg	60.0	60.0	
Pyridoxine	mg/kg	4.0	4.0	
Folic acid	mg/kg	0.8	0.8	
Biotin‡‡	mg/kg	0.07	0.07	
B$_{12}$	mg/kg	0.02	0.02	
Choline§§	mg/kg	2400.0	2400.0	
Taurine (extruded)	%	0.10	0.10	
Taurine (canned)	%	0.20	0.20	

DM, Dry matter; *ME*, metabolized energy.

*Presumes an energy density of 4.0 kcal/g ME, based on the modified Atwater values of 3.5, 8.5, and 3.5 kcal/g for protein, fat, and carbohydrate (nitrogen-free extract), respectively. Rations greater than 4.5 kcal/g should be corrected for energy density; rations less than 4.0 kcal/g should *not* be corrected for energy.

†Although a true requirement for fat per se has not been established, the minimum level was based on recognition of fat as a source of essential fatty acids, as a carrier of fat-soluble vitamins, to enhance palatability, and to supply an adequate caloric density.

‡If the mean urine pH of cats fed ad libitum is not below 6.4, the risk of struvite urolithiasis increases as the magnesium content of the diet increases.

§Because of very poor bioavailability, iron from carbonate or oxide sources that is added to the diet should not be considered as a component in meeting the minimum nutrient level.

¶Because of very poor bioavailability, copper from oxide sources that is added to the diet should not be considered as a component in meeting the minimum nutrient level.

‖Add 10 IU vitamin E above minimum level per gram of fish oil per kilogram of diet.

**Vitamin K does not need to be added unless diet contains greater than 25% fish on a DM basis.

††Because processing may destroy up to 90% of the thiamine in the diet, allowance in formulation should be made to ensure the minimum nutrient level is met after processing.

‡‡Biotin does not need to be added unless diet contains antimicrobial or antivitamin compounds.

§§Methionine may substitute choline as methyl donor at a rate of 3.75 parts for 1 part choline by weight when methionine exceeds 0.62%.

Choosing the correct diet for a puppy or kitten requires evaluation of the breed, age, activity level, and environmental conditions. Some breeds are less active than others, and a house-bound dog will likely use less energy than a farm dog. Large-breed dogs need a slower growth rate to help decrease skeletal abnormalities. Many breeds are predisposed to obesity. Puppies and kittens that develop a large number of adipose cells during growth may also be predisposed to obesity as adults. Clients should be educated well on preventing obesity by learning to score their pets' body condition to prevent a number of diseases related to obesity in the senior years.

Puppies

A healthy mother that is well nourished should be able to provide complete nutrition for a puppy for the first 3 to 4 weeks.

A healthy puppy will nurse actively and vigorously. A malnourished puppy will constantly cry, become inactive, and fail to gain weight. Pregnant and nursing mothers should be fed a high-quality puppy food; they use the extra protein, calories, and fats to nourish the puppies.

More neonates die from a lack of knowledge of husbandry and nutrition than from disease. Birth weight is the single most important predictor of neonate survival. Those that are less than 25% of the average birth weight are at a higher risk of hypoglycemia, hypothermia, and pneumonia. Hypothermia decreases the motility of the gastrointestinal tract, thereby slowing the digestion of nutrients. Body weight should be monitored daily to ensure normal weight gain.

Average birth weight for toy-breed puppies is 100 g to 200 g; large-breed puppies average 400 g to 500 g, and giant-breed puppies average 700 g. Low birth weight produces poor performance and increased morbidity and mortality rates; it can be caused by congenital cardiac and pulmonary defects. Inadequate nutrition leads to dehydration and muscular weakness. Puppies not gaining weight may not be receiving enough calories and therefore require supplementation.

In general, growing puppies need twice as much energy as adults for growth, activity, and body maintenance.

Occasionally, milk replacer may be needed because of the mother's refusal to care for the young, the death of the mother, or her inability to produce enough milk for the litter. Neonates that weigh less than 30% of their littermates or those losing weight after 48 hours may also need extra supplementation. Neonates that die when they are aged 48 hours or older most likely have died from starvation.

Successful hand-rearing of orphans can depend on several factors, including appropriate feeding schedule, selection of milk replacer, meeting the caloric needs of the neonate, and proper feeding methods.

Newborns should be fed every 3 hours for the first week. Once the puppy has doubled the birth weight, feeding can be decreased to every 4 hours. This can take 7 to 10 days for a normal healthy puppy and 14 days for a puppy receiving milk replacer.

Formulated puppy milk replacer is available from veterinary distributors. Both powder and liquid forms are available. Powder formula lasts longer, and the unused powder can be frozen for 6 months. Once formula has been reconstituted, it should be used within 48 hours; the unused portion should be refrigerated in a glass container. Liquid milk replacer should also be used within 48 hours once the can has been opened, refrigerating the unused portion. Formulated milk replacer is superior to homemade versions because it generally provides the correct balance of protein, fat, carbohydrates, vitamins, and minerals needed for growing puppies. Reconstituted milk replacer should be warmed to 95° F to 100° F in a warm water bath. Milk should never be placed in the microwave because it can become too hot, causing severe burns to the patient.

At 3 or 4 weeks of age, dry puppy food can be mixed with water and/or formula in a 1:3 ratio to form a gruel. If canned food is preferred, a 2:1 ratio can be made (canned food/formula and/or water). By 6 weeks of age, 50% of the puppies' diet should be from unmixed puppy food.

Water should be offered starting at 5 weeks of age. Puppies should still be receiving hydration from either their mother or the milk replacer, but water intake will increase once offered. Puppies should be allowed to play in the water at first; once they are acquainted with it, they will begin to drink it.

Puppies can be weaned at approximately 6 to 8 weeks. Early weaning is discouraged because it can lead to malnutrition, stress-related disease, and behavioral problems. It is important to watch the overall caloric intake because puppies can become obese, leading to a variety of diseases later in life. From the time of weaning until 6 months of age (9 months in large breeds), it is advised to feed puppies three times a day (more frequently for smaller and toy breeds). Thereafter, dogs should be fed twice daily on a regular schedule.

Large-Breed Puppies

Nutrition plays an important role in large-breed puppies and can lead to skeletal disease from an increased growth rate. Genetics and environmental components also play a role in disease development, but designing an adequate nutrition program can decrease the potential for a disease process.

> **PRACTICE POINT** Large-breed puppies should be fed a diet specific for large breeds; nutrients contribute to skeletal diseases commonly seen in large breed dogs.

Large-breed puppies require fewer calories per unit of body weight and mature more slowly than small-breed puppies. Rapid growth occurs in the first few months in all breeds but occurs over a longer period in large breeds. It is important to take into consideration the age, breed, gender, body condition, genetics, and environment. It is also important to understand how nutrients contribute to the expression of skeletal disease.

Excess dietary energy and caloric intake may support a growth rate that is too fast for appropriate skeletal development and that results in a higher number of skeletal abnormalities. Excess energy leads to increased growth rate; increased growth rate leads to increased skeletal abnormalities. Abundant caloric intake contributes to accelerated growth rate and excess weight gain.

Canine hip dysplasia is a genetic disorder of large and giant breeds but can be influenced by nutrition. Evidence suggests that rapid growth and weight gain in early development increase the risk for this condition.

Feeding methods can help control excess nutrient intake. Three methods of feeding include free-choice feeding, time-restricted feeding, and food-restricted feeding. Free-choice feeding allows the pet to eat ad libitum, thereby increasing the risk for excess nutrient intake. Time-restricted feeding allows the owner to feed two or three times per day for a set period. This may encourage the pet to eat ravenously, passing the normal satiety mechanism. Food-restricted feedings allow the owner to control caloric intake, maintaining optimal growth rate and body condition.

The body condition should be evaluated every 2 weeks. Food can be adjusted as needed to decrease excess fat, thereby decreasing the growth rate. Puppies should be scored on a 9-point scale as to how easy it is to palpate the ribs and spine. The ideal body condition score is an hourglass shape when viewed from above, with a definitive waist behind the ribs. Figure 23-14 demonstrates the appropriate technique for determining the body score of a canine.

Environment, genetics, and nutrient composition play key roles in skeletal development. The effects of skeletal disease in large-breed puppies can be minimized by regulating nutrient and caloric intake. The goal should be to regulate growth rate, not maximize it. Feeding an AAFCO-approved commercial diet is recommended to help achieve this goal.

Kittens

Normal, healthy kittens should be able to nurse vigorously. Healthy mothers can provide complete nutrition for kittens for the first 4 weeks of life. Signs of kittens receiving inadequate nutrition include constant crying, inactivity, and no weight gain.

◼ Nestlé PURINA
BODY CONDITION SYSTEM

TOO THIN

1 Ribs, lumbar vertebrae, pelvic bones and all bony prominences evident from a distance. No discernible body fat. Obvious loss of muscle mass.

2 Ribs, lumbar vertebrae and pelvic bones easily visible. No palpable fat. Some evidence of other bony prominence. Minimal loss of muscle mass.

3 Ribs easily palpated and may be visible with no palpable fat. Tops of lumbar vertebrae visible. Pelvic bones becoming prominent. Obvious waist and abdominal tuck.

IDEAL

4 Ribs easily palpable, with minimal fat covering. Waist easily noted, viewed from above. Abdominal tuck evident.

5 Ribs palpable without excess fat covering. Waist observed behind ribs when viewed from above. Abdomen tucked up when viewed from side.

TOO HEAVY

6 Ribs palpable with slight excess fat covering. Waist is discernible viewed from above but is not prominent. Abdominal tuck apparent.

7 Ribs palpable with difficulty; heavy fat cover. Noticeable fat deposits over lumbar area and base of tail. Waist absent or barely visible. Abdominal tuck may be present.

8 Ribs not palpable under very heavy fat cover, or palpable only with significant pressure. Heavy fat deposits over lumbar area and base of tail. Waist absent. No abdominal tuck. Obvious abdominal distention may be present.

9 Massive fat deposits over thorax, spine and base of tail. Waist and abdominal tuck absent. Fat deposits on neck and limbs. Obvious abdominal distention.

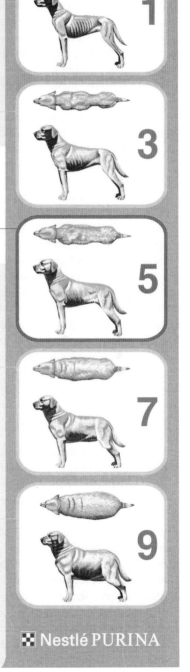

The BODY CONDITION SYSTEM was developed at the Nestlé Purina PetCare Center and has been validated as documented in the following publications:

Mawby D, Bartges JW, Moyers T, et. al. *Comparison of body fat estimates by dual-energy x-ray absorptiometry and deuterium oxide dilution in client owned dogs.* Compendium 2001; 23 (9A): 70

Laflamme DP. *Development and Validation of a Body Condition Score System for Dogs.* Canine Practice July/August 1997; 22:10-15

Kealy, et. al. *Effects of Diet Restriction on Life Span and Age-Related Changes in Dogs.* JAVMA 2002; 220:1315-1320

Call 1-800-222-VETS (8387), weekdays, 8:00 a.m. to 4:30 p.m. CT

VET 2897

◼ Nestlé PURINA

FIGURE 23-14 Determining body condition score in dogs. (Courtesy Nestle Purina, St. Louis, MO.)

The normal birth weight of healthy kittens is between 90 and 110 g. Kittens should gain 10 to 15 g per day and double their birth weight by day 10. Thereafter, kittens should weigh an average of 1 lb per month of age until 4 months. Formula-fed kittens grow more slowly, only doubling their body weight at 14 days, rather than 10, regardless of appropriate caloric intake.

Kittens require the most energy during their first 2 weeks of life, or 20 kcal/100 g/day. Kittens can begin to consume gruel at about 3 to 4 weeks of age. Gruel can be made of a dry kitten food mixed with formula and/or water (2:1) and fed in a saucer. They will increase consumption over the next 2 weeks, during which time the amount of water and/or formula added to the kitten food can be decreased, eventually weaning them onto kitten food.

Orphan kittens or kittens failing to gain weight can be fed a kitten milk replacer. Veterinary distributors carry a variety of replacers, as described in the canine section.

Vigorous orphans with a good suck reflex may be bottle fed in a sternal recumbency, with the head elevated, simulating a nursing position. Weaker kittens may need to be tube fed. Kittens that do not receive colostrum may be more susceptible to infection at about 35 days postnatal.

Neonates may need help to learn how to bottle feed. Some take to bottle feeding well, whereas others need assistance. The nipple should be proportionate to the kitten's size and fill its mouth. A drop of milk should readily form when the bottle is inverted. If not, enlarge the nipple opening with a hot 22-g needle. Kittens nursing from a too-small nipple may generate negative suction. Increasing the size of the nipple and/or the size of the hole helps weaker patients nurse more effectively.

The gag reflex does not develop until approximately day 10; therefore kittens should not be forced to bottle feed. Aspiration and/or pneumonia can be a fatal consequence.

Kittens should be fed every 2 to 4 hours for the first week, decreasing to every 4 to 6 hours the second week. Frequency can be decreased over the next 4 weeks while the amount being fed increases.

The urogenital area should be stimulated after every feeding to encourage urination and bowel movements. A moist, warm cotton ball can be used to stimulate movement. Kittens will begin to defecate and urinate without stimulation at about 3 to 4 weeks of age.

Kittens can be weaned at 6 to 8 weeks. Early weaning is not advised because separation from littermates can result in behavioral changes and a decline in social skills.

Kittens should be fed three times daily for 6 months, then twice daily for life. The label should be read on each food the kitten is eating to determine the correct amount to feed. If the kitten is eating both canned and dry food, the total caloric intake needs to be considered. As kittens mature, their energy requirements become less. At 10 weeks of age, the average daily energy requirement (DER) is 200 kcal/kg. By 10 months of age, the DER decreases to 80 kcal/day.

Kittens can become obese, leading to a variety of diseases later in life. Some cats will limit themselves and simply "graze" all day, whereas others will eat until they have a distended abdomen. The same rules apply for kittens and cats that apply to puppies and dogs; owners should be educated well on body scoring their pets for obesity. The ribs and spine should easily be palpable, with an hourglass shape from above and a trim waistline behind the ribs. Figure 23-15 demonstrates the appropriate technique to determine the body score of cats.

Adults

The same body condition score applies to dogs and cats as they mature to adults and seniors. In general, adult foods should be lower in calorie content because the adult pet does not have the same energy requirements as puppies and kittens. Research has shown that adults can benefit from higher protein diets with less carbohydrates and fat. This is especially true for cats. Cats are carnivores, meaning meat is their main source of protein. Carbohydrates are not a high requirement by cats and can significantly contribute to the obesity problem seen in adults. Dogs are omnivores; they use both meat and vegetables for their sources of protein, carbohydrates, minerals, and fat.

> **PRACTICE POINT** Any patient that has been spayed or neutered will have a decrease in metabolism up to 30%; therefore diets should be modified accordingly.

Seniors

Traditionally, senior patients were thought to need lower levels of protein because high levels of protein were thought to contribute to renal disease. Newer research has shown, however, that senior patients need higher levels of protein to help maintain muscle mass with low to moderate levels of fat to help maintain body mass.

Conditions that can be Treated or Maintained by Diet

Many conditions are diet responsive, whereas others must have medical management as well. Many diets can treat multiple diseases; the characteristics of a particular diet are vital to the treatment or maintenance of a disease or condition.

Allergies

Food allergies can be difficult to diagnose in patients because many different ingredients may contribute to the offending allergen. The goal, when determining what type of protein the pet may be sensitive to, is to eliminate all protein and carbohydrate sources for 8 weeks. A food trial of a hypoallergenic diet must be initiated with no other treats, trash, or snacks. A truly hypoallergenic diet is one that hydrolyzes (reduces the size of) the proteins to less than 18,000 Daltons (the size of the proteins). Once the pet's allergenic symptoms have subsided, the introduction of proteins can begin, one by one. Because hydrolyzed diets have been modified, the resulting protein is a medium-chain triglyceride, enabling the body to digest a higher amount of the nutrients. Diets with these protein modifications can also

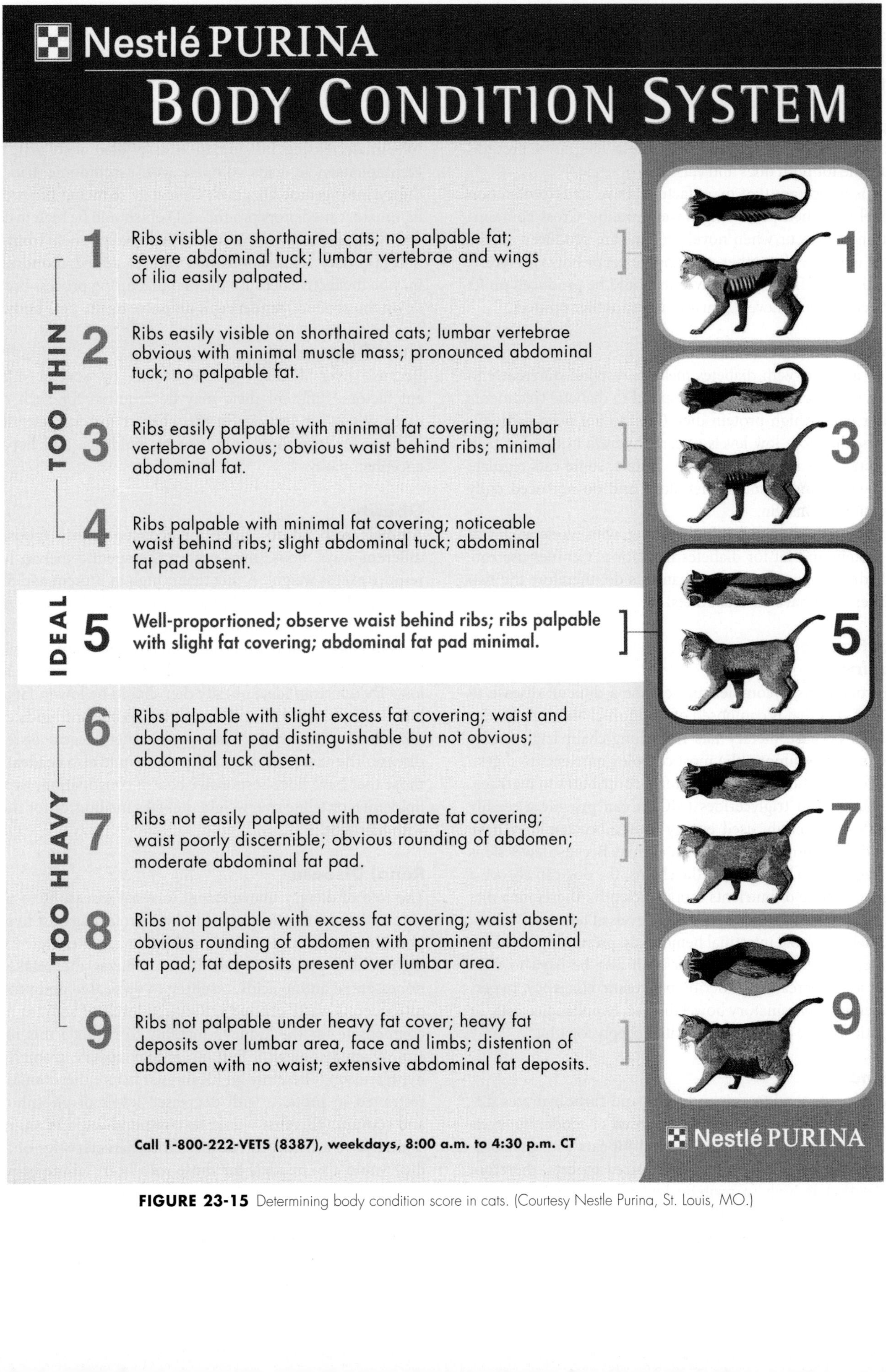

▣ Nestlé PURINA
BODY CONDITION SYSTEM

TOO THIN

1 Ribs visible on shorthaired cats; no palpable fat; severe abdominal tuck; lumbar vertebrae and wings of ilia easily palpated.

2 Ribs easily visible on shorthaired cats; lumbar vertebrae obvious with minimal muscle mass; pronounced abdominal tuck; no palpable fat.

3 Ribs easily palpable with minimal fat covering; lumbar vertebrae obvious; obvious waist behind ribs; minimal abdominal fat.

4 Ribs palpable with minimal fat covering; noticeable waist behind ribs; slight abdominal tuck; abdominal fat pad absent.

IDEAL

5 Well-proportioned; observe waist behind ribs; ribs palpable with slight fat covering; abdominal fat pad minimal.

TOO HEAVY

6 Ribs palpable with slight excess fat covering; waist and abdominal fat pad distinguishable but not obvious; abdominal tuck absent.

7 Ribs not easily palpated with moderate fat covering; waist poorly discernible; obvious rounding of abdomen; moderate abdominal fat pad.

8 Ribs not palpable with excess fat covering; waist absent; obvious rounding of abdomen with prominent abdominal fat pad; fat deposits present over lumbar area.

9 Ribs not palpable under heavy fat cover; heavy fat deposits over lumbar area, face and limbs; distention of abdomen with no waist; extensive abdominal fat deposits.

Call 1-800-222-VETS (8387), weekdays, 8:00 a.m. to 4:30 p.m. CT

▣ Nestlé PURINA

FIGURE 23-15 Determining body condition score in cats. (Courtesy Nestle Purina, St. Louis, MO.)

be used for dogs with dermatitis, pancreatitis, gastroenteritis, exocrine pancreatic insufficiency, protein-losing enteropathy, inflammatory bowel disease, lymphangiectasia, and hyperlipidemia.

"Allergy diets" made of proteins the pet has never been exposed to before may also provide relief for food allergies. Trout, duck, venison, and rabbit are a few novel proteins available for both dogs and cats.

It is important that manufactures have strict production guidelines when producing novel proteins. Cross contamination can occur when novel proteins are produced on the same equipment as other proteins (novel or not). Therefore, if a diet is hydrolyzed or novel, it should be produced on its own equipment, never "sharing" with another product.

Diabetes

Dogs and cats with diabetes mellitus respond differently to diets. Cats, being carnivores, respond to diabetic treatments better with a high-protein diet. Cats do not need carbohydrates; therefore low levels of carbohydrate in the diet help regulate the cat more efficiently. In fact, some cats regulate well with a high-protein diet alone and do not need daily injections of insulin.

Dogs must have a diet high in fiber, with moderate levels of protein and fat for diabetes regulation. Canines use carbohydrates for energy more than cats do; therefore the two species must have different diets.

Gastroenteritis
Canine

Gastroenteritis is complex and can be a difficult disease to treat. A diet that is composed of medium-chain triglycerides is ideal because dietary fats from long-chain triglycerides (LCTs) can be among the most complex nutrients to digest. The fermentation of undigested fats contributes to diarrhea. Medium-chain triglycerides (MCTs) can provide a readily digested and easily used energy source because they have already been broken down for the animal. Because fewer steps are required to break down the chains, the dog can absorb a higher volume of nutrients more efficiently. Therefore a diet composed of MCTs, with moderate levels of fat and low fiber, will help promote intestinal hemostasis, preventing diarrhea. A diet with these characteristics can also be used to treat dogs for pancreatitis, exocrine pancreatic efficiency, hyperlipidemia, inflammatory bowel disease, lymphangiectasia, or hepatic disease not associated with encephalopathy.

Feline

Because cats tend to respond to fat and carbohydrates differently than dogs do, a diet composed of moderate levels of fat and low carbohydrates is ideal for cats with gastrointestinal issues. High protein is required by cats; therefore a diet that is high in protein, low in carbohydrates, and moderate levels of fat is ideal. These characteristics will also provide a diet for those with hepatic lipidosis. Contraindications for this diet include cats with renal failure or hepatic encephalopathy.

Heart Disease

Patients with heart disease must consume a diet low in sodium to decrease the workload of the heart.

Joints and Arthritis

Research has shown that omega-3 fatty acids play a large role in decreasing inflammation associated with arthritis. Eicosapentaenoic acids compete with arachidonic acid for the cyclooxygenase enzymes, ultimately reducing the proinflammatory mediators produced. Diets should be high in cold water fish sources to allow dogs to maximally benefit from the omega-3 fatty acids. Foods that contain added chondroitin may be ineffective because the manufacturing process breaks down the product, rendering it unusable by the pet's body.

Liver Disease

Because liver disease can be caused by several different factors, different diets may be required for such diseases. See other sections in this chapter for characteristics of diets for hyperlipidemia, hepatic lipidosis, and hepatic encephalopathy.

Obesity

Animals respond to "light" or reduced-calorie foods in different ways. Some may need a therapeutic diet to help remove excess weight. A diet that is high in protein and fiber will help the pet feel full, inducing satiety. High protein may also increase the metabolism of the pet. In addition, a high protein/calorie ratio promotes the loss of body fat while helping minimize the loss of lean body mass during weight loss. Therefore an ideal obesity diet should be low in fat and high in protein and fiber. This diet would be contraindicated for animals that require a low-protein diet because of renal disease. The characteristics of this diet would also be ideal for those that have fiber-responsive colitis, constipation, hyperlipidemia, or feline overweight diabetes mellitus or for those with hairballs.

Renal Disease

The role of dietary management in renal disease is to provide a diet low in phosphorus to help protect against hyperphosphatemia and associated renal damage. Restricted but high-quality protein in the diet minimizes the intake of nonessential amino acids, resulting in decreased amounts of nitrogenous waste products. Reduced levels of sodium help compensate for the kidney's inability to regulate this mineral, whereas omega-3 fatty acids may reduce glomerular hypertension. Therefore an ideal renal failure diet should be restricted in protein, with decreased levels of phosphorus and sodium. This diet would be contraindicated in animals that require a high-protein diet. The characteristics of this diet would also be ideal for those with heart failure or with hepatic disease associated with encephalopathy.

Urinary Stone Formation

A diet that effectively reduces the stone formation of both struvite and calcium oxalate uroliths will minimize the

risk of recurrence while maintaining urinary tract health. An ideal diet should produce urine with a pH of 6.2, with moderate levels of salt to promote water intake. High levels of protein satisfy the protein needs of cats. Cats with heart disease or renal failure should not consume diets with these characteristics. Dogs may need a urine acidifier depending on the type of stones diagnosed.

Parasites

Parasites may be internal or external and occur in small and large animals. Internal parasites in small animals include roundworms, hookworms, threadworms, whipworms, tapeworms, and heartworms. Internal protozoan parasites of small animals include coccidia and *Giardia*. Parasites of horses include roundworms, pinworms, strongyles, threadworms, and tapeworms. Ruminants are commonly infected by strongyles, lungworms, tapeworms, coccidia, and *Trichomonas*. Pigs are often infected with stomach worms, ascarids, *Strongyloides, Oesophagostomum,* whipworms, lungworms, and kidney worms. External parasites include fleas, ticks, lice, and mites.

Parasite prevention programs should be implemented where possible because many parasites are zoonotic. Controlling parasites in large animals can be difficult; however, a program should be established to provide the most protection possible.

Common Small Animal Emergencies

Emergencies come in all sizes. Everyone needs to be prepared to handle an emergency at any time. Once the receptionist accepts the call, the owner's name, pet's name, and a phone number should be noted. The receptionist should ask as many questions as possible: what the emergency is, when it happened, and the current condition of the pet. Many clients will not be able to answer all the questions and may be in too much of a hurry to talk. The receptionist can then provide the information to the assistants, technicians, and doctors.

Anaphylactic Reaction

This is an immediate type of hypersensitivity reaction in which death may occur rapidly from respiratory and circulatory collapse. Causes of anaphylactic reactions include (but are not limited to) vaccines, bee or wasp stings, and medications.

Antifreeze Ingestion

Unfortunately, once a pet has ingested antifreeze, it may be too late to save its life. Unless the ingestion has occurred very recently, there is no effective treatment. Many people do not know when their pets have ingested antifreeze. Pets will not show symptoms for up to 12 hours after ingestion. They may be lethargic. A urine sediment sample can be checked to determine if any monohydrate crystals are present (this is a definitive diagnostic tool), or an ethylene glycol test can

be run. The patient can be supported with IV fluids while monitoring the blood urea nitrogen and creatinine values. Antifreeze basically shuts down the kidneys and does not allow the pet to produce urine.

> **PRACTICE POINT** Antifreeze is a sweet-tasting liquid that attracts pets and is fatal when consumed.

Bleeding

Frequently, the location of an active bleed can be difficult to determine, especially in patients that are active or in pain. In general, application of pressure directly to the site can induce clot formation, which will slow the bleeding. Once the bleeding has slowed, identification and a treatment plan can be initiated.

Blocked Cat

Many owners do not realize that a blocked cat is an emergency. Once a cat is blocked and cannot urinate, the blood urea nitrogen and creatinine levels increase dramatically. The cat may present with a distended abdomen, lethargy, and lack of appetite. These cats need to have a urinary catheter put in immediately. They may need to be sedated for the procedure, but if lethargic enough, it may be possible to advance a catheter without sedation. Vinegar may help the advancing of the catheter. Once a catheter has been placed, a urine sample needs to be collected and a urinalysis performed. The cat needs to be put on IV fluids to help flush the system out, and the urinary catheter needs to be left in place for 12 to 24 hours. An Elizabethan collar must be applied to the cat so it cannot pull the catheter out. A closed urinary tract system (an empty IV line and bag) can be put on the catheter to collect the urine. The amount of urine produced by the cat can then be measured and recorded. After the urinary catheter has been pulled, the cat should be observed for appropriate urination (straining, blood in the urine, etc.). Blood values of urea nitrogen and creatinine must be rechecked in 48 hours to make sure they have come down. The cat will need to be placed on a special diet and remain on the diet for the rest of its life because blockage can recur at any time.

Cardiopulmonary Resuscitation

When an animal is in cardiorespiratory arrest, everyone must be available to assist. When performing cardiopulmonary resuscitation (CPR), one person performs chest compressions, one person must breathe for the pet, another technician maintains the ECG machine, and someone needs to be available to get medications as needed.

Dyspneic Animal

An animal having difficulty breathing should be put into the oxygen cage (or have an oxygen mask put on) immediately. The gums will generally be a purple or blue color in this situation.

Dystocia

Difficult labor occurs in both the dog and cat but is far more common in the dog. Several conditions result in the diagnosis of dystocia:

- No fetus present within 4 to 6 hours from the onset of labor or from when the last time a fetus was born.
- No attempt to deliver a fetus despite the presence of fetuses in the uterus.
- Weak or infrequent contractions.
- Depression, weakness, and signs of toxemia.
- No puppies born by 72 days of gestation.
- No puppies born after 2 to 3 hours of active labor.

Gastric Torsion

Several factors may predispose dogs to gastric torsion. Older, large, and giant purebred dogs with a deep and narrow thorax are at a higher risk. Some studies indicate dogs that eat fast, are fed one meal a day, and have a nervous temperament may also be at a higher risk. It is associated with pain and stress and swallowing large amounts of air. The stomach distends with air and often twists 180 degrees on its axis. Signs include nonproductive retching and a distended abdomen that sounds air filled when thumped. The animal can die quickly from blood not being returned to the heart. The first priority is to relieve the air-filled stomach, then surgery to correct the torsion.

Car Accident

Having a pet be hit by a car is a very traumatic experience for the owner. Often, the best option for the veterinary practice is to take the animal to the treatment area and place the client in an exam room. This allows the team to evaluate the patient without the client. Once the pet has been evaluated, the veterinarian can provide information to the owner. It is important to try to determine where the pet has been hit by the car; the chest, abdomen, extremities only, or the whole body. If the pet is severely injured, it will most likely go into shock; the temperature will drop, oxygen circulation will decrease, and the system will try to compensate for the damage. A pet in shock should be warmed immediately and started on IV fluids. Caution should be used when moving the pet until the extent of its injuries can be determined. The veterinarian can then make recommendations for therapy and treatment of existing wounds.

Heatstroke

Heatstroke can be caused by a pet being left outside in extreme heat with no shade or water or by being left in a car with closed windows. Heatstroke patients often suffer irreversible damage that may go undetected for several days. Heatstroke patients present with temperatures in excess of 104° F, panting, and are usually in a lateral recumbent position. Although the goal when treating these patients is to decrease the temperature, it should be done slowly to prevent sudden hypothermia.

Proptosed Eye

A proptosed eye is when the globe of the eye has popped out of the socket. This is also a very traumatic experience for owners who can hardly look at the pet's face. Proptosed eyes are usually the result of trauma and commonly occur in small breeds with short noses. Pekingese, Pugs, and Boston terriers are the most common breeds to experience this trauma, although other breeds are susceptible. If the eye has just proptosed, and there is minimal damage to the muscles and tendons around the globe, it can occasionally be replaced into the socket and sutured shut. The majority of the time, the eye will have to be enucleated (removed) and the socket sutured closed.

Seizure

A seizure can have many different etiologies. Toxicity, head trauma, tumors, and epilepsy are only a few causes. Many breeds are predisposed to seizures. Some seizures only last for a few seconds; others may last for minutes. A seizure is characterized by the pet lying in a lateral recumbent position with the legs and body stiffening and shaking uncontrollably. The pet may lose control of its bowels during the seizure. Once it has finished shaking, it may be disoriented for several hours. Seizures can be controlled with medication.

> **PRACTICE POINT**   A seizing pets is extremely traumatic for its owner; therefore they may be unable to recall details of the event

Toxicities

Toxicities can result from a variety of different things, including plants, chemicals, and medications. Animals may present with shaking, disorientation, impaired balance, seizures, or lethargy. If the owner knows what product the pet ingested, Animal Poison Control can be called. Be sure to have the correct product name and, if possible, the package or container. Animal Poison Control charges a fee; however, it has information relating to animal toxicities, treatments, and protocols. If a pet has *just* ingested a toxin, vomiting should be induced immediately. Apomorphine, as directed by the veterinarian, can be administered into the corner of the eye to induce vomiting. After most of the stomach contents have been emptied, the apomorphine should be rinsed from the conjunctival area and charcoal should be given. This will help absorb any toxins left in the stomach.

Rodenticides

Different rodenticides have different chemical compositions. Each product should be called in to Animal Poison Control to get the specific details. The most common product is Decon, which causes an animal to become anemic. These animals are treated with an injection of vitamin K and released with a minimum 30-day supply of oral vitamin K.

Tylenol

Tylenol (acetaminophen) is toxic to both dogs and cats. The animal's body cannot break down the active ingredient in Tylenol, which therefore causes toxicity. If the pet has just ingested Tylenol, vomiting should be induced with

apomorphine. The pet should be started on intravenous fluids and continue treatment at the discretion of the veterinarian.

Common Equine Emergencies

Colic

Colic is a general term that encompasses abdominal pain and is most commonly associated with gastrointestinal pain. Colic can be due to gas distension, torsion of the intestines, or nephrosplenic entrapment (the intestine can become obstructed in the space between the kidney and spleen). Symptoms can range from mild (kicking at belly) to severe discomfort (rolling and unable or unwilling to walk). Treatment can be either medical or surgical. Medical treatment consists of sedation to help control pain, nasogastric intubation to check for reflux, and the administration of mineral oil and fluids. The veterinarian may or may not recommend IV fluids. If the horse does not respond, surgery is advised. Uncontrollable pain is one of the most important signals for surgery. Surgery consists of an exploratory laparotomy to determine the cause of the pain and should be performed in an appropriate facility where sterility can be maintained.

Laceration

Lacerations can be caused by a number of things, including wire fencing, stalls, or loading accidents.

Common Bovine Emergencies

Down Cow

A "down cow" is one that is unable or unwilling to stand. Down cows may be suffering from hypocalcemia, also known as *milk fever* (especially likely in high-producing cows that have just begun lactation) or *obturator nerve paralysis*. Hypocalcemia is treated with intravenous calcium gluconate. Nerve paralysis is treated with dexamethasone (if a cow is pregnant, dexamethasone can lead to abortion; therefore caution should be used in its administration).

Dystocia

Cows may have difficulty in calving because of the size or malpresentation of the calf. Dystocia can sometimes be easily corrected by a veterinarian repositioning the calf; obstetric chains may be needed to help pull the calf out. Dystocia can lead to a cesarean section if the calf cannot be removed. If the calf is dead or too large to be pulled, a fetotomy (cutting the calf and delivering in pieces) may be performed.

Uterine Prolapse

A prolapse of the uterus often occurs shortly after calving. A cow may present with a large, red, and bloody body of tissue protruding from the vagina. The cow rarely appears in distress but may be straining (unable to urinate). Treatment consists of trying to put the uterus in its proper location.

Common Ovine and Caprine Emergencies

Sheep commonly suffer from both dystocia and hypocalcemia, similar to cows. The treatment is the same.

Pregnancy Toxemia

Pregnancy toxemia is seen in late-term ewes. The ewes may appear depressed, stagger around, or may be down. Pregnancy toxemia is caused by a nutritional deficiency leading to ketosis, ketoacidosis, and fatty liver. It is often associated with a sweet smell (ketones) on the breath. Ketones can be observed in the urine, and glucose levels in the blood may be low. Ewes can be treated with propylene glycol via stomach tube and with intravenous fluids with added dextrose. If the lambs are dead or the ewe is valuable, a cesarean section can be performed.

Common Canine Disorders

Dogs can present with a variety of ailments; some are breed specific and others are species specific. It is imperative that the receptionist, assistant, and technician team be well informed on the most common diseases to provide clients with information about and be able to answer their basic questions.

Allergies

Allergies are a common problem among dogs and can be related to food or environment. Food allergies are a response to certain proteins in the diet; allergies to beef, chicken, or salmon are common. Pets with food allergies may suffer from vomiting, diarrhea, sensitive skin, and/or anal gland infections. To rule out suspected proteins as the source of allergic symptoms, pets must be placed on a food trial and fed a truly hypoallergenic diet. A hypoallergenic diet is one in which the proteins have been hydrolyzed (reduced in size), which prevents the pet's immune system from recognizing the protein and mounting an allergic response to it. A food trial must last for a minimum of 8 weeks; the pet cannot receive treats of any kind (this includes heartworm preventive if it is in the form of a flavored tablet). If the symptoms clear, then the pet has a true food allergy. If the symptoms do not completely clear, then the pet may have some existing environmental allergies as well. If the pet responded to the food trial, then individual proteins may be reintroduced to the diet one at a time to determine which protein the pet is allergic to. Once the symptoms return, a diagnosis can be made. The pet should not eat any food with that type of protein on the ingredient list.

> **PRACTICE POINT** Allergies in companion animals are very frustrating for owners. Take time to educate clients, using both visuals and printed materials to enhance the client's learning experience.

Pets can have environmental allergies to grass, pollens, or molds and can be treated with antihistamines to relieve the

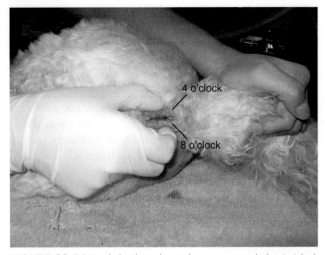

FIGURE 23-16 Anal glands are located at approximately the 4 o'clock and 8 o'clock positions around the anus.

symptoms. Just as with humans, some antihistamines may not work with an individual pet; therefore other antihistamines should be tried. Blood tests can also determine which environmental conditions a pet may be allergic to. Allergy injections can be formulated to help alleviate the symptoms. A variety of companies can compound allergy injections.

Anal Gland Impaction and/or Infection

Anal glands are located near the rectal area at approximately the 4 o'clock and 8 o'clock positions. These glands are used for scenting the pets' stool and frequently become impacted or infected. Smaller breeds tend to have more difficulty with these glands and often need assistance to express them. Many dogs will scoot on the carpet, expressing them and infuriating the owner with the horrible smell left behind. It is a common myth that dogs that scoot have worms; in fact, a majority of the time the anal glands are full or impacted (Figure 23-16).

Normal material from the anal glands should have a liquid consistency, with a slight brown color. Dark, thick material is not normal and may indicate that the pet needs to have its glands expressed more regularly. White liquid debris can indicate infection. Often, infected anal glands will rupture, becoming an anal gland abscess. At this point, the pet may need antibiotics and regular flushing of the draining tract.

Fiber can be added to the diet of some pets; by increasing the bulk in the stool, natural expression of the glands will occur. Others may need to have the glands expressed on a regular basis, either by the groomer, veterinary assistant, or veterinary technician.

Ear Infection

Ear infections are common in all breeds of dogs, especially those with ears that flop over. The warm, dark, and moist environment attracts yeast and bacteria. Pets may present with symptoms of scratching their ear or tilting their head, or the ear may be tender to the touch or have debris emanating from it.

It is advised to perform a cytology study of the ear to determine what type of bacteria or yeast may be residing in the ear canal. This can determine the appropriate treatment that will be recommended by the veterinarian. Cytology must be completed before the ear is cleaned; therefore technicians and assistants may want to gather the appropriate equipment to complete it. Once the appropriate medication has been dispensed, owners should be advised of the appropriate way to clean ears (described later in this chapter).

Ear infections may start as a result of allergies and are also more frequent in pets that swim in pools and lakes and in dogs that are hypothyroid. Cocker Spaniels are the most common breed to have both allergies and hypothyroidism, predisposing them to recurring ear infections.

Gingivitis

Gingivitis is inflammation of the gum line around both the inside and outside of teeth. Gingivitis can create a terrible odor, as bacteria live in and around the plaque buildup. Gingivitis can be prevented by regular teeth brushing. Many pets learn to enjoy their teeth being brushed, but it takes time and patience from the owner. Educating owners to brush their pets' teeth is an excellent puppy and kitten education topic. Animals learn to accept it when they are young; starting young prevents the disease later in life.

Gingivitis and dental disease are very common in smaller breeds of dogs because they do not chew on toys, bones, or sticks as they age. Larger breeds of dogs always find something to chew on. The actual mechanism to help keep teeth clean is similar to flossing; the simple scraping of an object against the teeth scrapes off plaque and bacteria. Once plaque builds up and calcifies, it turns to tartar, which requires a dental prophylaxis to remove. Without a dental treatment, gingivitis leads to periodontal disease, which ultimately leads to tooth loss. As bacteria build in the mouth, they begin to circulate in the bloodstream and can affect such organs as the kidneys and heart. Gum and dental disease prevention is key to maintaining a healthy body for the pet's life.

Hypothyroidism

Hypothyroidism is underproduction of thyroid hormone and most often occurs in dogs older than 2 years. Presenting symptoms include lethargy; obesity; dull, dry hair coat; and ear infections. A blood test is performed to diagnose the disease. Hypothyroid dogs are then started on a thyroid supplement, which is generally given twice daily. The thyroid levels are then checked 4 to 6 weeks later and 4 to 6 hours after the pill is given. A pet's activity level generally improves, along with the hair coat, once supplementation has started.

Kennel Cough

Kennel cough, usually caused by *Bordetella*, is a common bacterial or viral infection that is extremely contagious to other dogs. It is very common in boarding facilities, pet shops, and animal shelters. Symptoms include a dry, hacking cough that

can be induced upon palpation of the trachea. Dogs usually feel normal otherwise and continue to eat, drink, and play as normal. An antitussive agent (anticough) can be prescribed to relax the muscles of the trachea if needed. Antibiotics may be needed if the veterinarian feels that a secondary infection is starting or that the cough is due to a bacterial infection. Viral kennel cough must run its course because antibiotics will not kill a virus.

Owners of pets with kennel cough should be advised to confine their pets to a restricted area to prevent contact with other dogs until the symptoms have subsided. If pets are presented to the practice with symptoms of kennel cough, they should be placed into an exam room immediately, offered an isolation room, or asked to wait outside. This will prevent the further spread of this contagious disease.

Ocular Discharge

Ocular discharge is important to treat. Allowing eyes to drain excessively may increase the chance of permanent damage. Clear discharge may be normal for some smaller breeds and may be due to a blocked tear duct. Colored discharge, such as green or yellow discharge, can indicate an eye infection or damage to the surface of the eye. When clients call and are concerned about possible drainage from their pet's eye, they should be advised to come in to be seen as soon as possible.

Skin Diseases

Skin diseases can be due to a variety of ailments. The most common skin diseases seen are caused by allergies, infections, or mites. Allergies may cause a "hot spot," an area that has become irritated as the pet continues to lick and chew at it. Hot spots are localized, red lesions and are generally larger than the owner anticipates. Skin infections are characterized by scabby areas, with a small amount of purulent discharge oozing from the area. Both hot spots and infected lesions should be clipped and cleaned with a broad-spectrum cleaner. Antibiotics may be started, as well as shampoo or antihistamines to relieve skin irritation.

Mites can be difficult to diagnose, depending on the type of mite. *Demodex*, the common mite of mange, can be easily diagnosed with a skin scrape. Mites can be seen under the microscope and are easily treated. Dogs with mange usually present with patches of missing hair. Sarcoptic mange can be more difficult to diagnose because this mite resides in the hair follicles. Deep skin scrapes must be taken, which rarely yield *Sarcoptes*. Pets present with hair loss and intense pruritus (itching). A diagnosis is usually made when the pet's symptoms begin to remit with treatment.

Ringworm is a fungal skin disease that is zoonotic to people and other pets. The most common characteristics of ringworm include red, raised lesions on the face, nose, and ears, with hair loss on the rest of the body. Dermatophyte test medium (DTM), or fungal cultures, must be performed to rule out ringworm. If the DTM is positive, the client must be educated on proper eradication methods because ringworm can be difficult to eliminate.

Obesity

Obesity is a common disease that is on the rise. Many owners feel that they need to give their pets extra attention and love and do so by feeding too many treats. Obesity decreases a pet's life span and increases diseases such as osteoarthritis, heart disease, and hip dysplasia.

> **PRACTICE POINT** Leaner pets live an average of 1.8 years longer than those that are overweight.

Clients must be educated that leaner pets live longer lives, cost less to maintain, and are happier pets. Obesity programs may need to be instituted in the practice to decrease the number of obese patients. More importantly, if the owner is obese, instilling an activity program for the pet may increase the activity of the owner, ultimately increasing the health level of the client. Obesity must be tackled in America for both pets and clients.

Tumors

Tumors can be benign or malignant and must be removed to confirm the diagnosis. Fine-needle aspiration may be performed to attempt to view the cells that make up the tumor; however, trained pathologists that read such samples on a daily basis should make the diagnosis. A tumor may look benign or feel like a lipoma (fatty tumor) when, in reality, a smaller malignant mass may lie within.

Benign tumors are localized and do not metastasize to other regions of the body. Malignant tumors can metastasize to other parts of the body. Mast cell tumors, round cell tumors, and transitional cell carcinomas are just a few types of malignant tumors. Benign tumors do not generally require any treatment other than complete excision; malignant tumors require excision, along with chemotherapy or radiation treatment. A pathologist can recommend the best treatment when a mass has been submitted to the lab. Further consultation can occur with an oncology specialist in the area.

Common Feline Disorders

Cats present with a variety of diseases or problems, many of which can be difficult to diagnose and manage.

Abscesses

An abscess is a large pocket of pus and debris that has sealed over, retaining the bacteria inside. Many abscesses start from a cat bite wound or puncture that immediately seals over. The bacteria are left inside and replicate, causing an infection. Many cats present with fever, lethargy, and tenderness to touch in a specific area. Others may present with a ruptured abscess; the wound has opened, draining its contents. An abscess, if not already ruptured, will need to be opened and drained. The wound will then need to be flushed and the cat placed on antibiotics. Always wear gloves when cleaning abscesses. The threat of infection by methicillin-resistant *Staphylococcus aureus* (MRSA) is real and must be prevented in every way possible.

Asthma

Cats with asthma present with upper respiratory distress; they cannot breathe normally and are gasping for air. Most cats can only sit on their chests during an asthma attack because this is the only position that is comfortable. Cats may also "open mouth breathe"; they are trying to obtain more air by breathing through their mouths instead of their noses.

Cats with asthma generally need a radiograph to rule out other diseases. Asthma can be treated with a combination of several drugs, and cats can live long lives with asthma.

Feline Lower Urinary Tract Disease

Feline lower urinary tract disease (FLUTD) is common in male cats from 2 to 10 years of age. FLUTD is the blockage of the urinary tract between the bladder and the penis; the cause is unknown but is thought to be genetic or food related. Cats present with a painful abdomen, straining to urinate and meowing in discomfort. This is an emergency because the cat is unable to urinate. Most cats must be sedated immediately, have a urinary catheter placed that must remain in place for 12 to 24 hours, and be started on intravenous fluids. Many cats suffer kidney damage; therefore blood urea nitrogen and creatinine values must be evaluated and monitored.

FLUTD can be severe and life threatening. Once cats have become unblocked, the owner must be aware that the condition can recur at any time. Many cats are difficult to unblock and may reblock within a short period. Cats should be observed for normal urination for the rest of their lives. A special diet should be recommended that will maintain the urine pH within a neutral zone.

Hyperthyroidism

Hyperthyroidism is common in cats. Affected pets present with weight loss and vomiting. Cats look anorexic but have a vigorous appetite. The thyroid gland overproduces thyroid hormone, resulting in an excessive metabolism. Blood work determines if a cat is hyperthyroid. Medication is usually an effective treatment. Methimazole is the most common drug given and can be given once or twice a day, depending on the cat. If the cat does not easily take a pill, then a transdermal gel is available that can be applied to the ear pinnae.

Once a cat has been on the medication for 4 to 6 weeks, the thyroid level can be tested again to ensure the cat is receiving the correct dose.

Thyroid disease unfortunately can mask other diseases. Often, once the thyroid disorder has been treated, other diseases, such as renal and cardiac disease, will manifest.

Megacolon

Megacolon in cats is just as it sounds; it is an enlarged colon that often constipates cats. Many cats present with a distended and painful abdomen. Radiographs can be taken to diagnose megacolon. Enemas are often given to relieve the constipation. Medications must be given to the affected cat for life, and they must eat a special diet. Cats not receiving medication will reblock with feces and will need to have future enemas. Some cats block severely and must be anesthetized to perform a warm water enema to release the contents.

Ringworm

Ringworm is a common disease of cats, which can be symptomatic or asymptomatic carriers. Symptomatic is defined as showing lesions or hair loss, allowing areas to be cultured on a DTM. Asymptomatic carriers do not have any symptoms and are simply carriers of the fungus.

If one household has a cat that is positive for ringworm, it is recommended to test other cats in the house as well to determine if all must be treated. Cats can be orally medicated and bathed to treat the fungus.

Ringworm can be especially difficult to eradicate in the household setting. Strict cleaning procedures must be initiated and involve the carpet, upholstery, vents, and vacuum.

Housekeeping

It is imperative that the practice stay in immaculate condition at all times. Odors travel quickly through the practice; therefore urine, feces, anal gland secretions, and other unpleasant odors must be removed immediately. Odors are also absorbed into the walls, baseboards, and tile grout; once the odors have permeated, they may be impossible to remove.

> **PRACTICE POINT** Take pride in the practice, and ensure that the facilities are clean and well maintained on a daily basis.

Chemicals used to clean floors should never be mixed. The label on bleach products recommends that it be diluted to a 10% or 20% solution and warns not to mix it with other products. Caustic vapors may be produced, which can harm patients and team members. Labels must be read clearly to dilute the product to the correct strength to have a solution that kills viruses, fungi, or bacteria, whichever the product is designed to eradicate.

Trash should be emptied several times a day. Trash cans absorb odors that can also travel through the practice. Rooms must be cleaned after every patient, preventing the transmission of odors and diseases.

Walls should be cleaned weekly, if not more often; blood, hair, and dirt collect on walls and cabinets and must be cleaned off as soon as they are spotted.

Potted plants that sit on the floor must be cleaned frequently because animals often urinate on them. The entire pot must be cleaned. It should be moved each night while cleaning the practice, removing hair and dirt that has collected under the plant.

Blinds, fans, vents, baseboards, and door frames must be dusted weekly. Dirt collects in these locations quickly, and clients notice the dirt as they are waiting in the examination rooms.

The outside of the practice must remain clean as well. Feces must be removed daily, and common urination areas must be scrubbed with a dilute Clorox solution. Urine stains

walls and sidewalks and produces a terrible smell. Trash must be removed from the parking lot, including cigarette butts and cans. Windows should be washed weekly and dirt swept away from the entrance and exit areas. The outside of the building must be as presentable as the inside of the practice.

Boarding

Some practices allow their clients to leave their pets at the hospital when they leave town. Other practices may have a boarding facility that is separate from the practice. It is ideal to have separate facilities to allow hospitalized patients to recover in a quieter, cleaner environment. It also prevents boarding patients from being exposed to diseases or pathogens that hospitalized patients may be harboring.

Admitting

Admitting procedures for boarding animals are critical. The goal of any facility is to provide a safe, well-monitored, and caring environment. Every animal that is admitted must be reviewed for medications, feeding schedules, special diet, exercise requirements, and any other special needs. See Chapter 2 for examples of boarding admission forms. Release forms should include the above-mentioned information, and the owner should sign the bottom of the release. Release forms are absolutely critical when accepting patients for boarding. The release form must include the client's name, pet's name, and all available emergency contact information. If anything happens to the pet while the client is away, the practice must be able to contact the owner. The practice should also have established guidelines and the owner's consent that emergency procedures will be administered if and when an event should happen.

Release forms should also ask specific questions regarding the pet: What food does the pet eat and how often? What medications does the pet receive and how often? Has the pet had any vaccine or drug reactions in the past?

All patient blankets, collars, leashes, toys, and food must be clearly marked with the patient's name and owner's last name. All products left with the animal should be indicated on the release sheet. If a patient soils a blanket during the stay, it must be returned to the cage once washed. Kennels and cages may have a plastic holder on each to accommodate all personal items, preventing misplacement during the pets stay.

Facilities cannot be overcrowded, unsanitary, or loud; these factors can produce a stressful atmosphere for animals and team members. Boarding facilities or practices should have a boarding reservation software management system that allows the control of patient intake. Reservation management systems are similar to hotel reservations; they allow the team member to review available cages for a specific length of time.

The boarding center must be staffed by a kennel assistant as much as possible, allowing for the cleaning of cages as soon as patients defecate or urinate. Animals cannot be allowed to lie in their urine or feces for long periods. Animals boarded should always receive a bath before returning home because the odor of the facility will be present on the pet when it is discharged. This can be an unpleasant odor that leaves a client with a negative perception of the facility.

Every consideration should be given to the patient's dietary needs. If the practice does not carry a patient's food, clients should be advised to bring their own food. Changing the diet can cause a pet to have diarrhea; adding a stressful situation increases the chances of the pet experiencing stress colitis, a condition that also causes diarrhea. Medications should be administered as close to the normal times as possible, especially if insulin is being administered to a diabetic patient. Once the release sheet has been completed by the owner and team member, a treatment sheet should be filled out for the patient, indicating specific instructions for the kennel attendant. This allows each patient to receive individual care in a kenneled situation.

Isolation should be available for those patients with diseases that can be contagious to other patients in the boarding facility. Every precaution should be taken for patients to prevent the cross-contamination of disease; however, it can still occur. Kennel cough, or infectious tracheobronchitis, and feline upper respiratory diseases are spread through respiratory secretions and fomites. A fomite, or fome, is any object or material on which disease-producing agents can be conveyed. It is imperative that all bowls, litter pans, and blankets be washed in a warm, diluted bleach formula to prevent the spread of disease. If a dog is observed coughing or a cat is observed sneezing, it should be moved to an isolation area immediately.

Patients that are boarding may have options to receive treatments and special care while they are at the facility. It is important to always ask the client for permission before performing any service. Spa days are becoming very popular. Pets are pampered with a day of bathing, grooming, nail trims, ear cleaning, and anal sac expression; some may receive a massage!

Nail Trims

Nail trims should be offered to all patients because clients often cannot trim them at home. Long nails can have detrimental effects on the patient; altered gait, potential lameness, and ingrown nails are just a few. Resco-type nail trimmers work great. On white or clear nails, the quick can be visualized. The quick is the vein that runs midway through the nail; it is generally pink. If the quick is trimmed, it is extremely uncomfortable to the pet and causes the nail to bleed. Kwik Stop powder can be applied to the nail, or a silver nitrate stick can be used. The quick should be dabbed to absorb excess blood, and then the stick can be rolled in the quick bed. This can also be painful to pets. Short, quick actions can minimize the discomfort. Black nails can be hard to trim without cutting the quick because it cannot be visualized as easily as in white nails. It is advised to only trim the hook of the nail on black toenails. The quick will recede with each nail trim the pet receives. If a pet has excessively long nails, they can be

trimmed a small amount every 2 to 3 weeks until the desired length is achieved. Owners with sensitive skin should be warned that freshly trimmed nails are sharp and can scratch their skin easily. For elderly clients, patients' nails may be rounded off with a Dremel tool to decrease the sharpness of the nails.

Condo Facilities

Many facilities offer condominium-like housing for patients. Cat condos have several tiers available so that cats can move around. Toys may be available, or owners can bring their own. All toys and condos must be disinfected before exposure of the next patient. Canine condos may have themes associated with them (e.g., a cowboy room). This room may have painted walls, a step-up cot with a blanket, and a horse trough for water. Others may have water fountains or stereos to play music for the pets. Televisions may loop dog or cat videos to entertain patients.

Blankets and/or cots should be provided for pets to rest on; this can add comfort to the pets' stay, especially older and arthritic patients. Raised cots lift patients off the floor during colder times of the year. Blankets need to be watched; some patients love to chew on them. If a patient is known as a chewer, discretion should be used when allowing blankets to remain in the cage. All blankets should be washed in hot water with a dilute bleach solution. Blankets should be changed every day, regardless of whether they appear clean. Blankets can harbor odors, which penetrate the pet's hair coat. Blankets may also still look clean even when patients have urinated on them, leaving patients to lie in their own urine.

With the newest updated technology, web cameras can be installed in kennels, allowing owners to see their pets anytime on the computer. This is an added benefit for owners, and they love the ability to check in. Practices and facilities must be diligent about cleaning and ensure that the facility appears clean and friendly at all times.

Owners seek veterinary practices to board their patients for security and a guarantee that their pets will receive the treatment required while they are gone. This is especially true for patients that are unhealthy. Diabetics, senior patients, or those that receive any special medications must be monitored and medicated daily. All boarding patients must be monitored for urination, defecation, appetite, and activity. Increased water intake and urination must be noted, as well as any diarrhea, anorexia (lack of appetite), or lethargy (lack of energy). All the previously mentioned issues should be noted on the treatment sheet, and a doctor should be notified. If patients are seen limping, an exam by the veterinarian may be warranted; with the owner's consent, an NSAID may be administered.

Clients may elect to have procedures completed on the patient while boarding. Dentals, ovariohysterectomies, and castrations can be completed early in the boarding time, and the incision can be observed throughout the pet's stay. If a pet becomes too active in the kennel, drugs may be administered to calm the pet.

When releasing patients to owners, they should smell clean, look clean, and have all their personal items. If any procedures were performed during the stay, a release sheet should be provided to the owners with follow-up instructions, including permitted activity and when to give the next dose of medication. A report should also be generated regarding the pet's stay in the facility. Clients love to receive "report cards" of their pets; this is an excellent marketing tool and allows clients to feel that their pet is special.

VETERINARY PRACTICE and the LAW

Medications have the potential to treat conditions or induce harm. Many lawsuits are medication related, so the veterinary assistant and technician have a tremendous responsibility to follow all procedures to avoid doing harm.

Many patients are prescribed various medications at different stages in their life; a dog may receive a thyroid supplement and an anti-inflammatory (NSAID) for arthritis. If it was to experience an immune-related disorder, a veterinarian may place the pet on a steroid. The dog should not receive the steroid and NSAID together. Owners also add medications and herbs to their pets diet, hoping to improve the pets quality of life. Clients should be asked if any additional vitamins, minerals, or herbs are being supplemented, preventing the possibility of a toxic interaction.

When administering and dispensing medications, one must review the record, checking for all medications that have been dispensed. The assistant or technician should verify the medications with the veterinarian ensuring that the new medication is not contraindicated because of other medications.

Before administering the medication, the drug, dose, and route of administration must be verified. Labels should be verified for correct information and the client should be read the instruction.

REVIEW QUESTIONS

1. Why are informed consent forms so critical in veterinary medicine?
2. What is a carnivore?
3. What are the characteristics of an effective allergy diet?
4. Why is the admitting procedure for patients that are boarding so important?
5. What information is required on a medication label?
6. Interpret the following prescription: Diphenhydramine; 1 cap PO EOD × 21d.
7. Give an example of a nonsteroidal anti-inflammatory drug.
8. Why should all communication with the client be documented in the record?
9. Why should a receptionist double-check medication that is dispensed to clients?

10. What is a vasodilator?
11. Vital signs that should be obtained during the history-taking process include all of the following except:
    a. Body condition scoring
    b. Respiratory rate
    c. Heart rate
    d. Capillary Refill Time
12. A rabies vaccine is considered to be:
    a. Modified live vaccine
    b. Killed vaccine
    c. Live vaccine
    d. None of the above
13. A urine specific gravity indicates:
    a. A urinary tract infection
    b. The ability of the kidneys to concentrate urine
    c. The ability of the bladder to concentrate urine
    d. Diabetes mellitus
14. Patients undergoing anesthesia must have a physical exam:
    a. 12 hours before anesthesia
    b. During anesthesia
    c. 12 hours postoperatively
    d. Within 12 hours of anesthesia

15. Cerenia is considered which type of drug?
    a. Gastric
    b. Cardiac
    c. Nervous
    d. Respiratory

Recommended Reading

AAFCO guidelines. Available at www.fda.gov/AnimalVeterinary/Products/AnimalFoodFeeds/PetFood/default.htm.

Case LP: *Canine and feline nutrition*, ed 3, St Louis, MO, 2011, Elsevier.

Han CM, Hurd CD: *Practical diagnostic imaging for the veterinary technician*, ed 3, St Louis, MO, 2005, Mosby Elsevier.

McCurnin D, Bassert JA: *McCurnin's clinical textbook for veterinary technicians*, ed 8, St Louis, MO, 2013, Saunders Elsevier.

Sirosis M: *Principles and practices of veterinary technology*, ed 3, St Louis, MO, 2011, Mosby Elsevier.

Tear M: *Small animal surgical nursing*, ed 2, St Louis, MO, 2012, Elsevier.

Calculations and Conversions

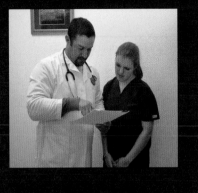

OUTLINE

Monthly Statement Fees, *435*
   Practice Set: Monthly Statement Fees, *435*
Accounts Receivable Percentages, *435*
   Practice Sets: Accounts Receivable
     Percentages, *436*
Inventory Turns Per Year (Turnover
  Rate), *436*
   Practice Sets: Turnover Rate, *436*
Determining Effective Reorder
  Quantities, *436*
   Practice Sets: Reorder Quantity, *437*
Determining Effective Reorder Points, *437*
   Practice Sets: Reorder Point, *437*
Putting it All Together: Turnover, Reorder
  Quantity, and Reorder Points, *438*
   Practice Sets, *438*
Determining if a Bulk Order is the Right
  Choice, *438*
Developing Effective Inventory Pricing
  Strategies, *439*
   Break-Even Analysis, *439*
   Markup, *439*

Dispensing Fees, *439*
Labeling Fees, *439*
Injection Fees, *439*
Putting it All Together: Break-Even
  Analysis, Markup, Dispensing,
  Labeling, and Injection Fees, *440*
   Practice Sets, *440*
Developing an Effective Service Markup, *440*
   Practice Sets: Developing an Effective
     Service Markup, *441*
Payroll Calculations, *442*
   Practice Set: Determining Gross Pay
     per 2-Week Pay Period, *442*
Drug Calculations, *442*
   Explanation #1, *443*
   Explanation #2, *443*
   Percentage Solutions, *444*
   Practice Set: Drug Calculations, *444*
   Teaspoons and Tablespoons, *444*
Intravenous Fluid Calculations, *445*
   Practice Set: Intravenous Fluids, *445*
Acknowledgments, *445*

LEARNING OBJECTIVES

When you have completed this chapter, you should be able to:

1. Calculate monthly finance charges.
2. Calculate accounts receivable percentages.
3. Calculate inventory turns per year.
4. Develop an effective product markup.
5. Develop an effective service markup.
6. Calculate cost/benefit ratio.
7. Calculate a break-even analysis.
8. Calculate payroll.
9. Calculate drug doses.
10. Calculate intravenous fluid doses.

Every team member should be familiar with the common calculations that are used in veterinary practice. Receptionists and office managers are generally responsible for determining finance and statement charges for client account receivables. They may also be responsible for product markup when products are special ordered for a client. Office managers may be responsible for payroll and for determining the cost/benefit ratio of special promotions or the purchase of equipment. Each team member must be familiar with drug calculations and equations because every team member must double-check medications before they leave the premises; this can prevent a fatal mistake.

The following equations have been covered in previous chapters. The purpose of this chapter is to allow the reader to become comfortable with equations used in everyday practice. The reader should practice the examples given, as practice results in improved skills. Math can be a difficult task, but with a little practice anyone can become proficient at conversions and calculations (see Box 24-1). Team members should memorize many of the conversions; this will allow tasks to be completed easily. A copy of the conversion table can be hung in a central location in the veterinary practice so that all team members can benefit. Conversion tables also provide a way to double-check work.

Monthly Statement Fees

Covered in Chapter 18.

Monthly statement fees must cover the cost of the statement being produced. This includes team member time, paper, ink, stamps, and envelopes. It may also be encouraged to add a finance fee; credit cards charge finance fees, why shouldn't a veterinary practice? State regulations must be verified as to what percentage of a bill is allowed as a finance charge.

 Veterinary practice managers are responsible for managing accounts receivable.

Items to consider when determining the cost of a statement fee:
- Number of statements to run
- Cost of invoice (paper, ink, envelopes, and stamps)
- Labor (pay rate of team member preparing statements, including taxes)
- Finance rate (if applicable)

Example A: What minimum dollar amount should be added in order to recover costs associate with monthly statements?
- 100 statements to run
- Supply cost per invoice is determined to be $0.99
- Labor: The team member's hourly salary is $12, and it takes 6 hours to complete the task. Taxes are approximately 20% of the pay rate.

$$\text{Labor: } \$12.00 \times 6 \text{ hours} = \$72.00 \times 20\% = \$14.40$$
$$\text{Total Labor: } \$86.40 \ (\$72.00 + \$14.40)$$
$$\text{Labor per invoice: } 0.86 \ (\$86.40 \div 100)$$
$$\text{Labor} + \text{Supply Costs} = \$1.85 \ (0.86 + 0.99)$$

A statement fee of at least $1.85 must be applied to each invoice to recover costs.

Practice Set: Monthly Statement Fees

Determine the minimum monthly statement fee and the new balance based on the following scenarios. Answers appear on the Evolve site accompanying this text.

1. 250 statements
- Set supply costs per invoice of $1.05
- Labor: 2.5 hours; hourly pay rate = $8.50/hr; 20% for taxes
- Set monthly statement fee of $6.50
- Client has a balance of: $563.09
2. 39 statements
- Set supply costs per invoice of $0.85
- Labor: 2.0 hours; hourly pay rate = $12.50/hr; 20% for taxes
- No monthly statement fee
- Client has a balance of: $54.09
3. *What minimum dollar amount should be added in order to recover costs associated with these monthly statements?*
- 50 statements
- Set supply costs per invoice of $1.85
- Labor: 4 hours; hourly pay rate = $19.50/hr; 20% for taxes
- Client has a balance of: $201.98

Accounts Receivable Percentages

What percentage of the gross revenue is tied up in accounts receivable?

Less than 1.5% of gross revenue should be tied up in accounts receivable. A practice that produces $100,000 per month should have a total of only $1500 in accounts receivable each month! If the amount were 3%, it would total $3000 per month. It should be the goal of every clinic to have the lowest accounts receivable possible.

Example A:

Gross revenue (GR) for a veterinary practice is $195,000 for the month of April. Accounts receivable (AR) total is $14,950. What is the percentage tied up in AR?

$$\$14,950 \div \$195,000 = 0.08 \times 100 = 8\%$$

The AR total is divided by the total GR to obtain a numerical amount (don't forget, to obtain a percentage, the numerical answer must be multiplied by 100).

Example B:

GR for a practice is $202,378.98. AR is 3%. What is the total dollar amount tied up in AR?

$$\$202,378.98 \times 0.03 = \$6071.37$$

Example C:

The predicted GR for a practice is $800,000 and the practice's goal is to keep accounts receivable less than 1%. What amount can the AR total to meet this goal?

$$\$800,000 \times 0.01 = \$8,000$$

Practice Sets: Accounts Receivable Percentages

Answers appear on the Evolve site accompanying this text.

1. GR is $495,958.02; AR totals 14%. What amount is tied up in AR?
2. GR is $2,891,098.04; AR totals $109,004.09. What percentage is tied up in AR?
3. GR is $355,758.72; AR totals 5%. What amount is tied up in AR?
4. GR is $1,564.642.98; AR totals $19,104.09. What percentage is tied up in AR?

Inventory Turns Per Year (Turnover Rate)

Covered in Chapter 15.

Turns per year is defined as the number of times an inventoried product turns over in a practice. This helps determine correct reorder quantities and points. Each practice should set a goal of eight to 12 turns per year, depending on the product (refer to Chapter 15 for more details). To determine the inventory turns per year, the beginning inventory is added to the ending inventory and the result is divided by two. This results in the average inventory per year. The total amount of product purchased during that year divided by the average inventory per year yields the number of turns per year for that product.

 Veterinary practice managers are responsible for maintaining appropriate inventory systems.

Example A:
- 35 bottles of Keflex 500 mg were purchased between January 1, 2012, and December 31, 2012,
- Beginning Inventory: 4
- Ending Inventory: 1

$$4 + 1 = 5$$
$$5 \div 2 = 2.5$$
$$35 \div 2.5 = 14$$

Keflex turned 14 times in 2012. To help decrease ordering costs, this number should ideally be 12.

Example B:
- 36 bottles of eye drops were purchased in 2012.
- Beginning inventory: 4
- Ending Inventory: 8

$$4 + 8 = 12$$
$$12 \div 2 = 6$$
$$36 \div 6 = 6$$

The eye drops turned 6 times in 2012. To help decrease holding costs and potential product expiration, this number should ideally be 12, if it is a top-producing product. Order quantity and reorder points should be evaluated closer in this case. If this is not a top-producing product, a turnover rate of 6 is acceptable.

Example C:
- Convenia was purchased 8 times in 2012.
- Beginning inventory: 1
- Ending inventory: 1

$$1 + 1 = 2$$
$$2 \div 2 = 1$$
$$8 \div 1 = 8$$

Convenia turned 8 times during 2012. This is an acceptable number.

Practice Sets: Turnover Rate

Answers appear on the Evolve site accompanying this text.

Determine the turnover rate for the following examples. Consider that these are the top 20% products of your hospital. Are these good turnover rates?

1. Baytril 22.7 mg tablets
- Beginning inventory: 22
- Ending inventory: 54
- Total purchased during 2012: 100
2. Nolvasan Otic
- Beginning inventory: 12
- Ending inventory: 10
- Total purchased during 2012: 120
3. Clavamox Drops
- Beginning inventory: 8
- Ending inventory: 12
- Total purchased during 2012: 144

Determining Effective Reorder Quantities

Three factors are presented when determining reorder quantities; average daily use, turnover goals, and product expiration.

When the *average daily use of product is calculated,* one can better determine the how many units will sell per day. Average daily use is determined by taking the number of units sold in the year, and dividing by the number of days the practice is open in a year.

Example of average daily use calculation: A practice is open 365 days per year, and sells 550 bottles of Rimadyl, 25 mg #180.
- $550 \div 365 = 1.5$
- Rimadyl 25 mg #180 sells on an average of 1.5 bottles per day

Turnover is important in this equation, because it must be known how long the quantity ordered should support sales (without running out or having excess product).
- Average daily use × Turnover goal (in days) = Reorder quantity

Example A:

- Rimadyl 25 mg #180 is a top producing product; therefore it has a turnover goal of 12 times per year (30 days). What is the reorder quantity of this product, if the average daily use is 1.5?

$$30 \text{ days} = 1 \text{ month}; 12 \text{ turns per year} = 1 \text{ turn per month}$$
$$1.5 \times 30 = 45$$

When this product is ordered monthly, 45 bottles should be ordered, which will decrease ordering costs. (This number may seem high to some; however, if 1½ bottles sell per day, and your supply must last for 30 days, then 45 bottles makes sense.)

Example B:

- Heartgard Plus (blue 6 mo) has an average daily use of 3.5 (3.5 boxes sell on a daily basis)
- The turnover goal for this product is 12 times per year (30 days)

$$3.5 \times 30 = 105$$

When this product is ordered, 105 boxes should be purchased at once (which is estimated to sell within 30 days.) Since Heartgard Plus (blue 6 mo) is supplied in 10 boxes per carton, then 11 cartons would be ordered.

Example C:

- A practice is open 259 days a year
- Revolution, feline 5 to 15 lb, sold 525 boxes during 2012
- Turnover goal: 12
- What is the reorder quantity of this product?

$$\text{Average daily use: } 525 \div 259 = 2$$
$$2 \times 30 = 60$$

When this product is ordered, 60 boxes should be purchased at once (which is estimated to sell within 30 days).

Practice Sets: Reorder Quantity

Answers appear on the Evolve site accompanying this text.

Determine the reorder quantity for the following examples. Consider that these are the top 20% products of your hospital.

1. Baytril 22.7 mg tablets
- Total purchased during 2012: 500
- Practice is open 284 days
2. Nolvasan Otic
- Total purchased during 2012: 220
- Practice is open 312 days
3. Clavamox Drops
- Total purchased during 2012: 144
- Practice is open 365 days

Determining Effective Reorder Points

Reorder points is defined as the point at which a product needs to be ordered, and takes into consideration lead time and average daily use.

Lead time is defined as the amount of time between when a product is needed, until it gets onto the practice shelf. For example, consider a practice that orders every Monday and the order is received on Tuesday. If a product is noticed to be low on Wednesday, and the next order will be placed the following Monday (to be received Tuesday), then the lead time is said to be 7 days.

- *Lead time × average daily use = Reorder point*

Example A:

- If a practice orders on the 1st and the 15th of each month, receives shipments in 2 days, and Heartgard is placed on the want list on the 10th, what is the lead time?
  - **7 days** (the product is needed on the 10th, the order will be placed on the 15th, received on the 17th)

Example B:

- If an order is placed on Mondays and Thursdays, received overnight, and DHPP vaccines are in short supply on Wednesday, what is the lead time?
- If the average daily use of DHPP is 15, what is the reorder point?

$$\text{Lead time: 2 days}$$
$$\text{Reorder point: } 2 \times 15 = 30$$

DHPP must be ordered when 30 vaccines remain.

Example C:

- A practice is open 300 days per year
- Rimadyl 100 mg #60 sold 281 bottles in 2012
- Rimadyl is placed on the want list June 20th
- An order is only placed on the 1st of every month
- Product is received in 2 days
- What is the lead time, average daily use and reorder point?

Lead time: 13 days *(the product is needed on the 20th, the order will be placed on the 1st and received on the 3rd)*

$$\text{Average daily use: } 281 \div 300 = 0.94$$
$$\text{Reorder point: } 13 \times 0.94 = 12$$

Rimadyl must be ordered when 12 bottles remain

Practice Sets: Reorder Point

Answers appear on the Evolve site accompanying this text.

Determine the reorder point for the following examples.

1. Baytril 22.7 mg tablets
- Total purchased during 2012: 500
- Practice is open 284 days
- Order is placed on: every Monday
- Product is placed on want list: Wednesday
- Product is received in: 2 days
- What is the reorder point?
2. Nolvasan Otic
- Total purchased during 2012: 220
- Practice is open 312 days
- Order is placed on: every Wednesday
- Product is placed on want list: Friday
- Product is received in: 1 day
- What is the reorder point

3. Clavamox Drops
- Total purchased during 2012: 144
- Practice is open 365 days
- Order is placed on: 15th of July
- Product is placed on want list: June 30th
- Product is received in: 2 days
- What is the reorder point?

Putting it All Together: Turnover, Reorder Quantity, and Reorder Points

Practice Sets

For the following examples, determine the turnover rate, reorder quantity, and reorder point. Is this turnover rate ideal? If not, what would you change to create the ideal turnover rate?

Answers appear on the Evolve site accompanying this text.

1. Heartgard Plus Brown, 12-month supply
- Beginning inventory: 45
- Ending inventory: 12
- Number of units sold in 2012: 780
- Top 20% item
- Days the practice is open: 300
- When the order is needed: 15th of August
- When the order is placed: Sept 1st
- When the order is received: 2 days

2. Otomax
- Beginning inventory: 12
- Ending inventory: 15
- Number of units sold in 2012: 144
- Top 20% item
- Days the practice is open 316
- When the order is needed: Monday
- When the order is placed: Monday
- When the order is received: Tuesday

3. Cephalexin 500 mg capsules
- Beginning inventory: 595 capsules
- Ending inventory: 1080 capsules
- Number of units sold in 2012: 20,000
- Top 20% item
- Days the practice is open 350
- When the order is needed: Wednesday
- When the order is placed: every Monday
- When the order is received: every Tuesday

Determining if a Bulk Order is the Right Choice

Some manufactures offer discounts when purchasing large quantities of items. Bulk orders can be a good decision, when purchased with the following in mind:
- Quantity is based off of historical sales within the period being measured
- The quantity ordered must sell before the delayed billing is due
- Product cannot have a short shelf-life

To determine an effective quantity for a bulk order, a manager would consider the average daily use of the product, the number of working days in the billing period, and the percent of growth (or loss) the practice may be experiencing.
- *(Average daily use)(# of working days in billing period) (% growth increase)*

Example A:
- ABC Veterinary Clinic has sold Trifexis for the last 2 years. Sales on the product have increased (3%), because only 2 prevention products are offered in this hospital.
- The promotion being offered to ABC is that if the hospital purchases 80 boxes of Trifexis, they will receive a 3% discount and delayed billing of 90 days.
- During 2012, 700 boxes of Trifexis were sold and the clinic was open 319 days.
  - Average daily use: 700 ÷ 319 = 2 boxes per day
  - Number of working days in billing period = 66 (90 days available to pay, but the practice is not open on weekends to sell product, therefore, the practice is only open 66 days)

    2 (avg. daily use) × 66 (working days) × 1.03 (percent increase in growth) = 136

It would make sense to purchase 136 boxes of Trifexis, to receive a 3% discount. The previous equation shows us we will sell the product before the payment is due.

Example B:
- Tampa Veterinary Hospital has sold Heartgard Plus (HGP) for the last 15 years. Sales on the product have remained steady in 2012.
- The promotion being offered to Tampa Veterinary Hospital is that if the hospital purchases 120 boxes of HGP, they will receive a 6% discount and delayed billing of 120 days.
- During 2012, 1020 boxes of HGP were sold and the hospital was open 365 days.
  - Average daily use: 1020 ÷ 365 = 3 boxes per day
  - Number of working days in billing period = 120 days

    3 (average daily use) × 120 (working days) = 360

It would make sense to purchase 360 boxes of HGP, to receive a 6% discount, even though the practice did not see growth in 2012. The previous equation shows the practice will sell the product before the payment is due.

Example C:
- All About Pets has sold Interceptor for several years, but sales on the product have decreased (3%), because more clients are switching to another product.
- The promotion being offered to All About Pets is that if the hospital purchases 80 boxes of Interceptor, they will receive a 3% discount and delayed billing of 90 days.
- During 2012, 280 boxes of Interceptor were sold and the clinic was open 269 days.
  - Average daily use: 280 ÷ 269 = 1 box per day
  - Number of working days in billing period = 66 (90 days available to pay, but the practice is not open

on weekends to sell product; therefore the practice is only open 66 days)

1 (average daily use) × 66 (working days) = 66

1 × 66 × 3% = 2 (Decrease in sales)

66 − 2 = 64 boxes would be the maximum order

It would not be effective for the hospital to purchase this bulk order.

Developing Effective Inventory Pricing Strategies

Break-Even Analysis

- *Unit cost + Hard cost + Soft cost + (Profit × SP) = Sales price*

  Recall : Unit cost = Original cost of product

  Hard cost = DVM production

  Soft costs = Holding and ordering costs

  Profit = In order to obtain profit once minimal costs have been covered, we take the profit % × the total of the unit cost, hard cost and soft costs

  SP = Sales price

 Veterinary practice managers conduct fee analysis and monitor and update fee schedules.

Example A:
- Rimadyl 25 mg #60: $28.59 (unit cost)
- DVMs are paid on production 15% (hard cost)
- Holding and ordering costs average 25% (soft costs)
- The practice has determined a 20% profit is necessary

$$\$28.59 \times 0.15 = \$4.29 \text{ (hard cost)}$$
$$\$28.59 \times 0.25 = \$7.15 \text{ (soft cost)}$$
$$SP \times 0.20 = \text{(profit)}$$
$$\$28.59 + \$4.29 + \$7.15 + (0.20SP) = \text{Sales price}$$
$$\$40.03 + 0.20SP = SP$$
$$\$40.03 = SP - 0.20SP$$
$$\$40.03 = 0.80SP$$
$$\frac{\$40.03}{0.80} = SP$$
$$\$50.03 = SP$$

Rimadyl must be sold at $50.03 in order to break even and obtain a 20% profit.

Example B:
- Cosequin - $18.29 (unit cost)
- DVMs are not paid on production
- Holding and ordering costs average 20% (soft costs)
- The practice has determined a 15% profit is necessary

$$\$18.29 \times 0.20 = \$3.66 \text{ (soft cost)}$$
$$SP \times 0.15 = \text{profit}$$
$$\$21.95 + (0.15SP) = \text{Sales Price}$$

$$\$21.95 = SP - 0.15SP$$
$$\$21.95 = 0.85SP$$
$$\frac{\$21.95}{0.85} = SP$$
$$\$25.82 = SP$$

Cosequin must be sold at $25.82 in order to break even and obtain a 15% profit.

Markup

Markup is a percentage added to the cost of the unit when determining the selling price. Markup percentages can be based on the number of inventory turns or a product category. Products with a higher turnover rate (10× to 12×) have a lower markup (140% to 175%); those with lower turnover rates (4× to 6×) have higher markups (200% to 275%) in order to account for the potential expiration of product.

Example A:
- Rimadyl 25 mg #60: $28.59 (Unit cost)
- *This product is competitively priced and is a high turnover item; therefore, markup is determined to be 100%.*

$$\$28.59 \times 1 = \$28.59$$
$$\$28.59 + \$28.59 = \$57.18$$

Sell price of this item is $57.18

Example B:
- Dasequin: $18.29 (Unit cost)
- *This product has a high turnover rate; therefore markup is determined to be 150%.*

$$\$18.29 \times 1.5 = \$27.44$$
$$\$18.29 + \$27.44 = \$45.73$$

Sell price of this item is $45.73.

Dispensing Fees

Dispensing fees are added after the markup has been determined. Dispensing fees cover the veterinary technician's time to count the medication, the vial to package the medication, prescription label, and label printer wear and tear. Average dispensing fees are $7.00 to $9.00.

Labeling Fees

Labeling fees are applied to products that are sold in the original container, and a team member does not have to count the medication. This fee covers the veterinary technicians' time to prepare the product, prescription label, and label printer wear and tear. The average labeling fee is 25% to 30% of the dispensing fee.

Injection Fees

Injections are priced differently than capsules or tablets. Injections are priced both as an inventory item and as a service item, because a skilled professional must give the injection. Injection fees will have the same product mark up the

practice has created for tablets or capsules, with a service fee for the injection. Injection fees range from $12.00 to $28.00.

Putting it All Together: Break-Even Analysis, Markup, Dispensing, Labeling, and Injection Fees

Practice Sets

For the following examples, determine the break even analysis, markup, dispensing, labeling or injection fees.

Answers appear on the Evolve site accompanying this text.

1. Determine the minimum analysis and client cost based on the markup and labeling fees.
- Dermazole Shampoo: Unit cost: $10.50
- DVM production: 15%
- Ordering cost: 15%
- Holding cost: 15%
- Desired profit: 20%
- Desired markup: 200%
- Desired labeling fee: $5.95
2. Determine the minimum analysis and the client cost based on markup and dispensing fees.
- XYZ Pet Vitamin: Unit: $3.06 per tablet
- DVM production: none
- Ordering cost: 10%
- Holding cost: 15%
- Desired profit: 20%
- Desired markup: 200%
- Desired dispensing fee: $11.95
3. Determine the minimum analysis and the client cost based on markup and injection fees.
- Salix Injectable; Unit cost: $1.23/ml
- DVM production: 20%
- Ordering cost: 15%
- Holding cost: 10%
- Desired profit: 30%
- Desired markup: 300%
- Desired injection fee: $16.95
4. Determine the client cost based on the following information.
- Product cost: $0.72 per tablet
- 200% markup
- 15 tablets dispensed
- Dispensing fee of $11.95
- Minimum prescription fee of $14.95

Developing an Effective Service Markup

Covered in Chapter 20.

(Fixed costs/minute + staff costs/minute) × (length of procedure in staff minutes)
+ (DVM costs/minute) × (length of procedure in DVM minutes)
+ (Direct costs × 2)
+ Profit

Recall:
- **Fixed costs per minute** are determined from the profit and loss statement (administrative and facility costs)

along with the number of billable minutes the hospital is open. Fixed costs are often referred to as overhead expenses.
- **Staff costs per minute** are determined by calculating all costs associated with paying all staff members. This number is then divided by the billable minutes the practice is open.
- **DVM costs per minute** are also determined from the profit and loss statement.
- **Direct costs** take into consideration of supplies used to produce the service, multiplied by 2 (covers soft costs associated with inventory items).
- **Profit!** Yes, a profit must be produced on services!

Calculating the number of billable minutes a practice is open:

The hospital is open from 8 AM to 8 PM and does not close for lunch; therefore it is available to produce services for 720 minutes per day (12 hours × 60 minutes per hour). That same practice is open Monday through Saturday (same hours every day). Therefore it is available to produce services for 4320 minutes per week (720 minutes × 6 days per week), which equals 17,280 minutes per month (4320 minutes per week × 4 weeks per month). A full month of billable minutes is used in this equation, because the fixed costs are calculated on a monthly basis (rather than a daily basis).

Example A:
- Service: Schirmer Tear Test
- Fixed costs per month: $28,615.27 (determined from Profit and Loss Sheet)
- Staff costs per month: $12,515.34 (determined from Profit and Loss Sheet)
- DVM costs per month: $24,446.10 (determined from Profit and Loss Sheet)
- Number of billable minutes the hospital is open to provided services: 17,280
- Direct costs associated with inventory: $3.54 (test, gauze, saline, syringes used to hold saline, exam gloves)
- Number of minutes a technician uses to complete the procedure: 10
- Number of minutes a DVM uses to complete a procedure: 10
- Expected profit: 20%

Fixed costs per minute: $28,615.27 ÷ 17,280 = $1.66
Staff costs per minute: $12,515.34 ÷ 17,280 = $0.72
DVM costs per minute: $24,446.10 ÷ 17,280 = $1.41

Fixed costs per minute + Staff costs per minute × time

$$(\$1.66 + 0.72) \ (10 \text{ minutes}) = \$23.80$$

DVM costs per minute × time

$$\$1.41 \times 10 = \$14.10$$

Direct costs: $3.54 × 2 = $7.08

Profit: 20%

$$\$23.80 + \$14.10 + \$7.08 = \$44.98$$
$$\$44.98 \times 0.20 = \$9.00$$
$$\$44.98 + \$9.00 = \$53.98$$

This client must be charged $53.98 for this service.

Example B:
- Service: Local mass removal
- Fixed costs per month: $18,666.27 (determined from Profit and Loss Sheet
- Staff costs per month: $9333.34 (determined from Profit and Loss Sheet)
- DVM costs per month: $7466.67 (determined from Profit and Loss Sheet)
- Number of billable minutes the hospital is open to provided services: 12,480
- Direct costs associated with inventory: $14.54 (lidocaine, syringe used to hold lidocaine, surgery gloves, surgical prep materials, suture material)
- Number of minutes a technician uses to complete the procedure: 15
- Number of minutes a DVM uses to complete a procedure: 5
- Expected profit: 35%

Fixed costs per minute: $18,666,27 ÷ 12,480 = $1.50
Staff costs per minute: $9333.34 ÷ 12,480 = $0.75
DVM costs per minute: $7466.67 ÷ 12.480 = $0.60

Fixed costs per minute + staff costs per minute × time

$$(\$1.50 + 0.75) \times (15 \text{ minutes}) = \$33.75$$

DVM costs per minute × time

$$\$0.60 \times 5 = 3.00$$

Direct costs: $14.54 × 2 = $29.08
Profit: 50%

$$\$33.75 + \$3.00 + \$29.08 = \$65.83$$
$$\$65.83 \times 0.50 = \$32.92$$
$$\$65.83 + \$32.92 = \$98.75$$

This client must be charged $98.75 for this service.

Example C:
- Service: Skin Scrape
- Fixed costs per month: $32,806.12 (determined from Profit and Loss Sheet)
- Staff costs per month: $19,750.32 (determined from Profit and Loss Sheet)
- DVM costs per month: $26,789.75 (determined from Profit and Loss Sheet)
- Number of billable minutes the hospital is open to provided services: 20,160
- Direct costs associated with inventory: $0.20 (blade, microscope slide, mineral oil)
- Number of minutes a technician uses to complete the procedure: 5

- Number of minutes a DVM uses to complete a procedure: 3
- Expected profit: 50%

Fixed costs per minute: $32,806.12 ÷ 20,160 = $1.63
Staff costs per minute: $19,750.32 ÷ 20,160 = $0.98
DVM costs per minute: $26,789.75 ÷ 20,160 = $1.33

Fixed costs per minute + staff costs per minute × time

$$(\$1.63 + 0.98) \times (5 \text{ minutes}) = \$13.05$$

DVM costs per minute × time

$$\$1.33 \times 3 = \$3.99$$

Direct costs: $0.20 × 2 = $0.40
Profit: 50%

$$\$13.05 + \$3.99 + \$0.40 = \$17.44$$
$$\$17.44 \times 0.50 = \$8.72$$
$$\$17.44 + \$8.72 = \$26.16$$

This client must be charged $26.16 for this service.

Practice Sets: Developing an Effective Service Markup

For the following practice sets, use the following data, and determine the clients cost of the service listed. Answers appear on the Evolve site accompanying this text.
- Fixed costs per month: $25,920.34
- Staff costs per month: $24,300
- DVM costs per month: $40,500.12
- Number of billable minutes the hospital is open to provided services: 13,800
1. Service: Fine needle aspirate
- Direct costs associated with inventory: $1.23
- Number of minutes a technician uses to complete the procedure: 10
- Number of minutes a DVM uses to complete a procedure: 2
- Expected profit: 30%
2. Service: Clip and clean wound
- Direct costs associated with inventory: $3.54
- Number of minutes a technician uses to complete the procedure: 7
- Number of minutes a DVM uses to complete a procedure: 0
- Expected profit: 50%
3. Service: Corneal stain
- Direct costs associated with inventory: $2.15
- Number of minutes a technician uses to complete the procedure: 5
- Number of minutes a DVM uses to complete a procedure: 5
- Expected profit: 20%
4. Service: Anal gland expression
- Direct costs associated with inventory: $0.20
- Number of minutes a technician uses to complete the procedure: 3
- Number of minutes a DVM uses to complete a procedure: 0
- Expected profit: 20%

Payroll Calculations

Covered in Chapter 20.

 Veterinary practice managers manage payroll.

Example A:

Salary formula: Team member is paid by salary only.
- A veterinarian receives $60,000 in salary per year
- Payday occurs on the 1st and the 15th of each month

$$\$60,000 \div 24 = \$2500 \text{ gross pay per pay period}$$

The definition of gross pay is the total amount earned before taxes or other withholdings.

Example B:

Pro-sal formula: A combination of salary and production-based pay.
- A veterinarian is paid $60,000 base salary per year
- 10% production bonus once production has reached $10,000 per month
- Bonuses are paid monthly for the previous month's production
- Payday occurs on the first and the fifteenth of each month (24 pay periods per year)

$$\text{Salary pay: } \$60,000 \div 24 = \$2500 \text{ per check}$$

- The veterinarian produced $33,000 for the previous month

$$\$33,000 \times 10\% = \$3300$$
$$\$3300 - \$2500 = \$800$$

- The gross pay for the first is $800 + $2500 = $3300.
- The gross pay for the fifteenth is $2500.

Example C:

Production-based pay: An associate is paid by production only.
- A veterinarian is paid 20% production of all services and products.
- Payday occurs on the first and the fifteenth of each month.

The payroll manager should pull a report of production of that specific associate from the 1st to the 14th of the month.
- $15,000 was produced from March 1, 2014, to March 14, 2014.

$$\$15,000 \times 20\% = \$3000 \text{ gross pay}$$

The second pay period report runs from the 15th to the 30th or 31st of the month.
- $16,236 was produced from March 15, 2014, to March 31, 2014.

$$\$16,236 \times 20\% = \$3247.20 \text{ gross pay}$$

Example D:

Hourly-based pay: Employees are paid by the hour at a regular rate for the first 40 hours; anything over 40 hours is paid overtime.
  Regular rate calculations:
- Wanda is paid $10 per hour and works 34 hours per week.
- Payroll is paid every other Monday; therefore the workweek is Monday, 12 AM, through Sunday, 12:59 PM.

$$34 \text{ hours per week} \times 2 = 68 \text{ hours per 2-week period}$$
$$68 \text{ hours} \times \$10 = \$680 \text{ gross pay}$$

Example E:

Overtime rate calculations:
- Ann has worked 44 hours during week 1.
- She has worked 32 hours during week 2.
- She is paid $10 per hour.
- Overtime is paid at $15 (1½ times the regular rate).

$$\text{Week 1: } 40 \text{ hours} \times \$10 = \$400 \,;\; 4 \text{ hours} \times \$15 = \$60$$
$$\text{Week 2: } 32 \text{ hours} \times \$10 = \$320$$
$$\$400 + \$60 + \$320 = \$780 \text{ gross pay}$$

Example F:

- Alex accrues 44 hours in week 1.
- He accrues 52 hours during week 2.

$$\text{Week 1: } 40 \text{ hours} \times \$10 = \$400, \; 4 \text{ hours} \times \$15 = \$60$$
$$\text{Week 2: } 40 \text{ hours} \times \$10 = \$400, \; 12 \text{ hours} \times \$15 = \$180$$
$$\$400 + \$60 + \$400 + \$180 = \$1040 \text{ gross pay}$$

Practice Set: Determining Gross Pay per 2-Week Pay Period

Answers appear on the Evolve site accompanying this text.
1. Team member 1: $10 per hour; 12 hours in week 1; 52 hours in week 2
2. Veterinarian paid by production only, 35%: gross revenue 1st through 14th: $12,300.23; gross revenue fifteenth through thirtieth: $16,345.09
3. Team member 2: $15 per hour; 40 hours in week 1; 40 hours in week 2
4. Associate veterinarian paid salary only; $95,000 per year
5. Team member 3: $11.37 per hour; 52 hours in week 1; 41 hours in week 2
6. Veterinarian paid pro-sal: $50,000 base salary; 13% production bonus once production has reached $10,000 per month; bonus paid 1st of the month for the previous month's production. Production total: $26,524.67

Drug Calculations

Every team member should be able to easily calculate drug doses because double-checking dispensed drugs can prevent a potential fatal error (Boxes 24-1 and 24-2).

BOX 24-1 | Common Conversions

1 kg = 1000 g = 10,000 mg
1 kg = 2.2 lb
- kg to lb: multiply by 2.2
- lb to kg: divide by 2.2
1 g = 1000 mg = 0.001 kg
1 grain = 64.8 mg
1 lb = 0.454 kg = 16 oz
1 lb = 454 g
1 mg = 0.001 g = 1000 mcg
1 L = 1000 mL = 10 dL
- L to mL: multiply by 1000
- mL to L: divide by 1000
1 mL = 1 cc = 1000 mcL
1 mL = 15 gtt
1 T = 3 t
1 t = 5 mL
1 T = 15 mL
1 oz = 30 mL
1 gal = 3.786 L
1 gal = 4 qt = 8 pt = 128 fl oz
1 pt = 2 c = 16 oz = 473 mL
1 km = 1000 m
1 m = 100 cm = 1000 mm

c, Cup; *cc*, cubic centimeter; *cm*, centimeter; *dL*, deciliter; *fl oz*, fluid ounce; *g*, gram; *gal*, gallon; *gtt*, drop; *kg*, kilogram; *L*, liter; *lb*, pound; *m*, meter; *mcg*, microgram; *mcL*, microliter; *mg*, milligram; *mL*, milliliter; *mm*, millimeter; *oz*, ounce; *pt*, pint; *qt*, quart; *T*, tablespoon; *t*, teaspoon.

Explanation #1

Step 1

Convert the body weight in pounds (lb) to kilograms (kg). In the United States, the most common weight measurement is pounds. Medication doses are recommended in milligrams per kilogram (mg/kg). There is 1 kg per 2.2 lb; therefore the number of pounds the patient weighs divided by 2.2 will yield the kilograms of body weight.

Step 2

Calculate the drug dose. The recommended dose is generally given in milligrams per kilogram. Therefore if 22 mg of a drug is recommended for each kilogram of body weight, 22 mg multiplied by the body weight will give the total number of milligrams needed for the patient.

Step 3

Calculate the volume of drug needed per dose. The concentration of the product is generally given as 22 mg per tablet, or 25 mg per milliliter, and so forth. If the patient needs 22 mg, then one 22-mg tablet will be needed to treat the patient per dose. If the patient needs 11 mg, then the concentration supplied divided by the amount needed will yield the volume to give the patient. In this example, if the patient needs 11 mg and a 22-mg tablet is supplied, then half a tablet will be administered.

Step 4

Determine the total amount of product needed to dispense for the client. If the patient needs half a tablet twice daily for 7 days, then multiply ½ by 2; this yields 1 tablet per

BOX 24-2 | Examples of Drug Calculations

What volume of a drug solution should be given to a 25-lb dog if the advised dose is 5 mg/kg and the concentration of the solution is 50 mg/mL?

Step 1. Convert pounds to kilograms:

$$2.5\ lb \div 2.2 = 11.36\ kg$$

Step 2. Calculate the drug dose:

$$X\ mg = \frac{5\ mg}{kg} \times 11.36\ kg = 5\ mg \times 11.36 = 56.8\ mg$$

Step 3. Calculate the volume of solution needed:

$$\frac{50\ mg}{mL} = \frac{56.8\ mg}{X\ mL} = \frac{56.8\ mg}{50\ mg/mL} = 1.1\ mL$$

What volume of a drug solution should be given to a 7.9-lb cat if the advised dosage is 10 mg/kg and the concentration of the solution is 5 mg/mL?

Step 1. 7.9 lb ÷ 2.2 = 3.59 kg

Step 2.

$$X\ mg = \frac{10\ mg}{kg} \times 3.59\ kg = 10 \times 3.59\ kg = 35.9\ mg$$

Step 3. $\frac{5\ mg}{mL} = \frac{35.9\ mg}{X mL} = \frac{35.9\ mg}{5\ mg/mL} = 7\ mL$

How many 25-mg tablets should be dispensed for a 10-lb cat if the recommended dose is 5 mg/lb twice daily for 7 days?

Step 1. 10 lb × 5 mg = 50 mg/dose
Step 2. 50 mg ÷ 25 mg = 2 tablets/dose
Step 3. 2 tablets twice daily = 4 tablets/day
Step 4. 4 tablets/day × 7 days = 28 tablets

How many 500-mg capsules should be dispensed for a dog that weighs 55 lb and needs 20 mg/kg every 8 hours for 14 days?

Step 1. 55 lb ÷ 2.2 = 25 kg
Step 2. 25 kg × 20 mg/kg = 500 mg
Step 3. 1 capsule every 8 hours = 3 capsules/day
Step 4. 3 capsules/day × 14 days = 42 capsules total

day. One tablet per day × 7 days yields 7 tablets. Seven tablets must be dispensed to this client for treatment of the patient.

Explanation #2

$$\frac{Dose\ (D) \times Weight\ (W)}{Availabe\ concentration\ (C)}$$

D is the dose of the drug as recommended by the manufacturer, usually written in milligrams per pound or kilogram. The dose for a particular drug may vary by species or treatment. For instance, Torbugesic has one dose if used for pain and another if used for coughing.

W is the weight of the animal being treated; this value can be in pounds or kilograms.

D × ***W*** is the desired dose (how much drug should be given to the patient per dose).

C is the concentration of the available drug to be administered, usually written on the label in milligrams per milliliter for liquids or milligrams for tablets and capsules. Drugs may come in multiple concentrations. For instance, amoxicillin is supplied as 50-mg tablets, 100-mg tablets, and 50-mg/mL oral suspension.

(D × W)÷C therefore represents how much of the available medication to give.

Example A:

A pet needs 320 mg (desired dose) of a drug with a concentration of 50 mg/mL (available). How many milliliters should be administered?

$$320 \text{ mg} \div 50 \text{ mg per mL} = 6.4 \text{ mL}$$

Example B:

A pet needs 114 mg (desired dose) of a drug with a concentration of 100 mg/tablet (available). How many tablets should be given?

$$114 \text{ mg} \div 100\text{-mg tablet} = 1.14 \text{ tablets}$$

Because 1.14 of a tablet cannot be given, a team member would give one 100-mg tablet.

Percentage Solutions

Some injectable solution concentrations are written as a percentage instead of milligrams per milliliter. Atropine, for example, is a 2% solution. Therefore the solution in question contains 2 g of atropine for every 100 mL of solution. Because drugs are not typically administered in grams per 100 mL, this amount must be converted to something more familiar. First, it should be determined how many grams are in 1 mL. To accomplish this, divide 2 g by 100 mL to get 0.02 g/mL. In general, doses are given in milligrams per milliliter rather than grams per milliliter; therefore the next step is to convert 0.02 g to milligrams by multiplying by 1000 mg/g to get 20 mg. Therefore 2% = 20 mg/mL.

Shortcut: Unless you like doing all these calculations, you can simply multiply the percentage by 10 and change the units to milligrams per milliliter.

Example C:

- 3% solution = 3 × 10 = 30 mg/mL
- 0.2% solution = 0.2 × 10 = 2 mg/mL
- 1.5% solution = 1.5 × 10 = 15 mg/mL
  Now, put it all together:
- How many milliliters would be required for 274 mg of a 0.75% solution?

$$0.75\% = 7.5 \text{ mg/mL}$$

274 mg (desired dose) ÷ 7.5 mg/mL (available concentration) = 36.5 mL

- How many milliliters would be required for 485 mg of a 4% solution?

$$4\% = 40 \text{ mg/mL}$$

485 mg (desired dose) ÷ 40 mg/mL (available concentration) = 12.1 mL

To determine how many milligrams are in the number of milliliter of a solution that was administered:

$$\% \text{ Solution (in mg/mL)} \times \text{mL} = \text{mg}$$

Example D:

- How many milligrams were administered if 3.5 mL of a 1% solution were given?

$$1\% = 10 \text{ mg/mL} \times 3.5 \text{ mL} = 35 \text{ mg}$$

- How many milligrams were administered if 4.3 mL of a 10% solution were given?

$$10\% = 100 \text{ mg/mL} \times 4.3 \text{ mL} = 430 \text{ mg}$$

Practice Set: Drug Calculations

Answers appear on the Evolve site accompanying this text.
1. A pet needs 50 mg of a tablet, and the medication is available as a 100-mg tablet. How many tablets will be needed?
2. A pet needs 35 mg of a solution, and the medication is available as a 100-mg/mL solution. How many milliliters will be needed?
3. A pet needs medication at a dose of 5 mg/kg, and the medication is available in 25-mg tablets. The pet weighs 10 lb. How many tablets will be administered?
4. A pet needs a medication at a dose of 100 mg/kg, and the medication is available in a 100-mg/mL solution. The pet weighs 25 lb. How many milliliters will be administered?
5. A pet needs 25 mg of a 2% solution. How many milliliters will be administered?
6. A pet needs butorphanol for pain at a dose of 0.04 mg/kg, and the medication is available in a 10-mg/mL solution. The pet weighs 4 lb. How many milliliters will be administered?
7. A veterinarian writes a script for 25 mg of acepromazine to be given every 8 hours for 5 days, and the medication is available in 25-mg tablets. How many tablets will be dispensed?
8. Translate the following prescription so that a client would be able to understand it: Give 25 mg Benadryl PO TID × 2 weeks. Benadryl is available as 25-mg capsules. How many capsules would be dispensed?
9. A pet needs 5 mg/kg of Albon PO SID on day 1, then 2.5 mg/kg PO SID for 5 more days. The medication is available in 125-mg tablets and the pet weighs 25 lb. How many milligrams will the pet need? How many tablets will be dispensed for the owner?

Teaspoons and Tablespoons

Many over-the-counter products are labeled in teaspoons (t or tsp) and tablespoons (T or tbsp); the team must be able to give the client correct conversions.
- 1 t = 5 mL
- 1 T = 15 mL

BOX 24-3 | Examples of IV Fluid Calculations

Drip Sets
- 15 gtt/mL for patients >20 lb
- 60 gtt/mL for patients <20 lb

Fluid Rates (Can Vary Based on Patient Condition and Doctor Recommendation)
- Surgical rate: 11 mL/kg/hr
- Maintenance rate: 66 mL/kg/24 hr
- Twice (doubled) maintenance rate: 132 mL/kg/24 hr

Steps
1. Convert pounds to kilograms (2.2 lb/kg)
2. Calculate milliliters per hour
3. Calculate drops per minute

Example 1
- 45-lb dog, 15 gtt/mL drip set
- Maintenance rate = 66 mL/kg/24 hr
1. 45 lb ÷ 2.2 = 20.45 kg
2. 20.45 kg × 66 mL/kg/24 hr = 20.45 kg × 66 mL/kg = 1350 mL/24 hr

3. 1350 mL/24 hr = 56.25 mL/hr
4. Place on IV pump; if no pump is present, continue:
5. 56.25 mL/hr = 56.25 mL ÷ 60 min = 0.9375 mL/min
6. 0.9375 mL/min = 0.9375 mL ÷ 60 sec = 0.015 mL/sec
7. 0.015 mL/sec × 15 gtt/mL (drip set) = 0.156 mL × 15 gtt/mL = 0.234 mL/sec
8. 0.234 mL/1 gtt = Reciprocate = 1 ÷ 0.234 mL = 1 gtt/4 sec

Example 2
- 25-lb dog, 15 gtt/mL drip set
- Surgical rate = 11 mL/kg/hr
1. 25 lb ÷ 2.2 = 11.36 kg
2. 11.36 kg × 11 mL/kg/hr = 11.36 kg × 11 mL = 125 mL/hr
3. Place on IV pump
4. 125 mL/hr = 125 mL ÷ 60 min = 2.08 mL/min
5. 2.08 mL/min = 2.08 mL ÷ 60 sec = 0.035 mL/sec
6. 0.035 mL/sec × 15 gtt/mL (drip set) = 0.035 mL × 15 gtt/mL = 0.52 mL/sec
7. 0.52 mL/sec = Reciprocate = 1 ÷ 0.52 = 1 gtt/2 sec

Therefore if the label states that the concentration is 25 mg/t, then the product contains 25 mg/5 mL, or 5 mg/mL. If the label states that the product has 25 mg/T, then the product contains 25 mg/15 mL, or 1.67 mg/mL. Once the correct milligrams per kilogram has been verified with the veterinarian, the team can determine the number of milliliters to be administered.

Intravenous Fluid Calculations

Patients on intravenous (IV) fluids must be monitored throughout administration to ensure they are receiving the correct amount. Too much fluid could drown a patient; too little fluid might prevent the patient from improving.

Fluid administration sets are available in two sizes for small animals. Also called *drip sets,* these sets help control the amount of fluids delivered to the patient. A macrodrip is a 15 gtt/mL (drops per milliliter) drip set; a microdrip is a 60 gtt/mL drip set.

Fluids are administered at a rate determined by the veterinarian, which can depend on the patient's fluid loss (Box 24-3). Basic rates are as follows:
- Surgical rate: 11 mL/kg/hr
- Maintenance rate: 66 mL/kg/24 hr
- Two times maintenance rate: 132 mL/kg/24 hr

Practice Set: Intravenous Fluids

Answers appear on the Evolve site accompanying this text.
1. A 22-lb dog needs IV fluids at a maintenance rate. How many milliliters per hour will the patient receive?

2. A 7-lb cat will have a dental procedure and needs IV fluids at the surgical rate. How many milliliters per hour will the patient receive?
3. A 120-lb dog is experiencing vomiting and diarrhea and must have IV fluids at two times maintenance. How many milliliters will he receive per hour?
4. A 32-lb dog needs IV fluids at a surgical rate. How many milliliters per hour will the patient receive?
5. A 50-lb dog needs IV fluids at two times maintenance. How much fluid will the patient receive?
6. A 4.5-lb cat requires maintenance fluids. How many milliliters per hour will be administered in a 24-hour period?

Acknowledgments

I would like to thank Laurie Rankin for her invaluable advice regarding the explanations for drug calculations and conversions in this chapter.

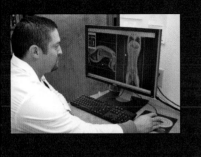

16 Personality Factors
Campbell Interest and
  Skill Survey
Career Planning
Cover Letter
Myers-Briggs Type
  Indicator
Personal Skills
Resume
Transferable Skills

Professional Development

OUTLINE

Self-Assessment, 447
  Myers-Briggs Type Indicator, 447
  Campbell Interest and Skill Survey, 447
  16 Personality Factors, 447
  Transferable Skills, 447
  Personal Skills, 447
Marketing Skills, 449
Employment Opportunities, 450

Preparing Employment Data, 451
  Cover Letter, 451
  Resume, 451
  Email and Internet Resumes, 453
Preparing for an Interview, 453
Follow-Up After the Interview, 455
Receiving Offers of Employment, 456
Retirement, 456

LEARNING OBJECTIVES

When you have completed this chapter, you should be able to:

1. Identify the importance of professional development.
2. Identify skills that one possesses.
3. Discuss career fields that are available.
4. Explain how to develop an effective cover letter.
5. Explain how to develop an effective resume.
6. Discuss how to email cover letters and resumes.
7. List methods used to prepare for an interview.
8. List questions to ask a potential employer.
9. Discuss how to follow-up after an interview.
10. Differentiate offers of employment.
11. Discuss retirement savings.

Professional development is vital to every career. There are many aspects of career and professional development, and all are vital to an individual's success. The successful development of an individual can lead to the development of a successful team. Individuals must first assess themselves and determine their strengths and weaknesses; they can then work on the weaknesses while striving to improve the strengths. They must determine what successes they want in life, define what success is, and set professional and personal goals. Professional and motivated individuals will seek out experiences to improve themselves as well as opportunities to improve others.

On average, individuals will change jobs every 3.6 years and change careers three times before retiring. Training and development in areas other than veterinary medicine are essential. Training in leadership, management, creativity, diversity, communications, and analytical skills will help even the most experienced individual. Many individuals change careers to veterinary medicine after being in another field for years, and the skills and knowledge they bring from other professions is essential for practice development. Each team member may possess a set of skills another does not; therefore everyone can benefit from one other.

Career planning is often intertwined with individual plans, goals, and successes. Career planning is the ongoing process of making career choices; these choices should be reviewed from time to time. Individuals may need to analyze themselves, their environment, and their occupation to determine if and when a change is needed. Goals can change as individuals mature, and enter different stages of life. For example, a young lady who marries and has children will have different goals once the kids are born, compared to when she entered college. As the kids grow, goals and career planning can change again.

When changes are needed, it is often overwhelming to start the process of looking for new employment. Self-confidence may falter, and suddenly the skills that once seemed so strong now seem useless. It is common to feel this way, but fortunately it is easy to turn that mind-set around. The skills that one has acquired over the years are essential for survival. Skills such as interpersonal and verbal communication, critical thinking, writing, and leadership are all valuable resources for any employer. In addition to these essential skills, self-discipline, excellent morals, outstanding ethics, and creativity are skills that should be reflected on to help rebuild confidence.

Self-Assessment

Knowledge of oneself can enhance personal strengths while helping become aware of unknown weaknesses, tolerances, or risks (Figure 25-1). Personalities, styles, and accomplishments will help guide personal assessment. The Myers-Briggs Type Indicator, Campbell Interest and Skill Survey, 16 Personality Factors, and transferable skills assessments are just a few self-evaluation tests.

PRACTICE POINT Self-assessment tests help individuals determine their strengths and weaknesses, which will help guide them in choosing a career.

Myers-Briggs Type Indicator

The Myers-Briggs Type Indicator (MBTI) is widely applied in the career development field to help individuals make more informed career decisions. This is an assessment of individual preferences, not a test of right or wrong answers. The goal of the MBTI in career planning is to assist an individual in gaining and understanding personal preferences and to use that information to explore various careers that will be supportive, challenging, and interesting.

Campbell Interest and Skill Survey

The Campbell Interest and Skill Survey (CISS) measures self-reported vocational interests and skills. Similar to traditional interest inventories, the CISS scales reflect an individual's attraction for specific occupational areas. However, the CISS instrument goes beyond traditional inventories by adding parallel skill scales that provide estimates of an individual's confidence in his or her ability to perform various occupational activities. Together, the two types of scales provide more comprehensive, richer data than interest scores alone. The CISS instrument focuses on careers that require postsecondary education and is most appropriate for use with individuals who are college bound or college educated.

16 Personality Factors

Since its introduction more than 40 years ago, the 16 Personality Factors (16PF) instrument has been widely used for a variety of applications, providing support for vocational guidance, hiring, and promotion recommendations.

Transferable Skills

Transferable skills are the skills that have been gathered through various jobs, volunteer work, hobbies, sports, or other life experiences that can be used in the next job or new career. In addition to being useful to career changes, transferable skills are also important to those who are facing a layoff, new graduates looking for their first jobs, and those re-entering the workforce after an extended absence.

Personal Skills

Team players seem to excel more in general and also more quickly than those who choose to work as individuals. This does not mean that people must depend on a team to succeed, but it shows that they have been successful in adjusting to a team environment as well as sharing and delegating responsibilities effectively.

Positive attitudes are contagious, and those with positive attitudes excel faster than those with negative attitudes. People prefer to be around happy, energetic, and enthusiastic individuals; they tend to be creative problem solvers and contribute well to a team environment.

Self-Evaluation Form

Name _____ Position _____

Date of employment _____ Date of promotion(s) _____

How long in present position _____

Attendance Record:

Number of days absent this year: _____ Approved days: _____ Unapproved days: _____

Number of days absent last year: _____ Approved days: _____ Unapproved days: _____

Number of days late this year: _____ Number of days late last year: _____

Attendance is: _____ Excellent _____ Good _____ Poor

Work Performance:

Rate your job performance by circling the appropriate letter.

Quality of Work:

A. Consistently performs quality work; requires little supervision.

B. Work is neat and accurate; requires some supervision.

C. Quality of work is good; makes some mistakes.

D. Produces work that is passable; needs improvement.

E. Makes frequent errors.

Comments: _____

Quantity of Work:

A. Superior work production. Completes tasks ahead of schedule and completes more than required.

B. Good producer; meets task deadlines and completes more than required.

C. Volume of work is satisfactory.

D. Requires close supervision to complete tasks; needs improvement.

E. Very slow. Does not complete tasks on time.

Comments: _____

Job Knowledge:

A. Understands all aspects of veterinary medicine. Masters tasks and skills extremely well.

B. Has a good knowledge base and performs tasks well.

C. Understands most procedures, tasks, and skills.

D. Shows understanding of job but requires help and instruction.

E. Lacks sufficient understanding of tasks and performs duties ineffectively.

Comments: _____

Staff Relations:

A. Goes out of the way to cooperate and assist all team members. Works well with others.

B. Willing to provide assistance to most team members.

C. Cooperates and works with others.

D. Usually helpful; may occasionally exhibit poor assistance.

E. Poor attitude.

Comments: _____

FIGURE 25-1 A self-evaluation form helps identify strengths and weaknesses.

A strong work ethic is an excellent attribute to possess. A strong work ethic is defined as striving for the best and excelling at finding tasks to complete. These tasks are completed quickly and efficiently, with excellent and consistent results. A strong work ethic cannot be taught; it is a trait that one possesses. Team members exhibiting a good work ethic in theory (and ideally in practice) should be selected for better positions, more responsibility, and ultimately promotion. Team members who fail to exhibit a good work ethic may be regarded as failing to provide fair value for the wage the employer is paying them and should not be promoted or placed in positions of greater responsibility.

Patient and Client Relations:

A. Extremely good at client relations and education; excellent patient care.

B. Consistently good at client relations and education; good at patient care.

C. Deals effectively with clients and patients.

D. Attitude and behavior not consistent.

E. Frequently rude or blunt.

Comments: _____

List four essentials that you are doing well:

1. _____

2. _____

3. _____

4. _____

List four essentials that need improvement:

1. _____

2. _____

3. _____

4. _____

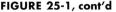

Signature _____ Date _____

FIGURE 25-1, cont'd

Education is essential for professional development. College courses enhance current skills, develop new skills, and teach independence. Continuing education is required of credentialed veterinary technicians, veterinarians, and certified veterinary practice managers to help them maintain the skills they have obtained as well as learn new techniques. Science, medicine, and laws continually change, and it is imperative to stay current with the new, up-and-coming trends and treatments.

Evaluating the surrounding environment may also be essential when evaluating oneself. Personal issues, family, health, and finances have a heavy impact on decisions to change or advance careers. For many, family comes first, and it is important for those who feel this way to find an occupation that agrees with and allows this philosophy. Health can be of concern for many, as employment positions with a high level of stress can cause increased blood pressure and a higher risk for heart attacks. Finances may be the highest of all concerns, especially in the veterinary community. Veterinarians and technicians are not paid very highly, which forces many out of the veterinary health care profession and into sales, marketing, or research.

Questions may be asked and researched every so often to determine if a career change or advancement is needed. Further questions can be asked of individuals in the field when examining the possibility of change (Box 25-1).

Individuals may re-evaluate the positions they currently hold. A manager may look to become certified by the Veterinary Hospital Managers Association. A technician may become specialized within a field such as internal medicine or emergency and critical care. A veterinarian

| **BOX 25-1** | Questions to Consider Before Applying for a New Job |

- Can this job change with the economy?
- Do I believe in the science the company produces and the products it develops?
- Do I have the ability to learn new topics, subjects, and fields?
- Does this job have a career track?
- How will a change benefit my family?
- If the job is in research or sales, does the company have excellent products?
- Is a change consistent with my values?
- What is my work style?
- What is the company's potential for growth?
- What traits do I have?
- What unique characteristics can I bring to this job?
- Will my family support a change?

may become board certified in a specialty. The possibilities are endless; it takes a motivated leader to find a niche that is a perfect fit.

Marketing Skills

All the previously mentioned skills help individuals market themselves as they look for employment. Team environments are going to look for a team-motivated individual to join their staff. Potential employers want a positive, smart, and motivated individual to join their team; confidence and

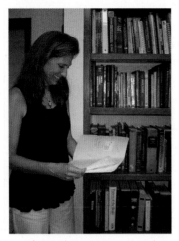

FIGURE 25-2 A professional appearance is a marketing tool that projects quality.

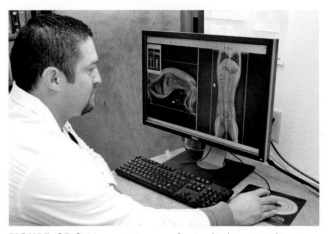

FIGURE 25-3 Many veterinary professionals choose teaching as a second career.

personality must be visible to the potential employer or a resume may be tossed aside.

Marketing starts with personal interactions within a profession or industry being investigated. Individuals must appear professional and confident as they explore employment opportunities (Figure 25-2). Many benign conversations can quickly change to an unscheduled interview once managers and representatives begin discussing employment opportunities.

Employment Opportunities

Team members must have personal goals as well as employment goals. It is important not to forget oneself and one's personal life, especially as dedicated and hardworking as many technicians are. They must make time for themselves; vacation, personal, or sick time, if awarded, should be used on a regular basis. It is imperative to take care of oneself to prevent burnout (see Chapter 6 for more information on stress and burnout).

> **PRACTICE POINT** Technicians can enjoy careers in general practice, specialty practices, sales, marketing, research, or management.

There are many different paths technicians can take in the field of veterinary medicine. Career opportunities include the many facets of clinical practice. General and specialty practice are very rewarding careers. General practice allows technicians to see a variety of animals, diseases, and treatments. Specialty practice limits the amount of diseases and species seen but allows specialization in specific areas such as internal medicine, surgery, dermatology, dentistry, or emergency and critical care.

Research and development can add challenges and rewards to any career by developing new products, foods, or treatments for a variety of species and diseases. Research has received negative attention in the past, and the media especially feels that research always involves harming animals. This is untrue and has been proven at excellent research facilities.

Veterinary manufacturers and distribution companies are always seeking the qualifications of credentialed and experienced technicians. Sales and marketing teams look for methods to target consumers, and technicians have the experience that these teams are looking for. Many companies require a bachelor's degree for employment; it is imperative to finish a bachelor's program in case a switch in careers is ever contemplated.

Management of a general or specialty practice takes time, patience, leadership, and independence. Technicians that have superseded expectations in practice are generally promoted to manage practices. While the technician portion is easy to manage, running an entire business is a whole new ballgame. Attending online courses and national conferences that focus on management (as well as learning from peers) will help the most inexperienced businessperson succeed.

Excellent technicians are also excellent educators. They have experience teaching clients as well as other team members about veterinary medicine. Those who take time to help others will find a very rewarding career in teaching. There is nothing more gratifying than seeing a student progress and become a distinguished individual in the veterinary profession; since they had an excellent teacher, they become an excellent teacher to others (Figure 25-3).

Many sources exist for locating employment opportunities. Large manufacturing companies post research and sales positions on their Web sites. Word of mouth is also a valuable resource; many representatives know when their company is or will be hiring. Veterinary practices may advertise locally, nationally, in schools, and at veterinary conferences. National publications such as the *Journal of Veterinary Medicine, Veterinary Economics,* and *Veterinary Practice News* list job announcements for all facets of veterinary medicine, including research, sales, and teaching opportunities.

WHAT WOULD YOU DO/NOT DO?

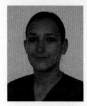

Julie has been a full time employee at ABC Veterinary Clinic for 5 years and has reached a plateau. She feels that her skills are not being used as much as they could, which has made her resent her position. She feels that it is time to look for another position at another practice. Upon submission of her resume to several other practices, one in particular has called for an interview. The interview seems to go well for both parties. The potential employer asks for a list of references, and asks permission to call her current employer. Julie is hesitant to give permission to call her current employer, as she feels he may be upset with her when she returns to the practice.

What Should Julie Do?

First, Julie may have discussed her dissatisfaction with the current employer before she decided to look for new employment. If Julie is a great employee, the current employer may simply need to make changes, using Julie's skills to her fullest potential. Should a change not occur, then the current employer has been made aware of Julie's dissatisfaction, and knows that she will be applying elsewhere.

Second, Julie should state to the potential employer that she prefer that the current employer be called as the last reference, as she feels the he will be extremely upset with her upon return to work, and she may suffer retribution as a result. It is important to be fair and honest with both individuals, preventing a shock from the current employer, while impressing the potential employer.

Preparing Employment Data

Many times, the only impression a potential employer can make about an applicant is from the cover letter and resume that are submitted. Care must be taken to develop a professional, error-free cover letter and resume conveying positive attributes and work ethic.

Cover Letter

Cover letters are an introduction of the applicant, without repeating information contained in the resume. Three basic goals should be achieved with a cover letter: create interest, describe abilities, and request an interview. Cover letters may be needed when a resume is sent to the human resources department or to someone who is not the decision maker. They may also be used when a type of action is required by either the reader or the applicant. For example, an applicant may notify the reader that a follow-up phone call will be made in a specified number of days.

PRACTICE POINT Prepare cover letters that are specific to the business in which you are applying; blanket cover letters are unacceptable.

A cover letter should be printed on the same type of paper the resume is printed on, with similar font type and size. Full contact information should be at the top of the page, similar to the resume, along with a date and the anticipated reader's name and address. If the applicant is unsure of the target reader's information, some research should be done to determine who it is; this adds a personal touch to the letter, identifying that the applicant has put extra effort into the cover letter.

A formal greeting is appropriate for the opening paragraph. A title such as Mr., Mrs., or Dr. should be used along with "Dear." Do not use "To whom it may concern," as this devalues the cover letter immediately. The first paragraph should let the reader know where the information was found to apply for the job; a newspaper article, a friend, or a co-worker can all be cited. The first paragraph should also stimulate interest about the candidate (Figure 25-4).

The second paragraph is the body of the letter. This section is used to promote and highlight the activities that qualify the applicant for the position. This may be the hardest paragraph to write, but it includes the most valuable information, information that may not be immediately visible on the resume. If the writer has difficulty writing this paragraph, a friend may be enlisted to state the positive attributes the candidate possesses. Those attributes can then be listed in this paragraph.

The final paragraph is an action paragraph; it states what the next step of either the applicant or the reader should be. If the applicant states that he or she will call and follow up, a specific date should be given. If the applicant is asking for an interview, a simple statement is appropriate, such as, "Please give me the opportunity to discuss my qualifications with you. My contact number is ____."

It is important to be proactive when searching for employment and it is essential to set one's resume apart from the rest. The applicant should call and follow up on the resume to ensure that it was received. If the target reader has not had a chance to review the resumes on file, the name of the applicant will be familiar once he or she does review the resumes, as the applicant's name has already been stated once, if not twice. If a call cannot be placed, an email or follow-up letter is appropriate. It is important not to be too aggressive, but it is imperative to be assertive and follow up.

The closing signature should be thoughtful: "Thank you for your time," or "Cordially," are appropriate, along with the applicant's name. Any degrees or titles should follow the name, along with the signature of the applicant.

Resume

A resume is a marketing tool that is tailored to the specific job the applicant has interest in. The goal of a resume is to be granted an interview; therefore as a general rule, resumes should be concise and limited to one or two pages in length. Abbreviations and acronyms should be avoided, and the font should be easy to read. Recommended fonts include Ariel, Times New Roman, or Tahoma and should not be smaller than 10 point or larger than 12 point size.

1000 Terrace View Apts.
Blackburg, VA 24060
987-654-3210
stevenmasonvt@fastwave.biz

Mr. John Wilson
Personnel Director
Anderson Veterinary Hospital
3507 Rockville Pike
Rockville, MD 20895

Dear Mr. Wilson:

I read in the most recent journal of Pet Product News of your need for an experienced veterinary technician in the Rockville area. I will be returning to the Rockville area immediately after graduation in May and believe I have the necessary credentials to fill your position.

I have worked at various veterinary hospitals prior to attending college. As you can see from my resume, I have also assisted graduate students with several research projects.

In addition to my practical experience, I will complete the requirements for my veterinary technician degree in May. As you know, Purdue is one of the leading universities in veterinary technology, specializing in business management. I am confident that my veterinary technician degree, along with years of experience, makes me an excellent candidate for your position.

I would welcome the opportunity to interview with you. I will be in the Rockville area during the week of April 12th and would be available to speak with you at that time. I will contact you in the next 10 days to answer any questions that you may have.

Thank you for your consideration,

Sincerely,

Steven Mason

Enclosure

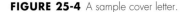

FIGURE 25-4 A sample cover letter.

As a resume is being created, the writer should keep a few things in mind. Potential employees should put themselves in the shoes of the potential employer. What is the potential employer looking for? What qualifications is the employer looking for? What attributes are needed? These qualifications and attributes can then be emphasized in the resume.

PRACTICE POINT   Use positive words when developing a resume, helping to improve the overall image of the candidate.

All resumes should have contact information listed first, centered at the top of the first page. This includes the applicant's name, address, telephone number, and email address. An objective statement follows, which is a brief description of the position that is being applied for and how the applicant's unique skills can contribute to the position. Education is cited next, listing schools by full name and address. Education should be arranged in reverse chronological order, listing the most current first. Degrees should be listed, along with any majors or minors, and the graduation date (Box 25-2).

Resumes can have a variety of arrangements, including reverse chronological (most common), skill, or mixed order. Reverse chronological order lists items starting with the most current position held. Education is generally listed first, followed by employment history. Job descriptions are included in the employment portion. Skills-based resumes may be used when changing careers. Education and work history are minimized, whereas the skills used to accomplish tasks are embellished. This may be of benefit when trying to match the target skills to the position available. Mixed resumes offer a combination of both chronological and skills-based resumes, allowing focus on individual skills.

BOX 25-2 | Resume Rules

- Avoid lengthy job descriptions or descriptions of nontransferable job duties.
- Be consistent. Use the same format throughout the resume.
- Construct a resume using action verbs, adjectives, and key words that describe skills.
- Describe accomplishments quantitatively where appropriate.
- Do not list unrelated personal information or include photographs.
- Do not make statements that cannot be backed up with examples or proof.
- Do not use the word "I" or indefinite or personal pronouns, and do not use articles such as "my," "our," "an," or "the."
- Do not include physical attributes such as age, weight, or height.
- Do not include salary information unless requested.
- Emphasize qualities and experience.
- Limit graphics.

- Limit the length. One page should be sufficient unless extensive professional experience is included.
- Make sure that it is free of spelling, grammatical, and typographical errors.
- Never handwrite a resume.
- Never print resumes double sided.
- Print the resume using a laser printer or very clear inkjet printer.
- Select resume paper that is light in color and has a fairly plain background so it can be copied, scanned, or faxed easily.
- Since computers and scanners vary, save a copy of the resume in a text-only format so it can be emailed easily or copied and pasted to a job Web site. Many companies scan resumes, but scanners have difficulty with lines, graphics, and some fonts.
- Use headings that allow the reader to find needed information quickly.

BOX 25-3 | Positive Words

- Accomplished
- Achieved
- Assisted
- Completed
- Conducted
- Coordinated
- Creative
- Demonstrated
- Dependable
- Enthusiastic
- Flexible
- Generated
- Have initiative
- Honest
- Implemented
- Improved
- Increased

- Initiated
- Instructed
- Listener
- Maintained
- Managed
- Motivated
- Organized
- Persuaded
- Prepared
- Produced
- Prompt
- Recruited
- Self-motivated
- Streamlined
- Team player
- Trained
- Updated

Employment history includes the name and location of the employer along with employment dates and responsibilities. Descriptions of job duties and responsibilities should be short and to the point (Box 25-3).

Volunteer experiences can be listed after employment history, especially if volunteering was a large part of a previous employment period. Previous volunteer experience may also be vital to the skills targeted for the open position. Just as for employment history, the name and location of the organization should be listed along with volunteer dates in chronological order. A brief description of duties should be included as well (Figure 25-5).

Membership organizations can be listed after volunteer experiences, especially if a leadership position has been held. A brief description of roles, responsibilities, and highlights should be documented.

References should be listed on a separate sheet of paper in alphabetical order. The applicant's contact information should be on the top of the sheet in case it becomes separated from the original resume. Reference information should include a full name, address, telephone number, and email address of each person listed. References should be reminded that they have been listed on the resume, preventing a shock when a potential employer calls.

If several jobs have been held, some related to career goals and some not, one might try creating a "Related Experience" section near the top of the resume to highlight career-related jobs. Other jobs could be listed under the headings "Other Experience" or "Supportive Experience" and have much more concise descriptions.

Every resume and cover letter should be meticulously read by a trusting friend or professional. The writer is bound to make typographical errors that will be overlooked; a fresh set of eyes will pick up the errors before the target reader does (who will then form a negative perception regarding the professionalism of the applicant). A good friend will also scrutinize the information and offer tips for improvement. If a good friend is not available for review, a local college is sure to have excellent resources and staff available for such tasks.

Email and Internet Resumes

Many companies now accept resumes online, either by the Internet or email. It is important to know that the Internet and email changes the configuration of resumes and cover letters. The resume can be saved as a PDF file; this will allow it to be viewed exactly as it was created. If a cover letter will be submitted via email, it may be easier to cut and paste the cover letter into the body of the email. An applicant does not want to submit a cover letter that is deformed and unreadable, especially when it is the first document the target reader will open.

Preparing for an Interview

Preparing for an interview is similar to completing homework for a college course. One must be prepared and present the homework in a professional, logical manner (Box 25-4).

Steven Mason

Current Address:
1000 Terrace View Apts.
Blackburg, VA 24060
987-654-3210

Permanent Address:
1650 Home Road
Rockville, MD 20895
123-654-0987

stevenmasonvt@fastwave.biz

Career Objective

Veterinary Technician: Seeking a challenging position in a dynamic environment that focuses on building strategic relationships with clients and promotes customer service while promoting high-quality veterinary medicine.

Education

Purdue University, Veterinary Technology Program
Bachelor of Science in Veterinary Technology

Expected graduation 5/10

Activities and Honors

- Captain, Intramural Softball Team; organized tryouts, selected team and coached an eight-week season
- President, Veterinary Technology Club; organized fundraisers as well as career days with local elementary schools

Experience

Animal Science Reproduction and Physiology Lab, Purdue University
08/09-present
Lab Research Assistant
- Researched, updated, and selected and more than 500 Holstein cows for a reproductive trial utilizing Lutalyse
- Drew blood, performed laboratory analysis on selected cows
- Assisted in calving

Animal Science Nutrition Lab, Purdue University
08/08-05/09
Lab Research Assistant
- Developed feeding protocols for calves
- Performed nutritional analysis on feedstuffs and fecal content
- Analyzed data, providing summary to graduate students

Ark Veterinary Hospital
08/07-08/08
Veterinary Assistant
- Assisted the veterinarians and veterinary technicians with restraint, examinations, and surgery
- Placed IV catheters
- Obtained blood samples
- Performed basic laboratory analysis utilizing Idexx Lasercyte and chemistry machines
- Completed urinalyses, fecal and microscopic examinations

FIGURE 25-5 A sample resume.

BOX 25-4 | Interview Rules

- Ask questions.
- Do not chew gum.
- Do not discuss salary immediately.
- Show enthusiasm.
- Do not talk excessively or appear too aggressive.
- Dress accordingly.
- Make eye contact.
- Use proper grammar.

Questions can be asked of oneself in preparation for an interview, and many additional questions asked during the interview may come from these basic questions (Box 25-5).

"Where are you at this time in your life?" This helps review the past and explains why the person is where he or she is today. Experiences, past employment, and lifestyle affect the development of an individual, including skills and attitude. Applicants should expect to answer questions about previous employment, gaps in employment history, or frequent changes in jobs. Skills, aptitudes, and responsibilities should be thought about when completing this section of the homework. (Where am I now? What changes need to take place? Why?)

BOX 25-5	Common Interview Questions

- Are you currently employed?
- Describe yourself.
- How did you learn about this profession?
- What are your goals? 5 years from now? 10 years from now?
- What can you bring to our team?
- What formal education have you received?
- What is your ideal job?
- What is your strongest asset?
- What is your weakest asset?
- What responsibilities have you enjoyed the least at your previous jobs, and why?
- What responsibilities have you enjoyed the most at your previous jobs, and why?
- What salary do you expect?
- Why are you interested in this company?
- Why do you feel you are qualified for this position?
- Why do you wish to change jobs?
- Why should our company hire you?

BOX 25-6	Questions to Ask Potential Employers

- Do you have an open-door policy regarding communications, problem solving, and personnel issues?
- Do you value your employees as team members or individuals?
- How many team members are employed?
- What are short-term goals for this company?
- What are the long-term goals of this company?
- What benefits are generally offered with this position?
- What is the biggest strength of this company?
- What is the staff turnover rate?
- What is the weakest attribute of this company?

"Where are you going?" A potential employer wants to know what the goals of the applicant will be. Where will this potential employee be in 1 year, 5 years, or 10 years? Will he or she benefit the company? Will the company waste money training a person for less than 1 year of employment? On a personal level, the individual must determine goals, understand that goals do change, and accept the challenges that come along the way.

"How are you going to achieve your goals?" Additional schooling, employment opportunities, or volunteering experiences may help achieve goals and dreams. A particular job may result in a dream or goal an applicant has; if so, it is important to take the right steps to obtain that goal.

"What are your strengths and weaknesses?" It is advantageous to determine one's strengths and weaknesses. These questions will certainly be asked in an interview, and the potential employer will want to know why. In many cases, a veterinary technician's greatest weakness is the inability to say no. They take on too many projects, become overwhelmed, and perhaps do not complete any of them on time or above the expected level. A great asset may be listening and talking. A great employee may talk a lot, but clients love team members who are social, listen, and reply with valuable knowledge.

"What type of benefits or salary would you be willing to accept?" Benefits and salary are generally a decisive factor when determining employment; therefore full thought and consideration should be given to this topic before an interview. The topic may or may not evolve during the interview process; it will, however, evolve by the time an offer of employment is made. Veterinarians, veterinary technicians, and practice managers can refer to the Veterinary Hospital Medical Association, American Animal Hospital Association, or National Commission on Veterinary and Economic Issues for standards of pay in the region in which they reside or will potentially reside. This can provide a guide of acceptable ranges of payment. Other considerations are benefits that are available to team members. Many times, benefits packages far outweigh salary; therefore consideration must be given to both. See Chapter 5 for benefits that are generally offered.

Applicants should learn about the business to which they are applying. Mission statements, values, or goals can be gained from Web sites for larger corporations; smaller practices may also have information available on their Web sites. If the applicant knows current employees of the company, questions can be asked about company policies, benefits, and promotional opportunities and procedures.

Depending on the type of company and position, wearing a suit may be appropriate. A suit may be overdressed for a veterinary assistant position; business casual dress may be considered. Appearances make an impression and can last forever; it is imperative to dress appropriately. If there is any question, dress a step above what might be expected.

Prepare questions for a potential employer (Box 25-6). An interview is for both the applicant and the employer. Applicants should want to know if they are an appropriate match for the practice or company. There is no need to waste the applicant's and employer's time if the morals, ethics, and goals do not match. A small notebook can be taken into the interview to remind the applicant of questions. Ask for a day to work in or observe the practice (if applicable). Learning about the environment is extremely important.

> **PRACTICE POINT** When interviewing for a position, be sure to interview the business and manager; interviews go both ways, and the potential candidate must ensure the position is a good fit for all involved. Candidates want to ensure they take a position with a professional, progressive company, and have a manager that they can work *with*.

Arrive early for an interview. Latecomers are automatically assessed a mental penalty; lateness may indicate that the interview is not important to the candidate.

Follow-Up After the Interview

A follow-up letter should be written 1 or 2 days after the interview. This is an indicator that the applicant is interested

in the position, which may help set the resume and interview apart from others. A letter may include a statement of thanks and once again highlight the qualifications of the candidate and how the applicant's assets will benefit the company. If, after the interview and observation of the practice, the applicant chooses not to pursue employment opportunities, a letter should be written stating so. This not only saves the employer time and money, but the applicant may need to return in the future for an interview with the practice.

Receiving Offers of Employment

It is important to remember the value one possesses. If more than one interview has taken place and multiple offers have been made, all offers should be considered before making a final decision. Potential employers should be told that several offers exist for employment, and that a response will be available in a stated time. (Be careful not to extend this time too far out, as potential employers may hire someone else.) Individuals must remember what their goals are: "What kind of employer do I want?" "What kind of work environment do I want?" "What is my goal for hours and salary?" Once a majority of expectations have been met, a decision can be made.

It is advisable to receive the offer in writing, including the agreed salary, the raise and evaluation structure, and any benefits that are offered at the time of employment. Some employees may be put on a trial period, which prevents benefits from immediately being offered; the rules of the trial period should also be clearly stated in the offer.

Retirement

Retirement should not be ignored while developing one's career. Whether an individual is changing to the veterinary profession, leaving the field, or creating a whole new dynamic, retirement is important to consider. Previous generations have had Social Security to rely on; although it does not produce a wealthy income, it at least provided enough money for food and shelter. Future generations may not have Social Security to depend on; if any money is left to distribute, it will not be enough for survival. It is therefore imperative to start planning as soon as possible.

If companies do not offer a retirement fund as a benefit, it is up to the individual to start one for himself or herself. One can contact a financial planning professional to determine what type of account would be best; it is best to find an advisor who is willing to educate and spend time finding the correct investments for each client. Co-workers, friends, and professionals in the community can offer recommendations.

It takes discipline to save money now, but it will be worth it later. Many practices or companies allow funds to be deducted directly from the payroll check and deposited into a savings or retirement account before the employee ever sees the money. This is helpful for enforcing a savings plan for those who lack the discipline to do so.

⚖️ **VETERINARY PRACTICE and the LAW**

When preparing for an interview, one should be aware of questions that cannot be asked of the applicant. The Equal Employment Opportunity laws are a collection of federal laws that prohibit job discrimination, both during the interview process and once the applicant has been hired. Questions regarding religious affiliation; citizenship or place of birth; pregnancy, family, or marital status; race; military affiliation; age; political affiliation; and holidays that are observed are off limits. If one feels that they have been discriminated against in the application process, reports can be filed with the U.S. Equal Employment Opportunity Commission.

REVIEW QUESTIONS

1. What is the MBTI?
2. Why should one prepare for an interview?
3. What is the purpose of a cover letter?
4. When would one use a skills-based resume?
5. Why should one ask potential employers questions?
6. How should one dress for an interview?
7. Why is professional development important to maintain?
8. What is the purpose of a follow-up letter?
9. Prepare a cover letter.
10. Prepare a chronological resume.
11. On average, individuals change jobs every:
    a. 1.5 years
    b. 2.5 years
    c. 3.5 years
    d. 4.5 years
12. Skills that have been gathered through various jobs and experiences are known as:
    a. Transferable skills
    b. Personal skills
    c. A skill survey
    d. Educational
13. Marketing oneself starts with:
    a. Cover letters
    b. Resumes
    c. Benign conversations
    d. Interviews
14. Cover letters are:
    a. Required
    b. Recommended
    c. Not needed
15. A successful interview encompasses all of the following except:
    a. Interviewing the potential employer
    b. Interviewing the potential candidate
    c. Answering questions with confidence
    d. Arriving to the interview late

Recommended Reading

Bolles RN: *What color is your parachute? 2009: a practical manual for job hunters and career changers,* Berkeley, CA, 2008, Ten Speed Press.

Green B: *Get the interview every time: Fortune 500 hiring professionals' tips for writing winning resumes and cover letters,* Chicago, IL, 2004, Dearborn Trade.

Abbreviations

ABBREVIATION	DEFINITION
AD	right ear
ad lib	freely as wanted
ARF	acute renal failure
AS	left ear
AU	both ears
BAR	bright, alert, responsive
BID	twice daily
BM	bowel movement
BP	blood pressure
BTT	blue top tube
BW	body weight
cc	cubic centimeter
CHF	congestive heart failure
CRF	chronic renal failure
d	day
d	diarrhea
D5W	5% dextrose in water
DIC	disseminated intravascular coagulation
DJD	degenerative joint disease
DM	Diabetes Mellitus
DOA	dead on arrival
Dx	diagnosis
ECG, EKG	electrocardiogram
ECHO	echocardiogram
EENT	eyes, ears, nose, throat
FB	foreign body
FeLV	feline leukemia virus
FIP	feline infectious peritonitis
FPV	feline panleukopenia virus
FUO	fever of unknown origin
FUS	feline urologic syndrome
FVR	feline viral rhinotracheitis
Fx	fracture
g, gm	gram
gal	gallon
GDV	gastric dilatation volvulus
gtt	drops
h	hour
HBC	hit by car
HR	heart rate
Hx	history
ICH	infectious canine hepatitis
ID	intradermal

ABBREVIATION	DEFINITION
IM	intramuscular
IN	intranasal
IP	intraperitoneal
IT	intratracheal
IV	intravenous
IVD	intervertebral disk disease
IVP	intravenous pyelogram
kg	kilogram
L	liter
LN	lymph node
LRS	lactated Ringer solution
LTT	lavender top tube
MAP	mean arterial pressure
mcg, μg	microgram
mEq	milliequivalent
mg	milligram
MI	mitral insufficiency
mL	milliliter
MLV	modified live virus
mm	mucous membrane
NPO	nil per os
NSF	no significant findings
OCD	osteochondritis diseccans
OD	right eye
OFA	Orthopedic Foundation for Animals
OS	left eye
OTC	over-the-counter
OU	both eyes
OVH, OHE	ovariohysterectomy
PM	postmortem
PO	per os
ppm	parts per million
PPN	partial parenteral nutrition
prn	as necessary
PTS	put to sleep
PTT	purple top tube or lavender top tube
q	every
qd	every day
qh	every hour
qid	four times a day
qod	every other day
R/I	rule ins
R/O	rule outs

ABBREVIATION	DEFINITION
RTT	red top tube
Rv	rabies vaccination
S/R	suture or staple removal
SC, SQ	subcutaneous
sig	label
Sx	surgery
tab	tablet
tid	three times a day

ABBREVIATION	DEFINITION
TPR	temperature, pulse, respiration
Tx	treatment
UA	urinalysis
URI	upper respiratory infection
UTI	urinary tract infection
v	vomiting
WNL	within normal limits

Glossary

16PF An instrument that is used to support vocational guidance, hiring, and promotional recommendations.

401(k) A retirement fund that employees contribute to; employers are not required to contribute, but may do so if they wish.

Accountability The ability of individuals to take responsibility for tasks and duties.

Accounts payable Amounts owed to suppliers that are payable in the future.

Accounts receivable Money owed to a practice for services rendered or products sold that is not paid at the time of service or when the product is dispensed.

Accrual-based accounting A system that recognizes income as it is earned and expenses as they are incurred, rather than when the actual cash transaction occurs.

Adjuvant An additive added to vaccinations to increase the immune response from the animal.

Administrative ethics Involves the action by administrative government bodies that regulate veterinary practice and activities in which veterinarians engage.

Adware A program or software that installs itself onto the computer without the user's knowledge. Adware plays a role in advertising; it collects information about the user, as well as Web sites visited, and uses this information to display pop-up advertisements that may interest the user.

Aerobic Bacteria that requires air or oxygen for growth.

Allowance The maximum amount available for a specific diagnosis in pet health insurance.

Anaerobic Bacteria that do not need air or oxygen for growth.

Anesthesia An agent that produces a loss of feeling or sensation.

Anesthetic release form A form signed by the client accepting risks associated with surgical and treatment procedures.

Anger A stage of grief that people experience.

Annual deductible An amount a client chooses to pay out before receiving benefits from pet health insurance.

Annual payout limit The maximum amount a pet health insurance company will pay out over the year for a pet's policy.

Anorexia Lack of appetite.

Anticoagulant Chemical added to a blood tube to prevent blood clot formation.

Appointment book template The outline of the appointment book.

Appointment cards Cards given to clients stating their scheduled appointment date, time, and patient name.

Appointment scheduler The appointment book.

Appointment units The specified amount of time that correlates to 1 unit. For example, 15 minutes equals 1 unit, 30 minutes equals 2 units.

Assertive marketing Provides the clients with the information they need in order to accept the practice recommendations.

Assets Any property owned by a business or individual. Cash, accounts receivable, inventory, land, buildings, leasehold improvements, and tangible property are examples of assets.

Average client transaction Revenue per client visit, calculated by dividing the income by the number of clients or patients seen.

AVMA The American Veterinary Medical Association: an organization developed to improve and set standards for veterinary medicine.

Backup devices Device that copies information from the central processing unit and stores it in the event of computer malfunction. Backup devices can be either internal or external.

Balance sheet A financial report detailing practice assets, liabilities, and owners equity.

Bargaining A stage of grief that people experience; they generally bargain to extend the life of their pet.

Benchmarking The process by which a practice compares itself to others (especially those known for outstanding performance) in an attempt to improve performance.

Benefit The payment made for a specific diagnosis in accordance with an insurance plan.

Better Business Bureau Also known as the BBB; accepts complaints of unhealthy business practices from consumers.

Billing cycle The period between statements produced for clients.

Biohazard A needle, glass or sharp object that is contaminated with vaccinations, pathogens or human blood, and must be disposed of in a leakproof container. The container must be incinerated by an approved company.

Blogging The practice of creating the `new' newsletter that must be linked to the practice's webpage; can detail the everyday happenings around the veterinary office.

Body language Posture, stance, and position that communicates messages to a listener.

Bookkeeper Generally a self-taught accountant that maintains payroll and books.

Brand An identifying symbol, words, or mark that distinguishes a company from its competitors.

Break-even analysis The process used to determine how much money or service must be recovered or performed in order to cover the cost of purchasing equipment or adding a service to the practice.

Broadband High speed Internet connection that can transmit information 40 times as fast as telephone and modem connection.

Bucky unit The portion of the x-ray machine that holds the cassette, under the table.

Budget An estimate of revenues and expenses for a given period.

Burnout Physical or emotional exhaustion, especially as a result of long-term stress or dissipation.

Calipers Instrument used to measure the thickness of the pet in centimeters (cm) for a radiograph; cm are then used to help determine peak kilovoltage (kVp) for the x-ray beam.

Campbell Interest and Skills Survey (CISS) measures self-reported vocational interests and skills.

Capital The rights (equity) of the owners in a business enterprise.

Capital inventory Equipment that is purchased for use in business.

Carcinogen A chemical or substance that is known to cause cancer.

Card reader A card reader/writer is useful for transferring data directly to and from a removable flash memory card. Examples of flash cards are those used in a camera or music player.

Career planning The ongoing process of making career choices that are reviewed from time to time.

Carnivore An animal whose diet is primarily meat.

Cash-based accounting A system that recognizes income as it is received and expenses as they are paid, rather than when the income was earned or the expense was acquired.

Cash flow statement Report on the sources of cash and its use during a period of time.

CD/DVD Device for storing data; a CD stores approximately 650 to 700 MB of information, a DVD stores approximately at least double that.

Central inventory location A central location within the practice where excess inventory is stored; often a locked location.

Chronic condition A condition of a pet that progresses over time.

Civil law Relates to the duties between people and the government.

Claim A submission for a request of payment in pet health insurance.

Client communication Listening and understanding to client needs, then delivering the information needed to ensure complete understanding.

Client compliance A key performance indicator monitoring the level of clients accepting recommendations made by the practice team.

Client discharge instructions Instructions that are given to a client upon the release of a pet from the hospital giving explicit instruction for post release care, including activity, food, and medication instructions.

Client grievances Client complaints.

Client patient information sheet A sheet that is filled out by the client, requesting client contact information, along with patient data.

Client retention A key performance indicator determining the number of clients that are retained in a practice between two set dates.

Client survey A survey asking clients of their thoughts and opinions of the services received in a practice.

COBRA Consolidated Omnibus Budget Reconciliation Act. It requires employers to continue insurance coverage for a specified time. COBRA requires employers to continue coverage for former employees who have a medical condition that would be prevent them from obtaining immediate coverage from a new employer.

Code of ethics Developed to help members of the veterinary profession achieve high levels of behavior through moral consciousness, decision making and practice

COGS – Cost of goods sold The expense incurred to purchase merchandise sold during a period.

COPS – Cost of professional services The direct costs associated with producing a product or service.

Collections agency A business that has been hired to collect funds from non-paid accounts.

Community service The donation of time to a non-profit organization.

Company supported Web site A Web site typically created by a design company; the practice may have little or no access to the content provided.

Compliance rate The measure of whether pets actually receive the care that has been recommended by the veterinary team.

Computer hacker A person or person(s) with intentions to illegally access a computer system and cripple its function.

Computerized medical records Medical records that are kept on the computer; all images, signed consent forms, and blood work are stored in the computerized medical record.

Conceptual skill The ability to sense how the leadership style affects the practice, and making change in a positive way.

Conflict management The process and management of resolving a dispute or disagreement.

Congenital condition Generally referred to as an abnormality present at birth, whether apparent or not, that can cause illness or disease.

Consent The voluntary acceptance or agreement to what is planned or is done by another person.

Contract employee An individual that has established a business for themselves and contracts out services to other businesses; relief veterinarians, groomers, and consultants can be contract employees.

Contract law Deals with duties established by individuals as a result of contractual agreement.

Controlled substance log A log or record used to manage all controlled substances dispensed.

Controlled substance A drug that has been deemed by the DEA as having the potential to be abused.

Controlled Substance Act of 1970 An act passed to reduce drug abuse by identifying substances that have high abuse potential.

Cookies Cookies are messages given to the browser, with information that has been collected about the user when visiting Web sites. When the user returns to the Web site, the browser remembers the user, and can present the user with a customized Web site.

Co-pay A specified dollar amount of covered services that is the policyholder's responsibility.

Cost analysis Breaking down the costs of some operation and reporting on each factor separately.

Cover letter A letter placed with a resume showing interest in employment.

CPA – Certified Public Accountant A college trained accountant professional that has attained certification in the state that he or she resides, by passing a comprehensive exam and maintaining continuing education.

CPU The brain of the computer; located in the main unit.

Cremation The incineration of a body.

Criminal law Prosecutes crimes committed against the public as a whole. Most criminal laws focus on acts that injure people or pets.

CRT – capillary refill time Provides an estimation of tissue perfusion and oxygenation, as well as an indication of cardiovascular tone. CRT should be 2 to 3 seconds.

Cystocentesis The insertion of a sterile needle into the bladder to obtain a urine sample.

Cytology The viewing of cells on a microscope slide, under high magnification.

Data Information stored on a computer, DVD or CD.

Data conversion The conversion of data from one software version to another.

DEA – U.S. Drug Enforcement Administration Provides approved means for proper manufacturing, distribution, dispensing, and use of drugs through licensed handlers.

Debit transactions Transactions paid with a credit card that is linked to the customer's checking account.

Deductible The dollar amount an individual must pay for services before the insurance company's payment. Clients may have a choice of per incident deductible or annual deductible.

Delegation Authorizing subordinates to take assigned responsibilities and make decisions.

Denial A stage of grief a person experiences in which they are in disbelief that a pet is injured, sick, or deceased.

Dependence The persistent use of a drug that involves physiologic dependence with symptoms of tolerance.

Deposit Placing or transferring funds into a savings or checking account.

Depression A stage of grief that a person experiences with the loss of a pet; symptoms include lethargy, sadness, and isolation from others.

Desktop Computer that sits on the top of a desk; not considered a portable unit.

Digital camera A camera that can capture images without the use of film. Images are then transferred to the computer with a connection wire. Photos can then be printed from the computer or stored for future use. Digital cameras come in a variety of megapixels. The higher the megapixel count, the better the resolution of the photo. A digital camera can be an effective marketing tool in a veterinary practice.

Direct deposit An automatic transaction that places money into an employee's checking account for payroll.

Direct expense An expense that can be directly related to a patient, client, or revenue center.

Direct marketing The most popular form of marketing and has been around for years. The Yellow Pages are a classic example of direct marketing.

Directive management Task-oriented style of management.

Distributor representative A representative of a company that sells products of larger manufacturing companies.

Docking station Stationary device that allows a tablet to function as a desktop computer.

Domain name A name given to a Web address that is recognizable, as Web addresses are provided in numeric format.

DSL High-speed internet connection that uses the same wires as a telephone.

EDTA Ethylenediaminetetraacetic acid is an anticoagulant that is added to a lavender top tube, preventing clotting of the blood.

Effective communication Communication to both clients and team members that is clear, conceptual, and easy to follow.

Electrocardiogram A record of the heart's electrical activity.

Embezzlement The fraudulent appropriation of funds or property entrusted to your care when it is actually owned by someone else.

Emotional intelligence The ability to identify, assess, and control the emotions of oneself.

Employee manual A manual explaining the terms and conditions employees must operate under while working for a given business.

Employee Polygraph Protection Act The EPPA prohibits most employers from using lie detector tests for either pre-employment screening or during the course of employment. Employers cannot discriminate against employees who refuse to take a lie detector test.

Employee procedural manual A manual explaining the procedures employees must follow while working for a given business.

Empower The act of sharing managerial power with subordinates. It is the concept of encouraging and authorizing workers to take initiative to improve operations, reduce costs and improve customer service.

End-of-day reconciliation The process required to close the business books at the end of the day; cash, credit cards, and checks must balance with the computer-generated report.

Enucleated Removal of the eye and the orbital tissues.

Equity The rights or claims to properties. Assets = Equities + Liabilities

Equal Employment Opportunity Prevents the discrimination against race, color, sex, religion, and national origin. Employers cannot deny a promotion, terminate, or not a hire a potential employee because of any of the reasons just mentioned.

Ergonomics The science that studies the relationship between people and their work environments.

ERISA The Employee Retirement Income Security Act regulates retirement funds once established in a business.

Estimates A printed idea of the cost of services and products that a client will incur while their pet is treated.

Etiquette The rules that society has set for the proper way to behave in dealing with other people.

Euthanasia The induction of a painless death.

Euthanasia release form The owner's consent to perform euthanasia.

Evaluation A report provided to employees stating their work performance and any improvements that need to be made; generally performed on an annual basis.

Exclusion A condition that would be excluded from the coverage of a medical plan.

Exposure time The amount of time radiation exposes a film during the x-ray process.

External hard drive An external hard drive is a storage drive that allows programs to be stored outside of the computer. External hard drives are protected in heavy black cases and create an extra storage space, or can provide a complete backup of the computer system.

External marketing A marketing technique that targets potential clients.

Fair Credit Reporting Act A federal law that regulates prescreening reports issued to employers by outside agencies called credit reporting agencies.

Fair Debt Collection Practices Act An act that was passed to protect the public from unethical collection procedures.

FDA – U.S. Food and Drug Administration An agency of the U.S. Department of Health and Human Services and is responsible for regulating and supervising the safety of foods, dietary supplements, drugs, vaccines, biological medical products, blood products, medical devices, radiation-emitting devices, veterinary products, and cosmetics.

Finance charge Money charged for payments that extend beyond an agreed-upon time limit. The amount of the finance fee must be clearly indicated on the clients invoice.

Firewall Device that regulates what comes in and out of the computer. The device will reject nonvalid programs.

First notice of accident The initial reporting of an accident to the owner or practice manager, as required by OSHA.

Fixed cost A cost that does not change with the variation of business. Rent, mortgage and utility costs remain the same, regardless of how busy the practice is.

Flowmeter A regulator that regulates the amount of oxygen flowing to a patient.

FLSA – Fair Labor Standards Act Federal law that sets minimum wage and overtime regulations.

FMLA – Family and Medical Leave Act Federal law that allows employees to take up to 12 weeks of unpaid leave to attend to a family member.

Focal-film distance This is the measurement in inches between the tube and film cassette.

Fomite Any object or material on which disease-producing agents can be conveyed.

Form W-2 IRS form that reports income paid and taxes withheld by an employer for a particular company during a calendar year.

Form W-4 IRS form that determines the amount of federal taxes the employer will withhold from a persons paycheck each pay period.

Formalin A chemical that preserves tissue for histopathology. Formalin is a known carcinogen; therefore, caution must be used while handling it.

FTP – File Transfer Protocol The process of uploading Web site information to the actual Web site.

FUTA – Federal Unemployment Tax Act Tax required to be paid by the employer.

Gas sterilization A chemical sterilization technique that uses ethylene oxide to sterilize products.

General administrative expenses All executive, organizational, and clerical expenses associated with the general management of and operations of a practice, rather than with delivery of patient care.

General anesthesia Controllable and reversible loss of consciousness induced by intoxication of the central nervous system.

Gigabyte Measure of computer data storage, approximately 1 billion bytes.

Gingivitis The inflammation associated with gum disease.

Graphics card Card inserted into the main unit of a computer that determines how detailed video images will appear on the monitor.

Grid Prevents scatter radiation before it hits the cassette, and is placed between the film and the table.

Groomer A professional that bathes, clips, and styles the hair of pets.

Gross income Income resulting from all veterinary operations before any cost or expenses deductions are made.

Gross profit A monetary amount, computed by subtracting the total cost of professional services from gross income.

Hacker An individual or group of people that intentionally attempt to break into computer systems and install worms, viruses, or other dangerous software. They may also alter information, cause damage, and erase programs.

Handwritten recognition Technology that allows the computer to convert touch screen writing into printed words.

Hard drive A hard drive stores all computer data.

Hardware Refers to the actual physical equipment of a computer. The central piece of hardware in the information system is the computer.

Herd health records Records that pertain to an entire herd; if one cow is treated for a disease, they may all be treated, on the same record.

Hereditary conditions An abnormality that is transmitted by genes from the parent to the offspring, whether apparent or not, that can cause disease or illness.

Histopathology The study of tissue or cells.

Hospital safety manual A manual required by OSHA listing hazards associated with the job, training topics and procedures in case of an emergency.

Host A computer that is connected to a network or the internet. Each host has a unique IP address.

Host-the-site website A website that is developed and maintained by the practice, which can be done with the practice server or by renting space on another server.

Human-animal bond A description of the emotion humans feel toward animals.

Human skill The ability to understand people and what motivates them, and to be able to direct their behavior through effective leadership.

Hypothyroidism A disease that results from underproduction of thyroid hormone from the thyroid gland.

Incident An individual accident, illness, or injury, including those that may require continual treatment until resolution.

Income statement Report on financial performance that covers a period of time and reports incomes and expenses during that period. Income statements are also known as profit and loss statements.

Indemnity insurance A system of pet health insurance in which the client is reimbursed for services after they have been provided.

Indirect expense An expense that contributes to the delivery of patient care, but cannot be tied directly to a patient, client, or revenue center.

Indirect marketing A marketing technique that is used by practices on a daily basis; clean facilities, genuine service, and excellent customer care are a few examples.

Informational brochure A marketing piece of material informing existing and potential clients of the services offered by the practice.

Informed consent A person's agreement to allow something to happen, such as a medical treatment or surgery that is based on full disclosure of the facts necessary to make an intelligent decision.

Injection site sarcomas A tumor common in cats that is thought to be caused by any injection given; vaccines, fluids, and antibiotic therapies may induce such tumors.

Intangible property Nonphysical property that has value; franchises, copyrights, client lists, goodwill, and covenants not to compete are examples of intangible property.

Intensifying screens Screens within a radiograph cassette that reduce the amount of radiation needed to take an x-ray.

Interest The cost of borrowing money, assessed by the lender over time, usually expressed as a percentage of the principle amount borrowed.

Internal marketing A marketing technique that targets current or existing clients for services offered within the practice.

International health certificates An official letter stating that an animal appears healthy for international travel.

Internet A network that connects millions of users to various Web sites.

Intervention A process that helps a drug addict recognize the extent of his or her problem.

Intrastate health certificates An official letter that states a pet appears healthy for travel within the Untied States.

Inventory Extra merchandise or supplies that the practice keeps on hand to meet the demands of customers.

Inventory management software Veterinary software that produces reports, PO numbers, and develops a list of needed items when requested.

Inventory turns per year The number of times an item must be reordered within a stated period. 8–12 turns per year should be a goal of each practice.

IP address A specific number that identifies the user's computer.

IRCA The Immigration Reform and Control Act prohibits employer discrimination against any employee or potential employee because of their national origin.

Just-in-time ordering The process of ordering and receiving product just as it is needed, rather than storing excess inventory.

Kennel assistant A team member that cleans kennels, aids in medical treatments, and observes hospitalized patients.

Key performance indicators Statistics that can be generated from client transaction data and reviewed for performance data.

Keyboard The keyboard is one of the most important devices used to communicate with the computer. It should have at least 101 keys on it and have a USB connection to plug into the computer. Some users prefer wireless keyboards, especially when a smaller desk space is being used. For team members that use the keyboard for a majority of the day, an ergonomic keyboard may be considered.

Killed vaccine A vaccine that introduces a killed bacteria or virus into the body, inducing an immune response.

Kilocalorie The amount of heat necessary to raise the temperature of 1 kilogram (kg) of water by 1 degree Celsius.

kVp Peak kilovoltage, defined as the level or penetrability of the resulting x-ray beam.

mAs A milliampere-second is the unit of measurement for the energy of x-rays produced at the set voltage.

Label printer Printers designed to produce labels for bottles, containers, or envelopes.

Laboratory log A log used to keep track of the tests performed in house or samples submitted to an outside laboratory.

Laptop Portable computer.

Lateral recumbency The placement of an animal on the side for an examination or completion of a procedure. Can be either right or left lateral recumbency.

Law Bodies of rules that are developed and enforced by government to regulate human conduct.

Lead time The amount of time between placing an order and receiving the order.

Ledger cards An older accounting method used to record client transactions.

Legibility The degree at which glyphs and vocabulary are understandable or readable based on appearance.

Lethargy Fatigue or exhaustion.

Liabilities Obligations resulting from past transactions that require the practice to pay money or provide service. Accounts payable and taxes are examples of current liabilities.

Lifetime limit The maximum dollar amount a company will pay out on one policy, for the lifetime of the pet.

Local anesthesia Anesthetic that deadens the sensory nerves.

Maintenance diet A food that is developed for a pet in which the requirements needed to maintain a perfect body condition score have been met.

Malpractice A limiting term specifically describing a professional's failure to practice the quality of medicine set by similarly situated veterinarians in a given geographical area, if the accused is a general practitioner.

Managed care A health care system under which health care professionals are organized into a group or network in order to manage the cost, quality, and access to health care.

Manufacturer representative A representative of a large company that produces products for businesses. Manufacturers may have distributors distribute product for them.

Markup The amount or percentage added to a product or service to cover the cost of the product or service, including a percentage of overhead expenses, and produce a profit. Most products are marked up 150% to 200%.

Master problem list A list placed in the front of a client record indicating all of the diseases, conditions, medications, and vaccinations a patient has had.

Medical records Daily written reports by veterinarians and technicians on each animal that is treated. Records must be legible and complete.

Megabyte Measure of computer data storage; approximately 1 million bytes.

Meyers-Briggs type indicator An assessment tool to help understand behavior preferences.

Microphone Used to record audio.

MISC-1099 A form a company issues to independent contractors, citing all money paid to the individual on an untaxed basis.

Mission statement A statement of the role or purpose, by which a practice intends to serve its stakeholders. It can clarify the way in which a practice plans to achieve its goals.

mm – mucous membranes Used to estimate tissue perfusion and oxygenation. Mucous membranes are normally pink, indicating adequate respiratory and cardiovascular function.

Mobile media Mobile media implies that webpages are mobile (smart phone) friendly. Mobile media supports the immediate connection clients want to have with a practice.

Modem A device used to connect to the Internet, as well as send and receive faxes via the phone line. The modem converts digital data to analog to send to the end user; the modem also converts analog information back to digital when it is received.

Modified live vaccine Uses a virus or bacteria that has been passed in culture to reduce its virulence.

Monitor The monitor is used to view documents, read email and view pictures. A minimum of a 17-inch screen is advised; however, if digital photos will be reviewed, a 19- or 21-inch monitor is recommended. Flat panel screens are excellent space savers and provide a high quality picture.

Monofilament suture Suture that uses one string instead of two or three (as in multifilament suture).

Monthly statement A statement produced for those with outstanding accounts; may include finance charges and/or statement fees.

Motion economy Eliminating unnecessary steps or tasks, rearranging equipment, organizing procedures, and simplifying tasks.

Mouse A mouse allows the navigation through applications on the computer. The mouse allows the user to point and click. A mouse can be purchased cordless, which may benefit some users. Others prefer a mouse with an ergonomic design and an optical sensor. An optical sensor allows the mouse to be used without a mouse pad, which may be useful if working in a small desk space.

SDS – Safety Data Sheet Detailed explanations about each drug or chemical providing all important information regarding the use of a substance or chemical.

Multifilament suture Suture that is made of multiple strings, producing a stronger holding capacity than that of monofilament suture.

NAVTA – National Association of Veterinary Technicians in America A nonprofit organization dedicated to improving the knowledge and professionalism of veterinary technicians.

NCCLS - National Committee for Clinical Laboratory Standards An organization that promotes the development and use of voluntary laboratory.

NCVEI – National Commission on Veterinary Economic Issues A nonprofit organization dedicated to improving the economic base of the veterinary profession, ensuring that the delivery of veterinary care and service meets the needs of society.

Negligence Performing an act that a person of ordinary prudence would not have done under similar circumstances, or, the failure to do what a person of ordinary circumstances would.

Net income A calculation determined when the expenses are subtracted from the income, with the desire of having a positive number.

Net profit The funds available to an owner after all expenses have been met.

Network card A network card allows connection to a network or DSL for internet connection. If a server is in use for the practice software system, each computer will need to have a network card to allow the computers to communicate with each other.

Neurotransmitters Chemicals that relay, amplify, and modulate signals between a neuron and another cell. Neurotransmitters are packaged into vesicles that cluster beneath the membrane.

Noncompete agreement An agreement made between two professionals limiting the ability to practice medicine within the established area, for a specified time, if one should leave the practice.

Normative ethics Refers to the search for correct principles of good and bad, right and wrong, justice or injustice.

NSF checks Checks that are returned to the business because of lack of funds or a closed client checking account.

Office manager A manager of a practice that oversees the reception area and possibly also accounts receivable.

Omnivore An animal whose diet consists primarily of meat and carbohydrates.

On-site hosting Web site A predesigned Web page that allows practices to change information on-site.

One-way door lock A lock placed on a door that allows exiting at any time but prevents entry when locked.

On-hold messaging Messages that are played while clients are placed on hold, marketing products or services that the practice provides or recommends.

Open house An event inviting clients to view the practice during nonworking hours. Tours, lectures, or the introduction of a new veterinarian may encourage this internal and external marketing technique.

Order book A book that provides distributor and manufacturer information as well as the order history for products purchased.

Organizational behavior The development, improvement, and effectiveness of an organization; it includes the culture, values, system, and behaviors of the practice.

OSHA – Occupational Safety and Health Administration Developed in 1970 to protect the safety of employees. Every employee has the right to know all of the hazards associated with their employment.

OSHA Form 300 A form required by OSHA to be filled out and maintained that states the facts of an injury that has occurred. The form must be kept for several years.

OSHA Form 300A A form required by OSHA to be posted each year from February 1st to April 30th, summarizing all injuries that occurred while on job premises.

Otic disease Infection, inflammation, or condition of the ear and ear canal.

Owner equity Owners interest or claim in the practice assets.

Oxygen pressure regulator A gauge that regulates the amount of pressure leaving the oxygen tank, before entering the anesthetic machine.

Paper medical records Handwritten medical records that are kept in a file folder and include all lab work results, consent forms, or correspondence with the owner.

Parthenogenesis The female has the ability to reproduce without fertilization.

PC – A personal computer The most common type of computer.

Per-incident deductible The dollar amount that the policyholder is responsible for before the insurance company will begin to pay out, for each incident that a claim form is submitted.

Per-incident limit The maximum dollar amount an insurance company will pay out, per incident filed.

Perimeter lighting The lighting on the outside of the practice; excess lighting provides a safer environment for team members and clients.

Permissible exposure limits The maximum exposure amount listed as being safe, before harmful side effects may occur.

Personal ethics Defines what is right or wrong on an individual basis.

Personal protection device A device used to protect oneself; may include mace, a Taser, or a personal gun.

Personal skills The skills or attributes an individual possesses; they are achieved through practical experience, education, and personal life lessons.

Pet portals A Web site designed to assist veterinary practices with the marketing of OTC products, foods, and prescription services.

Petty cash Cash that is held on the premises for purchasing miscellaneous items that may be needed for business; examples include pizza for the staff, special lunch meat for a picky patient, or cat litter.

Plasma The liquid portion of blood that has anticoagulants added to prevent blood clotting.

POMR medical record The most commonly used medical record format that is followed by veterinary health care teams. Each entry follows a distinct format; the defined database, the problem list (also referred to as master list), the plan, and the progress section. Within the progress section, a standard SOAP format is followed.

Pop-ups Windows that pop onto the user's screen, soliciting unwanted information.

Positive pressure relief valve Also referred to as a pop-off valve; prevents excess pressure in the rebreathing circuit and allowed removal of excess waste gases.

Postdated checks Checks that are written by a client on the current date, yet dated to be deposited on a future date.

PPE – Personal protective equipment Equipment provided by the practice that individuals must wear to provide protection from direct or indirect contact with hazardous substances. Examples include eyewash stations, lead gowns and thyroid collars, and safety goggles.

Practice manager An administrative position that oversees the practice's financial condition, organization, and training.

Preexisting condition Injury or illness contracted, manifested, or incurred before the policy effective date.

Premium The amount paid annually or monthly for a policyholder to maintain an insurance policy.

Preoperative instructions Instructions for clients to follow before a patient's procedure.

Primary complaint The main reason a client visits the practice with their pet.

Principle cost Initial cost of equipment when purchased.

Printer Laser and inkjet printers are available. Laser printers print faster with higher quality than an inkjet printer, and the ink generally costs less for a laser printer. Photograph printers are more expensive and print with a higher resolution. Printers should have a USB connection.

Privacy Act of 1974 An act that states, in part: No agency shall disclose any record which is contained in a system of records by any means of communication to any person, or to another agency, except pursuant to a written request by, or with the prior written consent of, the individual to whom the record pertains.

Problem-Oriented Medical Record (POMR) The medical record format most commonly used by veterinary health care teams. Each entry follows a distinct format: the defined database, the problem list (also referred to as master list), the plan, and the progress section.

Processor speed The processor speed is the rate at which the brain of the computer can sort information and produce results.

Professional ethics Developed by the professionals of a particular discipline; they include rules, codes, and conducts for the profession to follow.

Profit and loss statement Summary of the practices income, expenses, and resulting profit or loss for a specified period of time. Also known as the income statement.

Prognosis The estimated result or condition of a patient.

Purging records The act of separating inactive clients from active clients and placing them in another location of the practice that can be easily accessed.

Rabies certificate A certificate that provides proof of vaccination for rabies.

Rabies neutralizing antibody titer Titer levels in response to a rabies vaccination.

Radiology log A log that tracks radiographs that have been taken in the practice; it includes measurements of kVp, mAs, and exposure time.

RAM The short-term memory of a computer. RAM plays a vital role in the speed of the computer.

Recalls The process of making phone calls to follow up with clients regarding procedures that were performed in the practice.

Reception area The area of the practice that welcomes clients and provides a comfortable seating area while they wait to be seen by the veterinarian.

Receptionist A team member that greets clients, answers phones, makes appointments, and provides excellent customer service to clients.

Recombinant vaccine A vaccine that inserts a microorganism or engineered protein into a nonpathogenic vector to induce an immune response.

References People listed within a resume that can provide feedback on the performance of the applicant.

REM A normal stage of sleep characterized by rapid movements of the eyes. REM sleep is classified into two categories: tonic and phasic.

Reminders The generation of cards or letter reminding clients that their pet is due for a procedure.

Reorder point The inventory level at which additional product is ordered.

Reorder quantity A set amount of product that is reordered.

Resume A marketing tool that sells the applicant to the potential employer; it should be tailored to the specific job the applicant has interest.

Return on investment The income that investment generates, return on investment is a measure of how effectively a firm uses capital to generate profit.

Revenue centers The areas of the practice that generate revenue; dentistry, pharmacy, laboratory, etc.

Rider An extension of coverage that can be purchased and added to a base medical policy.

Role-playing A training technique that simulates situations and allows the proper response to be practiced.

Scanner A scanner can be used to scan documents or photos into the computer. Scanners are generally flatbed and should have a color depth of at least 48 bits and a resolution of at least 1200×2400 dpi. The higher the color depth, the more accurate the color. A higher resolution picks up more subtle gradations of color.

Scavenger system A system designed to scavenge excess anesthetic gases to increase the safety for the team members. Active, passive, and adsorbent scavengers are examples.

Security system A system designed to protect the practice from theft after-hours. Alarms, video surveillance, and pager systems are examples that may be used.

SEPS Simplified Employee Pension Plans (SEPS) are similar to a profit sharing plan, and is appropriate for small organizations. It is funded by tax deductible employer contributions, and employees are not allowed to contribute.

Serum The liquid portion of blood without cells.

Server A server stores information to the computers it connects to. When users connect to a server, they can access programs, files, and other information from the server.

sIRA – SIMPLE IRA – Savings Incentive Match Plan for Employees, Individual Retirement Plan A retirement plan in which employees and employers contribute pretaxed money to an established account.

SOAP medical record An acronym that identifies the most common data entry formats used by veterinary practices (subjective, objective, assessment, and plan).

Social ethics The consensus principles adopted by or accepted by society at large, and codified into laws and regulations.

Software The system or program the computer follows.

Sound card Sound cards are responsible for playing sounds and recording audio. Most sound cards available today are capable of recording and playing digital audio. If the computer will be used extensively for game playing or as an entertainment system, the sound card can be upgraded.

Spam Information including emails that are not considered useful and can be damaging to the user.

Spam filter A device that filters spam, preventing it from infiltrating the user's computer.

Speakers Speakers emanate sound, and as mentioned previously, if the computer will be used for game playing or used for presentations, the speakers can be upgraded for a higher quality sound.

Species A basic unit of biological classification and a taxonomic rank.

Spinal anesthesia A form of anesthesia that interrupts the function of the nerves.

Spyware Software that secretly gathers information from the user's computer and transmits it to the source.

Standard of care Statements of what a practice believes in and recommends for its patients for wellness testing, pain management, nutrition, senior pet care, and other aspects of patient care.

Statement A document that advises clients of their balance and indicates charges, payments, and the balance of their account for the month that has just concluded; also a request for money.

Steam sterilization The use of heat and moisture to sterilize objects.

Stress The reaction(s) of people and animals to deleterious forces that disturb homeostasis initially provided in nature.

Stressors Produced as a result of stress, and may be internal, external, or environmental.

Substance abuse The use of drugs or alcohol that violates social standards or is self-destructive by nature.

Supportive management Management theory that supports discussion, opinions, and delegation.

Surgical log A log used to record surgeries and controlled substances administered to patients.

System backup Recording the computer data nightly onto another disk or system off premises.

SWOT analysis An internal analysis of a company's strengths, weaknesses, opportunities, and threats.

Tablet Portable computer that allows touch screen and handwriting recognition.

Tangible property Physical property such as desks, chairs, equipment, computers, software, and vehicles that has value.

Target marketing A type of marketing in which a particular segment is picked to received a specific marketing plan.

Technique chart A chart developed for radiographs using the measurement of the animal's thickness in centimeters to determine the correct peak kilovoltage (kVp) setting.

The Right to Know OSHA's standard that every employee has the right to know the hazards associated with their job.

Therapeutic diets Diets recommended by a veterinarian to aid in the treatments of diseases or conditions.

Time and motion Refers to the amount of time and degree of motion required to perform a given task.

Tort A civil offense to an opposing party in which harm has occurred.

Transaction A purchase that must be recorded.

Transferable skills Skills that have been gathered through various jobs, volunteering, work, hobbies, sports, or other life experiences that can be used for career changes.

Travel sheet A sheet that is kept with (travels with) a client record at all times and lists all of the transactions a patient is to be charged for.

Trojan horse A destructive program that inhibits the computer and is generally attached to emails.

URL – Uniform Resource Locator The address of the Web site on the World Wide Web.

USB The most common type of computer port used to connect keyboards, printers, scanners, the Internet, or external drives.

USERRA The Uniformed Services Employment and Reemployment Rights Act was created to protect individuals who are enrolled in any branch of the military service; employers cannot discriminate against past, present, or potential duties that an employee or potential employee serves with the armed forces.

Values Guiding principles that are not to be compromised during change; they provide ethical guidance and will not be violated.

Vaporizer A component of an anesthetic machine that turns liquid into gas.

Variable cost Any cost that varies with the volume of business for the practice. Medical supplies and drugs increase or decrease, depending on the volume of business.

Verbal image The professional image that a person portrays while educating clients. Knowledge of the procedure, clarity of the communication, and correct pronunciation contribute to verbal image.

Veterinarian A professional that has attended a 4-year AVMA accredited program to receive their DVM degree.

Veterinary assistant A team member that assists the veterinarian and technician with animal restraint, procedures and client education.

Veterinary ethics Four branches of veterinary ethics exist: descriptive, official, administrative, and normative ethics.

Veterinary Practice Act Law established within each state outlining veterinary medicine.

Veterinary technician A team member that has attended a 2- or 4-year AVMA accredited program and obtains licensure. This team member assists the veterinarian and may provide client education as needed.

Video graphics card A video graphics card (VGC) enables the computer to display high quality and clear graphics. If the computer will be used for extensive graphic work, the VGC may be upgraded for enhanced performance.

Virus A man-made program that is loaded into a computer and runs against the users wishes. Viruses generally replicate and send themselves to other sites. Viruses tend to use up all of the memory available on a computer, decreasing the processing speed or stopping the system.

Vision The desired future of the practice.

Voice recognition Technology that allows a computer to input information from spoken commands.

VSPN – The Veterinary Support Personnel Network An online, veterinary support staff working with, for, or in the field of veterinary medicine, under the direction of a licensed veterinarian.

VTNE – The Veterinary Technician National Examination The national exam administered to those that have graduated from an AVMA accredited school and who wish to receive credentials within the state they wish to practice.

WAG – Waste anesthetic gases Anesthetic gases that are eliminated from a patient that should be expelled into an anesthetic machine for scavenging.

Waiting period The time between when an application for health insurance has been accepted and the date when the plan goes into effect.

Want list A list developed of needed inventory items.

Web site A site developed on the Internet to market the services available for the practice.

Wireless LAN access point A wireless LAN access point allows several computers to access a network or Internet connection through a single cable modem or DSL connection. Each device requires a wireless card.

Workers' compensation insurance Insurance required by many states that covers accidents that occur on the job site. Some states do not require workers' compensation insurance, but must contribute to a state fund that pays out for accidents that occurred while working.

Worm A program that replicates itself over a computer network and performs malicious actions that can shut the computer system down.

X-ray transformer Controls the amount of radiation emitted from the tube.

X-ray tube Emits radiation and contains the light housing that outlines the area of the radiograph on the table. The light housing allows collimation of the radiograph.

Zip drive A zip drive allows the back up of data and important files. An alternative to backing up files on a zip drive is to back up files on a CD-RW or DVD-RW.

Index

A

AAEVT. *see* American Association of Equine Veterinary Technicians and Assistants (AAEVT).
AAFCO. *see* Association of American Feed Control Officials (AAFCO).
AAHA. *see* American Animal Hospital Association (AAHA).
Abandoned animals, 82
Abbreviations, 271, 271b
  labels, 414b
Abscesses, common feline disorders and, 429
Academy, definition of, 7
Academy of Internal Medicine for Veterinary Technicians (AIMVT), 7b
  requirements for veterinary technician specialties and, 8
Academy of Veterinary Dental Technicians (AVDT), 7b
Academy of Veterinary Emergency and Critical Care Technicians (AVECCT), 7b
Academy of Veterinary Technician Anesthetists (AVTA), 7b
Acceptance, stages of grief and, 234
Accident reporting, 106
  and investigation, 384–387, 384b–387b
Accomplishments, employee, evaluations and, 60–63, 62f
Accountability, team member, 66
Accounting, 330–331
  basics of, 331–336, 331b
Accounts, chart of, 338, 338b, 339f–340f
Accounts payable, 334
Accounts receivable (AR), 307–316, 435
  accepting payment on, 309
  computerized, 309
  definition, 308
  goals for, 308, 308b
  percentages of, 435–436
  report, 311f
  summary of, 332–333, 333b, 333f
Accrual-basis accounting, 331–332, 331b
Acetaminophen. *see* Tylenol.
Acoustics, ergonomics and, 148, 149f
Action paragraph, cover letter and, 451
Active scavenger system, waste anesthetic gases and, 377–378
ADA. *see* Americans with Disabilities Act (ADA).
Adaptation, stress response and, 139
Administrative tasks, in veterinary practice safety, 363, 363b

Administrative veterinary ethics, 77
Admitting procedures, for boarding animals, 431
Adults
  dogs and cats, 422, 422b
  lifetime care and disease prevention for, 406
Advertising
  AVMA Principles of Veterinary Medical Ethics and, 73b–76b
  definition of, 73b–76b
  external marketing and, 194, 194b
Adware, 163b
Aerobic samples, 168
Age Discrimination in Employment Act of 1967, 93
Age requirement. *see also* Age Discrimination in Employment Act of 1967.
  employees and, 89
Agenda, meeting, 59
AIMVT. *see* Academy of Internal Medicine for Veterinary Technicians (AIMVT).
Airborne transmission, 362
Airlines, health certificates and, 25–28, 34f
Alarm, stress response and, 139
Allergies
  canine, 427–428, 427b
  food, 422–424
"Allergy diets," 424
Allowance, insurance and, 319b
Alphabetical filing, 257
  use of color and, 257, 259f
American Animal Hospital Association (AAHA)
  abbreviation summary and, 262
  benchmarking and, 337
  controlled substance log book and, 295
  employment benefits and, 455
  pay scale benchmarks and, 125
American Association of Equine Veterinary Technicians and Assistants (AAEVT), 7b
American Veterinary Medical Association (AVMA), 361
  benchmarking and, 337
  ethical marketing and, 191–194
  ethics and, 73
  open house and, 190
  Principles of Veterinary Medical Ethics, 73, 73b–76b
  veterinary technicians and, 6
  veterinary technologist accredited program and, 7

Americans with Disabilities Act (ADA), 152b
Amphetamines, drug schedule for, 292
Anaerobic cultures, 168
Anal gland impaction and/or infection, 428, 428f
Analgesics, nervous system and, 415
Anaphylactic reaction, 425
Anesthesia, 411
Anesthesia log. *see* Surgical log.
Anesthetic gases, 377–378, 377b–378b
Anesthetic release forms, 23–24, 26f–32f
Animal abuse, 79b
Animal behavior, 368
Animal bites, zoonotic diseases and, 362
Animal care attendants. *see* Kennel assistants.
Animal health technologist (AHT), 6
Animal instinct, basic, 15
Animal Poison Control, 426
Annual deductible, 319–320, 319b
Annual limits, 320
Annual payout limit, 319b
Annual policy, 320
Annual revenue per patient (ARPP), 333
Answering machine, 19
Antacids, gastric drugs and, 415
Anti-inflammatories, 414
Anticoagulants, 167
Anticonvulsants, nervous system and, 415
Antidiarrheals, 415
Antifreeze ingestion, 425, 425b
Antimicrobials, 414
Antiparasitics, 414
Antiseptics, 415
Antitussives, respiratory system and, 416
Antiulcer drugs, gastric drugs and, 415
Antivirus software, 163
Any occupation disability insurance, 103
Apomorphine, toxicities and, 426
Appearance
  and code of conduct, 105
  of practice brochure, 201
Appointment, 240
  entering of, 249–253
  length of time of, 244–246, 245b
  management of, 237–254, 240b, 248b
  no-show, 249, 249b
  preparing for, 253, 253b
  reminding clients of, 251
  scheduling, factors in, 244–247
  turning phone calls into, 19–20, 20b
  type of, 247, 249f
  units for schedule, 251, 251f
  of veterinary technician, 244, 245f

Note: Page numbers followed by *f* indicate figures; *t* indicate tables; *b* indicates boxes.

Appointment book template, designing of, 241–244, 243b
Appointment cards, 249, 249b, 249f–250f
Appointment scheduler, software programs and, 241
Appointment software, benefit of, 247
Appointment system
    goals of, 240
    training new employees for, 251–253
Appreciation, of client, 224
AR. *see* Accounts receivable (AR).
Arthritis, diet and, 424
Arthropods, as vectors, 362
Ashes. *see* Remains.
ASP Tactical Baton, 396, 396f
Assessment, SOAP format and, 265, 266f
Asset, 331b
Association of American Feed Control Officials (AAFCO), 416–419
    large-breed puppies and, 420
    nutrient requirements and, 417t–419t
Asthma, common feline disorders and, 430
Attending veterinarian, 73b–76b
Attitude
    negative, burnout and, 142
    positive, 447
Autoclaves, safety protocols and, 387
AVDT. *see* Academy of Veterinary Dental Technicians (AVDT).
AVECCT. *see* Academy of Veterinary Emergency and Critical Care Technicians (AVECCT).
Average client transactions (ACTs), 333
Average doctor transaction, 334
AVMA. *see* American Veterinary Medical Association (AVMA).
AVMA Code of Ethics, in emergency animal care, 80–81
AVMA Judicial Council, 73b–76b
AVTA. *see* Academy of Veterinary Technician Anesthetists (AVTA).

B
Back injury
    in ergonomics, 369
    lifting and, 371, 371f
Back order, 283–284
Background check, 111
Backing up, 164, 164b, 272
    to CD or DVD, 162
Backup device, 157b–159b
Backup system, 159b
Bacterial infection, zoonotic diseases and, 360t–361t
Bad debt, 313
Bad news, 215
Balance sheet, 331b, 338
Balancing accounts, 39
Bandannas, internal marketing and, 189, 189f
Bang's disease. *see* Brucellosis (Bang's disease).
Barbiturates, drug schedule for, 292
Bargaining, stages of grief and, 234–235
Bathing, safety protocols for, 387
Bayer Veterinary Care Usage Study (BVCUS), 325, 325b, 325f

Bedding, animal, chemotherapeutic agents and, 377
Behavior, substance abuse and, 141
Benchmarking, 337, 337b
Benefit
    insurance and, 319b
    of pet health insurance, 321, 321b
Benefits, employee, 101–102, 102b
    continuing education (CE) and, 104, 104b
    interview questions and, 455
Benefits statement, employee, 102, 102b
Billing cycle, 309
Biohazards, in veterinary practice, 381–382, 381f, 382b
    containers, 381, 381f
    materials, 382f
Birth weight
    of kittens, 422
    of puppies, 419–420
Bites. *see* Animal bites.
Biweekly payroll, 124–125
Blankets, condo facilities and, 432
Bleeding, emergencies and, 425
Blocked cat, emergencies and, 425
Blogs, 198–199
Blood pressure, 408
Blood tubes, 167f
Blood work, 407, 407t
    preanesthetic documentation and, 411
Board of Veterinary Medicine, common complaints to, 83–85, 84b
Boarding
    facility for, 431–432
    forms for, 29, 35f–36f
    written communication and, 211, 212f
Body bag, 231, 231f
Body condition score
    in cats, 422, 423f
    in dogs, 420, 421f
Body language, 213–214
    marketing programs and, 206
Body positioning, 147–148, 148f
Body posture, nonverbal skills and, 214, 214f
Bonus
    employee rewards and, 127
    production, 125
Bookkeeper, 330–331
Bookkeeping, 330–331
Bordetella, kennel cough and, 428–429
Borrowing money, 353
Bottle feeding, of neonate kittens, 422
Bovine viral diarrhea (BVD), 405b
Branding, 184
Breach of duty, 81–82
Break-even analysis, 286, 353, 353b, 439
    example of, 286b
Breaks
    burnout prevention and, 142
    coping with stress and, 141
Broadband, 157b–159b
Brochure, practice, marketing and, 201–202, 201b, 202f–203f
Bronchodilators, respiratory system and, 416
Brucellosis (Bang's disease), 405b

Buddy system, team member security and, 395
Budget
    creating a, 348–354, 349b
    for hardware, 160
    as management tool, 330, 331b
    raises and, 127
    for software, 161
    steps, 349–352
Bulk order, 284, 438–439
    example of, 284b
Burnout, prevention of, 142–143, 142b–143b, 142f
Business cards, 200–201, 201b
Busy times, management during, 248, 248b
Buzzers, at front doors, 394
BVD. *see* Bovine viral diarrhea (BVD).

C
"C," controlled substance identification, 292, 292f
Calculations, 434–445
    drug, 443b
    IV fluid, 445b
Call center, 19, 19f
Call tag, returning products and, 285
Calories
    adult foods and, 422
    growing puppies and kittens and, 404
    large-breed puppies and, 420
    unit of measurement, 416
Cameras, and recording devices, 395, 395f
Campbell Interest and Skill Survey (CISS), 447
Candidates, hire, using social media to review, 110
Canine disorders, common, 427–429
Canine hip dysplasia, 420
Canine parvovirus (CPV), 403b
Capital inventory, 288, 289f
Car accident, emergencies and, 426
Carbohydrates
    cats and, 422
    nutrient requirements and, 418
Carcinogen
    sample submission and, 167–168
    special chemicals and, 376
Card reader/writer, 157b–159b
Cardiac drugs, 415
Cardiopulmonary resuscitation (CPR), 425
Cardiorespiratory arrest, 425
CareCredit, 35–39, 308
Career days, community service and, 194
Career instability, substance abuse and, 141
Career planning, 447
Caring, clients and, 214
Carnivores, 422
Carpal tunnel syndrome, 369
Cash
    embezzlement and, 135
    theft of, 347
Cash-basis accounting, 331–332, 331b
Cash drawer, 41, 41f
Cash flow, 354–355
    statement, 331b

Cash payments, 37
deposits of, 41
Cashier's check, 38
Cat, bags for, 401–402, 402f
Cattle, diseases of, 405b
CBC. *see* Complete blood count (CBC).
CD, 157b–159b
backing up medical records and, 261
on-hold messaging and, 203–204
CD drive, 157b–159b
CE. *see* Continuing education (CE).
Central inventory locations, 282
Central processing unit (CPU), 157b–159b
Centrifuge, 167
Certified letter, 313
Certified public accountant (CPA), 331
Chair, ergonomic design guidelines for, 150f
Chamber of Commerce, 196–197
Change, resistance to, 57
Charcoal, adsorption scavenger and, 378
Check machine, fraud and embezzlement and, 348
Check payments, 37–38, 41
machines for, 37–38, 41, 41f
Check-writing programs, computerized, 349
Checks and balances system, 41
Chemical hazards, in veterinary practice, 373–378, 373b
Chemical inventory list, in veterinary practice, 373–374, 374f
Chemical name, for drugs, 412
Chemical spills, 379–381
cleanup procedures for, 380, 381f
Chemistries, laboratory tests and, 168t
Chemotherapeutic agents, 376–377, 376f, 377b
Children
death of pet and, 235
reception area and, 14–15
Choice, stress and, 138–139, 138b
Chronic conditions, 321, 321f
Chronological order, resume and, 452
Chute, large animal safety protocol and, 387
CISS. *see* Campbell Interest and Skill Survey (CISS).
Civil law, 78, 78b
Civil Rights Act of 1964, Title VII, 93
Claim, insurance
definition of, 319b
filing of, 321–324, 322f–323f
Claim payment delay, 321–324
Class I drugs, 292
Class II drugs, 292
Cleaning chemicals, housekeeping and, 430
Client collection, pricing and, 326
Client communication, 211–226, 211f
barriers to, 214–215
Client complaints, 224–226, 224b
Client compliance, 216–220, 216b
marketing and, 185, 186f, 207
Client discharge instructions, 83, 267–270, 268b, 269f–270f

Client education, 218f, 220f
ensuring understanding and, 222
length of time for, 246, 253b
Client grievances, 224–226, 225b
Client identification numbers, 259
Client instructions, Web page and, 197
Client/patient information sheet, 22f–23f, 262
Client relations, 21–22, 22f
Client retention, 226–227, 226b
Client service manual, client questions and, 213
Clients
angry, 31
arriving on wrong day, 249
copy of record and, 261
credit cards, fraud and embezzlement and, 348
drugs or alcohol and, 32
as factor in appointment scheduling, 247, 247b
grieving, 31
habitually late, 247–248
indirect marketing and, 184
invoices review and, 33, 36f
laboratory analysis costs and, 175, 175b
nonpayment and, 309
and patients, active/new, number of, 334, 334b
personal contact information and, 22
phone techniques with, 16–17, 17f
prospective, external marketing and, 190
role of receptionist and, 8
special situations with, 29–33, 32b
surveys, 224, 224b, 225f, 334, 334b, 335f
understanding, 218f, 222–223, 222b–223b
visits, managing of, 346, 346b
waiting, 42–43, 43b, 43f
Clinic tour, in Web page, 198
Clinical assisting, 399–433
Closed bottle sheet, 295–296
Closed-ended questions, 110–111
Clostridial infection
in cattle, 405b
in sheep and goats, 405b
Co-pay, 319b, 320
Coagulation, laboratory tests and, 168t
COBRA. *see* Consolidated Omnibus Budget Reconciliation Act (COBRA).
Code of conduct, 105
Code of ethics, 73–77, 77b
of National Association of Veterinary Technicians in America (NAVTA), 77, 77b
Colic, equine emergencies and, 427
Collection letter, 313–314, 313b, 314f
Collection procedure, 311–313, 312f
Collections agency, 314–315, 314b
Collimation, 382
Color, ergonomics and, 149, 151b
Common emergencies
bovine and, 427
equine and, 427
ovine and caprine and, 427
small animal and, 425–427

Communication
of groomers, 4
ideas to increase, 57b
methods of, 57–63, 57b
poor, complaints and, 83
reducing expenses, 346
in teamwork, 3
veterinary clients and, 211–212, 211f, 214b, 215
written, 211
client compliance and, 216
Community service, 194, 194b–195b
Compassion fatigue, 143–145, 143b, 143f
impact of
on individuals, 144
on practice, 144, 144f
management of, 144–145, 145b
signs and symptoms of, 144
Competition, salary and, 126
Competitive intelligence information, 182–183
Complaint, 83
Complete blood count (CBC), 167
Compliance rates, 334–335, 336f
Compliment, employee retention and, 123
Computed tomographic (CT) scanning, 410
Computer access, paperless records and, 260
Computer hacker, 393
Computer hardware, local support and, 162
Computer system
backing up of, 272, 272b
costs of, 162
security of, 393, 393b
Computerized medical records, 258–261, 259b–260b, 260f
Computers
hardware and, 159, 159b
location of, 160, 160b
software and, 159
types of, 160
Conceptual skill, 50
Condo facilities, 432
Conduct, correct, 83
Confidence, of team member, 215
Confidentiality, employee manual and, 101b, 105
Conflict
extent of, 63b
issues that cause, 63
with manager, 64
Conflict management, 63–64, 63b
Conflict resolution, 64b
Congenital conditions, 320–321
Congestion, in reception area, 149
Consensus, 59, 59b, 59f
Consent, 79
Consent forms, 23–24, 26f–32f, 79, 80f–81f
medical record inclusions and, 262
Consequences, stress and, 138–139, 138b
Consolidated Omnibus Budget Reconciliation Act (COBRA), 123
Consultation rooms, 152
Consulting veterinarian, 73b–76b
Contact information, resume and, 452

Continuing education (CE), 104, 104b
  burnout prevention and, 142, 142f
  employee retention and, 122
  as factor in appointment scheduling,
    247
  manufacturer and distributor
    representatives and, 276
  providing all levels of, 121–122, 122b
  software training and, 163
Contract employee *versus* employee,
  131–135, 132b
  Form 1099-MISC and, 135
Contract law, 79
Control, stress and, 138–139, 138b
Controlled substances, 291–300, 292f
  Employee Polygraph Protection Act,
    exemptions and, 93
  expired, 285
  fraud and embezzlement and, 348
  law, 300b
  loss reporting, 298, 298b
  management of, 295–298, 295b, 297b
  record keeping, 295
  registration, 293
  schedules of drugs, 292–293,
    292b–293b, 293t
  security and protection, 295, 295b
  substance disposal, 298–300
Controlled Substances Act of 1970, 292,
  293t
Controlled substances log, 302, 302b
Conversions, 434–445, 443b
Cookies, 163b
Copiers, 165
Coping, with stress, 140–141, 140b
Coronavirus, 403b
Correction, of medical record, 257, 257b
Cost analysis, 162, 162b
Cost-benefit analysis, 191
Cost-benefit ratio, 188
Cost of goods (COGs), 334
  expenses, 341b
  fees, reducing expenses and, 346–347
  variable expenses and, 339
Cost-of-living, raises and, 127
Cost of supplies, 349–350, 351f–352f
Cots, raised, condo facilities and, 432
Counterfeit money, 37
Cover letter, 451, 451b, 452f
CPA. *see* Certified public accountant
  (CPA).
CPR. *see* Cardiopulmonary resuscitation
  (CPR).
CPV. *see* Canine parvovirus (CPV).
Credit bureau, 312, 312b
Credit card payments, 35
  storage of slips for, 41
Credit card slips, 41
Credit cards charges, reducing expenses
  and, 346
Credit reporting agencies, 111
Cremations, 231–234
Crime, 79
Criminal intent, 393–394
Criminal law, 78, 79b
Critical competencies
  accounts receivable, 307
  appointment management, 239–240

Critical competencies *(Continued)*
  client communication and customer
    service, 210–211
  controlled substances, 291–292
  finance management, 329–330
  interacting with grieving client, 228
  inventory management, 274–275
  marketing, 181–182
  medical records management, 255–256
  pet health insurance and wellness
    plans, 317–318
  practice design, 146
  safety in veterinary practice, 358–359
  security, 392
  stress, burnout and compassion fatigue,
    137–145
  technology in office, 155–156
Cross-training
  invoices review and, 33
  reception desk and, 19
CT scanning. *see* Computed tomographic
  (CT) scanning.
Cultural differences, barriers to client
  communication and, 214
Culture samples, 168
Cultures, creating positive, 53–54, 53b
  preventing burnout, 54
  understanding diversity, 53–54, 53t–54t
  work and life balance, 54, 54b
Current Veterinary Therapy, 320
Customer service, 3, 226, 226b, 346
  client compliance and, 216–220
  marketing and, 183
Customization, computer software and,
  160
Cyanotic mucous membranes, 401
Cystocentesis, urinalysis and, 407
Cytology, 407
Cytology samples, submission of, 168,
  168b

D
Daily energy requirement (DER), of
  kittens, 422
Daily reconciliation, 39–41, 39b, 39f–41f
Daily routine, death of pet and, 235
Data conversion, 162
DEA. *see* Drug Enforcement
  Administration (DEA).
DEA form 106, 298, 299f
DEA form 222, 292–293, 294b, 294f
  schedule II drugs and, 298
DEA license, 293
Deadbolts, 393
Death
  in hospital, 231
  stress response and, 139
  unexpected, 83
Debit transactions, 33, 35
Decision making, 59, 59f
Declined transactions, 38–39, 38b
Deductibles, insurance and, 319–320,
  319b
Defense, methods of, 396, 396b
Degree, resume listing and, 452
Delegation, 56–57, 56b–57b, 56f
Delinquent checks, 308–309
Demodex, 429

Demonstration, selecting software and,
  161
Denial, stages of grief and, 234–235
Dental procedures, as factor in
  appointment scheduling, 246, 246f
Dependence, substance, 141–142
Deposit slip, 41, 42f
Deposits, 41
  check payment and, 41
Depression, stages of grief and, 234, 234b
DER. *see* Daily energy requirement
  (DER).
Descriptive ethics, 77
Desktop, 157b–159b
Diabetes, diet and, 424
Diagnosis report, medical record
  inclusions and, 262
Diagnostic flow sheet, laboratory, 262
Diagnostic imaging, 408–411
Diagnostic laboratory, 166–180. *see also*
  Outside laboratory.
  choosing of, 167
Diagnostics, 407–408
Diarrhea, fecal analysis and, 408
Diet
  conditions that can be treated/
    maintained by, 422–425
  frequently asked questions for, 18
  homemade, 418, 418b
  hypoallergenic, 422–424, 427
Digital camera, 157b–159b, 164–165,
  164b
Digital subscriber line (DSL), 157b–159b
Digital versatile disc (DVD), 157b–159b
Digoxin, laboratory tests and, 168t
Dipping, safety protocols for, 387
Direct costs, 344, 440
Direct deposit, 128
Direct supervision, 6
Directive management, theory of, 52
Disability insurance, 103
Discharge
  client instructions for, 83, 267–270,
    268b, 269f–270f
  complaints and, 83
Discharge sheets, 83, 268, 271b
Discount clubs, 324
Discounts, 344–345
  employee, 104–105, 105b
  per veterinarian, 334, 334b
Discrepancies
  drug, 296
  potential causes of, 287–288
Discrimination, 93
Disease prevention, and lifetime care,
  402–407
Disease transmission, 362
Diseases, 403–404, 403b
  common canine infectious, 403b
  common feline infectious, 404b
  common large animal, 405b
  tests available for common, 406t
  vaccinations and, 402–403
Disinfectants, 415
Dispensing, definition of, 73b–76b
Dispensing fees, 287, 439
Disrespect, team member complaints
  and, 83

Dissatisfaction, owner complaints and, 83
Distemper
    in canine, 403b
    in equine, 405b
Distributor representatives, 276–277
Diuretics, 415
DLH. *see* Domestic longhair (DLH).
DMH. *see* Domestic medium hair
    (DMH).
Docking station, 157b–159b
Doctor compensation, 328
Domain name, 196
Domestic longhair (DLH), 22
Domestic medium hair (DMH), 22
Domestic shorthair (DSH), 22
Donations, as external marketing, 205, 205b
Dosimeter, 383, 383f, 409
Dosimetry
    badges, radiation exposure and, 383
    reports, 383, 384f
Down cow, common bovine emergencies
    and, 427
Driver's license number, 309
Drop-off, patient, 249
Drug calculations, 442–445, 443b
    common conversions in, 443b
Drug Enforcement Administration
    (DEA), 285, 292
    controlled drug loss or theft and, 298
    controlled substances log and, 302
    record inspection and, 295
Drug intervention, 141–142, 141b
    steps of, 142
Drug logs, 295
Drugs, 415b
    categories of, 414–416
    expired, *see* Medication, expired.
    inventory management of, 276
    names for, 412
    theft of, 394
Dry matter basis, 416
DSH. *see* Domestic shorthair (DSH).
Duties
    delegation of, 56–57
    of team members, 107, 108b
DVD, internal marketing and, 189
DVD drives, 157b–159b
DVM costs per minute, 343–344, 440
DVM expenses, 334
Dyspneic animal, 425
Dystocia
    common bovine emergencies and, 427
    small animal emergencies and, 426

E
Ear infection, common canine disorders
    and, 428
Eating habits, coping with stress and, 140
ECG. *see* Electrocardiogram (ECG).
EDTA (ethylenediaminetetraacetic acid),
    167
Education
    client, 202b
        compliance and, 218, 218f, 222
        euthanasia process and, 230
        materials for, 197, 197f, 202–203, 204f
        newspaper ads and, 194
    for professional development, 449

Educational information, 218–220,
    218b–219b, 218f–220f
Effective listening, leaders and, 51
Effective practices, design and function
    of, 149
Ehrlichiosis. *see* Potomac horse fever
    (ehrlichiosis).
EHV-1. *see* Rhinopneumonitis (EHV-1).
Electrical safety, in veterinary practice,
    368, 368f
Electrocardiogram (ECG), 408
    preanesthetic documentation and, 411
Electronic medical records (EMRs), 66
Email address, 199
Email etiquette, 215–216
Embezzlement, 135–136, 309
Emergencies
    adapting schedule for, 247
    bovine, 427
    equine, 427
    ovine and caprine, 427
    small animal, 425–427
Emergency action plan (EAP), 368–369,
    369b
Emergency calls, security and, 395
Emergency care, 79–81
Emergency clinic, safety precautions and,
    394
Emergency pay, 126
Emergency situations, kennel assistant
    and, 5
Emotional intelligence (EI), 51–52, 52b
Employee
    accounts, fraud and embezzlement and,
        348
    accounts receivable, 315, 315b
    development, 88
    empowerment of, 55–56, 56b
    responsibilities, in veterinary practice
        safety, 363
    survey, 62–63, 62f
        guidelines for creating, 63b
    theft, 393, 394b
Employee manual
    code of conduct, 105
    developing of, 100–106, 100b–101b,
        112b–113b, 113, 114f–116f
    implementing of, 113–114, 114b
    laws of importance and, 106–107
    updating of, 114–115
    workplace problem solving and, 99,
        99f–100f, 100b
Employee Polygraph Protection Act, 93, 93b
    required poster for, 96f
Employee Retirement Income Security
    Act (ERISA), 104
Employer
    questions to ask potential, 455b
    responsibilities, in veterinary practice
        safety, 363
Employment
    data, preparation of, 451–453
    eligibility verification form. *see* Form
        I-9 (employment eligibility
        verification).
    history, 453
    opportunities, 450–451, 450b–451b, 450f
    receiving offers of, 456

Empowerment, 55–56, 56b
Encephalomyelitis, 405b
End-of-day reconciliation, 39, 45t
    fraud and embezzlement and, 347–348
Endocrine drugs, 415
Endocrinology, laboratory tests and, 168t
Endotracheal tubes, 411, 412f
Enthusiasm, leaders and, 51
Entrances, protection of, 393
Entries, blocked, 371
Environment, evaluating oneself and, 449
Equal Employment Opportunity (EEO)
    policy, 93, 93b
    required poster for, 97f
Equine diseases, 405b
Equipment
    budget for, 352–353
    capital inventory, 288
    inventory of, 335, 336f
    moving, 371
Equity, 331b
Ergonomics, 148, 369, 369b
ERISA. *see* Employee Retirement Income
    Security Act (ERISA).
Escaping animals, safety protocol and,
    369–370, 369f
Estimates, 220–222, 221f
    medical record inclusions and, 262
Ethical product, definition of, 73b–76b
Ethics, 73
Ethylene oxide, 376, 376f
Ethylenediaminetetraacetic acid. *see*
    EDTA.
Etiquette
    definition of, 15
    of receptionist team, 15–16, 15b
Euthanasia
    AVMA Principles of Veterinary
        Medical Ethics and, 73b–76b
    definition of, 230
    etiquette during, 15
    procedure for, 230–231, 231f
    release form for, 23–24, 26f–32f, 230
    understanding of, 230, 230b
Evaluations
    employees and, 60–63, 61b, 62f, 63b
    raises and, 127
Event calendar, in Web page, 198
Exam room, 206, 206b
    creating comfortable, 150–152, 151f
    report card, internal marketing and,
        190, 192f
Examinations, 401–402, 402b
Exceptional finale, creating an, 43–44, 43f
Exclusion(s), 319b, 321
Exemptions, from FLSA, 89
Exercise
    burnout prevention and, 142
    coping with stress and, 140, 140f
Exhaustion, stress response and, 139
Exit signs, 370f
    and lighting, 370, 370b, 370f
Exits, blocked, 371
Expenses, 338–339
    administrative, 341b
    areas of, 352–354
    budget and, 349–350, 350f–352f
    cost of goods, 341b

Expenses *(Continued)*
  facility, 341b
  staff, 341b
  veterinary related, 341b–342b
Expiration date, 284
External hard drive, 157b–159b
Eye contact, nonverbal skills and, 214
Eyewash stations, 380–381, 380b, 381f

F

Facial expressions, nonverbal skills and, 214
Facilitator, meeting, 58
Facility budget, 354, 354b
Fair Credit Reporting Act, 111
Fair Debt Collection Practices Act of 1996, 313, 315b
Fair Labor and Standards Act (FLSA), 89, 89b, 93, 93b
  required poster for, 94f
Family and Medical Leave Act (FMLA), 89, 93, 93b
  required poster for, 95f
FAQs. *see* Frequently asked questions (FAQs).
Fatigue, compassion, 143–145, 143b, 143f
Fats, nutrient requirements and, 418
FCV. *see* Feline calicivirus (FCV).
FDA. *see* Federal Drug Administration (FDA)
Fecal analysis, 408
Federal Drug Administration (FDA), expired medication and, 284
Federal income tax withholding form. *see* Form W-4.
Federal Insurance Contribution Act (FICA), Social Security and Medicare and, 129
Federal tax deposit (FTD) system, 129
Federal Unemployment Tax Act (FUTA), 129, 129b
Fee schedule, 343–344, 343b
Fee setting, appropriate, 66–68, 67b
Fee splitting, 73b–76b
Feedback, 191
Feeding, 404–405
  of kittens, 405
  methods of, 420
Feelings, expressing of, coping with stress and, 140–141
Fees, laboratory, 175, 175b
Fees and remuneration, AVMA Principles of Veterinary Medical Ethics and, 73b–76b
Feline calicivirus (FCV), 404b
Feline disorders, common, 429–430
Feline immunodeficiency virus (FIV), 404b
Feline infectious peritonitis (FIP), 404b
Feline leukemia virus (FeLV), 404b
Feline lower urinary tract disease (FLUTD), 430
Feline panleukopenia (FPV), 404b
Feline pneumonitis chlamydia, 404b
Feline viral rhinotracheitis (FVR), 404b
Felony, 79
FeLV. *see* Feline leukemia virus (FeLV).

Feral animals, safety precautions and, 369–370
Fetotomy, dystocia and, 427
FICA. *see* Federal Insurance Contribution Act (FICA).
FICA Form 8109, 130f
Fight or flight, stress response and, 139
File system, 257
File transfer protocol. *see* FTP.
Finance charge, 310, 314b
Finance management, 329–357
Financial reports, creating of, 337–338, 338b
FIP. *see* Feline infectious peritonitis (FIP).
Fire codes, 370
Fire extinguishers, 370–371, 370f
Fire prevention, 370–371
Fire response, 371, 371b
Fire safety, 370–371
Firewalls, 163, 163b
First Notice of Accident or Injury and Illness Incident Report, 383–384
FIV. *see* Feline immunodeficiency virus (FIV).
Fixed costs, 331b
  per minute, 343, 440
Fixed expenses, 339, 339b
Flea and tick preventive, frequently asked questions for, 18
Floors, wet, safety hazards and, 373
Floppy disk drive, 157b–159b
FLSA. *see* Fair Labor and Standards Act (FLSA).
Fluids, medical records and, 266
Fluoroscopy, 410
FLUTD. *see* Feline lower urinary tract disease (FLUTD).
FMLA. *see* Family and Medical Leave Act (FMLA).
Folded arms, nonverbal skills and, 213–214, 213f
Follow-up letter, 455–456
Fomite (fome), boarding and, 431
Food and Drug Administration (FDA), 284
  laboratory guidelines and, 167, 167b
Food-restricted feedings, 420
Foodborne diseases, contaminated food and, 362
Form 940, IRS, 131f
Form 941, IRS, 132f
Form 1099-MISC, 128f
  independent groomers, 127
Form I-9 (employment eligibility verification), 89–93, 90f–92f, 93b
  IRCA and, 89–93
Form W-2, 129, 135f
Form W-4, 129, 133f–134f
Formal greeting, of cover letter, 451, 452f
Formaldehyde, 376, 376b
Formalin, tissue transport and, 167
Forms
  boarding and, 29, 35f–36f
  consent forms and, 23–24, 26f–32f
  controlled substance
    DEA form 106, 298
    DEA form 222 and, 292–293, 294b, 294f

Forms *(Continued)*
  downloadable, 198
  euthanasia release forms and, 23–24, 26f–32f
  "first report of injury," 129
  health certificates and, 25–28, 34f
  laboratory, 168–173, 169f–173f
  medical record and, 22, 24f–25f
  patient history and, 24–25
  payroll tax
    FICA Form 8109, 130f
    IRS Form 940, 131f
    IRS Form 941, 132f
  rabies certificates and, 24
  release form and, 28–29, 29b
  vaccination release forms and, 23–24, 26f–32f
  in veterinary practice, 22–29, 22b
Four R's of team management, 55
Foursquare, 199
FPN. *see* Feline pneumonitis chlamydia (FPN).
FPV. *see* Feline panleukopenia (FPV).
Fraud and embezzlement, 347–348, 347b–348b
  decrease practice risk of, 348, 348b
Free catch, urine collection and, 407, 408f
Free-choice feeding, 420
Free doses, 288
Frequently asked questions (FAQs), 17
Front desk chaos, 42
FTD. *see* Federal tax deposit (FTD) system.
FTP (file transfer protocol), 195
Full paper records, 257
Full-time employment, 101
  benefits and, 101–102
Full-time students, FLSA exemptions and, 89
Fungal diseases, zoonotic diseases and, 360t–361t
FUTA. *see* Federal Unemployment Tax Act (FUTA).
FVR. *see* Feline viral rhinotracheitis (FVR).

G

Gag reflex, of neonate kittens, 422
Gastric drugs, 415
Gastric torsion, emergencies and, 426
Gastroenteritis, 424
  canine, 424
  feline, 424
Gastrointestinal tract, gastric drugs and, 415
GB. *see* Gigabyte (GB).
Gender, determination of, 411
Generations, in veterinary practice
  personal and lifestyle characteristics of, 53t
  workplace values as seen, 54t
Generic name, for drugs, 412
Genetic defects, 73b–76b
Gift certificates, 205, 205f
Gigabyte (GB), 157b–159b
Gingivitis, in canine, 428
Gloves, 382, 383f
Glucocorticoids, 414

Glutaraldehyde, 376
Goals
    of drug intervention, 141–142
    marketing strategy and, 183
    mission statement and, 101
    personal, 450
Goats, diseases of, 405b
Goodwill, practice, intangible property
        and, 105
Gossip, 63
Gouging, production salary and, 126
Graphics card, 157b–159b
Green-topped tube, with serum separator,
        167f
Grief
    children and, 235
    five stages of, 234
    understanding and dealing with, 229b,
        234–235
Grievances, handling of, 224–226
Grieving clients, 31
    interacting with, 228–236
Gripe session, 59
Groomer
    as career, 4, 4f
    independent, 127
    payroll and, 127
    responsibilities of, 4b
    as veterinary team member, 4
Gross pay, 442
    definition of, 126
Gross revenue, accounts receivable and,
        308, 308b, 435
Guardian ad litem, 82
Guilt, over animal death, 235

H
Hacker, 163b
Hallucinogens, drug schedule and, 292
Hands-on training, 116
Handwriting recognition, 157b–159b
Hard costs, 286, 286b
Hard drive, 157b–159b
Hard skills, 107
Hardware, 159, 159b
    selection of, 160
Hazard analysis, 363–365
    example of, 365f
Hazard Communication Standard, 363
Hazardous items, mailing of, 179b
Hazardous materials identification system
        (HMIS II) label, 378
Health certificates, 25–28, 34f
    international, 28
    interstate, 25–28, 34f
Health insurance
    employee benefits and, 103
    reducing expenses, 346
Health maintenance organization (HMO),
        health insurance and, 103
Health plans, suggested, 326b
Hearing protection, 372, 372b
Heart disease, diet and, 424
Heartworm preventative, frequently asked
        questions and, 18
Heating/cooling, ergonomics and, 148
Heatstroke, emergencies and, 426
Hematology, laboratory tests and, 168t

Hepatitis, 403b
Herd health records, 266
Hereditary conditions, 320–321, 320f
Heroin, class I drugs and, 292
Hiring, 109–112, 109b–110b
Histopathology
    preanesthetic documentation and, 411
    tissue samples for, 167
History taking, 262–264, 263b
    examinations and, 401
HMO. see Health maintenance
        organization (HMO).
Holding checks, 309
Holiday
    community service and, 195
    as factor in appointment scheduling, 247
Holiday pay, 104
Hospital administrator
    sample job description for, 108b
    as veterinary health team member, 10
Hospital safety manual (HSM), 390
Hospitalization sheets, 265, 268f
Host
    computer, 163b
    in disease transmission, 362
Hot spots, allergies and, 429
House calls, euthanasia and, 230
Housekeeping, clinical assisting and,
        430–431, 430b
Human-animal bond, 229, 235b, 318
    children and, 234, 234f
    understanding of, 206, 229–230, 229b,
        229f
Human resources, 86–136
    contract employee versus employee,
        131–135
    employee manual of, 93–107
    employee procedure manual of,
        112–115
    hiring the perfect team of, 109–112
    job descriptions and duties of, 107–109
    laws requiring familiarity, 88–93
    organizational behavior of, 88
    payroll of, 124–129
    personnel files of, 129–131
    social media policy of, 107
    standards of care (SOCs), 115
    team training, 115–123
    termination, 123–124
    theft and embezzlement, 135–136
    workers' compensation insurance, 129
Human skill, 50
Humane Society of the United States,
        24–25
Hyperlinks, 196
Hyperthyroidism
    common feline disorders and, 430
    endocrine drugs and, 415
Hypothyroidism
    in canine, 428
    endocrine drugs and, 415

I
IBR. see Infectious bovine rhinotracheitis
        (IBR).
ICANN. see Internet Corporation for
        Assigned Names and Numbers
        (ICANN).

IM (intramuscular), medication
        administration and, 413
Immigration Reform and Control Act
        (IRCA), 89–93, 93b
    form I-9 and, 89–93
Immune system, compromised, zoonotic
        diseases and, 362
Immunology, laboratory tests and, 168t
Impending laws, in veterinary practice, 82
In-house laboratory, 167
In-house use, discrepancies and, 288
Inability to pay, emergency treatment
        and, 81
Incident, insurance and, 319b
Income, budget and, 350–352, 352f,
        353b
Income centers, 334, 338, 338b, 340f–341f
    development and management,
        345–346, 346b
    vs. expense centers, 342–343, 343b
Income statement, 331b
Incorporeal property. see Intangible
        property.
Indemnity insurance, 318–321, 319b
Independent contractor, 132
Index card records, 257, 258f
Indigent account, 308
Individual Retirement Account (IRA). see
        SIMPLE IRA (sIRA).
Indoor air quality, 371
Infectious bovine rhinotracheitis (IBR),
        405b
Influences on judgment, AVMA
        Principles of Veterinary Medical
        Ethics and, 73b–76b
Influenza, 405b
Information
    informed consent and, 79
    manufacturer and distributor, 276
    for safety protocol, 390
Information age, 156
Information systems, 156–159,
        157b–159b
Informed consent, 79
Ingredients, diet and, 416
Injection fees, 287, 287b, 439–440
Injuries
    prevention of, 149
    reporting of, 106
    workers' compensation insurance and,
        129
Inkjet printer, 160
Innovation, awareness on, leaders and, 51
Inpatient charge, missed, 66
Insufficient funds, 308–309, 308f
Insulin, endocrine drugs and, 415
Insurance, 103, 103b
    fraud, 328b
    terminated employee and, 123
Insurance agents, 103
Insurance company
    brochures for, 325
    diseases, coverage of, 321
Insurance rates, 319b
Intangible property, 331b
    goodwill and, 105
Intentional tort, 78–79
Interest rate, 310

Internal Revenue Service (IRS)
  cash-basis accounting and, 332
  employee discounts, 104
  payroll and, 124
International health certificates, 28
Internet, 163b
  educational information and, 218–219
  as information source, 3
  safety practices, 164b
  terms for, 163b
Internet Corporation for Assigned Names
    and Numbers (ICANN), 196
Internet security, 163
  terms for, 163b
Interstate health certificates, 25–28, 34f
Intervention
  drug addiction and, 141
  steps of, 142
  substance abuse and, 141–142, 141b
Interview
  follow-up after, 455–456
  preparing for an, 453–455, 455b
  questions, 455b
  rules, 454b
Interview questions, hiring
  to ask, 110–111, 110f, 111b
  not to ask, 111, 111b
Intravenous drip, medical records and,
    266
Intravenous fluid calculations, 445, 445b
Inventory, 289b
  consolidating, 280, 280b
  of controlled substances, 295
  fraud and embezzlement and, 348
  fundamentals of, 275–276, 275b–276b
  on hand, 336
  hidden holding costs associated with,
      286b
  hidden ordering costs associated with,
      286b
  large, disadvantages of, 280b
  manual, 276, 276b, 276f
  policies manual topics, 276b
  pricing strategies, 439–440
  protection, 287–288
  software, 282
  storage, 282
  turns per year, 281b, 436
Inventory management, 66, 274–290
  capital inventory, 288
  decreasing loss, 288–289
  designing an, 277–280
  distributors and manufacturer
      representatives, 276–277
  effective pricing strategies, 285–287
  expiration date, 284
  fundamentals of, 275–276
  handling expired medications, 284–285
  inventory protection, 287–288
  keys to, 276b
  losses associated with poor, 276b
  outsourcing products, 287
  preparing orders, 282–284
  receiving orders, 284
  reorder points, 281
  reorder quantities, 281
  safety data sheets, 288
  storage, 282

Inventory management (Continued)
  system, 275, 276b, 277–280, 277f–279f
  turnover rates, 280–281
Invoices
  client complaint and, 83
  controlled substance, 295
  example of, 37f
  insurance claim and, 321–324
  internal marketing and, 190, 191f
  owners review of, 33, 36f
IP address, 163b
IRCA. see Immigration Reform and
    Control Act (IRCA).
IRS. see Internal Revenue Service (IRS).
Isolation, boarding and, 431
IV catheter and fluids, preanesthetic
    documentation and, 411
IV (intravenous), medication
    administration and, 413

J
Job change, 447
Job descriptions, 107–109, 108b–109b
Job enrichment, 68–69
Joint health, diet and, 424
Journal of Veterinary Medicine,
    employment opportunities and, 450
Jury duty, 105
Just-in-time ordering, 283–284, 284b

K
Kcal. see Kilocalorie (kcal).
Kennel assistants
  boarding center and, 431
  hearing protectors and, 148, 149f
  modules for, 116
  payroll and, 127
  responsibilities of, 5b
  sample job description, 108b
  as veterinary team member, 5
Kennel cough, 403b, 428–429
Ketamine, 292, 296
Key access, fraud and embezzlement and,
    348
Key performance indicators (KPIs),
    331b–332b, 332–336, 332f, 346
  to help analyze data, 342
Key words, web page design and, 196,
    196b
Keyboard, 150f, 157b–159b
Kg. see Kilogram (kg).
Killed vaccine, 403
Kilocalorie (kcal), 416
Kilogram (kg), 416
Kittens, 404–406
  AAFCO recommendations for,
      418t–419t
  nutrition of, 420–422
Know-it-all clients, 139–140

L
Label printer, 157b–159b
Labeling fees, 287, 439
Labels
  increasing legibility and, 257, 258f
  medication dispensing and, 414, 414b,
      414f
Laboratory fees, 175

Laboratory forms, 168–173, 169f–173f
Laboratory log, 304, 306f
Laboratory reports, 174, 262
Laboratory results, 174–175, 175f–178f
  internal marketing and, 190, 193f
Laboratory tests, 168t
Laceration, equine emergencies and, 427
Laptop, 157b–159b
Laser printer, 160
Laser safety, 383–384, 384f
Lavender-topped tube, 167, 167f
Law
  definition of, 78–79
  requiring familiarity, 88–93, 88b–89b
  veterinary practice and, 84b, 165b,
      179b, 235b
Law enforcement dog, death of, 235
Lawsuits, 81–82
Laxatives, gastric drugs and, 415
Lead time, 281, 437
Leaders, effective, 51b
  becoming an, 52–53
  characteristics of, 50b
  commitment, 52, 52b
  communication and, 51
  fundamentals that build, 50b
Leadership
  commitment, 52, 52b
  styles of, 52
  team, 47–71
  utilization of, 53
Ledger cards, 309
Legal document, medical record as, 257
Legal issues, 78–83, 79b–80b
Legend drug, definition of, 73b–76b
Legibility, of medical records, 257, 257b
Leptospirosis, 403b
Liabilities, 331b
  client falls and, 32–33, 36f
Liability insurance, 82, 103
Licenses, employee benefits and, 104
Lifetime limit, 319b, 320
Lifting, safety hazards of, 371,
    371f–372f
Lighting, ergonomics and, 148
Listening, marketing programs and, 206
Liver disease, diet and, 424
Lockout periods, 261
Log books, 302
  controlled substance, 295–296
Logs, 301–306
  controlled substances, 302
  laboratory, 304
  law, 304b
  learning objectives of, 301
  miscellaneous, 304–306
  radiology, 302–304
  surgical, 304
Long-chain triglycerides (LCTs), 424
Loss, decreasing, 65–68, 65b–66b,
    288–289
  inventory control and, 66
LSD, class I drugs and, 292
Lyme disease, 403b

M
Mace, personal protection and, 396
Macs, Apple Inc. software and, 159

Magnetic optical disk (MOD), digital radiograph storage and, 410
Magnetic resonance imaging (MRI), 410–411
Magnets, marketing and, 201
Mail, managing and processing of, 21
Mailing lists, client, 393
Maintenance diets, 152
Malpractice, 79, 81–82
    acts of, 79b
    medical records and, 256
    telephone calls and, 20–21
Managed care, 324
Management
    busy times and, 248, 248b
    of conflict, 63–64
    of controlled substances, 295–298, 295b, 297b
    delegation by, 56–57
    employee retention and, 122
    finance, 329–357
    four R's of, 55
    and improvement of programs, 328
    of inventory, 66, 274–290
    of medical records, 255–273, 257f
    passwords and, 393
    scheduling and, 240–241
    of walk-ins, 248–249
Manager
    decreasing loss and, 65
    inventory and, 275
    medical record check and, 256
Manual accounts receivable, 309
Manufacturer representatives, 276–277
Manufacturers, veterinary, open house and, 190
Marketing, 181–208
    assertive, 206
    budget for, 182
    definition of, 73b–76b
    direct, 185–186, 185b–186b
    external, 190–195, 190b, 194b
    indirect, 184–185, 184b, 185f
    internal, 186–190, 186b
    message, 200
    target, 188–189
        cost-benefit ratio of, 188
Marketing plan, creating and implementing, 207–208, 207b
Marketing programs, implementation of, 205–206, 205b
Marketing skills, for employment, 449–450
Markup, 439
    service, development of, 440–441
Markup percentage, 286
    average, 286b–287b
    example, 287b
Mass cremation, 231–232
Master problem list, 25, 33f, 262
Material Safety Data Sheets (MSDSs), 359
Maximizing revenue, 343–346
Maximum permissible dose (MPD), 409
MBTI. see Myers-Briggs Type Indicator (MBTI).
Medical and Genetic Aspects of Purebred Dogs, 320
Medical history, previous, 262

Medical record
    abbreviations, 271, 271b
    audit, 272, 272b
    AVMA Principles of Veterinary Medical Ethics and, 73b–76b
    criteria for, 261
    of each animal, 22, 24f–25f
    establishing of, 261, 262b
    inactive, 256
    inclusions for, 262, 262b
    initialing of, 265, 268b
    insurance claim and, 321–324
    legal ownership of, 82–83, 82b
    lost, 266–267
    malpractice and, 82
    management of, 255–273, 257f
        abbreviations, 271, 271b
        computerized medical records, 258–261, 259b–260b, 260f
        Herd health records, 266
        history taking, 262–264, 263b
        role in, 272–273
        SOAP and POMR medical records, 264–266, 265b
    patient information, 262
    purging of, 266–267, 267b
    radiographs, 271–272
    release of, 82, 261, 261b
    review of, 253
    rules for, 268b
    software, 261, 261b
    travel sheet and, 66
    violations, 270–271
Medical supplies, 288
Medicare, 102, 129
Medication
    administration of, 413, 413b
    calculations and conversions of, 413
    dispensing, 413, 414b
    expired, 284–285, 285f, 413
    and law, 432b
    medical records and, 265–266
    routes of administration, 268b
    toxic exposure to, 372
Medium-chain triglycerides (MCTs), 424
Meeting notes, 59
Meetings, 58b
    method of communication and, 58–60
    rules of, 58b
    team members and, 58b, 58f
Megabyte, 157b–159b
Megacolon, 430
Megapixel capabilities, of digital cameras, 164
Membership fees, employee benefits and, 104
Membership organization, resume and, 453
Mental changes, coping with stress and, 140
Merchandising, definition of, 73b–76b
Messages
    forming a, 212–215, 212b
    for veterinarians and technicians, 20, 21f
Messaging, on-hold, marketing technique and, 203–205

Metabolism, of spayed or neutered patients, 422b
Methimazole, hyperthyroidism and, 430
Microcomputer, 159
Microphone, 157b–159b
Microsoft Publisher, educational information and, 220
Microsoft Windows, 159
Microsoft Word, labels and, 257
Middle area, of veterinary practice, 152, 152b, 152f–153f
Military family leave entitlements, 89
Milk fever, bovine emergencies and, 427
Milk replacer
    formulated, puppy, 420
    kitten, 422
Minerals, nutrient requirements and, 418
Minicomputer, 159
Minimum wage, FSLA and, 89, 94f
Miscellaneous logs, 304–306
Miscommunications, prevention of, 215
Misdemeanor, 79
Missed charges, 288, 288b, 344, 345b, 345f
Mission, the vision, and the values (MVVs), 49, 49b
Mission statements, 101
    practice brochure and, 201
Mistakes
    leaders and, 56–57
    medical record correction and, 257
Mites, 429
Mobile media, Web page and, 199, 199b
Mobile practices, 395–396
MOD. *see* Magnetic optical disk (MOD)
Modem, 157b–159b
Modified live vaccines, 402–403
Monitor, 157b–159b
Monitoring badge, anesthetic, 378
Monthly ordering, 283
Monthly payment, 312
Monthly statements, 310
    fees, 435
Moraxella bovis infection (pinkeye), 405b
Morphine, class II drugs and, 292
Motion economy, 147, 147b
Mouse, 157b–159b
Mouth, medication administration and, 413
MPD. *see* Maximum permissible dose (MPD).
MRI. *see* Magnetic resonance imaging (MRI)
MSDSs. *see* Material Safety Data Sheets (MSDSs).
Multiple phone lines, management of, 18–19, 18b, 18f
Multitasking, 65
Muzzles, 401–402, 402b, 402f
Myers-Briggs Type Indicator (MBTI), 447

N
Nail trims, boarding and, 431–432
Name badges, 184
Name tags, wear by team members, 15–16
National Association of Veterinary Technicians in America (NAVTA), 77
    2011 demographics survey, 70, 70b
    code of ethics for, 77b

National Association of Veterinary Technicians in America (NAVTA) (*Continued*)
  open house and, 190
  veterinary technician specialties and, 7
National Board of Veterinary Medical Examiners, 73b–76b
National Commission on Veterinary Economic Issues (NCVEI)
  benchmark pay scales and, 125
  benchmarking and, 337
National Committee for Clinical Laboratory Standards (NCCLS), 167
National Dog Groomers Association, 4
National Fire Protection Association (NFPA)
  diamond labeling system, 378–381, 378f, 379b
  label, 379, 379f–380f
National Veterinary Technician Organizations, 11b
National Veterinary Technician Week, 6b
NAVTA. *see* National Association of Veterinary Technicians in America (NAVTA).
NCCLS. *see* National Committee for Clinical Laboratory Standards (NCCLS).
NCVEI. *see* National Commission on Veterinary Economic Issues (NCVEI).
Negative attitude, burnout and, 142
Negative reviews, handling, on internet, 226
Negligence, 79, 82b
  definition of, 81–82
Nervous system, drugs for, 415
Net income, 340, 340b
Network card, 157b–159b
Neurotransmitters, role of, 139
New hire
  benefit plan forms for, 111
  emergency contact information for, 111
  first day for, 111–112, 111b
  I-9 form for, 89–93
  state tax forms for, 111
  W-4 form for, 111
Newsletter, client communication and, 240, 240f–241f
Newspaper ads, 194
No-charge policy, 309, 309f
No-show appointment, 249, 249b
Noise hazards, 372, 372f
Noncompete agreement, 78b, 105–106
Nonprofit organization, donations and, 205
Nonproprietary name, for drugs, 412
Nonsterile procedures, as factor in appointment scheduling, 246, 246f
Nonsteroidal anti-inflammatory drugs (NSAIDs), 414
Nonverbal skills, 213–214, 213b
  improving, 214, 215b
Normative ethics, 77
Normosol, medical records and, 266
Notice of Contemplated Action, 83
NSAIDs. *see* Nonsteroidal anti-inflammatory drugs (NSAIDs).

Nutrients, 418
Nutritional instruction, kennel assistant and, 5

O
Obesity
  in canines, 429, 429b
  diet and, 424
Objective, SOAP format and, 264, 264f–265f
Obturator nerve paralysis, bovine emergencies and, 427
Occupational hazards, 365b, 365t
Occupational Safety and Health Administration (OSHA), 93, 93b, 359, 362–387, 362b–363b
  employee safety and, 93, 106
  form 300, 385f–386f
  form 300A, 389f
  inspections, 363
  Job Safety and Health, 364f
  Log 301, 388f
  required poster for, 98f
Ocular discharge, canine disorders and, 429
Odors, housekeeping and, 430
Office managers
  responsibilities of, 8b
  sample job description, 108b
  as veterinary health team member, 8
Official veterinary ethics, 77
Omega-3 fatty acids, 424
On hold, 18
One-way door locks, 393
Open-book management, 355
Open-ended questions, 19, 110–111
Open house, 190, 190b, 193f
Opiates, drug schedule and, 292
Order, receiving, 284, 284f
Order book, 275, 282–283
Organizational behavior, 88, 88b
Organizational development, 88
OSHA. *see* Occupational Safety and Health Administration (OSHA).
Outpatients, 3
Outside laboratory, 166–180
  client service and, 175–176
  specialties of, 179b
Outsourcing products, 287
Outstanding accounts, 309f, 310
  collection procedures for, 311–313, 312f, 315b
Over-the-counter (OTC) drug, 413
  definition of, 73b–76b
Overcrowding, in reception area, 149
Overtime pay
  Fair Labor and Standards Act, 89
  sick leave and, 103
  vacation and, 102
Own occupation disability insurance, 103
Owner's equity, 331b
Oxygen tanks, 387, 390f
Oxymorphone, class II drugs and, 292

P
Packing slip, 284
Painless death, 230. *see also* Euthanasia.
Panic buttons, security systems and, 394

Paper, *versus* software management schedule, 240–241
Paper appointment book, 240–241, 242f
  week-at-a-glance style of, 241
Paper records, 257–258, 258f, 261
Paperless medical records, 256
Parasites, 425
Parasitic infection, zoonotic diseases and, 360t–361t
Paraverbal skills, 213
Pareto principle, 280
Parking lot, perimeter lighting and, 395, 395b, 395f
Part-time employment, 101
Partial thromboplastin time (PTT), laboratory tests and, 168t
Passwords, computer system and, 393, 393b
Pasteurella sp., 362
Pathology samples, 168
Patient audit, 252f, 253
Patient drop-off, 249
Patient history, 24–25
Patient information, computerized records and, 260
Patient Protection and Affordable Care Act of 2014, 103
Patients, hospitalized, safety of, 396–397
Pay periods, 124
Pay scale, 125
Payment for services, 33–42, 35b, 37f, 38b
Payment plans, 308b
  third party, 308
Payment stickers, late, 312f
Payroll
  calculation of, 127–128, 442
  management of, 127–128, 127b
  process of, 124–129, 125b
  records of, 128
  reducing expenses, 347
  taxes of, 128–129, 129b
Payroll budget, 353–354, 354b
PC video camera, 157b–159b
Pentobarbital, class II drugs and, 292
Per-incident deductibles, 319–320, 319b
Per-incident limit, 319b, 320
Percentage solutions, 444
Perimeter lighting, 395, 395b, 395f
Perpetual inventory balance system, 295
Personal identification number (PIN), 33
Personal protection devices, 396
Personal protective equipment (PPE)
  evaluation of, 365, 366f–367f
  safety guidelines and, 408b–409b, 409–410, 409f
Personal skills, 447–449
  questions to consider before applying for a new job, 449b
Personalities, stress and, 139
Personnel files, 129–131, 131b
Pet elimination areas, 149, 149b
Pet health insurance
  benefits of, 321, 321b
  claim form, 322f–323f
  payment for services and, 38
  for practice, 324
  recommendations to clients, 324b–325b, 325
  and wellness plans, 317–328

Pet memorials, 231, 232f–234f
Pet portals, 197, 198b
    value of, 272–273
    web marketing and, 198–199, 198f
Pets
    depression and, 234b, 235
    living longer, 318, 319f
    reasons for visiting a veterinarian, 318b
    reception areas and, 14–15
    sick, frequently asked questions for, 18
    spaying and neutering, frequently asked
        questions for, 17–18
Pet's information, 22
Petty cash, 41–42
Pharmaceutical products, 73b–76b
Pharmaceutical violation, 83
Pharmacology, 412–416, 412b
Phase training, 116, 117b–121b
Phenobarbital, laboratory tests and, 168t
Philosophy, of practice, 101
Philosophy statements, 101
Phone calls
    to appointments, 19–20, 20b
    guidelines
        conversation control and, 16
        frequently asked questions and, 16
    liability of, 20–21, 21b
    personal, 21
    reminders and, 217
Phone techniques
    development of, 16–18
    multiple line management and, 18–19,
        18b, 18f
Photo albums, in reception areas, 150
Phrases, phone techniques, 17, 17b
Physical examination, 262
Physical inventory, 282
    annual controlled substance, 295–296,
        298f
PIN. see Personal identification number
    (PIN).
Pitch, human voice and, 16, 16f
Place, marketing and, 183
Plan development, 326, 327b
Planning, time management and, 65
Plants, housekeeping and, 430
Plasma, 167
POMR medical record, 264
Pop-ups, internet security and, 163b
Portrait photos, in reception areas, 150, 151f
Positive attitude, 447
    client compliance and, 216
Positive words, resume writing and,
    452b–453b
Postcard, 240, 240f–241f
    target marketing and, 188
Postdated check, 309, 309b
Posters, required, 93, 93b
Potomac horse fever (ehrlichiosis), 405b
PPE. see Personal protective equipment
    (PPE).
PPO. see Preferred provider organization
    (PPO).
Practice computers, main page for, 198
Practice design, 146–154
Practice manager, 10b
    leadership styles and, 52
    responsibilities of, 10b

Practice manager (Continued)
    sample job description, 108b
    as veterinary health team member,
        9–10, 10f
Pre-employment screening, 111
Preanesthetic documentation, 411
Preexisting health conditions, 320,
    320b–321b
Preferred provider organization (PPO),
    health benefits and, 103
Pregnancy, 106, 106b
    and maternity leave, 93, 106, 106b
Pregnancy toxemia, common ovine and
    caprine emergencies and, 427
Premises violation, 83
Premiums, 319, 319b
Preparing orders, 282–284, 282b
Prescribing, definition of, 73b–76b
Prescription, 412–413, 412f
    controlled substances and, 292
    diet, 416
Prescription drug, definition of, 73b–76b
Prescription fee, minimum, 287
Price, marketing and, 183
Pricing
    strategies, effective, 285–287
    wellness plans and, 326–328, 326b
Primary complaint, 262
Principal cost, 331b
Principles of Veterinary Medical Ethics, 73
Printer, 157b–159b
    selection of, 160
Privacy Act, 261, 396b
    release form and, 28
Private cremation, 231–232, 234f
Probationary period, 106, 106b
Problem solving, 55, 55b
Processor
    selection of, 160
    speed, 157b–159b
Product marketing, 183
Product shortage, 281
Production reconciliation hybrid, Pro-sal
    formula and, 125–126
Products
    incorrectly invoiced, 288
    returning to distributors, 285
Professional appearance, 450f
    client confidence and, 215
Professional behavior, 73b–76b
Professional development, 446–456
Professional fees, reducing expenses, 346
Professional incompetence, illegible
    record and, 257
Professional Liability Insurance Trust
    (PLIT), 82
Profit, 286, 286b, 344, 344b, 352, 352b
    analyzing, 354
Profit and loss statement (P&L), 331b,
    338–340
    fraud and embezzlement and, 348
    producing monthly, 340, 342f
    troubleshooting, 340–343, 342b
Profit-sharing plan, 103–104
Prognosis, medical record inclusions and,
    262
Promotion, marketing and, 183
Proprietary name, for drugs, 412

Proptosed eye, small animal emergencies
    and, 426
Pro-sal formula, 125–126
Protein, nutrient requirements and, 418
Prothrombin time (PT), laboratory tests
    and, 168t
Protocol, employee procedure manual
    and, 114
Protozoal infection, 360t–361t
Proximate cause, 81–82
Psychological harassment, 107
Public accountants (PAs), 331
Puppies, 404–406
    AAFCO recommendations for, 417t
    nutrition for, 419–420
        large-breed, 420, 420b
Purple heart, internal marketing and, 189,
    189f
Purpose statement, 101

Q
Quality
    of care, 64
    of life, 230, 230b
    of voice, 16
Quantity, reorder, 281
Questions
    client, 212–213
    interview, 110–111, 110f, 111b
Quick, nail trims and, 431–432
Quick response (QR) codes, 199, 199f,
    203b
QuickBooks, 338
    Intuit, 127

R
R/Is. see "Rule-ins" (R/Is).
R/Os. see "Rule-outs" (R/Os).
Rabies, 405b
    in canine, 403b
    in cattle, 405b
    in feline, 404b
Rabies certificates, 24
Rabies neutralizing antibody titer test
    (RNATT), health certificates and, 28
Rabies virus neutralizing antibody
    (RVNA), health certificates and, 28
Radiation safety, 382–383, 382b–383b
Radioactive iodine, feline
    hyperthyroidism and, 285b
Radiograph checkout log, 272f
Radiographs, 271–272, 271f
    digital, 410
    radiology log and, 302–303
    safety guidelines for, 408–409,
        408b–409b, 409f
Radiology checkout logs, 303, 303f
Radiology chemicals, 376
Radiology log, 302–304, 302f, 303b–304b
    checkout logs and, 303, 303f
Rainbow Bridge poem, 231, 233f
Raises, pay, determination of, 127, 127b
RAM (random access memory),
    157b–159b
Rapid eye movement (REM), 140
Rapport, management and, 55
Rate, of speaking, 16
Recall systems, 216–217, 217f

Recalls, patient follow-up and, 187–188, 188b
Reception area
　creating comfortable, 149–150, 149b, 151f
　isolated areas and, 32
　management of, 14–15, 14b
Receptionist
　client forms and, 22
　employee surveys and, 63b
　hostile clients on the phone and, 31
　increasing profits with, 19, 19b
　responsibilities of, 8b
　sample job description, 108b
　verifying identification and, 38
　as veterinary health care team member, 8, 8f
　wages for, 127
Receptionist team, 13–46
　client relations, 21–22, 22f
　etiquette, 15–16, 15b
　goal of, 14
　health and safety of, 149, 150f
　invoices with owners, 33, 36f
　mail, 21
　messages for veterinarians and technicians, 20, 21f
　multiple phone lines, 18–19, 18b, 18f
　payment for services, 33–42, 35b, 37f, 38b
　personal phone calls, 21
　phone techniques, 16–18
　reception area, 14–15, 14b
　special situations with clients, 29–33, 32b
　telephone calls, 20–21, 21b
Recognition, management and, 55
Recombinant vaccines, 402–403
Recommendations
　client compliance and, 222
　specific, assertive marketing and, 206
Reconciliation, 39. see also Daily reconciliation.
　of cash drawer, 41
　of checks, 41, 41f
Record, payroll, 128
Record keeping, violations of, 83
Recording devices, cameras and, 395
Red flags rule, 35, 356, 356b
Red-topped tube, 167, 167f
Reducing expenses, 346–347, 347b
Reference range, laboratory results and, 174
References
　hiring and, 110
　resume writing and, 453
　reviewing letter of, 110
Referral veterinarian, 73b–76b
Refrigeration
　safety protocols and, 382, 382f
　of samples, 168
Reinvestment, 352
Related experience, resume writing and, 453
Relationship building, 156
Release form
　boarding, 431
　medical records, 28–29, 29b

REM. see Rapid eye movement (REM).
Remains, picking up of, 232–234, 232b
Reminder systems, 217
Reminders, 186–187, 187b, 187f–188f, 216–217, 216f, 217b
Remodeling, computer system costs and, 162
Renal disease, diet and, 424
Reorder points, 281, 281b, 437–438
　determining effective, 281
　example of, 282b
Reorder quantities, 281, 281b, 437
　determining effective, 281, 436–437
　example of, 281b
Replacement cost, 285
Report card, 212f
Reports
　financial, 337–338, 338b
　laboratory, 174
Research and development, 450
Reservoir, disease transmission and, 362
Residual coverage, disability insurance and, 103
Resignation, employee, 123–124
Resilience, 156
Resourcefulness, 156
Respect, management and, 55
Respiratory system, drugs for, 416
Responsibility, management and, 55
Restraint, 368, 401–402, 401f
Restrictive covenant agreement (NCA). see Noncompete agreement.
Results, laboratory, 174–175, 175f–178f
Resume, 451–453, 452b, 454f
　email and internet, 453
　personnel files and, 131
　positive words used in, 453b
　reviewing of, 110
　rules, 453b
Retail area, 152
Retaining employees, methods for, 122–123, 122b
Retirement, 356, 456
Retirement funds, 103–104
　401(k) plans, 103
Retirement planning, 356
Return on investment, 352
Return policies, drug manufacturers, 284, 285b
Returned check, 308–309
Revenue and percent difference, from previous period or year, 334
Reviews, management of, 207, 207b
Rhinopneumonitis (EHV-1), 405b
Rickettsial diseases, zoonotic diseases and, 360t–361t
Rider, insurance and, 319b
Right to know, hazard communication and, 363–366
Ringworm, 429
　feline disorders and, 430
Risks, consent form information and, 23–24
RNATT. see Rabies neutralizing antibody titer test (RNATT).
Robbery, 394b
Rodenticides, toxicities and, 426

Role-playing, 122
　communication barriers and, 215
　developing effective phone techniques and, 17, 17b
　folded arms and, 213–214
　safety protocol and, 387
　verbal image and, 213
Routing number, bank, 128
"Rule-ins" (R/Is), 265
"Rule-outs" (R/Os), 265
Running, safety hazards of, 372
Running drug log, 296, 297f
RVNA. see Rabies virus neutralizing antibody (RVNA).

S
Safety, in veterinary practice, 358–391
Safety and security procedures, 106
Safety data sheets (SDSs), 288, 359b, 363b, 374–376, 375b
　descriptions, 375f
Safety hazard plans, OSHA and, 93
Safety officer, responsibilities of, 390b
Safety program, documentation of, 387
Safety protocols
　development of, 387–390, 387b, 390b, 390f
　implementation of, 390, 390b
Safety training program, 106
Salary
　employee retention and, 122
　production-only, 126
　for veterinarians, 126
Sales promotion, 277
Sample pickup, 174
Sample shipment, 168, 168b, 173–174, 174b, 174f
Sample submission, 167–168
Sarcoptes, 429
Savings Incentive Match Plan for Employees (SIMPLE). see SIMPLE IRA (sIRA).
Scanner, 157b–159b, 165
Schedules of drugs, 292–293, 292b–293b, 293t
Scheduling, for productivity, 247–249
Scrubs, 104. see also Uniforms.
SDSs. see Safety data sheets (SDSs).
Search engine optimization (SEO), 196–197
Seasonal employees, 101
Security, 106, 392–398
　cameras, fraud and embezzlement and, 348
　of computerized medical records, 261
　system, 394–395, 394f
Sedatives, nervous system and, 415
Seizure, small animal emergencies and, 426, 426b
Self-assessment, 447–449, 447b, 448f–449f
Self-confidence, leaders and, 50
Semimonthly payroll, 124–125
Senior patients, 406–407, 422
Sensory devices, security system and, 394
SEPs. see Simplified Employee Pension plans (SEPs).
Serum, 167
Serum separator tube (SST), 167, 167f

Server, 157b–160b, 160
Service dogs, death of, 235
Service pricing, equation to obtain, 343
Severe trauma, complaints and, 83
Sex discrimination, Civil Rights Act of 1964, Title VII and, 93
Sexual harassment, 106–107
Sheep, diseases of, 405b
Shrinkage discrepancies, 287–288
Sick leave, employee benefits and, 103
Signature cards, of controlled substances, 295
SIMPLE IRA (sIRA), 103
Simplified Employee Pension plans (SEPs), 103–104
sIRA. see SIMPLE IRA (sIRA).
Sixteen Personality Factors (16PF), 447
Skin diseases, canine disorders and, 429
Sleep, coping with stress and, 140
SMART system (specific, measurable, agreed, realistic and time bound), in delegation of tasks, 56, 56b
Smoke detectors, 371
SOAP medical record, 264
    plan, 265, 267f
Social media, 199–200, 200b
    developing plan, 200, 200b
    managing, 200
    policy, 107, 200
Social Security, 102, 129
Society, definition of, 7
Society for Human Resource Management, 88
Society of Veterinary Behavior Technicians (SVBT), 7b
Soft cost, 285–286
    example, calculation, 286b
Soft skills, 107
Software, 159
    appointment schedulers, 241, 243f–244f
    implementation of, 162–163, 162b
    integration, 326
    management schedule, paper versus, 240–241, 242f
    selection of, 160–162, 161b
    veterinary practice management, client education materials and, 202
Sound card, 157b–159b
Space efficiency, ergonomics and, 148–149
Spam, 163b
Spam filter, 163b
Spay and neuter certificates, 24–25
Spaying and neutering pets, 405–406
    frequently asked questions for, 17–18
Speakers, 157b–159b
Species, classification of, 22, 23b
Spill kit, chemical spills and, 379–380
Spreadsheet, 282
    creating a, 350
    example of, 283f
Spyware, 163b
SST. see Serum separator tube (SST).
Staff board, 185, 185f
Staff costs per minute, 343, 440
Staff education, programs to enhance, 11
Staff efficiency, 64–65, 64b
Stamps, 403, 403f
Standard laboratory services, 167

Standard of care, 115, 222, 345, 345b
    definition of, 82
Standards of conduct, ethics and, 73
State board of pharmacy, controlled drug loss and, 298
State law, employee manual and, 99
State veterinary medical board, 78
Statement fees, 310
    monthly, 435
Statements, monthly, 310, 310f
Stick urinalysis, 408, 408f
Stimulants, nervous system and, 415
Stock supply sheet, 295–296, 296f
Stool softeners, gastric drugs and, 415
Storage, of purged medical records, 267
"Strangles." see Distemper, in equine.
Stress
    coping with, 140–141, 140b
    factors affecting, 138, 138b
    negative, 138, 138b
    personalities and, 139
    positive, 138
    stages of, 139
Stress identification, 138–140, 138f
Stress management counseling, 141
Stressors
    career, 140
    client, 139–140
    environmental, 138–139
    external, 138
    identifying, 139–140, 139b
    internal, 138
    life-event, 139
    personal, 139
Student
    as veterinary team member, 3–4
    veterinary technology programs, 11
Subjective information, SOAP format and, 264, 264f
Substance abuse, 141–142
Supportive management, theory of, 52
Surgery
    complaints and, 83
    as factor in appointment scheduling, 246, 246f
    team member responsibility and, 411, 411b
Surgical log, 304, 304b, 305f
Surgical patients
    medical records and, 265
    written communication and, 211
Surgical report, 262
SVBT. see Society of Veterinary Behavior Technicians (SVBT).
SWOT analysis, 183–184, 183b
    opportunities in, 184
    strengths in, 183
    threats in, 184
    weaknesses in, 183
Symbol, branding and, 184

T
Tablespoon conversion, 444–445
Tablet, 157b–159b
Tangible property, 105, 331b
Tardiness, 248
Taser, personal protection and, 396
Tasks, delegation of, 56–57, 56b–57b, 56f

Tax identification numbers, independent groomers and, 127
Tax ledgers, 336
Taxes owed, 336
Team, veterinary health care members, 1–12
    advertisements and, 188
    calculations and conversions for, 434–445
    colored warnings stickers and, 257–258, 259f
    educating, 327
    empowerment of, 55–56
    fire extinguisher use and, 370–371
    hierarchy of, 3
    human-animal bond and, 229
    indirect marketing and, 184–185
    inventory management and, 283
    malpractice and, 82
    manager, 309b, 313b, 315b
    marketing and training program for, 205–206
    motivating and retaining, 68–70, 69b–70b, 69f
    new position for, 3, 4b
    pet health insurance, offering, 318b, 325
    responsibilities of, 3, 3b
    rights and responsibilities for, 3
    roles and duties of, 3, 10–11
    security and, 393
    structured hierarchy of, 3
    successful environments for, 11b
    termination of, 123–124
Team building, effective leaders and, 51
Team development, 88
Team interactions, 49b
Team leadership, 47–71, 49b
    conflict management, 63–64
    cultures, 53–54
    decreasing loss, 65–68
    delegation, 56–57
    empowering employees, 55–56, 56b
    empowerment, 55–56
    increasing staff efficiency, 64–65
    methods of communication, 57–63
    mission, 49
    motivating and retaining members, 68–70
    positive effect of, 54–55
    time management, 65
    values, 49
    vision, 49
Team management, four R's of, 55
Team morale, 52, 56f
Team newsletter, 60, 60f–61f
Team shortages, 105
Team training, 115–123, 116b, 366, 368b
Teaspoon conversion, 444–445
Technical skill, 50
Technician
    client communication and, 211, 211f
    credentialed, compensation for, 126–127
Technology terms, 157b–159b
Telephone calls
    liability of, 20–21, 21b
    outstanding accounts and, 313, 314b

Template, of appointment book, 241–244
Termination procedures, 106, 123–124, 123b, 124f
Testimonials
    definition of, 73b–76b
    ethical principles of, 191–194
Tests, laboratory, 168t
Tetanus, 405b
Textbook of Small Animal Internal Medicine, 320
"Thank you for the referral" letters, internal marketing and, 189
Theft, 135–136, 393–394, 394b
Theophylline, laboratory tests and, 168t
Therapeutic diets, 416–425, 416b, 416f
Third party payment plans, 308
Three-click rule, 196
Time, wasted, 65
Time and motion, principles of, 147, 147b
Time management, of leaders, 65
Time-restricted feeding, 420
Timing
    laboratory results and, 174
    and sample pickup, 174
Tissue samples, 167
To-do list, 65
Tone
    client perception and, 213
    human voice and, 16
Toothbrushes, pediatric, internal marketing and, 189–190, 190f
Tort, 78–79
"Toxic" topics, 14
Toxicities
    safety hazards of, 372–373, 373b
    small animal emergencies and, 426–427
    special chemicals and, 376
Trade name, of drugs, 412
Training
    empowered employees and, 56, 56b
    procedures, employee manual and, 105, 105b
    protocol, 117b–121b
        developing of, 116–121
Tranquilizers, nervous system and, 415
Transaction, 331b
Transferable skills, 447
Trash, housekeeping and, 430
Travel sheet, 66, 66f–69f
Traveler's checks, 38
Treatment area, 152–154, 153f–154f
Treatment plans, 220–222, 220b, 221f
    medical record inclusions and, 262
Treatment recommendation, medical record inclusion, 262
Triage, receptionist and, 15
Trojan horse, 163b
Troubleshooting, 55, 55b
Tumors
    benign, 429
    canine disorders and, 429
Turnaround time, sample submission and, 174–175
Turnover rates, 280–281, 280b, 436, 438
    determining effective, 280–281
Turns per year, 280
    inventory and, 436
Tylenol (acetaminophen), 426–427

U
Ultrasound, 410
Umbrella laws, 78
Understanding, client and patient needs and, 223–226, 224b
Unemployment tax, 129
Uniformed Services Employment and Reemployment Rights Act (USERRA), 89, 93, 93b
Uniforms, 104
Unintentional tort, 78–79
Units, appointment schedule and, 251, 251f
Unjust enrichment, law of, 80
Urinalysis, 407–408, 408f
Urinary stone formation, diet and, 424–425
Urine dipstick tests, 408b
Urine sediment evaluations, 408b
URL (uniform resource locator), 196
Urogenital area, stimulation of, 422
U.S. Department of Agriculture
    health certificates and, 28
    medical record release and, 82
U.S. Department of Labor, Wage and Hour Division, certificates of exemptions and, 89
USB (Universal Serial Bus), 157b–159b
USB flash (jump) drive, 157b–159b
USERRA. *see* Uniformed Services Employment and Reemployment Rights Act (USERRA)
Uterine prolapse, common bovine emergencies and, 427

V
Vacation
    burnout prevention and, 142
    employee benefits and, 102–103, 103b
    as factor in appointment scheduling, 247
Vaccination
    and diseases, 402–403
    history of, 262
    reactions, 403b
    release forms, 23–24, 26f–32f
Vaccine
    protocols, frequently asked questions for, 17
    types of, 402–403
Value
    emergency care and, 80
    in practice, 355–356, 355b, 356f
Variable cost, 331b
Variable expenses, 339
Vasodilators, 415
Vector, indirect disease transmission and, 362
Vehicle, indirect disease transmission and, 362
Verbal image, 212–214
Verbal skills, 212
Veterinarian-client-patient relationship, 73b–76b
Veterinarians
    as contract employees, 131
    definitions of, 73b–76b
    hiring and compensation of, 125–126

Veterinarians (Continued)
    pets visit, 318b
    professional behavior of, 73b–76b
    responsibilities of, 9b, 10f
    sample job description, 108b
    schools for, 9b
    seeing appointments, 244, 245f
    as veterinary health team member, 9
    zoonotic diseases and, 359
Veterinary assistants, 84b
    medication administration and, 413
    responsibilities of, 5b
    sample job description, 108b
    training modules for, 117b–121b
    as veterinary team member, 5–6, 6f
Veterinary Economics, employment opportunities and, 450
Veterinary ethics, 77
Veterinary health care, team members, 1–12
Veterinary Hospital Managers Association (VHMA), 73
    benchmark pay scales and, 125
    benchmarking and, 337
    code of ethics and, 77f
Veterinary Hospital Medical Association, employment benefits and, 455
Veterinary inventory software, 162
Veterinary management software, password protection of, fraud and embezzlement and, 348
Veterinary practice, 17b, 81
    biohazards in, 381–382
    branding and, 184
    building appearance for, 147, 147b, 147f
    chemical hazards in, 373–378
    conflict management and, 63–64
    design and function of, 149
    failure to issue Form 1099-MISC and, 135
    and law, 11b, 44b, 70b, 84b, 136b, 152b, 179b, 208b, 227b, 235b, 273b, 289b, 356b, 390b, 396b, 456b
    maintenance of records in, 257b
    marketing of, 182, 182b
    open communication and, 58
    physical hazards in, 368–373, 368b
    safety in, 358–391
    salary formula for, 126
    SDS and, 288
    signage of, 147f
    technology in, 155–165, 156b
Veterinary practice act, 78
    AVMA model of, 78b
Veterinary Practice News, employment opportunities and, 450
Veterinary prescription drug, definition of, 73b–76b
Veterinary schools, 9b
Veterinary software
    accounts receivable and, 310, 311f
    inventory system and, 277
    reminders and recall systems and, 217
    web addresses, 161b

Veterinary Support Personnel Network (VSPN), staff education programs and, 11
Veterinary technician
  body positioning and, 148, 148f
  continuing education requirements for, 6b
  credentialed, 84b
  licensed, 84b
  medication administration and, 413
  modules for, 116
  responsibilities of, 7b
  sample job description, 108b
  specialties of, 7–8, 7b
  training modules for, 117b–121b
  as veterinary team member, 6–7, 6b
Veterinary Technician National Examination Committee (VTNE), veterinary technician credentials, 6
Veterinary technologists
  responsibilities of, 7b
  as veterinary team member, 7
VetMedTeam, 11
VGC. see Video graphics card (VGC).
VHMA. see Veterinary Hospital Managers Association (VHMA).
Video graphics card (VGC), 157b–159b
Viral diseases, zoonotic diseases and, 360t–361t
Virus, 163b
Vision, of practice, 88
Vitamins, nutrient requirements and, 418
Voice
  human, components of, 16
  recognition, 157b–159b
Volume, of voice, 16
Volunteer experiences, resume writing and, 453
VSPN. see Veterinary Support Personnel Network (VSPN).

W
Wage and Hour Division, U.S. Department of Labor, certificates of exemptions and, 89
Wages, staff, 125, 125b
Waiting clients, 42–43, 43b, 43f
Waiting period, 320
Walk-ins
  euthanasia and, 230
  late for appointment, 247–248
  management of, 248–249
  scheduling and, 240
Wall cleaning, housekeeping and, 430
Want list, 282, 282b, 282f
Warning, of termination, 123, 124f
Warning stickers, colored, 257–258, 259f
Water
  nutrient requirements and, 418
  puppy diet and, 420
Weaning
  of kittens, 422
  of puppies, 420
Web browser, 163b
Web page, promoting the, 197–198, 197b
Web page design, 195–196, 195b
Web site address, 196
Web sites, 195–199, 195b, 203b
  company-supported, 195–196
  employment opportunities and, 450
  information on, 195–199, 195b
  marketing of, 190, 194b
  on-site hosting, 195
  organization tabs in, 197f
  safety on, 163
Week-at-a-glance style, appointment book, 240–241
Weekly pay periods, 124–125
Weight management hall of fame, internal marketing and, 189, 189b
Weighted hourly wage, 354

Well-Managed Practices (WMPs), benchmarking and, 337, 337f
Wellness exams, and recommendations, 404
Wellness plans, 325–328, 325b–326b, 326f
Wet floors, safety hazards of, 373, 373f
Wireless LAN access point, 157b–159b
Withdrawal, substance dependence and, 141
Work environment, turnover rate and, 53
Work ethic, personal skills and, 448
Work schedule policy, 105
Workers' Compensation Act, 103
Workers' compensation insurance, 129
  claim form, 384
Working interview, 111
Workplace rights poster, 364f
Workplace violence, veterinary practice safety and, 373
World Wide Web, 196
Worm, 163b
"WOW" service, creation of, 14, 14f, 42–44, 42b
Writing skills, 215–216
Written communication, 211
Written materials, 218, 218f
Wrong day arrival, 249

Y
Yellow Pages, 185–186, 194, 194b

Z
Zero tolerance policy
  psychological harassment and, 107
  sexual harassment and, 106–107
Zip drive, 157b–159b
Zoonotic diseases, 359–362, 360t–361t
  control of, 362, 362b
  transmission, 362